Jamieson & Kay's
Textbook of Surgical Physiology

Jamieson & Kay's Textbook of Surgical Physiology

Iain McA. Ledingham MB ChB MD (Hons) FRCS (Edin) FRCP (Glas) FRSE

Titular Professor of Intensive Care,
Department of Surgery,
University of Glasgow;
Honorary Consultant and Chairman,
Intensive Therapy Unit,
Western Infirmary,
Glasgow, UK

Colin MacKay BSc MB ChB FRCS(Eng) FRCS(Edin) FRCS(Glas)

Consultant Surgeon,
Western Infirmary and
Gartnavel General Hospital,
Glasgow

FOURTH EDITION

CHURCHILL LIVINGSTONE
EDINBURGH LONDON MELBOURNE AND NEW YORK 1988

CHURCHILL LIVINGSTONE
Medical Division of Longman Group UK Limited

Distributed in the United States of America by Churchill
Livingstone Inc., 1560 Broadway, New York, N.Y. 10036, and
by associated companies, branches and representatives
throughout the world.

First Edition 1959
Second Edition 1965
Third Edition 1978
Fourth Edition 1988

ISBN 0 443 026408

British Library Cataloguing in Publication Data
Jamieson, Robert Ainslie
    Jamieson & Kay's textbook of surgical
    physiology. — 4th ed.
    1. Physiology, Pathological   2. Surgery
    I. Title   II. Kay, Andrew Watt
    III. Ledingham, Iain McA.   IV. Mackay,
    Colin, *1936 Nov. 8-*
    612'.00246171   RB113

Library of Congress Cataloging in Publication Data
Jamieson, R. Ainslie (Robert Ainslie)
    Jamieson & Kay's textbook of surgical physiology.
    Includes bibliographies and index.
    1. Human physiology.   2. Physiology, Pathological.
3. Surgery.   I. Kay, Andrew Watt, Sir.   II. Ledingham,
Iain McA.   III. MacKay, Colin.   IV. Title.   V. Title:
Jamieson and Kay's textbook of surgical physiology.
VI. Title: Textbook of surgical physiology.   [DNLM:
1. Physiology.   2. Surgery.   WO 102 J32t]
QP34.5.J35   1988   612'.00246171   87-17658

Produced by Longman Group (FE) Ltd
Printed in Hong Kong

From the Preface to the First Edition

'Although there are several well-established texts dealing with surgical anatomy and surgical pathology, there is no familiar standard text dealing with surgical physiology. The lack of a suitable text is most sharply felt by the post-graduate student, and it is especially with his needs in mind that we have prepared our manuscript.

. . . Our aim has been to discuss only those aspects of applied physiology which are fundamental to the practice of general surgery. An occasional excursion into the realm of pathology, and more frequent excursions into the realm of clinical surgery, will, we trust, be readily condoned by the sympathetic reader who is making surgery his career.

. . . We owe both the inception and completion of the book to Professor (Sir Charles F. W.) Illingworth, and it is in token of our thanks that we dedicate it to him.'

1959

R. Ainslie Jamieson
Andrew Watt Kay

Preface to the Fourth Edition

In sympathy with the aims of the original authors of the *Textbook of Surgical Physiology*, the content of the Fourth Edition has been compiled to meet the needs of the modern surgeon-in-training. Each specialty demands knowledge of basic clinical physiology and our hope is that this book might also be of value of trainees in other disciplines.

The lengthy gap between the Third and Fourth Editions has made it necessary for most of the chapters to be rewritten and no chapter has escaped unscathed. We live in a day of advance and change and surgical physiology is no exception; to accommodate such advances a number of new authors have joined the existing team. We are pleased to welcome Sir A. P. M. Forrest, Dr R. A. Hawkins and Dr W. R. Miller (Breast), Dr T. E. Woodcock (Respiratory system), Professor K. M. Taylor (Heart), Dr J. G. Erskine (Blood and Spleen), Mr R. T. Mathie and Mr I. S. Benjamin (Liver), Mr W. R. Murray (Pancreas), Mr E. S. Glen (Bladder and Urethra), Mr T. B. Hargreave (Testis) and Mr J. A. Bradley (Immunology and Surgery).

In addition, some of the previous authors have been interchanged and thus bring a fresh brush to their new canvas. It is with sadness that we record the death of Mr L. Stuart Scott, who wrote with authority on the Testis.

It is a pleasure to record the readiness with which authors and publishers have given us permission to reprint illustrations. The source of each borrowed illustration is given either by a full reference in the legend to the illustration or by a name and date when the reference is listed in the Bibliography.

We are indebted to a number of colleagues for helpful discussions and in particular would like to thank Dr J. J. Brown (Western Infirmary, Glasgow) and Professor S. M. Jennett (University of Glasgow). Finally we wish to record our thanks to the publishers and printers of the Fourth Edition who have maintained their high standard of practice.

1988,
Glasgow

I. McA.L.
C. MacK.

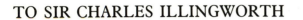

TO SIR CHARLES ILLINGWORTH

Contributors

William H. Bain MB ChB MD FRCS(Edin) FRCS(Glas)
Titular Professor, Department of Cardiac Surgery,
University of Glasgow;
Consultant in Charge, Cardiothoracic Unit,
Western Infirmary, Glasgow, UK

P. R. F. Bell MB ChB MD FRCS FRCSG
Professor of Surgery and Honorary Consultant Surgeon,
University of Leicester, UK

Irving S. Benjamin BSc(Hons) MB ChB FRCS
Senior Lecturer and Honorary Consultant Surgeon,
Royal Postgraduate Medical School and
Hammersmith Hospital,
London, UK

Leslie H. Blumgart BDS MD FRCS(Edin) FRCPS(Glas)
FRCS(Eng)
Professor of Surgery,
University of Bern;
Director, Clinic for Visceral and Transplantation Surgery,
Inselspital,
Bern, Switzerland

J. Andrew Bradley MB ChB PhD FRCS
Consultant Transplant Surgeon,
Western Infirmary,
Glasgow, UK

Kenneth C. Calman PhD MD(Hons) MB ChB FRCS FRSE
MRCP(Lon)
Dean of Postgraduate Medicine,
Professor of Postgraduate Medical Education,
The University,
Glasgow, UK

John F. Davidson MB FRCP(Edin) FRCPath
Consultant Haematologist,
Glasgow Royal Infirmary;
Honorary Clinical Lecturer,
Glasgow University, Glasgow, UK

A. S. Douglas BSc MD FRCP(Eng) FRCP(Edin) FRCP(Glas)
FRCPath Hon FACP
Emeritus Regius Professor of Medicine,
University of Aberdeen,
Aberdeen, UK

J. Gordon Erskine MB ChB MRCP(UK) MRCPath
Consultant Haematologist,
Area Laboratory,
Crosshouse Hospital,
Kilmarnock,
Ayrshire, UK

A. Fleck MB ChB PhD FRCPath FRCP(Glas) FRSE
Professor of Chemical Pathology,
Charing Cross and Westminster Medical School
University of London,
London, UK

Sir A. P. M. Forrest MD ChM FRCS(Edin, Eng, Glas) Hon
DSc(Wales) Hon FACS FRSE
Regius Professor of Clinical Surgery,
Department of Clinical Surgery,
The Royal Infirmary,
Edinburgh, UK

James C. Forrester ChM FRCS(Glas) FRCS(Edin) FRCS(Eng)
Consultant Surgeon and Senior Lecturer,
Department of Surgery,
Ninewells Hospital,
Dundee, UK

Iain E. Gillespie MD MSc FRCS(Edin) FRCS(Eng) FRCS(Glas)
Professor of Surgery, University of Manchester;
Honorary Consultant Surgeon,
Manchester Royal Infirmary,
Manchester, UK

Eric S. Glen FRCS(Glas) FRCS(Edin)
Consultant Urologist,
Southern General Hospital,
Glasgow;

Honorary Clinical Lecturer in Urology,
University of Glasgow,
Glasgow, UK

Andrew G. Graham MB ChB FRCS(Glas) FRCS(Edin)

Consultant Urologist,
Western Infirmary,
Glasgow;
Honorary Clinical Lecturer,
University of Glasgow,
Glasgow, UK

Keith E. Halnan MA MD FRCP FRCR FRSE

Honorary Consultant, Former Director,
Department of Radiotherapy and Oncology,
Royal Postgraduate Medical School,
Hammersmith Hospital,
London, UK

David L. Hamblen PhD FRCS(Edin) FRCS(Eng)

Professor of Orthopaedic Surgery,
Western Infirmary,
Glasgow, UK

Timothy Bruce Hargreave MS FRCS(Edin) FRCS(Eng) LRCP
(Lon)

Hon. Consultant Urologist,
Western General Hospital,
Edinburgh;
Senior Lecturer, University of Edinburgh,
Edinburgh, UK

R. A. Hawkins MSc PhD

Senior Lecturer, Department of Clinical Surgery,
The Royal Infirmary, Edinburgh, UK

Michael Jeffrey Hooper MBBS FRACP

Senior Specialist,
Department of Endocrinology,
Repatriation General Hospital,
Concord,
Sydney, Australia

Sir Andrew Watt Kay MB ChB MD FRCS(Glas) FRCS(Eng)
FRFPS(Glas) FRCS(Edin)

Formerly Regius Professor of Surgery,
Department of Surgery,
Western Infirmary,
Glasgow, UK

Iain McA. Ledingham MB ChB MD(Hons) FRCS(Edin)
FRCP(Glas) FRSE

Titular Professor of Intensive Care,
Department of Surgery,
University of Glasgow;

Honorary Consultant and Chairman, Intensive Therapy
Unit,
Western Infirmary, Glasgow, UK

Adam L. Linton MB FRCP(Eng) FRCP(Canada) FACP

Professor of Medicine,
The University of Western Ontario,
London, Canada

Colin MacKay BSc MB ChB FRCS(Eng) FRCS(Edin) FRCS(Glas)

Consultant Surgeon,
Western Infirmary and Gartnavel General Hospital,
Glasgow, UK

John MacVicar MD FRCOG FRCS(Glas)

Professor of Obstetrics and Gynaecology,
University of Leicester,
Leicester, UK

R. T. Mathie BSc PhD

Lecturer in Physiology,
Royal Postgraduate Medical School, London, UK

J. Douglas Miller MD PhD FRCS(Glas) FRCS(Edin) FACS
FRCP(Edin)

Professor of Surgical Neurology,
Department of Clinical Neurosciences,
University of Edinburgh,
Edinburgh, UK

W. R. Miller BSc PhD

Lecturer, Department of Clinical Surgery,
The Royal Infirmary,
Edinburgh, UK

W. R. Murray BSc MB ChB MD FRCS

Senior Lecturer in Surgery,
Western Infirmary,
Glasgow, UK

R. O. Quin BSc(Hons) MD(Hons) MB ChB FRCS(Eng) FRCS(Glas)

Consultant Surgeon,
Gartnavel General Hospital,
Glasgow, UK

K. M. Taylor MD FRCS FRCS (Edin) FSA

British Heart Foundation Professor of Cardiac Surgery,
University of London;
Professor of Cardiac Surgery,
Hammersmith Hospital,
London, UK

Thomas E. Woodcock MBBS FFARCS

Consultant Anaesthetist,
Southampton and South-West Hampshire Health
Authority, Southampton General Hospital, UK

Contents

Wound healing and fibrosis

The survival of an individual depends on the integrity of his tissues and organs. If continuity is lost following disease or injury, a restorative process is rapidly initiated. In superficial abrasions and certain visceral injuries this is predominantly a regenerative process but elsewhere the end result is simple fibrous union by scar. This non-specific connective tissue is most easily recognized in a healing incision but is found wherever tissues are damaged. The same general process can be observed in organizing thrombus, granulating wounds and the reactive tissue around a slowly growing neoplasm. Usually scar formation is uneventful but sometimes it is excessive. The resulting fibrosis impairs function and may threaten life.

THE ORGAN OF REPAIR

Connective tissue is produced by granulation tissue. This delicate matrix of cells and capillaries heals the wound and should be accorded the status, albeit temporary, of the organ of repair (Fig. 1.1). Good healing is dependent on its healthy growth and development and when repair is over it disappears. Macrophages and fibroblasts are the key cells. The former initiate healing by stimulating fibroblast activity and new capillary ingrowth (Leibovich & Ross, 1976; Wahl, 1981). The fibroblast synthesizes collagen (the glycosaminoglycans of the ground-substance) and fibronectin (the glycoprotein that seems to help hold the whole structure together). The normal function of the fibroblast is critically dependent on a readily available supply of diffusible oxygen and the limiting level of 10–15 mmHg is found 50–80 μm from the nearest normally perfused capillary (Fig. 1.2) (Hunt et al, 1969; Silver, 1969, 1980). For this reason the fibroblasts and capillaries develop together as a unit, and anything interfering with the delivery of oxygen to the wound has adverse effects on the repair process.

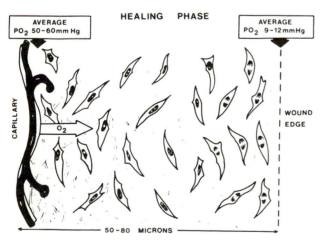

Fig. 1.1 The organ of repair or fibroblast-capillary system. Diagram showing P_{O_2} gradients in this healing granulation tissue. The activity of fibroblasts is limited at P_{O_2} 10 mmHg and they must therefore keep within 50–80 μm of the nearest functioning capillary. Healing cannot progress until new capillaries develop. (Reproduced by permission from Hunt T K et al, 1969)

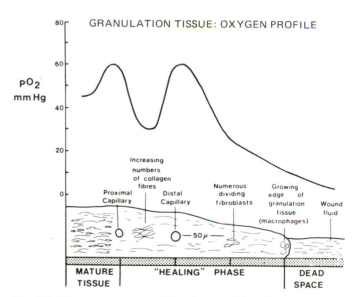

Fig. 1.2 Direct measurements of P_{O_2} in granulation tissue growing into a wound chamber. There is a steady fall from the normal mature tissue level of around 54 mmHg to anoxic levels in the centre of the wound. Macrophages have a lower oxygen requirement than fibroblasts and are found at the free edge of the growing granulation tissue. (After Silver I A, 1969, 1980)

THE REPAIR PROCESS

Mechanical aspects

The rate of gain of strength is of particular importance in many wounds and has proved to be one of the most useful indications of the progress of repair. The general form of recovery is the biological growth curve with three distinct phases. In the first few days there is no recordable tensile strength but enzyme and cellular activity is marked. This is the *phase of preparation* during which the foundations of repair are laid. After the fourth or fifth day collagen and ground substance appear in the wound in increasing amounts and strength rises rapidly. This is the *phase of proliferation* in which the fibroblast-capillary system is most active. After a month or so the wound activities moderate. Strength recovers more slowly and there is a progressive diminution of cell population and vascularity. This *phase of maturation* continues for many months.

Over 75% of the strength of the intact abdominal wall resides in its aponeurotic layers. Wounds in this tissue recover remarkably slowly. There is a rapid gain in strength during the first few weeks but after that progress is less obvious and by the end of a year there is only 70% recovery (Fig. 1.3) (Douglas, 1952). More recently, the same strength changes have been recorded in healing skin wounds, but this is of less moment since skin scar is protected from direct physical forces by its elastic surrounds.

Connective tissues are complex visco-elastic materials with time-dependent properties. Their true ability to resist rupture is therefore incompletely assessed by simple breaking-strength studies. A good scar has to be both strong and pliable. This is exemplified using bio-engineering techniques to analyse healing skin wounds (Forrester et al, 1970). Scar tissue is not only weaker but more brittle than normal. After 5 months it has only half the ability of normal tissues to resist rupture (Fig. 1.4).

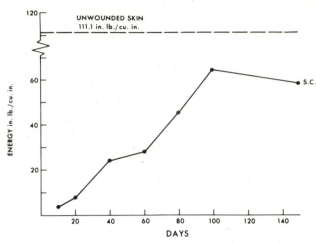

SKIN WOUNDS   ENERGY ABSORBED

Fig. 1.4 The ability of a wound to resist rupture expressed as its energy absorption. There is only a 50% recovery by 150 days. (Reproduced by permission from Forrester J C et al 1969 Journal of Surgical Research **9**: 207–212)

Histological aspects

Light microscopic studies show a characteristic sequence of events (Fig. 1.5). The fresh wound is rapidly united by a fibrin coagulum containing trapped red cells, debris and devitalized tissue. Neutrophils can be seen in increasing numbers after 8 hours and monocytes towards the end of the first day. Fibroblasts can be recognized after 24 hours but are not numerous till active microcirculation is established a few days later. At the end of a week the fibroblast-capillary system is actively synthesizing collagen and ground substance. The neutrophils play an important role in dealing with contaminating bacteria but apart from this are not directly involved in the process of wound healing.

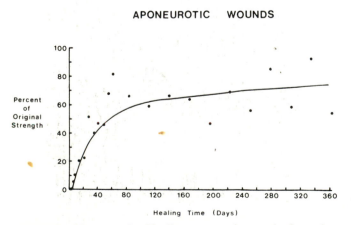

APONEUROTIC   WOUNDS

Fig. 1.3 Breaking strength of healing aponeurotic wounds. Strength increases rapidly for several weeks but then slows. There is only 70% recovery by the end of a year. (Douglas D M, 1952)

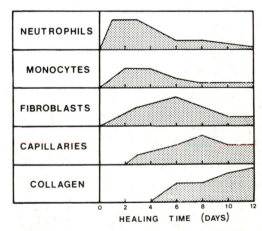

HISTOLOGICAL   EVENTS

Fig. 1.5 The characteristic sequence of events in the first few days of wound healing. Neutrophils and monocytes appear first. Collagen appears following development of a functioning fibroblast-capillary system.

When an animal is treated with antineutrophil serum, they disappear from the wound but healing is undisturbed (Simpson & Ross, 1972). The monocyte is the precursor of the macrophage but not the fibroblast. Macrophages have low oxygen requirements and are found at the free edge of the wound (see Fig. 1.2) (Silver, 1980). In addition to their scavenging activities they stimulate fibroplasia. When antimacrophage serum is used along with steroids to induce monocytopenia, collagen formation is delayed. A platelet factor is also known to be important in stimulating fibroblasts to synthesise collagen (Knighton et al, 1980; Devel et al, 1982).

The fibroblast is the surgeon's cell arriving on the scene to synthesize the collagen and ground substance of wound repair. When its work is done it disappears. Studies in parabiotic rats show it is of local origin from the perivascular areolar tissue (Ross et al, 1970). This is an important argument for avoiding unnecessary local trauma or tissue undermining during surgery.

Healing wounds have two striking physical abnormalities. First, the collagen bundles in the scar are distinctly narrower than those found in the mature tissue on either side. Secondly, normal collagen is markedly birefringent whereas wound collagen is not. This indicates a failure of organisation at the molecular or small fibril level (Douglas et al, 1969).

Scanning electron microscopy is particularly useful for demonstrating physical factors such as fibre shape and weave (Forrester et al, 1969). It provides a high magnification, three-dimensional image of large volumes of tissue and resolution is particularly good since it is determined by electron optical considerations. Normal skin has a well organized network of large collagen fibres (Fig. 1.6). Each large fibre is made up of a bundle of fine, cross-banded

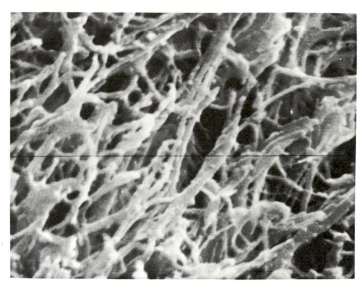

Fig. 1.7 Scanning electron micrograph of a 10-day sutured wound showing the randomly orientated collagen fibrils. They show little tendency to aggregate. Cross-banding is not apparent (× 9750). Compare with the normal skin shown in Figure 1.6 at the same magnification. (Reproduced by permission from Forrester J C et al, 1969)

fibrils. Wound collagen is quite different. At 10 days the collagen fibrils lie relatively haphazardly (Fig. 1.7). As time goes by the fibrils coalesce to form large irregular masses. However there is no evidence of fibril substructure and remodelling is minimal. It seems likely that normal collagen fibre patterns are not restored (Fig. 1.8).

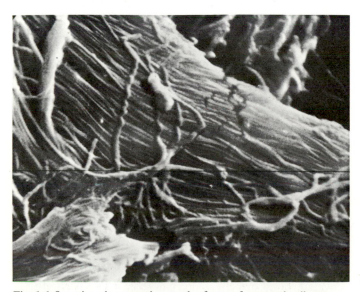

Fig. 1.6 Scanning electron micrograph of part of a normal collagen fibre showing that it is made up of bundles of cross-banded fibrils (× 9750). (Reproduced by permission from Forrester J C et al, 1969)

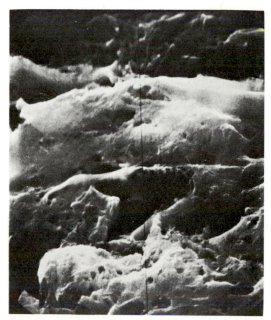

Fig. 1.8 Scanning electron micrograph of a representative portion of a 100-day wound. The collagen fibrils have aggregated to form large collagen masses but the network architecture of the normal has not been restored. Compare with the unwounded skin in Figure 1.6.

Biochemical aspects

Scar tissue is a matrix of cells and fibres embedded in a ground substance. There is little doubt that the physical properties of the wound are determined by their interaction as well as the quantity and quality of each. In practice, collagen is the main element contributing to wound strength and the permanent soundness of repair. Apart from being prominent in healing wounds it is the general support tissue of the body, forming some 30% of the total protein content of most animals. A knowledge of its formation and resorption mechanisms is fundamental to understanding normal growth and development and a variety of connective tissue disorders.

Collagen is formed in the endoplasmic reticulum of the fibroblast and excreted into the extracellular space in monomeric form (tropocollagen) (Prockop et al, 1979). When synthesis is upset, as in scurvy, precursor material collects and distorts the cell (Figs. 1.9 and 1.10) (Ross & Benditt, 1964). The collagen molecule is a rigid rod 300 nm long and 1.5 nm wide. Each is composed of three polypeptide chains (α chains) wound in a left-hand helix. The molecule itself is twisted the opposite way in a right-hand super-helix. There are five genetically distinct α chains and five types of collagen have now been identified (Bornstein & Sage, 1980). Type I predominates in mature skin, tendon and bone, Type II is found in cartilage, Type III features in cardiovascular structures, infant skin and the granulation tissue of healing skin wounds. Types IV and V are associated with basement membranes (Miller & Matukas, 1974).

Each α chain contains more than 1000 amino acids but glycine, proline and hydroxyproline together account for

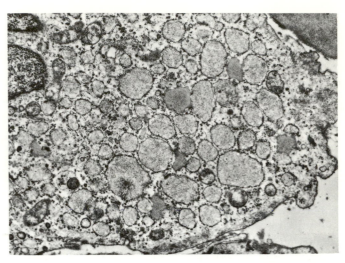

Fig. 1.10 Electron micrograph of part of a scorbutic fibroblast. Note the typical distended endoplasmic reticulum. There is no sign of collagen but it will appear within 24 hours of providing ascorbic acid. Electron micrograph, × 9000. (Courtesy of Professor Russell Ross, Seattle)

over half the molecule. The individual amino acids are assembled in the endoplasmic reticulum of the fibroblast beginning at the amino terminal end and proceeding towards the carboxy terminal end. Hydroxyproline and hydroxylysine are not incorporated directly into the collagen molecules. A proline- and lysine-rich collagen precursor molecule, protocollagen, is formed and then hydroxylation is carried out under the influence of protocollagen hydroxylase. This enzyme has the specific requirements of molecular oxygen, alpha-ketoglutarate, ferrous iron and ascorbic acid and is one reason why collagen synthesis is delayed in scurvy (Hutton et al, 1967). Iron deficiency has no practical importance but hypovolaemia and poor delivery of oxygen can markedly retard collagen synthesis (Heughan et al, 1974). Recent studies show that synthesis is enhanced when P_{O_2} is raised by increasing the oxygen in the inspired air to 45% (Fig. 1.11) (Hunt & Pai, 1972).

It should be stressed at this point that collagen synthesis does not equate with wound healing. Although many factors enhance individual components of the healing process no factor has as yet gained general clinical significance.

As soon as tropocollagen leaves the fibroblast it starts to polymerize and forms strong covalent crosslinkages with neighbouring molecules. Intramolecular and intermolecular crosslinking is initiated by oxidative deamination (lysyl oxidase) of amino groups of lysine and hydroxylysine to form aldehydes. An aldehyde can undergo an aldol condensation with a second aldehyde to form a strong covalent bond directly. Alternatively, it can react with an amino group and form a Schiff base (Grant & Prockop, 1972; Prockop et al 1979).

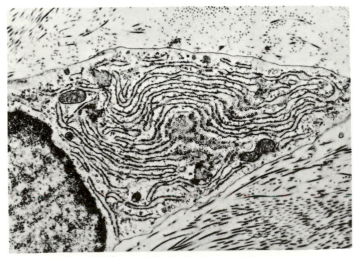

Fig. 1.9 Electron micrograph of part of a normal fibroblast. Note the characteristic well developed endoplasmic reticulum. The lining ribosomes, which are responsible for its 'rough' appearance, are the active site of collagen synthesis. New collagen fibrils are rapidly excreted and are seen here surrounding the cell. Electron micrograph, × 9000. (Courtesy of Professor Russell Ross, Seattle)

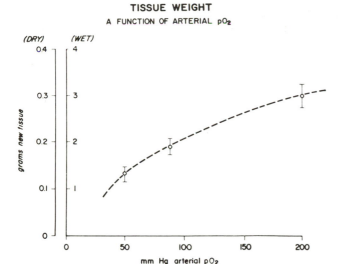

TISSUE WEIGHT
A FUNCTION OF ARTERIAL pO₂

Fig. 1.11 The amount of new tissue formed in a wound is considerably greater when arterial P_{O_2} is increased by changing the ambient oxygen from 14 to 20 to 45 per cent for 25 days. (Reproduced by permission from Hunt T K, 1970 J. Trauma **10**: 1001–1009)

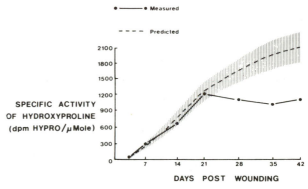

COMPARISON OF PREDICTED AND MEASURED COLLAGEN ACCUMULATION IN SKIN WOUNDS

Fig. 1.13 Comparison of scar collagen accumulation predicted from its rate of synthesis with that actually measured. Total collagen does not increase after 3 weeks even though it continues to be synthesised and deposited at a rapid rate. Collagen is now being removed as quickly as it is formed (collagenolysis). The difference between the curves represents scar collagen turnover. (Reproduced by permission from Madden J W & Peacock E E Jr 1971 Annals of Surgery **174**: 511–520)

At one time collagen was regarded as metabolically inert. In scar tissue this is far from the case (Madden & Peacock, 1968). Although the total amount of collagen in a wound may reach normal levels after 60–80 days, qualitative changes continue for a good deal longer (Fig. 1.12). These play a major role in determining the ultimate strength of wounds in fascia and skin. Specific studies of wound

collagen turnover using tritiated proline show how these qualitative changes may be brought about. Collagen synthesis and lysis continue to run at high rates long after the total amount of collagen in the wound has returned to normal (Fig. 1.13). The loss of collagen substance is not confined to the wound and is particularly marked in the mature collagen on either side (Fig. 1.14). As a result it temporarily becomes weaker and may hold sutures less well. The continued collagen turnover means that wound scar is less stable than normal. For example, in scurvy, collagen synthesis fails and if lysis continues the wound will weaken and possibly break. If lysis is less prominent than synthesis then a hypertrophic or keloidal scar may result (Craig et al, 1975). Enzymes other than collagenase are also active in the early phases of wound healing (Fig. 1.15) (Raekallio, 1972). Adenosine triphosphatase can be found within an hour of injury. Aminopeptidase is

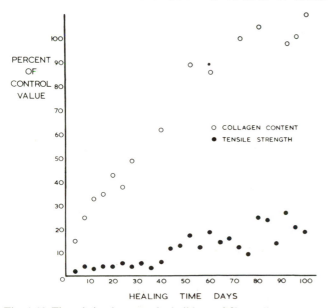

LATE STAGES OF HEALING OF INCISED WOUNDS
RELATION OF COLLAGEN AND TENSILE STRENGTH

○ COLLAGEN CONTENT
● TENSILE STRENGTH

Fig. 1.12 The relation between the build-up of fibre collagen and tensile strength in healing guinea-pig skin wounds. The collagen has reached its control value by 80 days when the wounds are still only 25% as strong as unwounded skin. (Reproduced by permission from Douglas D M et al, 1969)

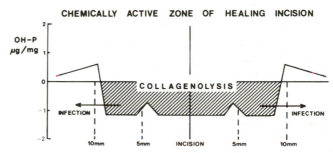

CHEMICALLY ACTIVE ZONE OF HEALING INCISION

Fig. 1.14 The chemically active zone of an incised wound extends for at least 5 mm on either side of it. Collagenolysis is prominent in the first week and is even more marked when infection is present. The zero line is the concentration in normal abdominal wall. (Adamsons R J et al 1966 Surgery, Gynecology and Obstetrics, **123**: 515–521)

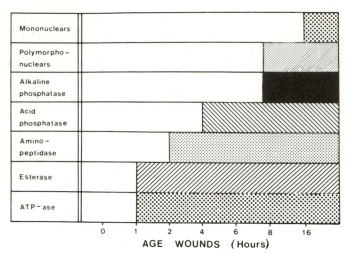

Fig. 1.15 Schematic diagram showing the histochemical estimation of the age of ante mortem skin wounds. (Reproduced by permission from Raekallio J, 1972)

present after about 2 hours and the phosphatases appear at 4 and 8 hours. This sequence can be detected histochemically and used together with the degree of leucocytic infiltration to determine the age of a wound. It also proves to be a useful way of assessing wound treatments and dressings and suture absorption mechanisms (Salthouse & Williams, 1969).

The ground substance

All connective tissues contain fibres and cells embedded in a variable quantity of ground substance. The chemistry of the ground substance is complex and incompletely understood (Bentley, 1967). In general, there are a number of related structural polysaccharides (glycosaminoglycans), of which chondroitin-4-sulphate is one of the better known. In wounds these are usually found as large protein-polysaccharide complexes called proteoglycans (mucopolysaccharides) (Jackson, 1975). The basic structure is a central protein core bordered by repeating disaccharide units. The current concept of these protein-carbohydrate complexes goes beyond that of a simple supporting role. They appear to have the capacity for determining the pattern of tissue growth in the wound.

Fibronectin is a recently discovered component of the extracellular matrix. This large glycoprotein is found in many tissues and in plasma. It has chemotactic effects on fibroblasts (over and above those of the macrophage and platelet) and plays a significant role in both intercellular adhesion and cell-to-matrix adhesion (Mosher et al, 1980; Postlethwaite et al, 1981).

Superficial wounds

Although epithelial and mesenchymal interactions are

prominent in embryonic life there is less indication of their relationship after birth. It is therefore not inappropriate to consider the healing of superficial or open wounds separately from the general process of connective tissue formation.

Superficial or open wounds heal by a combination of epithelialisation (Van Winkle, 1968) and contraction. The stimulus for epithelial repair is not clear but the loss of contact of one cell with another is of prime importance (Abercrombie & Heaysman, 1954). There is also evidence that intact epithelium produces an inhibitory local hormone or chalone (Bullough & Laurence, 1960). When epithelium is removed, chalone levels fall. Either way repair is accomplished by a combination of cell migration and multiplication which does not cease until edge-to-edge apposition of cells has been re-established. Epithelialisation is delayed by drying and scab formation, and proceeds most readily in moist areas, provided they can be kept free from infection. It now appears that in many apparently normal situations the oxygen supply is less than optimal, for epithelialisation has been accelerated using oxygen permeable wound covers and intermittent hyperbaric oxygenation (Winter, 1972).

The other mechanism by which an open wound closes is contraction (Van Winkle, 1967). This form of tissue migration involves the entire thickness of skin and subcutaneous tissues. The prime movers are specialized myofibroblasts in the wound margin (Ryan et al, 1974; Gabbiani 1981). It therefore proceeds independently of collagen formation but is readily disturbed by irradiation and cortisone. Although less important in man than many animals, it contributes significantly to wound closure where skin is slack, as on the abdomen and back of the neck. Elsewhere it is less effective. It is important to differentiate this physiological process from pathological fibrosis and wound contracture.

FACTORS AFFECTING HEALING

Although many factors affect healing few have attained general clinical significance. Studies of the metabolic response to trauma show that the wound has a compelling biological priority and usually heals satisfactorily even in ill patients. Many of the principles have been established in animal studies and may have less significance for man. For instance, guinea pigs die relatively quickly when ascorbic acid is withheld and rats do not tolerate starvation for more than a week or two. In both situations man can survive for months.

Age

Healing is at its most vigorous in the young and hyperplastic scars and keloids are more common then.

Protein

Experimental studies showed that protein starvation retarded repair unless sulphur-containing amino acids such as methionine were supplied. Recent work confirms the adverse effects of protein deprivation but does not support the claims made for methionine. In patients the situation is less clear. Uneventful healing is usually the rule and hypoproteinaemia is not always correlated with wound dehiscence (Keill et al, 1973). It seems that protein deficiency has to be associated with a body weight loss of about 20% before the chance of wound failure becomes significant.

Vitamin C

Although ascorbic acid is required for synthesis and maintenance of collagen, there is little evidence that it matters much in practice. However, following trauma and general bodily stress there is an enormous metabolic demand for it and daily supplements of up to one gram are fully utilised (Fig. 1.16). Therefore, when subclinical scorbutic states are suspected it would seem wise to supplement it (Booth & Todd, 1970). Recent studies show that the observed fall in leucocyte ascorbic acid level postoperatively is associated with the body's increased production of cortisol. It seems likely that the increased demand for ascorbic acid in the immediate postoperative period reflects the systemic response to injury rather than the local requirements of collagen formation in the wound. (Forrester et al, 1983).

Oxygen

Good healing is dependent on a readily available supply of oxygen. Although fibroblasts, neutrophils and macrophages do not necessarily die in low oxygen concentrations they are unable to perform their more specialised synthetic and bactericidal functions. Fortunately this hypoxic situation is self-limiting. There is increasing evidence that hypoxic macrophages produce angiogenic factors (Knighton et al, 1981). The fibroblast requires an ambient P_{O_2} of around 10 mmHg if it is to synthesize collagen and ground substance properly. Prior to the establishment of a functioning microcirculation wound P_{O_2} is well below this (Hunt et al, 1969). When wound perfusion is normal satisfactory P_{O_2} levels are found up to 70 μm from the nearest capillary (Silver, 1969). The delivery of oxygen depends on the natural vascularity of the tissue as well as the quality of blood flow. Wounds in highly vascular tissues such as the face heal more rapidly than those in relatively ischaemic areas. The single most important factor is maintenance of blood volume (Fig. 1.17) but blood viscosity, vasomotor activity and pulmonary and cardiac function can seriously impair oxygen supply and delivery. Experimental studies confirm the essential rate limiting role of oxygen in healing reactions. Collagen synthesis is increased by raising the concentration of inspired oxygen

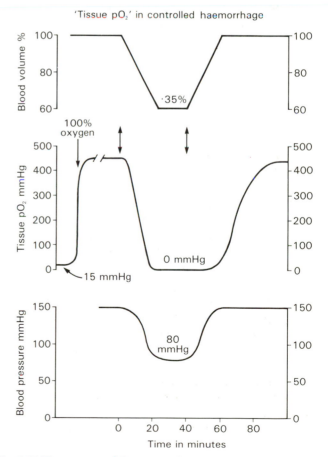

Fig. 1.17 Tissue oxygen falls to zero when an animal loses 35% of its blood volume. Replacement with dextran restores blood pressure promptly but tissue oxygenation recovers much more slowly (Reproduced by permission from Hunt T K 1970 Journal of Trauma 10: 1001–1009).

URINARY ASCORBIC ACID

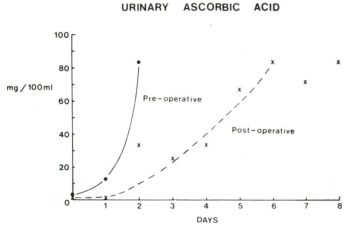

Fig. 1.16 The effect of trauma on the urinary excretion of a daily oral supplement of 1 g of ascorbic acid. Normally, tissue saturation is effected within 48 hours and urinary levels are high. Following operation the body's requirement for ascorbic acid appears to be considerably increased, and tissue saturation is not achieved for 5–6 days.

to between 35 and 70% (Niinikoski, 1969; Hunt & Pai, 1972).

Trauma

The wound that heals best is the sharp clean cut. Any further local injury delays healing by impairing the vitality of the tissues. This in turn encourages the development of infection which further interferes with healing. A severe injury elsewhere in the body may also upset healing and enhance infection by causing a generally impaired capillary flow and wound hypoxia. Restoration of blood volume reverses these effects (Zederfeldt & Hunt, 1968).

Metabolic diseases

Diabetes, jaundice and uraemia are associated with impaired healing of an unpredictable degree (McDermott et al, 1968; Lee, 1972). In diabetes the main problem is believed to be due to the upset carbohydrate metabolism in the wound. The poor tissue perfusion and increased susceptibility to infection simply make matters worse. In jaundice there is evidence of impaired fibroblast function and delay in angiogenesis. Uraemia retards connective tissue formation and slows epithelial repair.

Corticosteroids

Cortisone impairs collagen synthesis and enhances collagen lysis (Berliner et al, 1967). A minimal inflammatory response is required for satisfactory wound healing and because of this, anti-inflammatory drugs such as cortisone markedly impair healing when administered at the time of wounding. After 3 days, when healing is established, the effect is much reduced. In open wounds cortisone retards contraction at any time but healing has been restored to normal on several occasions by systemic or local applications of vitamin A (Ehrlich et al, 1973).

Radiotherapy and cytotoxic drugs

Since healing is primarily a cellular activity, agents causing cell damage should have a marked effect on it. Ionising irradiation destroys cells and irreversibly damages capillaries and small blood vessels. The effects are cumulative and progressive and fully irradiated tissue finishes up as a somewhat ischaemic materal with little potential for repair. Scars in irradiated areas are unstable and may break down or become neoplastic.

Although cytotoxic drugs interfere with cell proliferation they do not have a marked effect on wound healing. Topical nitrogen mustard impairs healing but intra-arterial injection has no effect (Newcombe, 1966) provided it is given before cell proliferation is prominent. Other studies are less easily interpreted since the picture is confused by general systemic effects such as weight loss and bone marrow depression. As a general rule, systemic administration of cytotoxic drugs in therapeutic doses causes less problems than their local application.

Beneficial irradiation

Radiotherapy is intended to damage or destroy tissue but other forms of radiant energy can improve healing. In 1927 Wood and Loomis studied the interaction betwen ultrasound and living tissue. More recently pulsed electromagnetic energy (PEME) and ultrasound appear to have stimulated healing in both hard and soft tissue wounds (Bassett et al, 1981; Fitton-Jackson et al, 1981).

Temperature

Vital processes involve chemical reactions. In cold blooded animals a very marked increase in healing rate results when the temperature is raised from 20° to 30°C. Likewise, the increased blood flow and warmth following sympathectomy has a markedly beneficial effect on healing in peripheral vascular disease. Recent studies show that both open wounds and incisions heal best when a thermoneutral state is maintained at environmental temperature of 30°C (Cuthbertson, 1970). Attempts to accelerate healing in other ways have met with little success.

Zinc

Small amounts of zinc are essential to life, and quite large oral supplements appeared to accelerate healing of pilonidal wounds and indolent leg ulcers (Pories et al, 1967). This role is still not clarified because the subject is exceedingly complex and a number of good studies have produced conflicting results. Recently there has been renewed interest. In areas of the world where zinc is naturally deficient, it limits growth and the onset of puberty in man. There is also evidence that it plays an important role in stabilizing macromolecules and biological membranes as well as in the biosynthesis of collagen. In silicotic lung disease, zinc appears to stabilize lysosomes and therefore reduces tissue necrosis and the resulting fibrosis. It also directly protects the macrophage from damage by silica (Chvapil, 1974). The daily nutritional requirement of 10–15 mg is easily met but the beneficial effects of further supplementation suggest that dietary zinc may yet be shown to have an important role in repair (Fell, 1985).

Wound dressings

Wounds heal best when undisturbed. Closed wounds give little trouble unless infected but open wounds usually require dressing and possibly packing. Changing the dressing is often painful and the procedure is likely to damage the delicate new cells and capillaries on the wound surface. Between changes a relatively unyielding material provides uneven support and abrasive damage. Two new materials go a long way to overcoming these objections. The first is suitable for raw surfaces. It is available as a wet gel made by polymerizing a mixture of agar and acrylamide. Provided it is kept wet it does not adhere to or damage the underlying granulations. Oxygen passes through it readily and it does not encourage bacterial growth (Myers, 1983). The second material is ideal for dressing deep open wounds. It is a foam elastomer which 'sets' in the wound to provide an exact fit. It too is inert and non-adherent (Wood et al, 1977). Between them these two synthetic materials provide, for the first time, a means of optimising healing in an open wound by providing gently conforming inert support.

FAILURE OF HEALING

When healing is progressing normally it gives little trouble but, when it is defective, life may be endangered. Although healing is a unified response to injury, failures usually present in the apparently distinct categories of infection, dehiscence and fibrosis. In practical terms, it is of inestimable value to be able to predict these problems before they arise and so avoid or minimize their effects.

Infection

Wound sepsis is the most important cause of defective healing. It retards collagen synthesis and enhances breakdown of pre-existing collagen. Although bacterial contamination is a prerequisite, several other factors help determine whether or not a wound suppurates (Altemeier, 1984).

The susceptible individual is often debilitated or suffering from a generalized disorder such as diabetes or leukaemia. Alternatively, his lowered resistance may be a side effect of immunosuppressive regimens, long-term corticosteroids or cancer chemotherapy. In cardiopulmonary disease, wound perfusion is often poor and local oedema makes matters worse.

Bacterial contamination may be exogenous or endogenous. The relative importance of each depends on the particular circumstances under consideration. Usually, endogenous organisms outnumber exogenous and the latter only become important when there is little or no endogenous component, as in the clean wound types associated with specialised orthopaedic, cardiac and neurosurgical procedures.

Exogenous contamination is minimized by strict attention to the established aseptic and antiseptic regimens. The importance of protective coverings for patient and staff is unquestioned although the enhanced bacterial transfer when these become wet is sometimes overlooked. Glove technique is important even when skin preparation is faultless. Examination of gloves shows that almost one-third become punctured or torn during surgery and up to 1000 staphylococci can pass through a single needle hole within a minute. Plenum ventilation with 12–18 changes of filtered air per hour suits most theatre requirements.

Ultraviolet irradiation reduces airborne contaminants by half and sterile laminar flow systems discourage mixing with air that may already be contaminated (Charnley, 1973). These measures can be important in ultra-clean surgery but have little relevance when endogenous organisms predominate. A simple and effective way to cut down aerial contamination is to keep physical activity to a minimum, avoid unnecessary conversation and adopt hand signals where possible. Staphylococcal carriage is only important in those who 'shed' the organism. Fortunately, shedding is usually from a single site and can be eliminated effectively if not permanently by prompt local treatment with appropriate topical antibiotics.

In general surgery, endogenous organisms are the principal contaminants (Shaw et al, 1973) and less than 5% of wound infection results from airborne bacteria. In the absence of active inflammatory disease the potential contaminants are to be found on the body surfaces so, when the skin is prepared effectively, the wound is not exposed to bacteria unless an internal epithelial surface is breached. Wounds for operations such as lumbar sympathectomy and thyroidectomy, in which there is no internal epithelial incision, are classified as 'clean' and should not become infected in more than 1 or 2% of cases. Elective gastric and biliary operations include internal epithelial incision and are classified as 'clean-contaminated' wounds. Their infection rate may be as high as 5 or 6%. When infection rates rise above these levels the likely causes are breaks in asepsis or poor surgical technique. When the operation site is acutely inflamed or purulent the wound is 'severely contaminated' and may have an infection rate as high as 40%.

Sometimes pathogens reach the wound following transient bacteraemia associated with bowel manipulations or the gentle rocking of an infected tooth in its socket. On other occasions there is an obvious septic focus elsewhere in the body. Recent studies have identified the particular hazard of contaminated intravenous catheters. This is most troublesome in long-term use but can be found to some degree at almost any time. In-line bacterial filters and local antibiotics deal with this problem very effectively (Wilmore & Dudrick, 1968).

Although infection rates can be predicted from these assessments of bacterial load, the fact remains that few contaminated wounds ever get infected. The healing wound is remarkably resistant to infection and factors that impair this resistance are almost as important as bacterial ones in determining whether or not sepsis occurs.

The susceptible wound is one in which tissue viability has been impaired by local trauma. Poor surgical technique is the prime example since the tissues may be subject to the repeated assaults of retraction and haemostatic manoeuvres with diathermy and ligature. Tight sutures compound the problem by impairing wound perfusion. Susceptibility is also enhanced when remote trauma is associated with hypovolaemia. Here too the defect is impaired perfusion of the wound with its attendant hypoxia (Fig. 1.18). Macrophages require oxygen to activate their peroxidase system and enable them to kill ingested bacteria. Hypoxia allows the bacteria to multiply and kill the cells.

The presence of extraneous material in a wound increases the likelihood of infection developing. A single piece of sterile silk has enhanced the infectivity of staphylococci several thousand times. When a ligature is tied the resulting local necrosis makes matters worse (Fig. 1.19). For these reasons it would seem wise to avoid sutures in contaminated wounds and this is borne out in practice. Further benefits accrue when the skin wound is left unclosed; the wound surface may become infected but invasive infection is very rare (Edlich et al, 1969). If, after 5 days or so, healthy granulation tissue is developing the wound may safely be closed with little loss of total healing time. This technique (delayed primary closure) is very effective but the 'fail-safe' way to preventing invasive infection in a heavily contaminated wound is to leave it open and let it heal by itself.

Although the majority of wound infections are due to organisms implanted before the wound is closed, it can be infected afterwards (Fig. 1.20). A primarily closed wound has no resistance to bacteria swabbed on its surface during the first 6 hours. Thereafter it becomes increasingly difficult to infect it. By 5 days it is as resistant as the surrounding skin. In practice the wound is not challenged

so severely and may be left without dressings after 24–48 hours provided it is dry and not exposed to an obvious local source of contamination.

The use of antibiotics was controversial. The overall incidence of surgical infections has not changed since their introduction; only the types of infection have altered (Altemeier et al, 1973). In the past, staphylococci accounted for almost two-thirds of the invasive infections. Now it is the Gram-negative ones which predominate. Recent work has clarified the position. Antibacterial regimes are highly effective when used properly. Burke (1964) drew attention to the necessity of starting antibiotic therapy as close as possible to the time of tissue contamination. Prophylactic antibiotics are of most value when they reach the wound at the same time as the contaminating organisms. They are not effective if started 2–3 hours later (Fig. 1.21). The routine administration of penicillin and tetracycline within 45 minutes of injury has

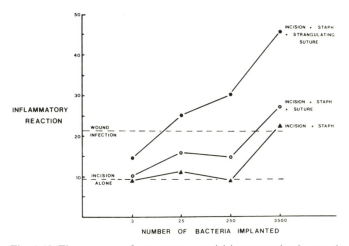

Fig. 1.19 The presence of extraneous material in a wound enhances the likelihood of infection developing. The presence of one tied silk suture doubles the chance of a contaminated wound becoming infected. (After Howe C 1966 Surgery, Gynecology and Obstetrics **123**: 507–514)

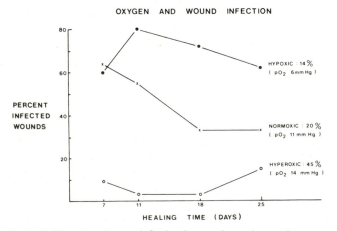

Fig. 1.18 Hypoxia enhances infection in experimental wounds. Increasing the oxygen in the inspired air has the reverse effect. (Reproduced by permission from Hunt T K et al 1972 Surgical Forum **23**: 47–49)

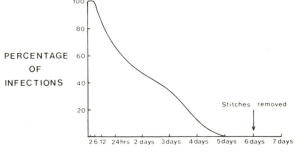

Fig. 1.20 The vulnerability of a healing incised wound to surface contamination with microorganisms. During the first 6 hours it has no resistance. Thereafter it becomes increasingly resistant to invasion, and by 5 days it is as resistant as normal skin. (After Du Mortier J J 1933 Surgery, Gynecology and Obstetrics **56**: 762–766)

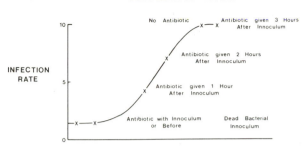

EFFECT OF SYSTEMIC ANTIBIOTIC ON A
CONTAMINATED WOUND

Fig. 1.21 Prophylactic antibiotics are really only effective if given immediately. When they are administered more than 3 hours after bacterial inoculation they do not influence the incidence of infection. (After Burke J F 1961 Surgery **50**: 161–168)

reduced the infection rate in traumatic abdominal wounds from 30% to 7%. In other clinical studies, cephaloridine has more than halved infection rate (Polk & Lopez-Mayor, 1969; Evans & Pollock, 1973). Antibiotics used in this true prophylactic fashion are not continued beyond the first or second day. As a result, resistant strains are not encouraged and possible side effects of treatment are minimized.

In clean wounds, there is little justification for using antibiotics. The infection rate is already minimal and any risk of side effects may well be unacceptable. In heavily contaminated wounds antibiotics do not influence the outcome greatly. A better routine is to leave the wound open (Edlich et al, 1969). A number of studies suggested that topical antibiotics were almost as effective as intravenous (Belzer et al 1975). However, recent work using cefuroxime prophylaxis has demonstrated the clear superiority of systemic administration (Hares et al, 1981). A major criticism of using prophylactic antibiotics is that they cannot be selected with absolute certainty of matching the bacterial sensitivities. Antiseptic routines are not open to this objection and iodine coupled with polyvinylpyrrollidone has proved its worth in several studies of contaminated wound management. The reduced infection rate is comparable to that obtained with antibiotics (Gilmore & Sanderson, 1975; Pollock & Evans, 1975).

Therapeutic antibiotics are required less often since the more direct measures of incision and drainage are usually sufficient. Sometimes a therapeutic and prophylactic problem present together. A patient being operated upon for a ruptured appendix has two problems, a therapeutic one in the abdomen (peritonitis) and a prophylactic one in the wound (sepsis). In this case the antibiotic regimen starts off as a combined therapeutic and prophylactic one and continues after 48 hours as a therapeutic one.

Wound drainage is required when infection is established but may become a hazard if it has to be prolonged. The exit point is colonized by pathogens and a fresh invasive infection may develop. Ideally drains should be placed well to the side of incisions to minimize contamination.

When the wound is the problem it should be left open rather than drained. A drain in the wound itself completely negates the beneficial effect of topical ampicillin following appendicectomy.

A good dressing protects the wound from postoperative contamination but if it becomes wet it does more harm than good. Local moisture and abrasion enhance infectivity. Biological dressings, like skin grafts, behave differently. They enhance local defence mechanisms and help sterilize the surface of infected open wounds.

Dehiscence

If a superficial wound breaks open it can safely be left to heal by itself. In most other sites secondary healing is unacceptable and immediate repair must be undertaken. Abdominal wound dehiscence serves to illustrate the problem but it is relatively unimportant compared with breakdown of colonic or vascular anastomoses.

A fresh wound has no strength of its own and requires artificial support with sutures (Forrester, 1972). If the support system fails before functional integrity is regained then the wound edges break apart (Reitamo & Möller, 1972; Keill et al, 1973). Although suture failure plays an obvious role the main problem is upset connective tissue formation in the scar. Local sepsis is the single most important factor delaying collagen synthesis and increasing collagen lysis. Softening of the wound edge is even more marked when local trauma has been excessive.

Although sutures are required for security they may contribute to dehiscence by enhancing the infectivity of wound pathogens. The determinants are the mass of implanted suture material and its natural irritating propensity. It is therefore important to ensure that unnecessarily heavy gauges are avoided and bland materials are used whenever possible. The synthetic sutures fit these requirements best and in monofilament form are particularly non-reactive. Absorbable sutures lose strength before they are absorbed and by the end of a month are behaving as a foreign body without helping support the wound. So far as 'cutting out' is concerned, this is minimized by ensuring that the sutures are placed through fascia and other condensed collagen layers. They are the only tissues with significant holding power for sutures.

Wound dehiscence often reflects an error of judgement on the part of the surgeon. That is, a failure to assess the risk of breakdown and adopt the appropriate wound closure technique to prevent it. In assessing risk, all factors that delay collagen formation and enhance its lysis are important. Prominent among these are starvation with loss of body weight, long-term corticosteroid treatment, sepsis and antimetabolites. The single most important factor is poor surgical technique and in particular tying the sutures too tight and compromising wound perfusion. Continuous sutures provide the most uniform support but interrupted sutures are more secure. Since there is initially quite marked softening of the wound edges, security is further ensured by placing the stitches well back (5–7 mm) from the wound edge (see Fig. 1.14).

Wounds in the abdominal wall require strength and since this develops slowly the continued support of non-absorbable sutures is necessary (Douglas, 1952) (Fig. 1.22). The moment a wound is sutured it has 40–70% of the strength of unwounded tissue. If non-absorbable sutures have been used, strength is maintained indefinitely and by 3 months the strength of the scar is sufficiently great that suture support can safely be removed. Absorbable material, on the other hand, loses strength rapidly and after 2 weeks is contributing very little to wound strength. If healing is delayed, say by infection, absorbable sutures cannot be relied upon to provide adequate support and the wound may break open.

Wound dehiscence with evisceration is rare. Immediate resuture is usually followed by rapid uneventful healing and if the true healing time is not taken into account it appears to be more rapid than normal (Fig. 1.23). The disruption is simply a mechanical event and no biochemical disturbances have been detected. Since the fibroblast-capillary system is active the resutured wound has a head-start and the preparatory phase of healing is not repeated. These active local changes persist throughout the period of fibroplasia and a similar rapid recovery of strength should be anticipated if a further operation has to be performed through the same scar. After several

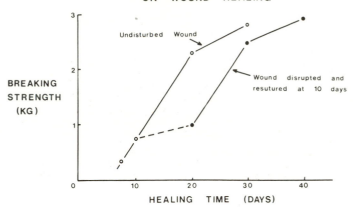

THE EFFECT OF RUPTURE AND RESUTURE ON WOUND HEALING

Fig. 1.23 If a healing wound is broken open and resutured it picks up strength rapidly. Ten days later it is stronger than a fresh 10-day wound, but still a good deal weaker than if it has been left undisturbed.

months when the scar has matured and devascularized this is no longer the case.

The colon does not have great natural strength. Following anastomosis, healing is rapid and full strength is recovered in 3 weeks. Despite this, rapid healing wound breakdown with anastomotic leakage is not all that uncommon (Irvin & Hunt, 1974). The unusually high turnover rate of collagen is responsible (Figs. 1.24 and 1.25). During the first 4 to 6 days up to 40% of the old collagen in the wound is lost as a result of marked collagenase activity (Cronin et al, 1968a; Cronin et al, 1968b). Normally strength is maintained by rapid synthesis of new collagen. However, with such high rates of turnover the balance is easily upset. Local factors such as trauma, foreign material and bacterial contamination have adverse effects and the mechanical effects of faecal abrasion compound the problem. When an anastomotic leakage is

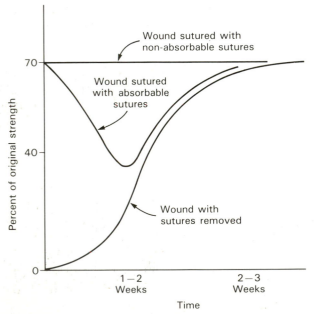

Fig. 1.22 Strength is recovered slowly in fascial wounds and suture support is required for about 3 months. The moment a wound is sutured it has between 40 and 70% of its original strength. This is maintained when non-absorbable sutures are used. Absorbable sutures lose their strength before the wound has fully recovered and dehiscence is more likely.

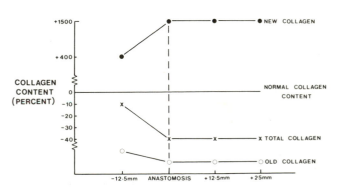

HEALING COLONIC ANASTOMOSIS

Fig. 1.24 Collagen is synthesized rapidly in colonic wounds but during the first 4 days there is extensive destruction of pre-existing submucosal collagen and net losses of up to 40% are found on either side. (After Cronin K et al 1968)

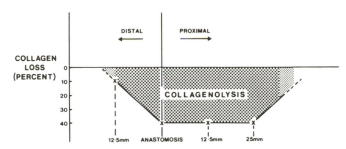

COLLAGENASE ACTIVITY IN HEALING COLON

Fig. 1.25 During the first few days of healing there is marked collagenolytic activity above and below the site of anastomosis. As a result sutures may become insecure. (After Cronin K et al, 1968)

believed to be likely the continued support of fine non-irritant non-absorbable sutures is recommended. In addition, tension-relieving hitch stitches to adjacent structures may be beneficial.

The connective tissue response in the cardiovascular system is limited and the continued support of non-absorbable material is essential if wound breakdown is to be prevented (Berger et al, 1972). In prosthetic grafts a pseudo-intima rapidly develops but longitudinal in-growth of fibrous tissue is limited to a few centimetres at either end. The graft proper is well supported by circumferential collagen. Surgical mobilization activates collagenase and may be responsible for rapid enlargement of aortic aneurysms following laparotomy.

Fibrosis

Healing is usually uneventful and may even proceed relatively normally when genetic disorders such as dermatosparaxis and Ehlers-Danlos syndrome are present. Physical integrity is best restored by the smallest amount of scar and attempts to improve repair by encouraging excessive scar formation are unsuccessful because it is an inherently weak material. When scar tissue is naturally over-produced it causes fibrosis. This abnormally contracting material is often a late sequela of injury or inflammatory disease and features a whole range of chronic fibrotic processes, from simple adhesions in peritoneum and tendon sheath to interstitial pulmonary fibrosis. Other troublesome examples are benign oesophageal strictures, mitral stenosis, hepatic cirrhosis and the post-traumatic cerebral scar. Attempts are now being made to control fibrosis by specific antifibrotic treatment of the scar and non-specific methods aimed at diminishing the inflammatory process that precedes fibroblast activation (Chvapil, 1974; Peacock, 1981).

Drugs which affect collagen metabolism have specific effects in scar because of its high rate of turnover. Collagen synthesis can be prevented by interfering with hydroxylation of protocollagen within the fibroblast. This is

accomplished by removing co-factors such as iron and ascorbic acid or disturbing the configuration of the unhydroxylated molecule with proline analogues. These techniques work in vitro but are disappointing in practice.

The most effective approach is to delay the maturation of the wound by preventing polymerization of tropocollagen. Simple accumulation of uncrosslinked collagen does not interfere with function. It is the development of rigid crosslinked collagen masses that causes fibrosis and deforming contractures. The abnormal physical behaviour appears to be associated with failure of soft tissue remodelling following irretrievable fixation of the random collagen fibril patterns by rapid intermolecular crosslinking. When physical forces are applied to the wound before polymerization is complete the fibrils are aligned and mechanical properties enhanced (Forrester et al, 1970). More useful effects follow if polymerization is arrested using B-amino-propionitrile (Peacock & Madden, 1972). This drug works by blocking aldehyde formation and crosslinking. Penicillamine has similar effects. It chelates newly formed aldehydes before they bond. Uncrosslinked collagen is free to organize in more physiological patterns and these are maintained when crosslinking is allowed to proceed. Since these new molecular patterns are reflected in the shape and weave of the collagen fibres themselves the physical properties of the scar should be nearer normal (Fig. 1.26) (Forrester, 1975).

Non-specific methods are aimed at controlling fibrosis by limiting the inflammatory process that precedes fibroblast activation. Anti-inflammatory drugs of steroid and non-steroid type prove useful here but more precise effects appear likely when the tissue mediators and activators of fibroblasts are properly identified. Following tissue injury

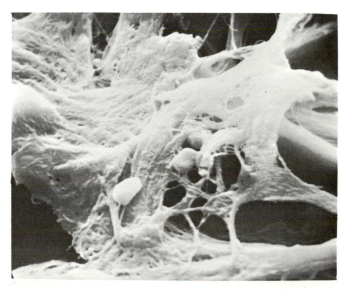

Fig. 1.26 Scanning electron micrograph of a 60-day penicillamine-treated wound (× 3250). The collagen fibre patterns are better organised than in the untreated wound (see Fig. 1.8). Large fibril bundles are well demarcated and a network structure is developing.

lipid peroxidases are activated and lysosomes break open. The lysosomal enzymes damage the macrophages and the damaged macrophages stimulate the fibroblasts to increase collagen production. In this way trauma creates necrosis, and fibrosis results. If necrosis is reduced, fibrosis is less. Studies in silicotic lung disease suggest that zinc may be useful here. It stabilizes lysosomes and protects macro-phages from damage by silica. There is a considerable reduction in necrosis and fibrosis (Chvapil, 1974).

The present methods of managing fibrosis are imprecise, relying on surgical excision and judicious use of cortico-steroids. The need for effective antifibrotic therapy is obvious. Until it is available the serious health hazard of excessive scar formation remains.

REFERENCES

Abercrombie M, Heaysman J E M 1954 Observations on the social behaviour of cells in tissue culture. II. Monolayering of fibroblasts. Experimental Cellular Research 6: 293–306

Altemeier W A, Hummel R P, Hill E O, Lewis S 1973 Changing patterns in surgical infections. Annals of Surgery 178: 436–445

Altemeier W A, Burke J F, Pruit B A, Sandusky W R (eds) 1984 Manual on control of infection in surgical patients, 2nd edn J B Lippincott Co, Philadelphia

Bassett C A L, Mitchell S N, Gaston S R 1981 Treatment of ununited tibial diaphyseal fractures with pulsing electromagnetic fields. Journal of Bone and Joint Surgery 63A: 511–523

Belzer F O, Salvatierra O, Schweizer R T, Kountz S M 1973 Prevention of wound infections by topical antibiotics in high risk patients. American Journal of Surgery 126: 180–185

Bentley J P 1967 Rate of chondroitin sulfate formation in wound healing. Annals of Surgery 165: 186–191

Berger K, Sauvage L R, Rao A M, Wood S J 1972 Healing of arterial prostheses in man: its incompleteness. Annals of Surgery 175: 118–127

Berliner D J, Williams R J, Taylor G N, Nabors C J 1967 Decreased scar formation with topical corticosteroid treatment. Surgery 61: 619–625

Booth J B, Todd G B 1970 Subclinical scurvy — hypovitaminosis C. British Journal of Hospital Medicine 4: 513–526

Bornstein P, Sage H 1980 Structurally distinct collagen types. Annual Review of Biochemistry 49: 957–1003

Bullough W S, Laurence E B 1960 The control of epidermal mitotic activity in the mouse. Proceedings of the Royal Society B151: 517–536

Burke J F 1964 Wound infection and early inflammation. Monographs of Surgical Science 1: 301–345

Charnley J 1973 Clean air in the operating room. Cleveland Clinic Quarterly 40: 99–114

Chvapil M 1974 Pharmacology of fibrosis and tissue injury. Environmental Health Perspective 9: 283–294

Craig R D P, Schofield J D, Jackson D S 1975 Collagen biosynthesis in normal human skin, normal and hypertrophic scar and keloid. European Journal of Clinical Investigation 5: 69–74

Cronin K, Jackson D S, Dunphy J E 1968a Changes in bursting strength and collagen content of the healing colon. Surgery, Gynecology and Obstetrics 126: 747–753

Cronin K, Jackson D S, Dunphy J E 1968b Specific activity of hydroxyproline-tritium in the healing colon. Surgery, Gynecology and Obstetrics 126: 1061–1065

Cuthbertson D P 1970 Intensive care — metabolic response to injury. British Journal of Surgery 57: 718–721

Devel T F, Senior R M, Huang J S, Griffin G 1982 Chemotaxis of monocytes and neutrophils to platelet-derived growth factor. Journal of Clinical Investigation 69: 1046–1049

Douglas D M 1952 The healing of aponeurotic incisions. British Journal of Surgery 40: 79–84

Douglas D M, Forrester J C, Ogilvie R R 1969 Physical characteristics of collagen in the later stages of wound healing. British Journal of Surgery 56: 219–222

Edlich R F, Rogers W, Kasper G, Kaufman D, Tsung M S, Wangensteen O H 1969 Studies in the management of the contaminated wound. I. Optimal time for closure of contaminated wounds. II. Comparison of resistance to infection of open and closed wounds during healing. American Journal of Surgery 117: 323–329

Ehrlich H P, Tarver H, Hunt T K 1973 Effects of vitamin A and glucocorticoids upon inflammation and collagen synthesis. Annals of Surgery 177: 222–227

Evans C, Pollock A V 1973 The reduction of surgical wound infections by prophylactic parenteral cephaloridine. British Journal of Surgery 60: 434–437

Fell G S 1985 The link with zinc. British Medical Journal 290: 242

Fitton-Jackson S, Jones D B, Murray J D, Farndale R W 1981 The response of connective tissue and skeletal tissue to pulsed magnetic fields. Transactions of the Bioelectrical Repair and Growth Society 1: 1–85

Forrester J C 1972 Suture materials and their use. British Journal of Hospital Medicine 8: 578–592

Forrester J C 1975 Collagen fibre patterns in penicillamine treated wounds: A tensiometric and scanning electron microscope study. In: Gibson T, van der Meulen J C (eds) Wound Healing. Foundation Int Co-op Medical Science, Montreux: 69–72

Forrester J C, Hayes T L, Pease R F W, Hunt T K 1969 Scanning electron microscopy of healing wounds. Nature 221: 373–374

Forrester J C, Zederfeldt B H, Hayes T L, Hunt T K 1970 Tape-closed and sutured wounds: A comparison by tensiometry and scanning electron microscopy. British Journal of Surgery 57: 729–737

Forrester J C, Ruckley R W, Browning M C K 1983 Leucocyte ascorbic acid and adrenal cortical function in patients having elective surgical procedures. Unpublished data

Gabbiani G 1981 The myofibroblast: a key cell for wound healing and fibrocontractive diseases. Progress in Clinical Biological Research 54: 183–194

Gilmore O J A, Sanderson P J 1975 Prophylactic interparietal povidone-iodine in abdominal surgery. British Journal of Surgery 62: 792–799

Grant M E, Prockop D W 1972 The biosynthesis of collagen. New England Journal of Medicine 286: 194–199 242–249 291–300

Hares M M, Hegarty M A, Warlow J, Malins D, Youngs D, Bentley S et al 1981 A controlled trial to compare systemic and intra-incisional cefuroxime prophylaxis in high risk gastric surgery. British Journal of Surgery 68: 276–280

Heughan C, Grislis G, Hunt T K 1974 The effect of anaemia on wound healing. Annals of Surgery 179: 163–167

Hunt T K, Pai M P 1972 The effect of varying ambient oxygen tensions on wound metabolism and collagen synthesis. Surgery, Gynecology and Obstetrics 135: 561–567

Hunt T K, Zederfeldt B, Goldstick T K 1969 Oxygen and healing. American Journal of Surgery 118: 521–525

Hutton J J, Tappel A L, Udenfriend S 1967 Cofactor and substrate requirements of collagen proline hydroxylase. Archives of Biochemistry Biophysics 118: 231–240

Irvin T T, Hunt T K 1974 Reappraisal of the healing process of anastomosis of the colon. Surgery, Gynecology and Obstetrics 138: 741–746

Jackson D S 1975 The interaction of collagen with glycoproteins and proteoglycans. In: Gibson T, van der Meulen J C (eds) Wound Healing. Montreux: Foundation Int Co-op Medical Science, p 76–80

Keill R H, Keitzer W F, Nichols W K, Henzel J, De Weese M S 1973

Abdominal wound dehiscence. Archives of Surgery 106: 573–577

Knighton D R, Thakral K K, Hunt T K 1980 Platelet-derived angiogenesis: initiator of the healing sequence. Surgical Forum 31: 226–227

Knighton D R, Silver I A, Hunt T K 1981 Regulation of wound healing angiogenesis — effect of oxygen gradient and inspired oxygen concentration. Surgery 90: 262–270

Lee E 1972 The effect of obstructive jaundice on the migration of reticulo-endothelial cells and fibroblasts into early experimental granulomata. British Journal of Surgery 59: 875–877

Leibovich S J, Ross R 1976 A macrophage-dependent factor that stimulates the proliferation of fibroblasts in vitro. American Journal of Pathology 84: 501–513

McDermott F T, Nayman J, DeBoer W G R M, Path M C 1968 The effect of acute renal failure upon wound healing. Annals of Surgery 168: 142–146

Madden J W, Peacock E E 1968 Studies on the biology of collagen during wound healing. I. Rate of collagen synthesis and deposition in cutaneous wounds of the rat. Surgery 64: 288–294

Miller E J, Matukas V J 1974 Biosynthesis of collagen. The biochemist's view. Federation Proceedings 33: 1197–1204

Mosher D R 1980 Fibronectin. Progress in Hemostasis and Thrombosis 5: 111–151

Myers J A 1983 Geliperm: a non-textile wound dressing. Pharmaceutical Journal 230: 263–264

Newcombe J F 1966 Effect of intra-arterial nitrogen mustard infusion on wound healing in rabbits. Formation of granulation tissue and wound contraction. Annals of Surgery 163: 319–329

Niinikoski J 1969 Effect of oxygen supply on wound healing and formation of experimental granulation tissue. Acta Physiologica Scandinavica, supplement: 334

Peacock E E 1981 Pharmacologic control of surface scarring in human beings. Annals of Surgery 193: 592–597

Peacock E E, Madden J W 1972 On the use of lathyrogens in human biology. Surgery 71: 922–924

Polk H C, Lopez-Mayor J F 1969 Post-operative wound infection: A prospective study of determinant factors and prevention. Surgery 66: 97–103

Pollock A V, Evans M 1975 Povidone-iodine for the control of surgical wound infection: A controlled clinical trial against topical cephaloridine. British Journal of Surgery 62: 292–294

Pories W J, Henzel J H, Rob C G, Strain W H 1967 Acceleration of wound healing in man with zinc sulphate given by mouth. Lancet i: 121–124

Postlethwaite A E, Keski-Oja J, Balian G, Kang A 1981 Induction of fibroblast chemotaxis by fibronectin. Journal of Experimental Medicine 153: 494–499

Prockop D J, Kivirikko K I, Tuderman L, Guzman N A 1979 The biosynthesis of collagen and its disorders. New England Journal of Medicine 301: 13–23 77–85

Raekallio J 1972 Determination of the age of wounds by histochemical and biochemical methods. Forensic Science 1: 3–16

Reitamo J, Moller C 1972 Abdominal wound dehiscence. Acta Chirurgica Scandinavica 138: 170–175

Ross R, Benditt E P 1964 Wound healing and collagen formation. IV. Distortion of ribosomal patterns of fibroblasts in scurvy. Journal of Cellular Biology 22: 365–389

Ross R, Everett N B, Tyler R 1970 Wound healing and collagen formation. VI. The origin of the wound fibroblast studied in parabiosis. Journal of Cellular Biology 44: 645–654

Ryan G B, Cliff W J, Gabbiani G, Irle C, Montandon D, Statkov P R, Majno G 1974 Myofibroblasts in human granulation tissue. Human Pathology 5: 55–67

Salthouse T N, Williams J A 1969 Histochemical observations of enzyme activity at suture implantation sites. Journal of Surgical Research 9: 481–486

Shaw D, Doig C M, Douglas D M 1973 Is airborne infection in operating-theatres an important cause of wound infection in general surgery. Lancet i: 17–20

Silver I A 1969 The measurement of oxygen tension in healing tissue. In: Herzog H (ed) Progress in Respiration Research, Karger, Basle, vol 3. p 124–135

Silver I A 1980 The physiology of wound healing. In: Hunt T K (ed) Wound Healing and Wound Infection, Appleton Century Crofts, New York p 11–28

Simpson D, Ross R 1972 The neutrophilic leukocyte in wound repair. A study with anti-neutrophil serum. Journal of Clinical Investigation 51: 2009–2023

Van Winkle W 1967 Wound contraction. Surgery, Gynecology and Obstetrics 125: 131–142

Van Winkle W 1968 The epithelium in wound healing. Surgery, Gynecology and Obstetrics 127: 1089–1115

Wahl S M 1981 Role of mononuclear cells in the wound repair process. In: Dineen P, Hildick-Smith G (eds) Lea & Febiger, Philadelphia p 63–74

Wilmore D W, Dudrick S J 1968 Growth and development of an infant receiving all nutrients exclusively by vein. Journal of the American Medical Association 203: 860–864

Winter G D 1972 Epidermal regeneration studied in the domestic pig. In: Maibach H I, Rovee D T (eds) Epidermal Wound Healing, Year Book Publishers, p 71–112

Wood R W, Loomis A L 1927 The physical and biological effects of high frequency sound waves of great intensity. Dublin Philosophical Magazine and Journal of Science 4: 417–436

Wood R A B, Williams R H P, Hughes L E 1977 Foam elastomer dressings in the management of open granulating wounds. British Journal of Surgery 64: 554–557

Zederfeldt B H, Hunt T K 1968 Availability of oxygen in tissue remote from major injury. Bulletin de la Societe Internationale de Chirurgie 27: 15–21

Biological effects of radiation

INTRODUCTION

This chapter describes the unique effects of the classes of radiation used medically in treatment of cancer and in diagnosis. Radiation of these kinds are referred to as 'ionizing', the process by which energy is transferred. The effects are not simply those of burning or freezing, like, for example, diathermy, laser beams and cryosurgery; they are those of selective 'cell killing' for neoplastic and normal tissues, as well as other important short- and long-term effects, genetic and somatic. The special advantage of 'ionizing' radiation in treating many kinds of neoplastic tissue is that it may be possible to give a suitable dose schedule of radiation so that all tumour cells are killed while the normal tissue bed receives no more than temporary, repairable, damage (the 'radiation reaction'). The main value of using ionizing radiation to treat cancer — radiotherapy — is that the treatment is selective, to a chosen volume of tissue; this compares with the general effect of hormones or of chemotherapy to the whole body, and in addition there is no need for any removal of tissue, the obvious main disadvantage of surgery.

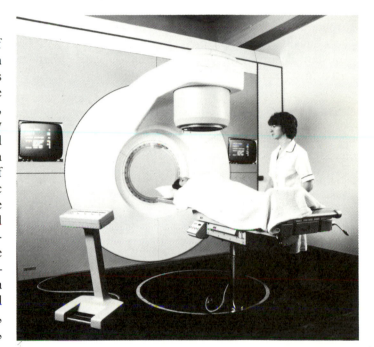

Fig. 2.1 Linear accelerator — 14 MeV

IONIZING RADIATION

History and physics

The main kinds of radiation used medically consisted until the 1940s of X-rays and of the rays emitted by radium. Both of these were discovered at the end of the 19th century.

Roentgen discovered and named X-rays in 1895. He found that when cathode rays (beams of negatively-charged electrons) struck the anode (or positive electrode) in an evacuated glass tube, rays were emitted which could fog photographic plates and could penetrate opaque materials. It was found at once that these X-rays would penetrate soft tissue more easily than dense tissue such as bone; radiographs could be taken of the body to show normal and pathological organs as well as foreign bodies. Modern X-

ray tubes have been made more reliable and powerful and the potential difference or voltage applied across the electrodes is still often used to describe the kind of unit in use. Diagnostic X-ray tubes usually operate at up to 140 kV (kilovolts). Therapy tubes will not only have a higher output quantitatively but will also use higher voltages, producing more penetrating X-rays. Superficial X-ray therapy units suitable for treating skin conditions will operate at 50–150 kV. The common 'deep' X-ray therapy tube or 'orthovoltage' will produce 200–500 kV (usually 250–300 kV) X-rays of medium penetration; these tubes which used to be the mainstay of radiotherapy departments are now considerably superseded by linear accelerators (Fig. 2.1). These use high frequency radio waves which are fed into a wave guide (an evacuated metal tube) and accelerated to nearly the speed of light. A beam of electrons is also fed in and in effect 'surf-ride' on the crests of the radio waves to a very high energy. The electrons then strike a metal target and are converted into megavoltage (million volt) X-rays, with a very high output, so that individual treatment times are only a few minutes and large numbers of patients can be treated.

Radium was isolated by the Curies in 1902 and was found to emit three kinds of ionizing radiation: alpha rays, charged helium atoms; beta rays, electrons; and gamma rays which are high energy X-rays under another name. Radium is the main natural radioactive isotope, the gas radon being another. Many artificial radioactive nuclides (usually but incorrectly called only 'isotopes') are now available from nuclear reactors and from cyclotrons. All will disintegrate, giving off radioactivity, or 'decay', with a constant exponential half-life. The radiation emitted is occasionally α-rays but more commonly β- and γ-rays of constant energy, expressed in a 'decay-scheme'. Many are used in medicine for diagnosis and therapy (Table 2.1).

Table 2.1 Radio-nuclides used commonly in radiotherapy

Isotope	Half-life	Radiation (MeV energy)		
		α	β	γ
Caesium-137	27 yr	—	0.52, 1.2	0.67
Cobalt-60	5.2 yr	—	0.32	1.2, 1.3
Gold-198	2.7 days	—	0.96	0.41
Iodine-125	60 days	—	—	27–35 keV
Iodine-131	8 days	—	0.25–0.81	0.08–0.72
Iridium-192	74 days	—	0.66	0.14–0.65
Phosphorus-32	14 days	—	1.7	—
Radium-226	1620 yr	4.6, 4.8	—	0.19
decays to				
Radon-222	3.8 days	5.5	—	—
decays to				
Radium-C-214	19.7 min	5.5	1.6, 3.1	0.4–2.4
Strontium-90	28 yr	—	0.54	—
decays to				
Yttrium-90	64 h	—	2.2	—
Tantalum-182	111 days	—	0.52	0.07–1.2

'Interstitial' treatment by implants of needles or wires remains of value when localized irradiation is required, for example to intra-oral tumours (Fig 2.2) and small carcinomas of the bladder. Radium and radon seeds are still used, though obsolescent, and 'grains' or wires (often as 'hairpins') of gold-198, iridium-192, tantalum-182 or iodine-125 are becoming more commonly used.

Intracavitary treatment is mainly used for gynaecological cancer, especially of the cervix (Fig. 2.3) and body of the uterus. Radium tubes are now commonly replaced by caesium-137 or cobalt-60 and are frequently loaded by remotely controlled units such as the 'Cathetron', 'Selectron' and 'Curietron' with no radiation at all to staff. The most important unit however is the telecobalt unit (Fig. 2.4), using a small high specific activity source of cobalt-60–1000 curies or more — in a shielded head with

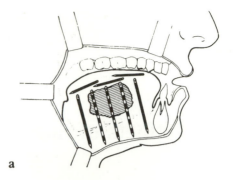

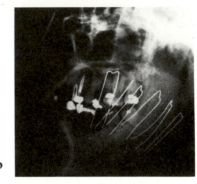

Fig. 2.2 (a) A radionuclide needle implant for carcinoma of the tongue. (b) A modern iridium-192 'hair-pin' implant for a long superficial tongue carcinoma.

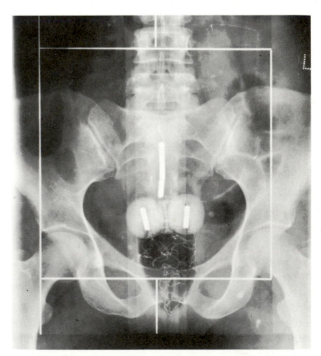

Fig. 2.3 Treatment of carcinoma of the uterine cervix by insertion of radionuclide tubes into the cervical canal and the lateral fornices of the vagina, as shown on a verification X-ray film.

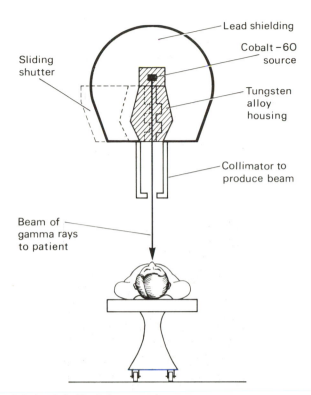

Fig. 2.4 A cobalt-60 teletherapy unit.

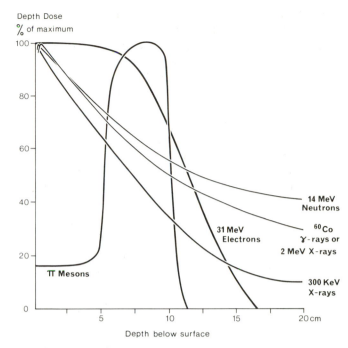

Fig. 2.5 'Depth dose' curve.

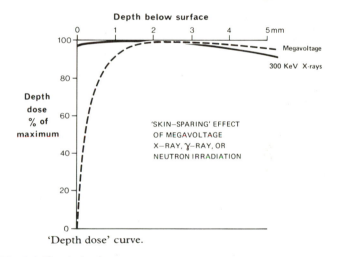

Fig. 2.6 'Depth dose' curve.

a shutter and collimator system; this gives a beam similar to that from a linear accelerator.

All external beam units, whether X-ray or γ-ray, are constructed with a collimation system of interchangeable applicators or a continuously variable diaphragm so as to give square or rectangular beams ranging from about 4 × 4 to 30 × 30 cm (superficial units giving even smaller fields, often circular and down to 1 cm diameter circles). The depth dose in the body (Figs. 2.5 and 2.6) will depend firstly upon the f.s.d. or s.s.d. (focus- or source-skin-distance) — the dose falling inversely as the square of the distance. A long f.s.d. of 100 cm is therefore desirable. Secondly the penetration will vary according to the energy of the radiation used.

X- and γ-rays are not the only rays used in modern radiotherapy. Several charged particles can be used, such as the small subatomic particle called a π-meson, and the common uncharged particle, the neutron, that is a major component of the atomic nucleus.

Electrons and other charged particles are absorbed in a way different to that of X- and γ-rays and neutrons which are absorbed gradually as the rays penetrate tissue. In contrast, charged particles are mainly absorbed at a specific tissue depth (dependent on their energy) and then penetrate *no further*, i.e. they are stopped and have a maximum *range of penetration*. This interesting contrast is well shown in Figure 2.5 which shows that π-mesons and 31 MeV electrons are completely absorbed by about 11 and 17 cm respectively, compared with the more gradual and

continued decrease in depth dose of neutrons, γ- and X-rays. Low energy electrons may therefore be very useful for treating skin tumours, such as mycosis fungoides; higher energy electrons (from a betatron) may be useful in treating head and neck tumours, sparing the spinal cord. The most interesting new units treat tumours by fast neutrons or π-mesons, with the main object of avoiding the oxygen-effect, as explained below. Neutrons of high energy and penetration can be produced by cyclotrons, such as the three in Britain, at Hammersmith Hospital, at Edinburgh (Fig. 2.7) and at Clatterbridge Hospital, near Liverpool. π-meson generators are even more sophisticated

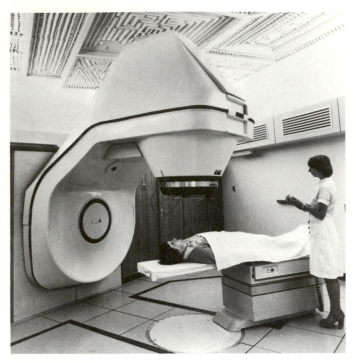

Fig. 2.7 A medical cyclotron used to treat human cancer by neutrons.

and expensive but may give the advantages of very accurate localized dose-distribution as well as avoidance of the oxygen-effect.

The only important method of radiotherapy remaining to be described is the systemic administration of radioactive isotopes. The principal isotopes are *radio-iodine* to irradiate the thyroid for thyrotoxicosis and thyroid cancer, and *radio-phosphorus* to treat blood diseases — polycythaemia rubravera, thrombocythaemia, and chronic leukaemia. *Absorption of radiation* needs brief mention since it differs with different radiation sources and there are clinical consequences. Low energy X-rays are absorbed more heavily in dense tissues and this can lead to over-irradiation of bone and consequent damage. High energy megavoltage X-rays are absorbed mainly uniformly, of great clinical importance since the doctor can then be confident that the dosage is similar in both tumour and normal tissues. They also penetrate so rapidly that there is a 'skin-sparing' effect and an undesirable skin reaction can therefore usually be avoided (see Fig. 2.6).

Radiation dosage and units

Radiation dosage can be very precisely measured and specified and it is important to understand the units used, since dosage in this context is different to the common usage in clinical pharmacology or therapeutics and unfortunately has three quite different meanings. A dose of radioactive isotope refers to the quantity measured in terms of radioactivity. The old unit is the *curie* (activity giving 3.7×10^{10} disintegrations per second, nearly equivalent to 1 g of radium) and the new S.I. unit, now in widespread use, is the becquerel (activity giving 1 disintegration per second), a very small quantity. Test doses of isotopes have been measured in microcuries, treatment doses in millicuries, and treatment sources in curies (see appendix, p. 32).

Dose in this first sense, quantity of radioactivity given, will not correspond to radiation effect since this relates to the energy absorbed. This second and more important usage is defined in terms of energy absorbed per gram of tissue. This is not the same as the original *exposure* dose — the roentgen — which was defined as the quantity of radiation (X or γ) which produces ionization of 1 electrostatic unit in 1 ml of air at normal temperature and pressure and was much easier to measure. The modern units, the rad and the gray, relate well to their effect on tissue. The rad is the unit of absorbed dose corresponding to absorption of 100 ergs per gram of material. The new S.I. unit, the gray, is defined as the dose of radiation giving 1 joule per kg and is therefore 100 times larger. It should be repeated finally that dose of radiation corresponds to energy absorbed per gram; it is *not* the total energy absorbed which is termed 'integral dose'. Examples of radiation dosage and a summary of definitions are given for reference in the appendix at the end of this chapter (p. 32).

Ionization and transfer of energy

The process of ionization or the very similar 'excitation' is the method by which energy is transferred when radiation is absorbed in tissue. The physical details vary but the common process is the displacement or disturbance of one or more orbital electrons of the atoms in the track of the radiation, and this takes about 10^{-16} seconds. If biological material is involved, the ionization will next cause chemical damage — the production of free radicals, most commonly in water which is split into OH and H radicals in 10^{-14} to 10^{-3} seconds. There will next be both direct damage to organic biological molecules and also indirect damage from radicals formed in water. This will lead to biomolecular damage over succeeding seconds or hours especially to important compounds such as proteins and nucleic acids and finally, much later, the biological damage will be seen after a period of time ranging from hours to years. This brief and simple explanation covers very complicated processes of radiochemistry which, because of their extreme rapidity, are very difficult to investigate. It can at least be accepted that the energy transfer is peculiarly effective, since the energy needed for death in man (say 10 gray) would not produce a measurable temperature rise if converted into heat (10 gray would cause a rise in temperature of 0.0025°C).

RADIATION EFFECTS ON CELLS

The beginnings of radiobiology

Ionizing radiation was first consciously applied to living tissues by Roentgen in 1895 for diagnostic purposes. Biological effect on the skin was soon observed, in April 1896, by an American professor who attempted to demonstrate gunshot in the head of a colleague and therefore gave a long exposure because of the low penetration of the X-rays then in use. Twenty-one days later both the doctor and the patient were astonished to find that all the hair in the exposed scalp was dropping out. The first recognition of a biological effect from radium was probably the description given by Henri Becquerel and Pierre Curie to the French Academy in 1907: 'Monsieur Becquerel carried a small sealed tube containing a few centigrams of radioactive barium chloride. The radioactive substance was wrapped in paper and kept in a small cardboard box. On April 3 and 4 this box was placed several times in the waistcoat pocket for times not exceeding in all 6 hours. On April 13 it was noticed that the radiation through the tube, the box, and the clothes had caused on the underlying skin a red mark which became darker during the next few days and had the oblong shape of the tube.'

It was soon recognized that both X-rays and radium could cause damage to the skin and in Hamburg in 1902 the first case of radiation-induced skin cancer occurred in an X-ray tube factory worker. The use of radiation to cure cancer was being discovered at the same time; the first cure of skin cancer by X-rays was in 1899 (the patient, a Viennese lady, survived for over 20 years) and the first successful use of radium for skin cancer was in Russia in 1903.

Clinical and experimental radiation biology expanded rapidly and modern radiotherapy of cancer began to develop, but remained empirical for many years. It used to be said that the main rationale for radiotherapy was the unique selective action of ionizing radiation on rapidly dividing less differentiated cells, which were thought to be more radiosensitive as shown by Bergonié and Tribondeau as long ago as 1906. Modern cell biology and kinetics have shown that cellular radiosensitivity is a much more complicated subject.

Cell survival curves

The technique described by Puck and Marcus (1956) was extremely important, and is still the basis of a large proportion of much experimental work in cellular radiobiology. The method (Fig. 2.8) consists of pipetting a known number of single cells, suspended in liquid nutritive medium, on to Petri dishes in which the cells spread out and attach to the bottom of the dish. Next, the dishes can be given different doses of radiation from zero for controls up to several hundred gray. The dishes are then

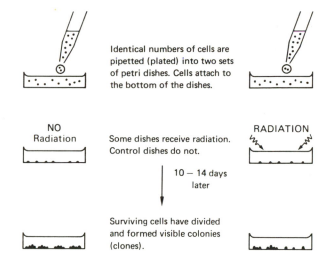

Fig. 2.8 Puck and Marcus cloning technique for obtaining *in vitro* cell survival curves.

incubated at 37°C for 10–14 days and after this time surviving cells will have grown into easily visible colonies of say 50 cells, which are called 'clones' and can be counted.

It is important to understand the meaning of this cell survival which is being measured. Cell death can have several meanings. Non-proliferating, well-differentiated cells such as nerve, muscle or secretory cells might be said to die when they lose a specific function. It is, however, loss of the capacity for sustained proliferation — *reproductive integrity* — which is the appropriate definition for the patient with cancer. For a tumour to be eradicated it is only necessary to prevent further division of the malignant cells resulting in no further spread or metastasis. Cells may still be physically present and superficially intact; they may even be able to synthesize proteins or DNA and to struggle through one or two mitoses, but if they are unable to proliferate indefinitely, to be 'clonogenic', they can be regarded as dead in this sense.

This point is of great importance to the surgeon and pathologist. It is essential to realize that the persistence of histologically normal tumour cells, which can appear morphologically intact and can stain normally, does *not* neccessarily indicate the probability of regrowth of a tumour which has been irradiated (Suit & Gallagher, 1964). Lack of understanding of this can lead, for example, to unnecessary laryngectomy after a misinterpreted biopsy.

The first cell survival curves were derived from hamster lung cells but the curves are similar for very many mammalian cells, both benign and neoplastic.

The typical cell survival curve (Fig. 2.9) will usually consist of a 'shoulder' at the beginning of the curve followed by a straight exponential line. The initial shoulder is caused by sublethal damage and may be characterized by alternative measurements — the 'extrapolation number' n, found by extrapolating the straight portion of the

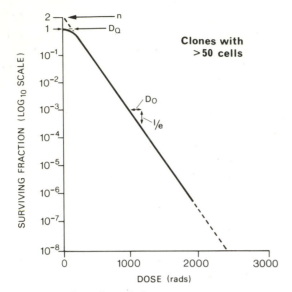

Fig. 2.9 A mammalian cell survival curve.

survival curve back to the surviving fraction axis, or the 'quasithreshold dose' D_Q, the dose at which the extrapolated straight portion of the curve cuts the dose axis. This shoulder becomes smaller with increase in density of the radiation until it may appear non-existent. The slope of the straight portion will be a measure of radiosensitivity and is usually expressed as D_O, the dose required to reduce the number of cells by $1/e$ or 0.37; it is the dose which on average produces one lethal event in every unit of volume equal to that of a sensitive 'target' region in a cell (perhaps 5–100 nm diameter).

In vitro cell survival curves were at first viewed with considerable scepticism. Some critics suggested that they were quite different from clinical radiotherapy of man, indeed one of the pioneer radiation biologists, Dr F. G. Spear, even suggested that the behaviour of an isolated cell in vitro might be 'no more typical of its behaviour in the parent tissue than Robinson Crusoe on his desert island was representative to social life in York in the mid-17th century'. However, curves have now been obtained for several different cell lines, for example, HeLa cells from a human carcinoma of uterine cervix or lung, ovarian cells from newborn Chinese hamsters, human kidney cells, and mouse connective tissue cells. In addition, ingenious techniques have now been devised to measure in vivo cell survival curves for mouse leukaemia cells, skin, bone marrow and jejunal crypt cells, and others.

The response of human tumours to clinical radiotherapy cannot yet be entirely explained but there is at least considerable relevance now between experimental and clinical work; most of the newer ideas for radiotherapy, such as use of hypoxic cell sensitizers, fast neutrons and variation in timing of fractionation, have good experimental bases.

Linear energy transfer and radiobiological equivalence — radiation quality

Dose, time and volume are not the only relevant parameters that determine the biological effect of radiation. The kind or *quality* of radiation is very important. The major factor is the density of ionization of the radiation track and this can be expressed in physical terms as 'linear energy transfer' (LET), the energy transferred per unit length of track. In practice many radiation tracks are not straight lines and the energy deposition can be in clusters rather than uniform. However, it remains true that LET is lowest for megavoltage and γ-rays (as from cobalt-60), intermediate for orthovoltage (250–300 kV) X-rays, and highest for fast neutrons and the more esoteric particles such as π-mesons and alpha particles. The biological effect is usually specified in relation to the classical orthodox X-rays, 250 kV orthovoltage, and is termed relative biological effectiveness (RBE). The RBE will be about 0.8 for 4 MeV X-rays, whereas it will be as much as 3.0 for fast neutrons given in a fractionated course, since recovery and the time factor are also of importance.

Time factor — recovery and fractionation

Time is the next important factor to be considered; a simple clinical example will make this clear. If one treats a small basal cell carcinoma of skin by a single treatment, about 20 gray will be a lethal dose, but if the treatment is spread out into five daily fractions, a total of about 35 gray will have the same effect; if the treatment is given 5 days per week for 6 weeks about 60 gray will be required.

The first good correlation of such data was by Strandquist in 1944 and modern 'iso-effect' curves are little different (Fig. 2.10).

These curves show very clearly that the slope for cure of squamous carcinoma is flatter than that for normal tissue effects. It follows that a long fractionated course of X-ray therapy will result in a better ratio between tumour cure rate and normal tissue damage. This is of course the main basis for using fractionated courses of treatment, the second advantage being the avoidance of very severe acute

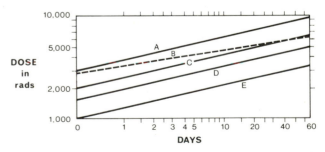

Fig. 2.10 Iso-effect curves relating total dose to overall treatment time for A, skin necrosis; B, cure of skin carcinoma; C, moist desquamation of skin; D, dry desquamation of skin; E, skin erythema.

reactions, such as nausea and vomiting, that depend upon the magnitude of an individual treatment. In these curves 'time' involves the effects both of overall time and of the number of fractions and it is the latter which is the more important. The relative importance of numbers of fractions and overall time can be seen very clearly from the simple classical experiment of Fowler (1966) who determined the equivalent doses on pigskin for 1, 5 and 21 fractions over 1, 4 and 28 days (Table 2.2).

Table 2.2 Typical time and fractionation effects: Equivalent doses to give moist desquamation in pigs

Time schedule	Equivalent dose (gray)
Single	20
5 fractions over 4 days	36
5 fractions over 28 days	42
21 fractions over 28 days	55

It will be seen that the necessary increase between 4 and 28 days for the same number of fractions was only 6 gray compared with an increase of 16 gray in changing from 1 to 5 fractions in 4 days, or with 13 gray from 5 to 21 fractions over 28 days.

Ellis (1969) has devised an empirical equation to relate normal tissue effects, usually called the 'tolerance dose' (D), to both the overall treatment time (T) and the number of fractions of treatment (N).

The Ellis equation is

$$D = (NSD)T^{0.11}N^{0.24}$$

where NSD is the 'nominal standard dose'. This equation is specifically based on the iso-effect curve for normal skin but has been widely used for comparison of many different fraction schemes and for effects on other tissues and indeed on tumours. It is of course no more than a mathematical convenience and has no clear theoretical rationale. The NSD can be expressed in units called rets (rad equivalent therapy) and is *not* a nominal *single* dose, because the equation is least accurate for less than four fractions. The system has been expanded to take account of volume treated and of gaps in treatment courses and has been rewritten in a much more sophisticated form by Kirk, Gray and Watson (1971) using another term, cumulative radiation effect (CRE).

The main explanation for this fractionation time-dose effect is of course the recovery from sub-lethal damage that has already been seen in typical cell-survival curves, with particular relevance to the 'shoulder' at the origin of the curve. If there is only a small shoulder, as is the case for fast neutrons, there will be a much smaller fractionation effect, as is shown in Fig. 2.11 for four fraction treatment by X-rays and by neutrons.

The oxygen effect

Gray et al (1953) showed that the sensitivity of anoxic mouse tumour cells to X-rays could be increased 2.6 times by raising the partial pressure of oxygen to normal tissue levels; further increase of oxygen tension has only slight effect (Fig. 2.12). This difference in sensitivity is known as the 'Oxygen Enhancement Ratio' (OER).

Almost all tumours are poorly organised and poorly vascularized. Even tiny tumours often have hypoxic or anoxic centres and this can be confirmed both by direct

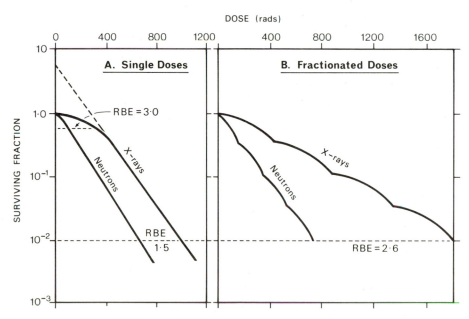

Fig. 2.11 Cell survival curves for X-rays and neutrons. (a) single doses; (b) four fractionated doses. Note the 'shoulder' for X-rays and the consequent different fractionation effect for X-rays and for neutrons.

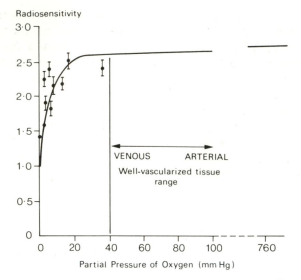

Fig. 2.12 L. H. Gray's classical demonstration of the oxygen effect for mouse Ehrlich ascites tumour cells.

measurement of oxygen tension by electrodes and by the histological appearance of tumours. Thomlinson and Gray (1955) showed clearly that tumour cells more than about 180 μm from capillary vessels become anoxic and necrotic.

This oxygen effect can obviously be the major explanation for the unexpected failure of radiotherapy when the correct dose has been given and yet there is local recurrence or regrowth within the treated volume. The effect is demonstrated very well by cell-survival curves (Fig. 2.13), when there will be an alteration in slope corresponding to the reduced sensitivity for anoxic compared with normally oxygenated cells.

There are several theoretical methods of overcoming the oxygen effect. Some are quite impractical, such as treating the patient under complete anoxia (so that all cells will have equal, even though reduced, sensitivity), though this has been tried for limb tumours, which can be made almost completely anoxic by tourniquet. There are only two practical methods in widespread clinical use. The first is to improve tumour oxygenation by treating the patient in a hyperbaric oxygen chamber. The method is now standard, using a pressure of 3 atmospheres of oxygen in the 'Vickers' transparent plastic double cylinder chamber. Clinical trials have been in progress for many years but only recently have small but significant improvements in survival been shown for 'head and neck' cancer and advanced carcinoma of the cervix and bladder (Dische, 1978). The other method is to use particles for which the oxygen effect is much reduced or non-existent, such as fast neutrons or π-mesons. Cell survival curves show clearly that the OER is much reduced for fast neutrons, and also that the shoulder is smaller and that there is less fractionation effect (see Fig. 2.13).

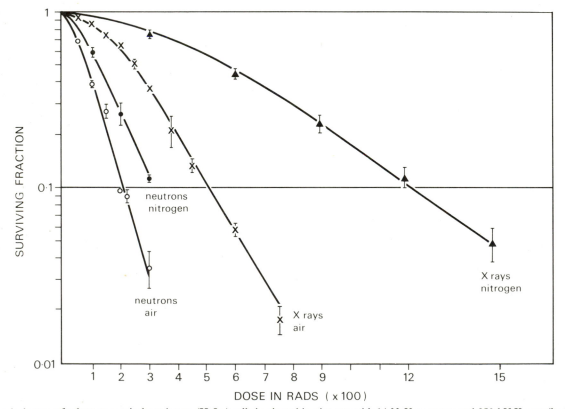

Fig. 2.13 Survival curves for human cervical carcinoma (HeLa) cells in air and in nitrogen with 14 MeV neutrons and 250 kV X-rays (by kind permission of A. H. W. Nias).

Fast neutrons for medical use can be obtained from cyclotrons and from 'd-t' generators. The d-t reaction between deuterons (^{2}H) and tritium (^{3}H) yields 14 MeV neutrons and clinical units are being tested in Manchester and Glasgow in Britain, as well as in the Netherlands, Germany and the USA. The most encouraging initial clinical results came from the Medical Research Council cyclotron at Hammersmith Hospital (Catterall & Bewley, 1979), where much of the basic radiation biology had also been done. The Hammersmith work has not been confirmed in Edinburgh on a second low energy MRC cyclotron, but new work has begun in 1986 in Clatterbridge near Liverpool, where a new high energy MRC cyclotron has been installed. Cyclotrons are also being used clinically in East Berlin and in the USA. π-mesons are much more expensive and difficult to use clinically, but preliminary work has started at Los Alamos and Stanford University in the USA, at Vancouver, Canada and at the Swiss Institute for Nuclear Research. Fast neutron treatment of cancer may yet be a worthwhile technical advance in radiotherapy, but its final value remains to be proven with the newer cyclotrons.

Chemical modifiers of sensitivity

Since the beginning of radiation biology it has been hoped that a chemical radiosensitiser could be developed. In fact there has been much more progress in the development of cytotoxic drugs which directly affect tumour cells rather than merely sensitising them to radiation. However, experimental work has been done on many agents that modify the radiation response; these agents are termed 'protectors' or 'sensitisers' according to whether they diminish or potentiate the effects of radiation.

Many sulphydryl compounds can be shown experimentally to have a protective effect, cysteine and cysteamine especially, but no clinical application has been shown. A new protective agent WR-2721 is believed to protect normal tissues but not tumours and its effect is being tested in clinical practice (Yuhas 1980).

Oxygen is of course the most important sensitizer to the common low LET types of radiation, X- and γ-rays. Some cytotoxic drugs such as actinomycin-D, methotrexate, and 5-fluorouracil act as apparent sensitizers but their action may be no more than an additive effect. One very important action of actinomycin-D especially, and of some of the newer cytotoxic drugs, is the potentiation of normal tissue radiation effects, such as renal damage; they may even bring back or 'recall' a radiation reaction on the skin or elsewhere. Synkavit (vitamin K) and the halogenated pyrimidines such as 5-iododeoxyuridine have been shown experimentally to be true sensitizers but no effective clinical exploitation has yet been possible.

The latest sensitizers mimic the effect of oxygen and are known as electron-affinic sensitizers. Experimental work has been more convincing than in the past and it is particularly interesting that one of the main classes of compound is the nitrofurans, some of which are already well known and well tested in clinical pharmacology as anti-bacterial drugs.

Metronidazole ('Flagyl') was the first found to be effective and a more powerful compound, 'Misonidazole', is now being investigated in clinical trials. Neurotoxic side-effects can occur at high dosage (Adams et al 1978). Newer sensitizers are being investigated but cannot yet be taken into routine clinical radiotherapy.

Cell kinetics

Mammalian cells divide by mitosis. This can easily be seen by normal light microscopy and the continual procession of division or proliferation is known as the cell cycle. Cell division, continually repeated in each generation, can be represented as a circle, whose circumference will represent the mitotic cycle time, the period of mitosis itself only taking a small part of the cycle, as shown in Figure 2.14. Modern autoradiographic techniques show that the remainder of the cell cycle can be further subdivided. If cells are fed with radioactive tritiated thymidine, a precursor of DNA, this will be incorporated into cells actively synthesizing DNA; and these cells will be visible on autoradiographs because of their radioactivity. This phase of DNA synthesis can be called the S phase. It can then be shown that synthesis itself only occurs during a well-defined fraction of the cell cycle and that there are intervals or 'gaps' between the S- and M-phases. These are termed G_1, the gap between mitosis and synthesis, and G_2, the second gap after synthesis and before the next mitosis. Some cells do not go on dividing and will temporarily pass into a resting phase; this is called G_0. The mean generation or cycle time will vary from about 12 hours to as long as several months or more.

Most cells are dividing at random, and at any one time in a culture there would be a mixture of cells at all phases of the cell cycle. Techniques are now available, however,

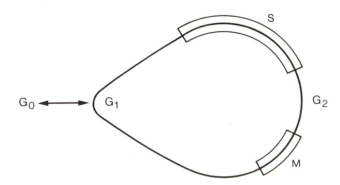

Fig. 2.14 The cell mitotic cycle, determined by autoradiography. M-mitosis S-DNA synthesis G_1 and G_2, the gaps between M and S and G_0 representing a temporary resting phase.

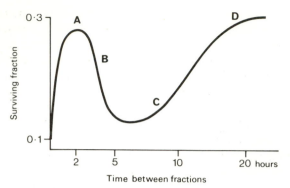

Fig. 2.15 The fluctuating 'Elkind' recovery curve of cells given two doses of radiation at different time intervals: A, phase of intracellular recovery; B, phase when predominantly resistant cells become more sensitive to the second dose as they begin to move round the cell cycle again; C, phase where the semi-synchronized cells begin again to become more resistant; D, final phase where cells have lost synchrony and are beginning to multiply normally again.

to obtain populations of cells synchronized at the same stage of the cycle, all dividing together. It can then be shown that cells in mitosis are most sensitive to radiation, with intermediate sensitivity at the beginning of synthesis, and least sensitivity in early G_1, late S and G_2. This variation in phase sensitivity is less for high LET radiation. There is also some variability between different cell lines. One very important demonstration of this variation in sensitivity was made by Elkind and Sutton (1959) who investigated the effect of two doses of radiation given at time intervals up to 24 hours (Fig. 2.15).

The first dose of radiation kills the most sensitive cells leaving a population in the most resistant parts of the cycle, and also temporarily inhibiting movement round the cycle. The remaining cells become synchronized and move into more sensitive phases before becoming more resistant again and finally, once again, becoming desynchronized.

When tumours are investigated by cell labelling it is found that only a proportion of cells are dividing regularly and this proportion is called the 'growth fraction'. It is also found that a further proportion of cells are lost from the tumour — the cell loss fraction — by necrosis, phagocytosis, metastasis and exfoliation (Fig. 2.16). The oxygen-

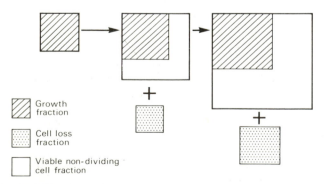

Growth fraction

Cell loss fraction

Viable non-dividing cell fraction

Fig. 2.16 The change in tumour growth as its size increases.

ation or vascularization will affect the growth and cell loss fraction. Radiation need not necessarily reduce the number of viable cells to zero since host immunological factors and the effects of radiation on the stroma of the tumour bed may also cause growth restraint.

RADIATION EFFECTS ON TISSUES

Clinical radiobiology

There is a considerable body of knowledge on the effect of radiation on cells — this is of relevance to clinical radiotherapy but does not yet provide answers to all the problems. When we consider the more obvious gross effects on tissues we begin to explore more familiar ground.

The skin

Normal and abnormal skin are easily visible and radiation effects can be well seen and measured. Let us follow the effects of a large single dose — 200 gray of superficial X-rays — to a circular field of diameter 3 cm to treat a small basal cell carcinoma of about 1 cm diameter (Halnan, 1962).

The first significant point is that there will usually be no visible effect at all for about 10 days. This *latent period* makes it very clear that the effect of ionizing radiation is unique, quite different to the more rapid unselective damage that would have been observed after heat, cold light (diathermy, cyrosurgery, laser beams, etc.), and other damaging agents used surgically to remove or destroy tissue. Both the normal skin and the tumour will then be seen to undergo damage. The skin rapidly becomes pink and then deep red ('skin erythema') followed at this dose level by so much destruction that there is exudation of serum which will then form a scab over much of the treated area. The tumour will disappear rapidly, within 2 or 3 weeks whereas the surrounding skin will heal over the succeeding 4–8 weeks. Biopsy would show no surviving basal cell carcinoma cells at all and the patient should be permanently 'cured'. The normal skin however is at the same time capable of permanent and complete repair. This is of course the ideal result of radiotherapy for cancer; although not always achieved, it is frequently worth attempting, with special care needed for all the correct treatment factors — tumour dose, time pattern, quality of radiation and dose distribution.

The patient must be followed up carefully to ensure that there is no recurrence of the tumour, or that it is detected and treated early. After a period of about 2 years changes will gradually be seen in the treated skin. It will become depressed, atrophic and pale or depigmented and tiny superficial blood vessels will begin to appear — telangiectasis. These skin changes are often called 'radiation stigmata' and may be difficult to see, their severity being dependent both upon the radiation dose and volume and also upon individual variation. It is often said that skin radiosensitivity lessens with pigmentation but it may perhaps be equally correct that the pigmentation makes the radiation changes less easily seen. Overdosage may of course lead to permanent, irreparable skin damage — an indolent ulcer that will not heal, often called 'radiation necrosis'. Damage of this kind may equally well occasionally occur in irradiated skin years after treatment, as a result of infection, trauma, or both.

One important radiation effect is epilation, which can occur after low doses of about 3 gray or more. The hair will usually regrow, often with a different pigmentation, unless a much higher dose is given.

General time pattern of radiation effect

The skin changes just described fit well into a more general pattern of change (Fig. 2.17) that can be observed in almost all tissues.

After radiotherapy, or after the beginning of a course of treatment, there will be a latent period of 10 days or more, before any reaction is evident. The length of this period will vary with the tissue, the dose and the time, and of course this reaction may not be evident at all with many modern treatments. Subclinical damage will be occurring during and after this time and it may only be after a second latent period of a year or more that late changes such as telangiectasis in the skin or lung fibrosis will be detected. Tumours suitable for treatment by radiotherapy will have a much lower potential for repair and recovery and so will in suitable cases and after optimum treatment, be 'cured' with no clonogenic tumour cell remaining within the treated volume. The tumour may of course continue to grow for a short time before response is seen, and inflam-

matory oedema, particularly in the closed cranium, chest and upper respiratory tract, may also occur and mask any early tumour response.

A very early normal tissue response may be seen within hours or a day or two, particularly after high doses, but this is the exception rather than the rule.

The two main tissue components particularly involved in radiation damage are vascular and connective tissue. Late damage results in gradually increasing sclerosis of capillaries and arterioles; there is thickening and degeneration of the walls, with gradual obliteration and replacement by very poor thin-walled new capillaries, which are fragile, easily distensible, and liable to break — telangiectasis. Poor vascularization results in poor nutrition and a liability to damage and even poorer response to further damage from tumour or infection. The more active and better differentiated tissues requiring a good blood supply will therefore be most susceptible. Fibrous tissue is relatively undifferentiated and 'resistant' to radiation and it will fill the gaps and play an important role in repair of radiation damage.

Gastrointestinal tract

Gut damage will follow the general pattern. Gastric secretion will be inhibited (indeed, radiotherapy has been used to treat peptic ulcer) and early damage to the small and large intestines will result in diarrhoea. The intestinal mucosa is rapidly dividing and especially sensitive but the late changes due to radiation of a smooth bowel with malabsorption, liability to stricture, adhesions, and even perforation, should not be common and only occur occasionally after high dose irradiation of the pelvis. One important instance is the rectal necrosis seen after badly positioned radium (or radio-isotope substitute) treatment of gynaecological cancer. This can occur after doses of about 50 gray or more to the rectum and the resultant indolent indurated ulcer can mimic a rectal carcinoma and indeed be misdiagnosed as such.

Like other glands the salivary glands can be indurated and fibrosed, as can their ducts, and this may result in dryness of the mouth and dental decay. Another special instance is sialitis, a painful swelling at meal times caused by stricture of the ducts, after high dose radio-iodine treatment for thyroid cancer (iodine is concentrated and secreted in saliva).

The liver can be affected, due to blood vessel changes, after perhaps 40 gray in 4 weeks and radiation of the *whole* liver to high dosage can lead to hepatic failure.

Urinary tract

Radiation 'nephritis' (strictly speaking nephropathy) is now well known, with histological appearances similar to idiopathic nephritis and with the same clinical course —

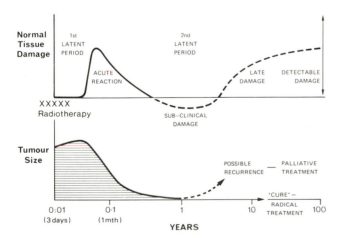

Fig. 2.17 Time patterns of radiation response of normal tissues and of tumour; there will be considerable variation between individuals and between different tissues, tumours, and dose, time and volume irradiated.

red cells, casts and protein in the urine, secondary hypertension and renal failure. The first signs, analogous to acute nephritis, can appear within 6–12 months; these may be mild and undetected, but lead to chronic changes later. Like any other radiation effect, renal damage is both dose- and volume-dependent and the significant threshold level is about 20 gray in 3 weeks to the *whole* of a kidney. Partial renal irradiation is less harmful, and part or the whole of a kidney can sometimes be excised before the process is irreversible.

High doses, at least 60 gray in 5 weeks, can cause stricture of the ureters. Changes can occur in the urinary bladder mucosa similar to those in skin; fibrosis and contracture of the whole bladder can occur, and telangiectasis can even result in severe uncontrollable bleeding. Bladder changes should not be important at doses of 60 gray or less in 5 weeks.

The prostate itself is relatively little affected by even high doses; the urethra, like the ureter, can become involved in fibrous stricture but only after high dosage.

Thoracic organs

The lungs also are well known to be vulnerable. The acute changes of pneumonitis occurring within weeks are not usually seen except after high dosage to the whole lung. The late changes of fibrosis can develop over about 2 years; the significant threshold level is of the order of 30 gray in 3 weeks to the whole lung, with the 'tolerance' level for irradiation of the whole thorax being about 25 gray in 4 weeks.

There is no more than anecdotal evidence of full scale cardiac infarcts being caused by normal radiotherapy but temporary, reversible, T-wave electrocardiographic changes can certainly occur at 2–6 weeks after 40 gray given over 4 weeks.

Breast and gonads

The testis and ovary are both radiosensitive. Permanent sterility in men and women can be caused by single doses of about 5 gray and temporary sterility by lower doses of perhaps 2.5 gray and upwards. Recovery from radiation is of course more likely in younger patients. It is very important to realize, and to explain to the patient, that much higher doses would be needed to alter hormone secretion and that men who may be sterile should *not* also be impotent.

Irradiation of the breast in prepubertal children, e.g. for thoracic tumours, may lead to hypoplasia.

Cartilage, bone and growing tissues

Most developing and growing tissues in children can be partially or completely inhibited by radiation with doses in excess of say 20 gray in 3 weeks. This applies particularly to growing epiphyses; to ensure minimal deformity, any epiphyseal damage should be symmetrical, for example, the whole of a segment of the spine rather than one half only should be irradiated.

Mature bone and cartilage are much more resistant, unless damaged by infection, trauma or tumour. The sinister reputation of irradiated bone comes from the historical use of orthovoltage (200–500 kV) radiation, whose absorption depends upon density, with consequent very high dosage to bone leading to vascular damage and necrosis. Modern megavoltage X-rays should not cause significant bone damage except in special circumstances where the need for cure justifies high dose irradiation of bone.

Central nervous system

The brain and spinal cord are most vulnerable to radiation. The volume irradiated is, as always, very important, and although damage may occur after irradiation of the *whole* brain to more than 45 gray in 3 weeks, smaller volumes, e.g. less than $8 \times 8 \times 8$ cm^3 may safely be given 55 gray in 3 weeks. Damage to the spinal cord may more easily be related to the length irradiated and permanent damage to a 20 cm length can be caused by more than 30 gray in 3 weeks, while a 10 cm length can tolerate 45 gray in 3 weeks.

Permanent damage can result in complete motor and sensory loss but it is important to note that there is a special instance of temporary damage, l'Hermitte's syndrome, consisting of bizarre paraesthesiae often described as 'electric shocks', brought on by flexure of the spine. This syndrome comes on 6–15 months after treatment of perhaps more than 2.5 gray in 3 weeks and is temporary; it does *not* imply later permanent complete cord damage.

Eye

The eye is particularly vulnerable to radiation. Radiation cataract, which can be dealt with like senile cataract, can be caused by single doses to the whole lens of 2 gray upwards, but if only a segment of lens is irradiated, 20 gray will be the threshold. Fast neutrons are even more cataractogenic. Other parts of the eye will be damaged only after much higher doses — 60 gray in 6 weeks or more — and haemorrhages in the vitreous and retina, keratinisation and conjunctivitis, epiphora and lid distortion are among the effects seen. The eye should not be regarded as a 'sacred' organ, never to be irradiated. Carefully planned radiotherapy to eyelid tumours will often result in no significant damage; even when it is necessary to radiate heavily an orbit invaded by, for example, an antral tumour, it must be remembered that most patients would prefer to be alive and free of cancer, although blind in one eye, than to die with full sight.

Whole body effects

Irradiation of the whole body is the extreme example of the importance of volume as well as of dose, and many general points can be illustrated.

The lethal dose (LD_{50}) varies widely between species and individuals. For man it is probably about 6 gray, though this estimate is based on relatively little good evidence from man, and is probably correct only if no medical treatment is given. There are three kinds of death. After very high doses of 100 gray or more, death occurs within hours from failure of the central nervous system — the 'CNS syndrome'. After intermediate doses, about 5–15 gray, death occurs within days, from extensive bloody diarrhoea with destruction of the gastrointestinal mucosa — the 'gastrointestinal syndrome'. At the lowest possible lethal levels, 2.5–5 gray, death may come several weeks after exposure because of bone marrow failure — the 'haemopoietic syndrome'.

The bone marrow is particularly sensitive to radiation damage and the changes seen in the peripheral blood are used as a monitor or index of radiation effect. After a single dose the changes seen (Fig. 2.18) correspond more to the life-span and turnover of the different cells concerned, than to sensitivity as such. Lymphocyte, granulocyte and platelet counts are in turn reduced with the relatively long-life red cells being last affected.

The familiar 'radiation sickness' and the prodromal radiation syndrome are really the same. Like 'sickness'

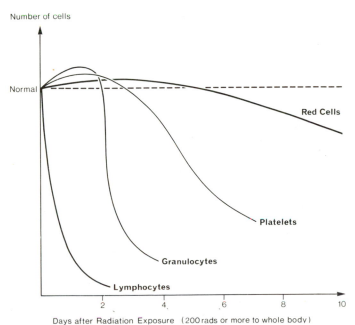

Fig. 2.18 Response of peripheral blood count to a large dose of radiation.

from pregnancy or motion, radiation sickness is difficult to investigate and may have psychological reinforcement. It is usually produced a few hours after substantial radiation to a large volume of the trunk and is related to the integral dose of radiation.

RADIATION HAZARDS

There are three dangerous biological effects of radiation to man. There is the immediate danger of damage to individual tissues from high exposure, there are long-term dangers of chronic damage with possible carcinogenesis, and there is the more remote but important danger of genetic damage that may affect subsequent generations. It should be remembered that none of us will ever be completely free from radiation exposure, from natural radioactivity within ourselves, our environment, the earth's crust, cosmic rays from outer space, and man-made sources (see appendix, p. 32).

The immediate danger of tissue damage has been described above and the relevant balance of damage and benefit has been well worked out for most clinical problems.

Carcinogenesis

Harmful long-term effects were first seen in occupational exposure. Early X-ray workers would often expose their hands, not only when screening a patient, but even deliberately to see whether the tube was working properly. The earliest changes seen in the fingers were brittleness and ridging of the nails, blunting and flattening of the skin ridges that show in finger-prints, dryness and loss of hair, and a loss of sensitivity to touch and temperature. After many years these changes led in some cases to skin cancer. Many early radiologists died from radiation induced skin cancer and the memorial to them erected in Hamburg listed 169 names from 15 countries, 14 from Great Britain.

Radiation cancer was first seen in the skin because the skin received the highest doses. Many other types of tumour occurred from radium and other natural radio-isotopes. Cancer of the lung from inhalation of radon has been known for many years in the uranium mines of Joachimstal in Czechoslovakia and Schneeburg in Germany. Radium salts have long been used in luminous paints and both leukaemia and bone sarcoma have occurred in the radium workers who used to lick their fine paint brushes to form good points.

Good quantitative estimates of risk have appeared more recently from well recorded and measured diagnostic and therapeutic medical irradiation (Doll, 1981) and from nuclear arms work, especially from the two atomic bombs exploded in Japan in 1945. The general position is exhaustively surveyed in the United Nations Reports in 1977 and

1982 from their Committee on the Effects of Atomic Radiation (UNSCEAR, 1977, 1982). Radiation-induced cancer induction is a long-term continual risk with a medium latent period of as long as 25 years. It must be appreciated that radiation-induced cancer is not in any way different to normal or 'spontaneous' cancer. There is no method of identifying it or picking it out from the general mass of cancer, all one can do is observe a statistically significant increase or 'excess' of cancer in a given population after a given event or hazard. Excess leukaemia began to appear in Hiroshima and Nagasaki in about 1947, with a maximum incidence between 1955 and 1959, when there was 3–4 times the expected incidence. Data on leukaemia has also come from the investigations initiated by Court-Brown on patients treated by X-ray therapy (with considerable benefit) for ankylosing spondylitis. 14 558 patients treated between 1935 and 1954 in 81 radiotherapy units in the United Kingdom were traced (a compliment to British radiotherapy standards of record keeping and follow-up); there were 52 cases of leukaemia compared with 5.5 expected, an incidence of 0.35%. From these and other data it has been estimated that the leukaemia risk is about 2 cases per 100 000 population per rad or centigray whole body radiation (the spontaneous incidence in the middle-aged population is about 1 in 25 000 per year). The second tumour in which we have substantial evidence is thyroid cancer, because it is uncommon and because there is a special risk seen after irradiating babies and children, especially in the United States, where numbers of infants were treated by X-ray therapy to the thyroid before and during the war. These radiation-induced thyroid carcinomas are, however, almost always successfully treated. There is further evidence on radiation causation of cancer in the breast, bone, lung and skin; much more doubtfully in other organs.

In summary, one can expect a risk of about 1 excess case of leukaemia or cancer in 10 000 people per rad or centigray radiation exposure, with a latent period of 25 years or more, up to the 40 years or so expectation of life after irradiation. This can be compared with the spontaneous incidence of cancer of 200 000 cases *per year* in our population of 50 million, or final cumulative incidence of 1 in 3, or mortality of 1 in 5 of the population. The risk is clearly significant but low, and the risk in radiotherapy of cancer will compare well with surgical operative mortality.

Genetic and fetal risks

Genetic hazards must be assumed to exist at the lowest radiation levels and yet are very difficult to evaluate. Ionizing radiation causes both major changes in chromosomes, usually lethal, and minor changes appearing as gene mutations, which are usually deleterious and recessive. It had usually been accepted that all radiation induced mutations are cumulative and irreversible, and similar to the spontaneous mutations which are always occurring. Work on mice, however, suggests that the different cell-stages of sperm and oocyte vary widely in mutation induction sensitivity, and that considerable apparent recovery may occur a few months after radiation exposure (Russell, 1965). There is very little good quantitative evidence in man; the Japanese atom bomb survivors are being closely followed but no significant mutation has been detected. The evidence we have from animals suggests that a dose of about 1 gray will double the spontaneous mutation rate in man. This means for example that the incidence of retinoblastoma might be 1 in 15 000 live births instead of 1 in 30 000, or that the incidence of Duchenne muscular dystrophy might be 1 in 5000 males instead of 1 in 10 000.

Risks to the developing fetus or embryo are quite different (Rugh, 1963) and radiation to the uterus of a pregnant woman is much more important. The first 3 months of pregnancy — especially the 9th to 40th days — are the most hazardous. A dose of 5 rads or centigrays will cause a 0.1% risk of malformation or developmental abnormality. It is therefore vitally important to be aware of early pregnancy, and if radiation of more than 10 centigray is given at this time then termination of pregnancy is quite justifiable. The long-term incidence of carcinogenesis from diagnostic X-ray examinations must be accepted as a very low risk that should only be taken when there is a strong medical indication for the examination concerned — it may often be reasonable to use an alternative method of examination such as ultrasound.

Interaction with cancer chemotherapy

Treatment of cancer by chemotherapy is now a very important and expanding field, though curative on its own in only a numerically small proportion of human tumours. Its interaction with surgery and with radiotherapy must not be forgotten. Different drugs will have effects not only on the bone marrow, the gastrointestinal tract, and the hair, but on most other tissues (Table 2.3). The vinca alkaloids can reduce intestinal motility so much that acute or subacute obstruction can be caused, with the patient at risk also at surgery because of impaired platelet and leucocyte concentration. Bleomycin can cause lethal lung fibrosis, adriamycin (doxorubicin) can cause lethal cardiac failure. Many drugs can cause additive and even synergistic increase in the radiation changes already described. Some can result in 'recall' of radiation changes, for example, radiation skin and gut changes being brought back or 'recalled' by adriamycin or dactinomycin. Chemotherapy, by alkylating agents especially, can be more carcinogenic than ionizing radiation, as has been shown in polycythaemia vera, myeloma, and ovarian cancer. Long term effects of chemotherapy have not yet been fully assessed in large numbers of long-term survivors (Schottenfeld & Fraumeni, 1982). Even hormone therapy is not

Table 2.3 Toxicity of Cancer Chemotherapy (main examples). Potentially lethal effects are italicised.

Target Organ	Toxicity	Drugs
Bone marrow	*Cytopenia*	Almost all except bleomycin, asparaginase and vincristine
Gastrointestinal tract	Stomatitis	Adriamycin, actinomycin-D, bleomycin, 5-fluorouracil, methotrexate
	Gastritis and vomiting Diarrhoea	Very many drugs Methotrexate, 5-fluorouracil
	Constipation or *ileus*	*Vincristine, vinblastine*
Skin	Pigmentation, alopecia or ulceration	Bleomycin, adriamycin, cyclophosphamide and others
Nervous system	Peripheral neuropathy Cerebral dysfunction Deafness	Vinblastine, vincristine methotrexate cis-platinum
Heart	Arrhythmia and *failure*	*Adriamycin, daunorobucin*
Lungs	*Fibrosis*	*Bleomycin*, methotrexate and alkylating agents
Bladder	Cystitis	Cyclophosphamide
Liver	*Impaired function*	*Methotrexate and others*
Kidney	*Impaired function*	Methotrexate, cis-platinum

necessarily free from risk, a good example being the substantial cardiac risks induced with stilboestrol treatment. The main moral of course is to make sure that harmful and helpful consequences of chemotherapy are both very carefully considered in the multi-disciplinary management of carcinoma, in comparison and combination with radiotherapy, and surgery.

Immunity and radiotherapy

Immunity in general is reviewed extensively in Chapter 27. There are misunderstandings regarding the effect of radiotherapy. It has to be accepted that immunological defenses play an important part in the control of human cancer. Two important pieces of evidence are the small but significant increased incidence of cancer in patients on immunosuppressive drugs to avoid rejection of organ transplants, and the high incidence of cancer in patients with the rare congenital immunological defects. It also has been suggested that ionizing radiation has a deleterious effect both locally and generally upon the immunological system although the only clear evidence of this is lymphopenia in the peripheral blood count. Some forms of chemotherapy and indeed surgery itself have a similar effect. So far, however, there is very little reliable evidence to support the hypothesis that any form of treatment, including radiotherapy, is harmful because of its immunosuppressive side effects.

Too little is at present known to justify any decision other than to remember immunity and to investigate its relevance to radiotherapy and to other forms of treatment.

CONCLUSIONS — THE RATIONALE FOR RADIOTHERAPY

We, the medical profession, surgeons and colleagues, like to think that our treatment of patients is based upon scientific evidence and that our management has a scientific rationale, but we are still often sadly wrong. Our knowledge of radiation biology provides a substantial basis for radiotherapy but our present knowledge is by no means complete, even though we attempt to exploit the latest advances in physics and biology.

The techniques of cell, organ, and tissue culture and quantitative measurements of survival and death have led to a better understanding of radiosensitivity and of the importance of the time factor. Detailed knowledge of tissue effects is leading to an appreciation of the relative importance of radiation effects on tumours and on normal organs and the tissue bed. The oxygen effect has been the single most important discovery in radiation biology, leading to the attempts to overcome it by hyperbaric oxygen treatment, by electron-affinic chemical sensitisers and by the new particle radiations, fast neutrons and π-mesons.

The success that radiotherapy has achieved so far has been caused by the better recovery of normal tissues from its harmful effects as well as from its immediate lethal effects on tumour cells. Radiotherapy will continue to be used mainly in the local sterilization of the main tumour bulk but will also play a part in the removal of microscopic and latent metastases as well as the treatment of large deposits. It will of course complement surgery, chemotherapy, hormone treatment and perhaps immunotherapy in the treatment of cancer.

APPENDIX

RADIATION DOSAGE (definitions and examples)

Units

Exposure

Roentgen (R) — produces 1 electrostatic unit of charge in 1 ml of air at normal temperature and pressure.

Absorbed dose

Rad — energy absorption of 100 ergs per gram ($\simeq$ 1R)
Gray (Gy) — energy absorption of 1 joule per kilogram (1cGy $\simeq$ 1R)

Quantity of radioactivity

Curie (Ci) — 3.7×10^{10} disintegrations per second ($\simeq$ 1 g of radium)

Becquerel (Bq) — 1 disintegration per second

'Dose equivalent' (for harmful effects)

Sievert (Sv) — for γ rays, β-rays and X-rays (1 Sv = 1 Gy)

Fractionation, time and dose

The biological effect from a given dose is related both to the number of fractions given and the overall time, corresponding approximately to the 'Ellis' formula:

$$D = (NSD) \, T^{0.11} N^{0.24}$$

D = total dose, NSD = nominal standard dose, T = days overall time, N = number of fractions

e.g. Typical equivalent lethal doses to a small squamous carcinoma.

Regimen	Total dose
1 fraction	2500 cGy
5 fractions/4 days	4250 cGy
15 fractions/3 weeks	5500 cGy
30 fractions/6 weeks	6500 cGy

Natural and occupational radiation exposure per year

Natural body radioactivity	0.4 mSv
Natural radiation from earth's crust, radon in the atmosphere and from cosmic rays at sea level	1.5 mSv
From cosmic rays in outer space	250 mSv
Maximum permissible for radiation workers	50 mSv
Average medical dosage in Britain (almost all from diagnostic procedures)	0.5 mSv

Hazards

Carcinogenesis — 1 case per 10 000 people exposed to 1 cGy to the whole body.

Genetic damage — Spontaneous mutation rate (e.g. 1 case of retinoblastoma in 30 000 births) doubled by 1 gy.

Lethal doses (LD_{50} whole body gray)

Viruses	10^4	Newt	300
Bacteria	10^5	Mammals	? 2–10
Amoeba	10^5	Man	? 6.

Diagnostic doses (Gray)

One chest film	0.001 to chest	0.00005 to gonads
One lateral film of pelvis	0.2 to skin	0.007 to gonads
Barium meal	0.05 to skin	0.00003 to gonads
Iodine-131 test (10 μCi)	0.15 to thyroid	0.00005 to gonads
Iodine-132 test (10 μCi)	0.002 to thyroid	0.00002 to gonads

Therapeutic doses (typical examples)

Megavoltage X-ray therapy

(a) 30 Gy/10 fractions/2 weeks to a bone metastasis from breast cancer
(b) 35 Gy/20 fractions/4 weeks to para-aortic nodes for seminoma
(c) 60 Gy/25 fractions/5 weeks to early carcinoma of larynx

Superficial X-rays

(a) 23 Gy single treatment for small basal cell carcinoma
(b) 35 Gy/5 fractions/4 days for 4 cm diameter basal cell carcinoma

Radio-Iridium-192 hairpin implant for tongue carcinoma

65 Gy over 7 days

Fast neutron therapy

15.6 Gy/12 fractions/26 days for superficial carcinoma

FURTHER READING

Duncan W, Nias A H W 1977 Clinical radiobiology. Churchill Livingstone, Edinburgh

Hall E J 1978 Radiobiology for the radiologist, 2nd edn. New York and London, Harper and Row

Halnan K E (ed) 1982 Treatment of cancer. Chapman and Hall, London

National Radiological Protection Board 1981 Living with Radiation, 2nd edn. H M S O, London

United Nations Scientific Committee on the Effects of Radiation 1977 and 1982 Sources and effects of ionizing radiation. H M S O, London

REFERENCES

Adams G E, Fowler J F, Wardman P (eds) 1978 Hypoxic cell sensitisers in radiobiology and radiotherapy. British Journal of Cancer 37 (Suppl. 111)

Bergonie J, Tribondeau (1906) Comptes Rendue, 143:983 (Modern English translation by G. Fletcher 1959 in Radiation Research 11:587

Catterall M, Bewley D K 1979 Fast neutrons in the treatment of cancer. Academic Press, London.

Court-Brown W M, Doll R 1965 Mortality from cancer and other causes after radiotherapy for ankylosing spondylitis. British Medical Journal 2: 1327–1332

Dische S 1978 Hyperbaric oxygen: the Medical Research Council trials and their clinical significance. British Journal of Radiobiology 51: 888–94

Doll R 1981 Radiation Hazards. British Journal of Radiology 54: 179–185

Elkind M M, Sutton H 1959 X-ray damage and recovery in mammalian cells in culture. Nature 184: 1293–1295

Ellis F 1969 Dose, time and fractionation. Clinical Radiology, 20: 1–7

Fowler J F 1966 Radiation biology as applied to radiotherapy. Current Topics in Radiation Research 11: 305–364

Gray I H, Conger A D, Ebert M, Hornsey S, Scott O C A 1953 Concentration of oxygen in tissues as a factor in radiotherapy. British Journal of Radiology 26: 638–648

Halnan K E 1962 The effect of corticosteroids on the radiation skin reaction. British Journal of Radiology 35: 403–408

Kirk J, Gray W M, Watson E R 1971 Cumulative radiation effect, part 1. Fractionated treatment regimes. Clinical Radiology 22: 145–160.

Puck T T, Marcus P I 1956 Action of X-rays on mammalian cells. Journal of Experimental Medicine 103: 653–666

Rugh R 1963 The impact of ionising radiation on the embryo and fetus. American Journal of Roentgenology 89:182

Russell W I 1965 Studies in mammalian radiation genetics. Nucleonics, 23: 53–56.

Schottenfeld D, Fraumeni J F 1982 Cancer epidemiology and prevention. W B Saunders, Philadelphia

Strandquist M 1944 Studien uber die kumulative Wirkung der Rontegenstrahlung bei Fraktionerung, Acta Radilogica. Supplement, 55: 1–300.

Suit H D, Gallagher H S 1964 Intact tumour cells in irradiated tissue. Archives of Pathology 78: 648–651

Thomlinson R F, Gray L H 1955 The histological structure for some human lung cancers and the possible implications for radiotherapy. British Journal of Cancer 9: 539–549

Yuhas J M 1980 A more general role for WR-2721 in cancer therapy. British Journal of Cancer 41: 832–34

Fluid and electrolyte balance

An awareness of the possible disturbances in fluid and electrolyte balance which may arise in the surgical patient is a major step towards preventing their occurrence and progression. In a few patients the nature of the underlying disease process, or its surgical sequelae, leads inevitably to more severe disturbances, the treatment of which may require the combined expertise of the surgeon and the clinical biochemist. The following brief summary illustrates the background to some of the more common of these problems including the frequently associated abnormalities in acid-base homeostasis.

In common with other metabolic processes, fluid and electrolyte balance is influenced by the intake and output of water and solutes, which in turn are regulated by various circulating hormones. External events such as trauma, surgical operations and disease all modify the normal homeostatic mechanisms.

A basic concept is that the concentration of any constituent of a body compartment, such as the blood, is determined by the factors illustrated in Figure 3.1. The four principal factors are (a) changes in the volume of the body compartment (e.g. blood or plasma volume) in which the concentration of the substance is being considered; (b) the input or rate of flow of substance (or precursor) into the body compartment; (c) the rate of excretion, loss or outflow of the substance or metabolic product; and (d) the rates of exchange of the substance in to extracellular

spaces, tissues etc. An important example of the value of this concept is the understanding of the causes of hyponatraemia which is more often due to an increase in body water than to a decrease in total body sodium.

TOTAL BODY WATER AND ITS PARTITION

A summary of the anatomical fluid compartments of the body is illustrated in Figure 3.2. This demonstrates that

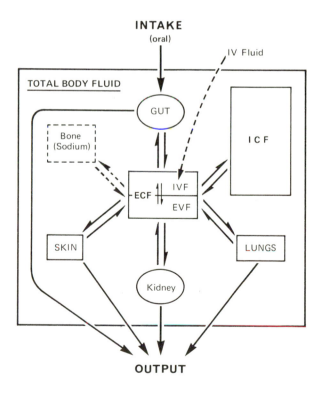

IVF = Intra vascular fluid   ICF = Intra cellular fluid
EVF = Extra vascular fluid   ECF = Extra cellular fluid

Fig. 3.2 The relationships of the body fluid compartments (not to scale).

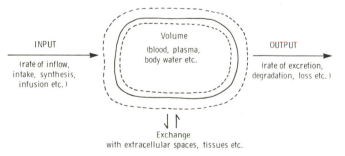

Fig. 3.1 Factors which determine the concentration of a constituent of blood, plasma, tissue fluid or body water.

water is freely exchanged between the extracellular fluid (ECF) and the intracellular fluid (ICF). In turn the intravascular fluid (IVF) and extravascular fluid (EVF) exchange and combine to make up the ECF. The role of the lungs, skin and kidney in water loss is also shown. The oral intake of fluid is absorbed from the alimentary tract which has its own fluid exchange (see Table 3.3).

The distribution of water in the body is summarized in Table 3.1. The body mass is composed of the mass of lean tissue (lean body mass) which is about 75% water, and the mass of body fat. The density (specific gravity) of lean body tissue is therefore only slightly greater than 1.000, while that of fat is rather less than 1.000. Consequently, the greater the proportion of fat in the body, the lower the specific gravity, and the lower the percentage of water in the body (Table 3.1) will be.

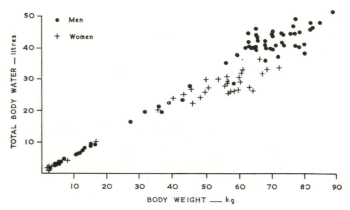

Fig. 3.3 Relationship between total body water and body weight. In boys and girls (body weights up to 40 kg) the relationship is linear. In men, the same relationship holds good on the average, but there is greater scatter. In women, body water accounts for a smaller proportion of the body weight. (Redrawn from Edelman et al, 1952)

Table 3.1 Fluid 'compartments' of the body

	Male % of Body Weight	Female % of Body Weight
Total body water	61 (43 litres)	51
Intracellular water	44 (31 litres)	35
Extracellular water	17 (12 litres)	16
Plasma water	4–5 (3.2 litres)	4
Blood volume	7 (5 litres)	6
Extravascular fluid	8–11 (7 litres)	6
Body fat	16 (11 kg)	30
Specific gravity	1.067	1.039

Note: 1. The values are approximate and for healthy adults.
     2. The values in brackets are those for the 'ideal' 70 kg man.

The relationship between total body water and body weight is shown in Fig 3.3. The good linear relationship at the lower body weights indicates the relative leanness of growing children. The scatter at higher body weights is to be expected in a population of adults in whom the body fat is individually determined and varies widely. Generally however, the contribution of body fat to the total body weight is greater in adult females than males, consequently the total body water expressed as a percentage of body weight is smaller in females than males, and the body specific gravity is less in females than males.

The amount of fat in the body can be determined in several ways. Experimentally, the most reliable method is to determine the body density or specific gravity using a specially constructed displacement tank. Alternatively, a radioactive isotope of the gas krypton which diffuses into body fat can be used.

Skinfold thickness calipers are being increasingly used to assess body fat in nutrition studies. Good calipers and care are required for accurate results.

The volume of the total body water can be determined using deuterium oxide ('heavy water' — D_2O) or by using tritiated water — ^3H_2O. The determination of the radioactive isotope of hydrogen — tritium — is simple using liquid scintillation spectrometers. To obtain an estimate of total body water it is only necessary to inject a known amount of isotopically 'labelled' water, allow a suitable time for complete equilibration in the body compartments (see Fig. 3.2) and then obtain a sample of plasma water to determine the activity. This is an example of an isotope dilution method. Using the same principle, ethanol, which is freely diffusible in the body fluid compartments, has also been used to obtain an estimate of total body water.

Blood volume can be determined from the plasma volume and the haematocrit. Plasma volume is simply measured using radioisotope (^{125}I or ^{131}I)-labelled albumin, commercial preparations of which are readily available. Determination of red cell volume by radioactive chromium tagged red cells can also be used to measure blood volume. If the patient is shocked or has unstable cardiovascular function, mixing of the labelled substance may be delayed so that care is necessary in interpreting the results of blood or plasma volume measurements in these situations.

Estimation of the extracellular fluid volume is not routinely performed and interpretation of results of, for example, the chloride or the inulin space is complex (Cohen, 1974).

The daily water balance is summarized in Table 3.2. The losses from lungs and skin are 'obligatory' in the sense that some loss always occurs during life. Similarly there is a minimum obligatory urine volume (300–500 ml) which a normal individual will continue to pass despite extreme fluid deprivation. Normally output is balanced by intake and by water produced by metabolism (e.g. oxidation of fat or carbohydrate). The intake is in two forms — that which occurs in food and that drunk. On a normal diet it is evident that the urine volume will roughly match the intake of oral fluids. In general, the daily fluid intake or output is equivalent to about 7% of the total body water.

A simple, practically useful point is that a 'normal' urine

Table 3.2 Daily water balance

Output (= losses) litres		Gains (= intake) litres	
Lungs	0.7	'Metabolic' water	0.3
Skin	0.7	In food	1.0
Faeces	0.1	Oral fluids	1.7
Kidney	1.5		
Total Out	3.0 l/day	Total In	3.0 l/ day

Note: 1. Output in urine tends to match oral intake.
2. Intake and output = turnover = approximately 3 litres = 7% of total body water per day.

output corresponds to 1 ml per minute or 60 ml/h. Excretion rates of less than half of this are usually a cause for alarm.

It will be evident that changes in total body water will be seen immediately as changes in body weight which is the most sensitive indicator of fluid balance. Although there are practical problems in weighing patients in bed, bed weighing machines are available and provide valuable information, especially in the management of patients who are severely burned or are being dialysed.

The alimentary tract makes a considerable contribution to body water exchange. The evidence for this is summarized in Table 3.3. The total volume of fluid secreted into the alimentary tract per day is about four times the usual oral intake of water and amounts to almost 20% i.e. one-fifth of the volume of the total body water. Although the volumes quoted in Table 3.3 may seem large in some cases, those who have seen the large volumes of gastric

Table 3.3 Fluid secreted into the alimentary tract per day (approx. 70 kg man)

	Litres	% Body Water
Saliva	1.0	2
Gastric secretions	2.5	6
Bile	0.7	2
Pancreatic secretion	0.9	2
Intestinal secretion	3.0	7
Total	8.1	19

aspirate in patients with pyloric stenosis or intestinal obstruction will agree that any error is not excessive. We have observed 1.5 l of saliva collected in 24 h from a 70-year-old patient with complete oesophageal obstruction due to carcinoma.

ELECTROLYTES

The term 'electrolytes' is usually used to include sodium, potassium, chloride and bicarbonate. Because the role of bicarbonate is intimately related to acid-base balance the present discussion will concern mainly the first three substances, the elemental cations sodium and potassium and the anion chloride.

The electrolytes are distributed among the various fluid compartments of the body in a similar fashion to water, as shown in Figure 3.2. One important addition is that bone forms a significant source of exchange for body sodium. The quantitative aspects of the exchange of electrolytes among the various body compartments are summarized in Table 3.4, which shows that 30% of the total body sodium is to be found in bone, although in 'exchangeable' terms the amount is rather less, 17% of the 'exchangeable' sodium being in bone. The term 'exchangeable' was introduced because when body sodium was measured using radioactive isotopes and the dilution technique, the values obtained for sodium in experimental animals were less than the values obtained by direct analysis. Some of the body sodium — almost 45% — appears to be 'fixed' or slowly exchangeable because equilibration with the radioactive isotope of sodium is not complete within about 24 hours after its administration. In contrast with water which is clearly diffusible throughout all compartments of the body, ions are usually not freely exchangeable. The 'sodium pump' mechanism maintains sodium largely as an extracellular ion and potassium as mainly intracellular (see Table 3.4).

When using isotopes of sodium to determine the total exchangeable sodium, at least 24 hours must be allowed for equilibration in normal individuals and rather longer is required in patients with congestive cardiac failure.

Table 3.4 Distribution of sodium, potassium and chloride in the body (approx. 70 kg man)

	Sodium	Potassium	Chloride
Total body	5250 mmol	3850 mmol	2300 mmol
'Exchangeable'	2900 mmol (55%)	3200 mmol (84%)	2300 mmol (100%)
Composed of:			
Extracellular	1785 mmol (34%)	3108 mmol (8%)	1770 mmol (77%)
Intracellular	210 mmol (4%)	2735 mmol (71%)	275 mmol (12%)
Bone	895 mmol (17%)	195 mmol (5%)	345 mmol (15%)
Note: total in bone	(30%)		
Daily intake	120 (4% of exchangeable Na$^+$)	120 (4% of exchangeable K$^+$)	230 (10%)

Note: All percentages are expressed in relation to the total body value, except for the intakes of sodium and potassium.

Table 3.5 Electrolytes secreted into the alimentary tract

	Sodium Daily Total mmol	% Exchangeable	Potassium Daily Total mmol	% Exchangeable	Chloride Daily Total	% Exchangeable	Bicarbonate Daily Total mmol
Saliva	20	0.5	30	1	35	1	10[a]
Gastric juice	115	4	25	1	300	13	0
Pancreatic juice	125	4	7	0.2	110	5	30
Bile	100	4	5	0.2	75	3	20
Intestinal secretions	350	12	15	0.5	270	12	[b]
Total	710	25	82	3	790	34	[c]

These data are modified from 'Documenta Geigy', 7th edn. (1975) and 'rounded off'.
[a] Variable, depending on rate of salivary secretion.
[b] It is likely that bicarbonate largely makes up the anion-cation balance. The pH of intestinal secretion can vary from acid to alkaline.
[c] The anion-cation discrepancy can be accounted for, in part, by secretion of calcium and magnesium.

Potassium, in contrast, diffuses among the body compartments more rapidly, taking about 6–8 hours for initial approximate equilibration. These observations on equilibration times or on the kinetics of distribution of the isotopes have important implications for the monitoring of replacement therapy and to some extent they justify the conventional 24 hour or daily assessment of fluid and electrolyte balance.

The exchange of sodium, potassium and chloride in the alimentary tract is summarized in Table 3.5. From the data it appears that approximately one-third of the total exchangeable sodium and chloride of the body are secreted into the alimentary tract and reabsorbed each day. As for fluid balance, this again illustrates the significant role of disturbances of the normal physiology of the alimentary tract in producing severe electrolyte upsets.

Those who have observed disturbances of fluid and electrolyte balance resulting from intestinal obstruction, fistulae or pyloric stenosis may have noted the apparent contrast between the severity of the hypokalaemia which frequently occurs in these conditions and the data of Table 3.5 which indicate that only an insignificant proportion (3.0%) of the exchangeable body potassium is secreted into the gut each day. It should be noted firstly that this small proportion represents 30% — a significant fraction — of extracellular fluid potassium. Secondly, when there is depletion of body fluid, an endocrine response occurs leading to increased secretion of antidiuretic hormone (ADH) and aldosterone (see pp 39, 40). The action of the latter tends to produce sodium retention with increased renal losses of potassium and hydrogen ions. Thus, in the conditions mentioned above, hypokalaemia results predominantly from renal losses of potassium rather than from the direct loss of potassium from the gut.

A renal mechanism also accounts for the occasional occurrence of a paradoxical secretion of an acid urine in severe alkalosis. This has been observed in patients with severe fluid losses due to pyloric stenosis. Initially, the homeostatic renal mechanisms to correct for alkalosis are to promote the excretion of sodium or potassium ions and retain hydrogen ions. However, if potassium and body water depletion becomes severe, then sodium and potassium are retained and hydrogen ion is excreted by the kidney, which gives the paradoxical secretion of an acid urine in severe, prolonged alkalosis.

Osmolality

The osmolality of the body fluids, including urine, can give a useful guide to the state of fluid and electrolyte balance, and renal function (Chapter 22). Normally in plasma and ICF the cations and anions approximately balance. This is illustrated for plasma in Figure 3.4 from which it is clear that the most significant cation in plasma is sodium and the most significant anion is chloride. Osmolality is determined by the sum of all the molecules present in a solution. Thus the osmolality of plasma is given approximately by 145 plus 133 (the combined sum of the anions and cations) plus 13 (the molar contribution of non-ionised substances such as glucose, urea, uric acid, proteins etc) giving a total osmolality of approximately 290. Hydrogen ions or changes in pH do not contribute to the osmolality of plasma because the normal pH of plasma corresponds to a hydrogen ion concentration of 40 nmol/l, about 1 million times less than that of sodium (140 mmol/l). The osmolality of a body fluid can be measured rapidly by determining the freezing point depression of a small volume of the fluid. Modern apparatus is available which is not very expensive, occupies little bench space and gives a direct read-out of the result.

In Figure 3.4 the concentration of substances has been expressed as moles/litre in SI units (Système International d'Unités). The relation between quantities expressed in the new SI units and the older convention of mass per unit volume (mg/100 ml) for several substances commonly measured in body fluids in fluid and electrolyte disturbances is given in the Appendix. A rough guide to the values usually found in 'normal' individuals is also given.

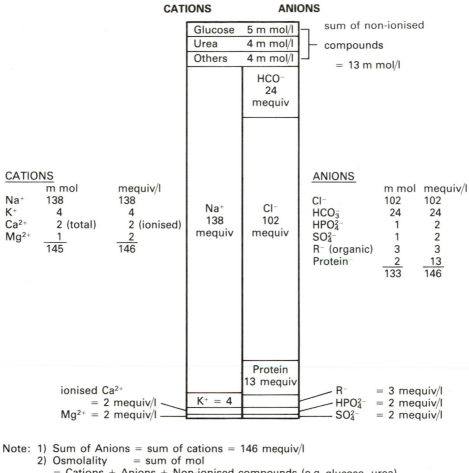

Fig. 3.4 The composition of plasma.

Control of water and electrolyte homeostasis

The control of water and electrolyte homeostasis in man is mainly effected by two hormones: arginine vasopressin (AVP) otherwise referred to as the antidiuretic hormone (ADH), and aldosterone. The renin-angiotensin system is also involved.

Our understanding of the mechanisms has been increased by developments in the quantitation of hormones. It is now possible to measure steroid hormones by the very sensitive radio immunoassay methods or in many cases, the hormones and their metabolites by chromatographic methods. Several techniques are available for the measurement of AVP: bioassay which is tedious; radioimmunoassay which renders the assay feasible on large numbers of samples; and cytochemical bioassay which, although requiring special skill and equipment, is exceptionally sensitive.

Arginine vasopressin is the main antidiuretic hormone for most mammals. It is a strongly basic, cyclic, peptide containing nine amino acids. It is synthesized mainly in neurons of the paraventricular and supraoptic nuclei of the hypothalamus in association with a carrier protein — neurophysin. Following synthesis, AVP molecules in association with their specific neurophysin travel along the axon of the neuron in which it was synthesized to the posterior lobe of the pituitary gland or to one of the other two terminations of the synthesizing neurons, the median eminence and the floor of the fourth ventricle. The hormone is released into the systemic blood by cleavage from its neurophysin and appears to circulate free, that is, not bound to plasma proteins.

The most important biological action of AVP is to conserve body water by reducing the rate of urine flow. Its secretion is in response to changes in tonicity (i.e. osmolality of blood), blood pressure and blood volume. The osmoreceptors are located in the anterior hypothala-

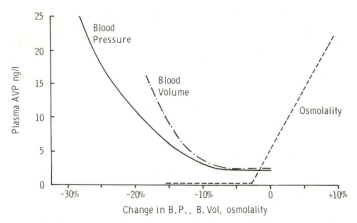

Fig. 3.5 The effects of changes in blood pressure, blood volume and osmolality on plasma arginine vasopressin (anti-diuretic hormone).

mus and the sensitivity is considerable — a change in plasma osmolality of less than 1% can produce a detectable increase in AVP above a threshold of 285 mosmol/kg (see Fig. 3.5). Below the threshold, which may differ slightly in individuals, the secretion of AVP is normally very low or undetectable. Figure 3.5 clearly shows that, above the threshold, increase in plasma osmolality leads to large increases in AVP secretion. This is in clear contrast to the relation between AVP secretion and changes in blood pressure or blood volume. In each case a fall in blood pressure or volume stimulates AVP secretion but only after a decrease of 10–15% from the normal pressure or volume. The increase in AVP secretion is more gradual with fall in pressure or volume. An additional notable stimulus to AVP secretion is nausea which may lead to increases in plasma AVP of several hundred times. Pain and hypoglycaemia may also stimulate AVP release.

The sensitivity of the osmoreceptors differs for different solutes. For example, the receptors are very sensitive to Na^+ and mannitol but less sensitive to changes in urea concentration; changes in plasma glucose have no effect. Because of its very short half-life in plasma (of the order of 5–10 minutes), plasma AVP concentration is determined mainly by its rate of secretion. Its clearance is mainly by the liver and kidney.

The effects of changes in blood pressure or volume and osmolality are largely independent and not antagonistic. For example, even if blood pressure falls sufficiently to stimulate AVP secretion, decreased osmolality is still likely to lead to a decrease in the elevated AVP.

Although at high blood concentrations AVP promotes the contraction of the smooth muscle of blood vessels, especially of the splanchnic bed, its main function is to reduce the rate of urine flow. It acts on the distal and collecting tubules of the nephron to increase their permeability to water and solutes, by a cyclic AMP-mediated mechanism, which implies a rapid response. In the absence of AVP urine flow reaches a maximum of

15–20 ml/min and extreme dilution of 60–70 mosmol/kg. The maximum concentration of urine is achieved by an increase in AVP of 10 times that at the greatest dilution of urine and is 1200–1400 mosmol/kg with urine flow reduced to 0.3–0.6 ml/min.

In summary, increases in plasma osmolality above a threshold in the region of 285 mosmol/kg lead to sharp increases in plasma AVP, while decreases in blood volume and pressure must be of the order of 10–15% to stimulate more gradual changes in AVP secretion. Consequently in these situations (i.e. increased osmolality, low blood pressure or volume) urine flow will decrease, fluid will be retained and osmolality, blood volume and pressure will tend to be restored.

Thirst is also stimulated by hypertonicity. Although the osmoreceptors may not be identical with those mediating AVP release, the specificity to various substances is similar in that, for example, changes in blood glucose have no effect. The threshold is higher than that promoting AVP release — 295 mosmol/kg. This corresponds to the plasma osmolality at which maximum concentration of the urine occurs and thus extends the mechanism protecting against dehydration.

Mineralocorticoids, the most significant of which is aldosterone (see Fig. 3.6) also have an important role in fluid and electrolyte homeostasis. The main site of action is the cortical collecting tubules of the kidney and the main effect is to promote reabsorption of sodium and the excretion of potassium and ammonium; the last being an important method of excreting acid, in effect, hydrogen ions. The response of the kidney to increased aldosterone is not immediate because the mechanism depends on cell receptors and RNA and protein synthesis, the lag being from 30 minutes to 2 hours. The duration of the effect is from 4–8 hours.

High levels of aldosterone secretion lead to increased total body sodium, loss of potassium and hence hypokalaemia and alkalosis. Fluid retention usually accompanies sodium retention. In mineralocorticoid deficiency such as Addison's disease, there is loss of sodium, retention of potassium and decreased excretion of acid by the kidney which together lead to the well-known syndrome of dehydration, hyponatraemia, hyperkalaemia and acidosis.

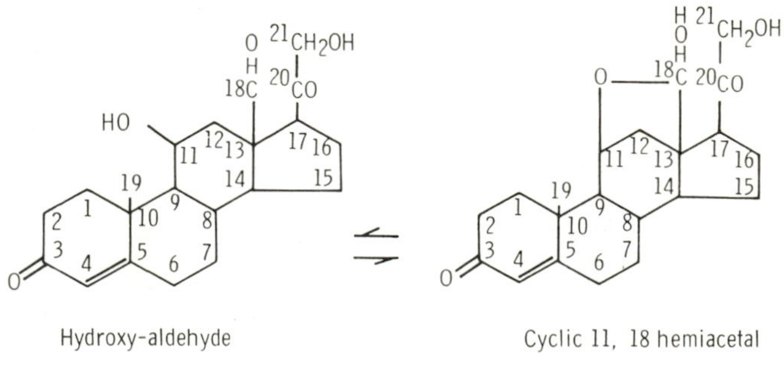

Hydroxy-aldehyde   Cyclic 11, 18 hemiacetal

Fig. 3.6 Aldosterone.

In normal subjects the retention of sodium in response to excess mineralocorticoids is limited, so that after an initial period of positive balance, less of the sodium filtered by the kidney is reabsorbed and a balance of intake and output is regained. This has been referred to as the 'escape' phenomenon. It does not occur in patients with cardiac failure, cirrhosis of the liver or nephrosis which may account for the secondary hyperaldosteronism, usually present in these conditions, contributing to fluid retention and oedema.

The secretion of aldosterone by the cells of the adrenal glomerulosa is mediated mainly by the renin-angiotensin system which is summarized in Figure 3.7. Renin is a protein of molecular weight about 40 000 daltons. It is synthesized in the juxtaglomerulosa cells of the afferent renal arteriole and stored in them. The release of renin is under the influence of renal baroreceptors, adrenergic receptors and ions and hormones which in turn are stimulated by a fall in blood pressure such as usually occurs in changing from the supine to erect posture, beta-adrenergic stimulation, salt depletion and some prostaglandins. The converse is also true, that is, renin release is inhibited by an increase in blood pressure (in normal individuals), salt loading, beta-adrenergic blockers and prostaglandin inhibitors such as indomethacin. The half-life of renin in plasma is 10–20 minutes and it is inactivated by proteolytic enzymes in the liver or plasma or excretion in the urine or bile.

The macula densa of the distal nephron also has a role in controlling the release of renin, by detecting changes in the composition of tubular fluid, especially in sodium and chloride. Reduced blood volume or lowered plasma sodium or chloride stimulate the production of renin. Renin substrate which is synthesized in the liver is a glycoprotein of molecular weight 50 000–100 000 daltons. Generally, the level of renin substrate in plasma is such that changes in its concentration will influence the amount of angiotensin produced, so that it may be important to note that its level is increased by glucocorticoids and by oestrogens (e.g. because of the relation between steroid excess and hypertension). Renin acts on renin substrate to produce angiotensin I.

Angiotensin converting enzyme is a glycoprotein which occurs in the endothelium of blood vessels, in the lung and plasma and in the proximal renal tubule. It converts angiotensin I to angiotensin II. It also inactivates bradykinin. In contrast with angiotensin I which has no significant physiological effects, angiotensin II is the most potent known vasoactive substance. It increases blood pressure by stimulating vasoconstriction of arterioles. It acts in a few seconds and the duration of effect is a few minutes. It inhibits the release of renin, but is a very potent stimulus of aldosterone production. In the normal, non-hypertensive person, angiotensin II promotes sodium retention although in those with hypertension the opposite, that is, natriuresis, has been found to occur.

The half-life of angiotensin II in plasma is only a few minutes and 50% or more of its activity is removed in a single circulation through the vasculature.

The concentration of angiotensin III in plasma is about

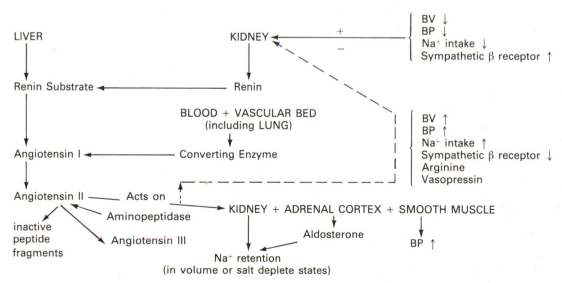

BV: blood volume; BP: blood pressure.

Renin Substrate is an α_2 globulin and glycoprotein of molecular weight (MW) 50–100 000 daltons.

Renin has a MW of 40 000 daltons, and is synthesized in the juxta glomerulosa cells of the afferent renal arteriole.

Fig. 3.7 The interactions of renin, the angiotensins and aldosterone.

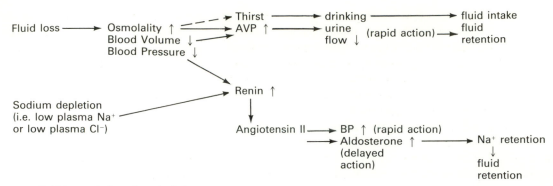

Fig. 3.8 Response to fluid loss and electrolyte depletion.

1/5 of that of angiotensin II so that although it has some physiological effects similar to those of angiotensin II, it is less significant.

It appears that the renin-angiotensin system is important in maintaining blood pressure in volume-depleted or sodium-depleted states but may be of little significance for the regulation of blood pressure when body sodium (or blood volume) is normal.

The overall response to fluid and electrolyte depletion including loss such as blood loss is summarized in Figure 3.8. Loss of water from the body will lead to an increase in osmolality of plasma, to very small changes in which the osmoreceptors are very sensitive with consequent stimulation of the secretion of arginine vasopressin, the antidiuretic hormone in man. This leads to a prompt decrease in urine flow and consequently conservation of fluid. This mechanism has a set-point or threshold about 285 mosmol/kg. If the plasma osmolality increases to about 295 mosmol/kg thirst is stimulated which normally leads to an increased intake of fluid. Reductions of blood volume or pressure also stimulate AVP secretion although the mechanism is very much less sensitive. They also stimulate the release of renin which is promptly converted to angiotensin II which can rapidly constrict arterioles and hence increase blood pressure in sodium depleted subjects. It also stimulates the production of aldosterone. This in turn, after a short lag, promotes sodium retention by the kidney which usually also indirectly leads to fluid retention. A low level of plasma sodium or chloride similarly stimulates the release of renin and consequently the secretion of aldosterone which again has the effect of increasing sodium retention by the kidney.

FLUID IMBALANCE

Excess fluid

Changes in body water correlate directly with changes in body weight so that when a patient gains a kilogram or more in a few days this is due to fluid retention, and certainly not to increased muscle mass. If the fluid reten-tion is of a sufficient degree to give rise to oedema, the measurement of plasma and urine osmolalities, electrolytes and rarely plasma albumin may assist in defining the cause of the fluid retention. Oedema may be local, as in the inflammatory response to an injury, including a burn. It may be due to the administration of large volumes of fluid. If saline has been given urine sodium will be high and osmolality normal, whereas if predominantly water has been given, the urine will be more dilute.

Congestive cardiac failure, chronic liver disease and nephrosis are all likely to be associated with oedema. In each of these, the low plasma sodium does not indicate sodium deficiency or a decrease in total body sodium. When the pathological process has progressed sufficiently far to lead to oedema the renin-angiotensin-aldosterone system is stimulated and consequently, excess sodium is being retained by the kidney (if sufficient renal function remains) and the 'escape' mechanism mentioned above does not operate to return the balance of sodium intake and output to normal. The humoral mechanisms which in the normal are homeostatic in these conditions operate to increase body sodium. Treatment in these cases should be aimed at eliminating the excess water and not at increasing the subnormal plasma sodium concentration by giving isotonic saline intravenously.

Water depletion

This is commonly known as dehydration and may result from a primary deficit of water or from a primary deficit of salt.

The two types of dehydration differ not only in cause, but in effects, in symptoms, and in treatment.

Causes of water depletion

A primary deficit of water results from intake failing to match loss. One cause is simple weakness, for the exhausted patient may only manage a few sips instead of slaking his thirst. Drinking may be prevented by nausea or vomiting, may be difficult because of painful lesions of the mouth or throat, and is impossible in the comatose.

A primary deficit of salt is more commonly due to increased loss and rarely from reduced intake. The deficiency may be of salt alone if the patient loses both salt and water and replaces the water by drinking, as may happen in diarrhoea, copious sweating, or Addison's disease. When dehydration is the result of vomiting there is a deficiency of both salt and water, for the vomiting prevents the replacement of water by drinking.

The distinction between primary water deficit and primary salt deficit is easily made in surgical patients in temperate climates where copious sweating is not in question and where diuretics have not been administered. If there has been no loss of intestinal secretions, the deficit will be predominantly of water. If intestinal secretions have been lost there must be a deficit of salt and water.

Effects of dehydration

A primary *deficit of water* leads to cellular dehydration. It might be thought that the water deficit should be shared proportionately between the intracellular and extracellular fluids, but this is not so. Black and others (1944), working with volunteers who refrained from drinking while continuing to eat a standard diet, found that after 3 to 4 days there was a deficit of about 3.5 litres of water. Nevertheless there was no increase in the haematocrit or in the concentration of haemoglobin or of plasma protein, indicating that there was no reduction in the blood volume. During the experiment very little sodium was excreted in the urine but there was a sharp increase in the excretion of potassium and nitrogen, presumably in response to the AVP, renin-angiotensin-aldosterone mechanisms outlined above. It is this response which permits the volume of the extracellular fluid to be maintained so that deprivation of water leads to cellular dehydration, but not to circulatory failure from a shrinking blood volume.

A primary *deficit of salt* has the opposite effect, and leads to a reduction in the volume of extracellular fluid (including a reduction in blood volume), but not to cellular dehydration.

When the deficit of salt arises from loss of intestinal secretions the loss of water and of sodium (and other electrolytes) is in about the same ratio as they occur in blood plasma, and consequently the osmotic pressure of the extracellular fluid does not rise. Because of this there is no tendency for water to be withdrawn from the cells, and the brunt of the depletion must be borne by the extracellular fluid alone. There is some conservation of the plasma volume at the expense of the tissue fluid (because of the oncotic pressure effect of the plasma protein), but both components of the extracellular fluid are much reduced in volume. The reduction in the volume of the tissue fluid can be demonstrated by the research methods mentioned earlier. The reduced plasma volume can be demonstrated

easily by simple routine tests: the red cell count, the haemoglobin concentration, the haematocrit, and the plasma protein concentration all increase by 10–20% or even more. As the blood volume shrinks there is increasing difficulty in maintaining an adequate circulation and death results from circulatory failure.

Clinical features of dehydration

The outstanding symptoms of water depletion are thirst and oliguria. Personality changes in the direction of either depression or euphoria occur early, but the patient remains capable of mental and physical exertion until relatively late.

The outstanding symptoms of salt depletion are mental and physical lassitude, followed by evidence of circulatory failure. Thirst is not a feature. There is no oliguria in the early stages of salt depletion, and there may even be polyuria if there is free access to drinking-water (as in salt depletion from diarrhoea or copious sweating).

The principal features of water depletion and salt depletion are contrasted in Table 3.6.

Treatment of dehydration

In treating dehydration, it is usually easy to decide what kind of fluid to give, and often difficult to know how much is required. A deficit of water calls for the administration of water (which can often be given by mouth). A deficit

Table 3.6 The contrasting features of water depletion and salt depletion

	Water depletion	Salt depletion
Cause	Deficient intake	Excessive loss (especially loss of intestinal secretions)
Dehydration	Cellular	Extracellular
Thirst	+++	Absent
Urine volume	Scanty	Normal (even increased till late)
Lassitude	+	+++
Weakness	Late	Early
Vomiting	Absent	+
Plasma volume	Normal till late	Reduced
Haemoconcentration	Late and slight	Early and severe
Blood pressure	Normal till late	Fall
Blood urea	Increased	Increased
Plasma sodium	Slight increase	Reduced
Plasma chloride	Slight increase	Reduced
Urine sodium	Reduced	Reduced
Urine chloride	Reduced	Reduced
Cause of death	Uncertain ? Rise of intracellular osmotic pressure	Peripheral circulatory failure

of salt calls for the administration of saline solution or Ringer's solution (a mixture containing NaCl, KCl, lactate, etc.) which must usually be given parenterally.

Treatment of a primary deficit of water

Good treatment is often synonymous with good nursing: weak patients can be induced to drink by encouragement. In patients who cannot be given water by mouth a 5% solution of glucose may be given parenterally. The amount of water given is judged to be adequate when thirst is relieved and the rate of excretion of the urine restored to normal. It is worth noting that the volume of the urine excreted per hour is a good guide to the requirement for water, but is not at all a guide to the requirement of salt (p. 43). The amount of water required, in patients who are unable to eat, is about 3 litres per day in addition to the amount required in the first instance to correct the initial deficit. Some idea of the magnitude of the initial deficit can be obtained from Table 3.7 (from Marriott, 1947).

Table 3.7 Magnitude of water deficit

Mild (about 1 day without water). Pronounced thirst without other effects: a deficit of about 2% of the body weight (about 1.5 litres in a 70 kg man)

Moderate (about 3 or 4 days without water). Severe thirst, dry mouth, oliguria, weakness, ill appearance, but nevertheless still capable of fair mental and physical work: a deficit of about 6% of the body weight (about 4 litres in a 70 kg man)

Severe (about 6 days without water). As above, with marked impairment of mental and physical capacity: a deficit of 7–14% of the body weight (about 5–10 litres in a 70 kg man)

In treating dehydration resulting from a simple deficit of water the common errors are to give too little water to obtain real benefit, and to add saline solution needlessly. The few conditions in which 'water intoxication' might be induced are: (a) after copious sweating, (b) during the 24–36-hour period of postoperative oliguria, and (c) in renal failure with oliguria or anuria.

Persisting dehydration calls for a determined effort to increase the amount of water ingested. The temptation to give saline solution in addition is to be resisted. It is to be remembered that saline solution does nothing to relieve the intracellular dehydration of a water deficit.

Treatment of a primary deficit of salt

Patients who are losing intestinal secretions are losing salt, and require to have the loss made good by the administration of saline solution or Ringer's solution. Patients who have had their adrenals removed surgically or destroyed by disease, or who have salt-wasting chronic nephritis, may

Table 3.8 Effects of salt depletion

Slight to moderate depletion. Lassitude, and perhaps giddiness and orthostatic fainting: a deficit up to about 4 litres of isotonic saline in a 70 kg man

Moderate to severe depletion. As above, with anorexia and perhaps vomiting, and with a fall in blood pressure but with the systolic pressure still exceeding 90 mmHg: a deficit of about 4–6 litres of isotonic saline in a 70 kg man

Severe to very severe depletion. As above, with apathy, stupor, vomiting and a systolic blood pressure less than 90 mmHg: a deficit of about 6–10 litres of isotonic saline in a 70 kg man

also require to be given salt, but such patients are few in surgical practice. The only common cause of salt deficiency is loss of intestinal secretions.

It is much easier to decide that salt is required than to judge how much should be given. Guidance on dosage can be obtained from the patient's clinical state, from measuring the volume of intestinal secretion lost, and from simple laboratory estimations.

The clinical state of the patient indicates deficits of the magnitude shown in Table 3.8 (Marriott, 1947).

It can be seen from this table that in treating extracellular dehydration large amounts of saline should be given. It is helpful to reflect that the volume of the extracellular fluid is about three times the blood volume, and the surgeon who willingly transfuses 3–4 units of blood in treating severe haemorrhage need have no hesitation in infusing 4–6 litres of saline in treating severe dehydration. The common errors of management are to give initially too little saline to be of real benefit, and to continue giving saline postoperatively when it is no longer needed. In view of the large volume of fluid that must be given rapidly, unless the concentration of electrolytes in the body of fluids can be monitored readily and appropriate potassium given, it may be best to give Ringer's solution rather than a simple solution of sodium chloride in order to avoid diluting the other electrolytes.

When a patient develops a salt deficiency in hospital, the volume of fluid lost from the intestine provides some guide to the amount of saline required for replacement, but it must be remembered that additional salt-containing fluid may be sequestered in the lumen and walls of the intestine and in the peritoneal cavity. A determined effort should be made to collect and measure the fluid lost, adding an allowance for the fluid which has soiled the bed linen and dressings, and for the amount sequestered in the abdomen.

Finally, input must be adjusted in the light of the patient's progress. Failure to improve and persistence of haemoconcentration call for more saline, and oedema and hypoproteinaemia indicate overloading.

The laboratory tests which are informative and helpful are extremely simple: they are tests of haemoconcentration. Measurements of the concentration of electrolytes in the serum are simply carried out but the interpretation of the results can be complex. In the ward, in seriously ill patients monitoring the central venous pressure (CVP) gives valuable guidance for the management of the patient, especially to changes in the circulating effective blood volume.

Tests of haemoconcentration

These include measurement of the packed cell volume, the red cell count, or the haemoglobin concentration. One or more of these measurements should certainly be made whenever salt deficiency is suspected. Quite often they indicate that dehydration is more severe than the clinical findings suggest. Measurement of osmolality can also give valuable information. In patients given saline over several days, the concentration of the plasma proteins may be a guide to fluid balance.

In cases of fluid deprivation or dehydration, the ratio of urine to plasma osmolality or urea can give a rapid indication of whether renal function is adequate (Chapter 22). The urine : plasma ratio of osmolality can be equally useful in assessing cases of possible fluid or water overload or inappropriate secretion of ADH (see below). Although, as mentioned above, the ratio of urine urea to plasma urea has also been used, this can give rise to some problems because the blood urea concentration is frequently raised postoperatively due to the metabolic response to trauma (see Chapter 4). It is mainly for this reason that osmolality is used.

Serum concentration of sodium and chloride

Although these concentrations are very often measured, the results can be difficult to interpret. Some of the difficulties have already been mentioned, and others are discussed in the next chapter; for convenience they are summarized here:

1. A deficit of sodium leads not to any striking reduction in sodium concentration, but to water excretion, and eventually to dehydration: a considerable loss of sodium is necessary to reduce the concentration from 140 mmol/l to 120 mmol/l.

2. An excess of sodium leads not to any striking increase of sodium concentration, but to water retention and eventually to oedema.

3. A slight decrease in the concentration of sodium in serum is the rule after operation or in fever even in patients who have no renal or extrarenal loss of sodium, and is due to migration of sodium into cells or into bone. In later convalescence the sodium is again extruded, and the serum concentration returns to normal even though no sodium has been administered.

4. An increase in the concentration of sodium in serum postoperatively is an uncommon finding, and suggests water deprivation in a patient unable to excrete sodium because he is in the stressed state.

Within recent years it has become customary to measure urine electrolyte concentrations and osmolality in conjunction with serum concentrations (see above). This has helped to rationalize therapy and along with haemodynamic measurements, such as central venous pressure, prevents gross degrees of overload, or indeed, the opposite.

ACID-BASE BALANCE

Disturbances of acid-base balance are discussed in this chapter because in surgical patients they commonly accompany fluid and electrolyte disorders.

Acids and bases

According to the theory developed by Lowry and by Bronsted, an acid is a substance which in solution tends to yield protons (hydrogen nuclei); a base is a substance which tends to accept protons (Bates, 1966). As the dissociation of an acid is reversible the following equations can be written:

Acid (H^+ donor)	$\rightleftharpoons H^+ +$ base (H^+ acceptor)
HCl	$\rightleftharpoons H^+ + Cl^-$
H_2CO_3	$\rightleftharpoons H^+ + HCO_3^-$
NH_4^+	$\rightleftharpoons H^+ + NH_3$
H proteinate	$\rightleftharpoons H^+ +$ protein

This short list is enough to indicate the heterogeneous nature of bases. It shows also that the ammonium ion, being a hydrogen donor, is included among the acids.

An acid is strong when it dissociates freely in solution, and weak when it dissociates only slightly. Further, the base present in a strong acid must itself be weak for it readily yields up its hydrion, whereas the base present in a weak acid, since it tends to retain its hydrion, must itself be strong. Thus:

HCl (strong acid)	$\rightleftharpoons H^+ + Cl^-$ (weak base)
H_2CO_3 (weak acid)	$\rightleftharpoons H^+ + HCO_3^-$ (strong base)

It is to be noted that the metallic cations (exemplified by Na^+) neither yield nor accept hydrogen ions, and are therefore neither acids nor bases. The anions (exemplified by Cl^-) are, by definition, bases but they are so feeble that they do not materially influence the reaction of the blood. Excess or deficit of sodium ions or chloride ions, important though they are in governing fluid balance, have no direct influence on acid-base balance.

NORMAL REGULATION OF THE HYDROGEN ION IN BLOOD

The reaction of the blood is stabilized by three mechanisms: the buffer systems, the respiratory excretion of carbon dioxide and the renal excretion of acids and bases.

Buffer systems

The buffer systems of the blood can be regarded as a first line of defence against a change of pH, coming into action at once and allowing time for the main defence by respiratory and renal excretion to become effective. Alternatively, the buffer systems can be regarded as responsible for maintaining an equable pH throughout the body, whereas the excretory mechanisms control only the acid-base balance of the body as a whole.

The buffers in the plasma are weak acids paired with their sodium salts. The chief buffer pair is carbonic acid and sodium bicarbonate. Next comes plasma protein paired with sodium proteinate. Last comes sodium dihydrogen phosphate (NaH_2PO_4) which can be regarded as a weak acid having disodium hydrogen phosphate (Na_2HPO_4) as its sodium salt: this phosphate pair is much less important in the plasma than in the urine (p. 47).

The principal buffer in red cells is haemoglobin paired with its potassium salt (the carbonic acid-bicarbonate pair is here unimportant). Haemoglobin also has properties which increase its buffering power in venous blood. First, by forming a carbamino compound, haemoglobin can remove carbonic acid from solution. Secondly, haemoglobin is an even weaker acid than oxyhaemoglobin: in the tissues, the change to haemoglobin (the weaker acid) helps to counteract the increase of carbonic acid that results from the influx of carbon dioxide; conversely, in the lungs, the change to oxyhaemoglobin (the stronger acid) helps to counteract the removal of carbonic acid.

Table 3.9 shows clearly the importance of haemoglobin as a buffer, and also indicates why the bicarbonate system is a useful guide to the total buffering power of the blood.

The theory of the action of buffers can well be left to the student of chemistry. There are, however, two properties of buffers which the clinician must grasp if he is to appreciate the significance of the various measurements used in the assessment of acid-base balance in patients, and estimations of hydrogen ion — usually expressed as pH, see below. Firstly, the buffering power of a buffer pair (such as carbonic acid and sodium bicarbonate) depends on the total concentration of these substances rather than their ratio: the greater the concentration the greater the buffering power. The second important property is that the pH of a solution containing a buffer pair (such as carbonic acid and sodium bicarbonate) depends wholly on their ratio. Provided this ratio remains unchanged, concentrating or diluting the solution leaves the pH unchanged.

Table 3.9 Approximate contribution of individual buffers to total buffering in whole blood (after Winters et al, 1967, p. 40)

Buffers	Buffering in whole blood %
Haemoglobin and oxyhaemoglobin	35
Plasma bicarbonate	35
Erythrocyte bicarbonate	18
Organic phophates	3
Inorganic phosphates	2
Plasma proteins	7

This can be demonstrated by applying the basic chemical 'Law of Mass Action' to the dissociation of hydrogen ion from an acid in solution:

$$K = \frac{[H^+]\,[Base]}{[Acid]}$$

in which the square brackets indicate concentration and K is the equilibrium constant. If this equation is rewritten:

$$[H^+] = K\,\frac{[Acid]}{[Base]}$$

it is obvious that the hydrogen ion concentration of a system is determined by the ratio of acid to base. If we note further that

$$CO_2 + H_2O \rightleftharpoons H_2CO_3 \rightleftharpoons H^+ + HCO^-_3$$

it is again obvious that CO_2 produced by metabolism and excreted by the lungs and its related bicarbonate buffering system plays an important role in acid-base balance. Retention of CO_2 due to impaired lung function will increase H_2CO_3, the acid component, and hence lead to respiratory acidosis. Changes in $[HCO_3^-]$, the base, are referred to as metabolic changes and the ratio of acid (H_2CO_3) to base (HCO^-_3) determines blood hydrogen ion concentration. Since pH is defined as the negative logarithm of $[H^+]$, applying logarithms to the above equation gives, after minor rearrangement, the Henderson-Hasselbalch equation:

$$pH = pK + \log_{10}\frac{[HCO_3^-]}{[H_2CO_3]}$$

in which pK is the negative logarithm (to base 10) of the equilibrium constant K. We must also note that $[H_2CO_3]$ is determined by P_{CO_2}, the partial pressure of the gas CO_2 in the solution.

Excretion of carbon dioxide by the lungs

The continuous influx of carbon dioxide from the tissues,

soon forming carbonic acid, introduces more acid into the blood than any other metabolic process. For this reason the transport and excretion of carbon dioxide can be regarded as the most important of the mechanisms which stabilize the reaction of the blood.

A small fraction of the carbon dioxide is transported in simple solution in the plasma, forming carbonic acid. About one-quarter of the carbon dioxide passes into the red cells, and is transported in the red cells as carbamino-haemoglobin. The rest of the carbon dioxide enters the red cells, is rapidly converted to carbonic acid under the action of carbonic anhydrase, and dissociates to hydrogen ions and bicarbonate ions: the hydrogen ions are removed from solution by combining with the haemoglobin while the bicarbonate ions migrate out of the red cells, their place being taken by chloride ions migrating in (the 'chloride shift').

In the lungs, these changes operate in reverse when the equilibrium is disturbed by carbon dioxide diffusing out of the blood into the pulmonary alveoli.

The amount of *bicarbonate* present in the plasma is controlled by the total amounts of other ions. The total cations (mainly Na^+) exceed the total non-volatile anions (mainly Cl^-) by about 27 mmol/l, (see Fig. 3.3), this difference must be made up exactly by HCO_3 — otherwise a colossal electrical potential would be set up. The amount of *carbonic acid* in the plasma depends on how much carbon dioxide is carried in simple solution. As the carbon dioxide dissolved in arterial plasma is in equilibrium with the partial pressure of carbon dioxide in the pulmonary alveoli, the P_{CO_2} of arterial blood is about 5.3 kPa (40 mmHg), and this is responsible for a concentration of carbonic acid of 1.35 mmol/l. It follows that the ratio of bicarbonate to carbonic acid is normally 27:1.35, or exactly 20:1 required to maintain pH 7.4 (p. 48).

Renal excretion of acids and bases

Most acids and bases are excreted as neutral salts and not in the free state. An exception of some practical importance is uric acid, some of which may be excreted in the free state and give rise to uric acid calculi.

The oxidation of protein, carbohydrate and fat gives rise principally to carbon dioxide, but may give rise also to non-volatile acids which must be excreted by the kidneys, for example, uric acid from purines, sulphuric acid from cystine and methionine, lactic acid from muscles contracting anaerobically, and keto-acids from fat during starvation. These acids, like all acids (p. 45), consist of hydrion plus a base. The base could be excreted, if need be, as a neutral salt in company with a cation such as sodium, but this would tend to leave in the blood an excess of hydrion and would also be wasteful of sodium. Accordingly, the normal task of the renal tubules is to find means of excreting hydrion and conserving sodium. Three mech-

anisms come into play, probably all ultimately dependent on the action of carbonic anhydrase within the tubule cells; these mechanisms include phosphate excretion, substitution of ammonium for sodium, and reabsorption of sodium bicarbonate.

Carbonic anhydrase plays its part within the cells of the tubules by speeding up the union of carbon dioxide with water to form carbonic acid. The carbonic acid dissociates to H^+ and HCO_3 , yielding a ready source of hydrion, some of which can migrate into the tubular urine.

Phosphate excretion

In the tubular urine, each molecule of disodium phosphate (Na_2HPO_4) can yield one sodium ion for reabsorption in exchange for one hydrogen ion made available from carbonic acid (Fig. 3.9), leaving monosodium phosphate (NaH_2PO_4) to be excreted. The ratio of monosodium to disodium phosphate is only 1:4 in the blood, but it is about 10:1 in normal urine and can be as high as 50:1. This preferential excretion of monosodium dihydrogen phosphate serves both to conserve sodium and excrete hydrion. The mechanism is limited by the availability of phosphate, but it can achieve the excretion of about 30 mmol/l of acid per day.

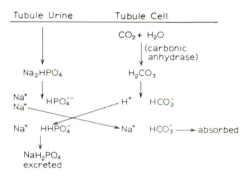

Fig. 3.9 Scheme of the substitution of dihydrogen phosphate for monohydrogen phosphate. This diagram and the next two illustrate mechanisms for excreting hydrion and conserving sodium and bicarbonate. The three mechanisms can all be blocked by carbonic anhydrase inhibitors.

Ammonium substitution

Each molecule of sodium chloride in the tubular urine can yield one sodium ion for reabsorption in exchange for one hydrogen ion made available from carbonic acid (Fig. 3.10). This exchange would form hydrochloric acid in the tubular urine were it not for the ability of the tubular cells to liberate ammonia from glutamine and other amino acids: this ammonia passes into the tubular urine and converts the hydrochloric acid to the neutral salt ammonium chloride. The mechanism achieves the conservation of sodium and the excretion of hydrion without leaving free acid in the urine. The daily excretion of

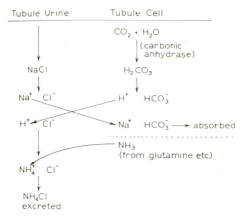

Fig. 3.10 Scheme of the substitution of ammonium ion for sodium ion.

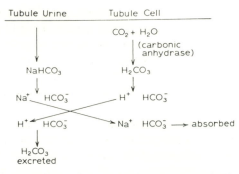

Fig. 3.11 Scheme of the substitution of carbonic acid for bicarbonate.

ammonium salts is very variable. It is normally about 0.5–1 g, but it can be reduced to zero when there is no need to excrete hydrion, and it can be as much as 4–5 g per day when the need for excreting hydrion is increased.

Bicarbonate excretion

The voided urine is normally about pH 5.5 to 6.0, and contains no bicarbonate. Bicarbonate is present however when the voided urine is alkaline. Most of the bicarbonate present in the proximal tubules is reabsorbed along with sodium and is not available for excretion. The small amount remaining in the distal tubules can be reabsorbed or excreted in accordance with needs. In the tubular urine the bicarbonate is present with sodium, but the sodium can be reabsorbed in exchange for hydrogen made available from carbonic acid in the tubule cells (Fig. 3.11). It is thus possible to conserve sodium and excrete carbonic acid instead of bicarbonate.

All three mechanisms discussed above can be blocked by drugs which inhibit the action of carbonic anhydrase. The carbonic anhydrase inhibitors therefore interfere with sodium reabsorption, increase the amount of sodium excreted, and have been used as diuretics.

Indices of acid-base balance

Hydrogen ion in the blood is expressed as pH, the negative logarithm of hydrogen ion concentration $[H^+]$ or as concentration (nmol/l). The interested reader is referred to the monograph by Siggaard-Andersen (1974) in which the relationship between hydrogen ion activity, concentration, potential and pH is discussed. The normal range is 7.36–7.43 units in fully oxygenated arterial blood at 37 °C. Blood pH depends on the relationship between the 'respiratory' and 'metabolic' components of acid-base metabolism and alterations in pH may result from disturbances in either of these components.

'Respiratory' disturbances are defined by changes in carbon dioxide tension ($P\text{CO}_2$). Changes in $P\text{CO}_2$ usually indicate some alteration in ventilatory function but the value is also influenced by the rate of production of carbon dioxide in the tissues. The normal range is 4.8–5.9 kPa (36–44 mmHg).

Both pH and $P\text{CO}_2$ are measured directly using an electrode system and although such measurements are usually the responsibility of the biochemical laboratory, the method is straightforward enough to be practised by clinical staff under appropriate supervision. The need for rapid and repeated blood gas data makes this mandatory in the intensive therapy unit. A small sample of arterial blood is withdrawn, under anaerobic conditions, either via a needle or indwelling catheter and placed immediately into the electrode system. The result is available within 3 minutes using modern apparatus.

The 'metabolic' or 'non-respiratory' component of acid-base balance is not measured directly but may be calculated from the Henderson-Hasselbalch equation described above ie:

$$pH = pK + \log \frac{[HCO_3]}{[H_2CO_3]}$$

pH is known; pK is termed the 'dissociation constant' although the value falls with temperature (at 38 °C, pK is 6.1); the carbonic acid concentration $[H_2CO_3]$ at body temperature is given as the product of $P\text{CO}_2$ and the 'solubility coefficient' (0.030); the concentration of bicarbonate ion $[HCO_3]$ is thus derived and is one of the indices used to describe metabolic changes.

This method of calculating the 'metabolic' component is tedious if done manually. Several nomograms have been devised to simplify the calculation, dating from the Henderson-Davenport diagram (Davenport, 1958) to the Siggaard-Andersen alignment nomogram, and a specially designed slide-rule, the blood gas calculator, has been produced which permits rapid derivation of the 'metabolic' component even when gross fluctuations of body temperature have to be taken into consideration (Severinghaus, 1966). Completely automatic calculation of the 'metabolic' indices is one of the many advances incorporated in the most recent models of blood gas apparatus, using microprocessors.

The indices in common use to describe the 'metabolic' component include plasma bicarbonate, standard bicarbonate, buffer base and base excess.

Plasma bicarbonate represents the total carbon dioxide extractable from an anaerobic sample of plasma at body temperature minus the carbonic acid concentration. Since this value changes with P_{CO_2} it does not truly differentiate between metabolic and respiratory disturbances. If respiratory dysfunction can be confidently excluded on clinical grounds, plasma bicarbonate may be considered to reflect predominantly metabolic changes. Total extractable carbon dioxide is the value normally reported in laboratory analyses of venous blood (mean — 24 mmol/l) and, in the absence of respiratory disease, approximates closely to plasma bicarbonate.

Standard bicarbonate is a more recently introduced term (Siggaard-Andersen, 1965). It represents the bicarbonate value derived when the blood is assumed to be fully oxygenated at a P_{CO_2} of 5.3 kPa (40 mmHg) and at a temperature of 37 °C. The normal range is 21.3–24.8 mmol/l.

Buffer base is the sum of the buffer anions in blood (see Table 3.9). The normal mean is about 48 mmol/l. Base excess represents the change in buffer base concentration of blood in the presence of surplus acid or base. The normal mean is zero and the range is from −2.3 mmol/l to +2.3 mmol/l. A negative base excess indicates a trend towards increased hydrogen ion activity and may be alternatively termed base deficit.

Disturbances of acid-base balance

'Acidosis' and 'alkalosis' are the terms conventionally used to describe disturbances in acid-base equilibrium, although they have no universally agreed meaning and are not dependent upon actual blood pH changes (Morgan, 1969). Gain or loss in the form of carbonic acid is described as a 'respiratory' acidosis or alkalosis. Otherwise gain or loss of hydrogen ion is termed a 'metabolic' or 'non-respiratory' acidosis or alkalosis.

Acid-base disturbances may be considered as having two phases: the initial physicochemical or 'uncompensated' phase and the secondary physiological or 'compensated' phase. A set of acid-base data is only capable of being intelligently interpreted when viewed against the clinical background. In this way, the initiating factors may be separated from the body's normal compensating mechanisms.

Acidosis

'Respiratory' acidosis is associated with a rise in arterial carbon dioxide tension (P_{CO_2}) above 6.0 kPa (45 mmHg). Initially this produces a reduction in the ratio of bicarbonate to carbonic acid (p. 48) and pH tends to fall. This type of disturbance can result from hypoventilation as, for example, following surgery or drug overdosage, or from reinhalation of exhaled carbon dioxide as in a faulty breathing circuit. The rate of rise of P_{CO_2} in either of these instances cannot exceed 0.66 kPa (5 mmHg) per minute. Only by inhalation of exogenous carbon dioxide can rates of rise in P_{CO_2} exceed this value — a largely theoretical hazard of anaesthetic circuits (Prys-Roberts et al, 1967).

Compensation for respiratory acidosis takes the form of increased renal tubular reabsorption of bicarbonate and excretion of hydrogen ion in the form of dihydrogen phosphate and ammonium salts. The ratio of bicarbonate to carbonic acid is thus restored to the 20:1 required to maintain a normal pH. Base excess will then be substantially positive. The fully compensated state may be seen in patients with long-standing chronic respiratory disease. When patients of this type present for surgery a preoperative evaluation of their acid-base state can be of considerable value, particularly if a postoperative complication produces further acid-base disturbances.

'Metabolic' acidosis is a common accompaniment of surgical problems (Norman & Clark, 1964). It is associated with a fall in base excess which becomes increasingly negative. There is an initial reduction in the bicarbonate carbonic acid ratio and pH tends to fall. This type of disturbance is seen most commonly in surgery when there is a significant degree of hypoxaemia or generalized hypoperfusion. Tissue hypoxia leads to an accumulation of lactic acid. In the extreme case of cardiac arrest it has been shown that organic acid accumulates at the rate of about 1.1 mmol/l/min at 37 °C (Ledingham & Norman, 1962). The accumulation of organic acids leads to a raised 'anion-cation gap', which is expressed as the difference between the sums of the anions and cations usually measured in plasma (see Fig. 3.4). It is usual to combine the values of chloride and bicarbonate and to subtract the result from either the sum of sodium and potassium or sodium alone. Figures significantly greater than 20 m equiv. may indicate the accumulation of unmeasured anions such as lactate or those of the ketoacids. Metabolic acidosis may also result from small bowel fistulae and profuse diarrhoea because of loss of alkaline intestinal fluid, in renal failure because of failure of hydrogen ion excretion, and in diabetic states because of the accumulation of keto acids. A rare form of acidosis ('hyperchloraemic acidosis') follows the absorption of chloride from the colon in a few patients who have undergone ureterocolic transplant.

Physiological compensation for metabolic acidosis takes two forms. The first occurs rapidly and consists of an increase in the rate of excretion of carbon dioxide by hyperventilation. The second comes into play more slowly. The excreted urine is acid, about pH 5. The ratio of monosodium to disodium phosphate increases, the excretion of ammonium salts increases, and the excretion of bicarbonate stops. Both mechanisms restore the ratio:

$$\frac{[HCO_3^-]}{[H_2CO_3]}$$

and therefore pH, towards normal.

Treatment of acidotic state should always be directed towards eliminating the underlying cause but in certain circumstances it may be considered advisable to act rapidly to avert a critical fall in blood pH. In the case of respiratory acidosis such treatment may take the form of a short period of intermittent positive pressure ventilation to reduce $PaCO_2$. Metabolic acidosis may be corrected using alkaline solutions, usually sodium bicarbonate. It is possible to quantitate the degree of a metabolic acidosis. This is usually expressed as 'base deficit' and computed as;

Base deficit = 0.3 × body weight (kg) × base excess (mmol/l)

for example, in a 72 kg man with a base excess of −10 mmol/l;
base deficit = 0.3 × 72 × 10 = 216 mmol

Such deficits can be treated using molar sodium bicarbonate solution, i.e. 8.4% w/v, which contains 1 mmol $NaHCO_3$/ml. In practice, correction of metabolic acidosis is rarely required unless very severe, and it is unnecessary and usually hazardous to correct an acidosis completely. There are many reasons for this, including the administration of an equal number of sodium ions with the bicarbonate with consequent expansion of the extracellular volume, which carries a risk to the patient in cardiac or renal failure. There is also a risk of 'overshooting' because during recovery, the metabolites such as lactate or ketones causing the acidosis are metabolised to CO_2, part of which appears in solution as bicarbonate, thus increasing the base excess.

Although 'respiratory' and 'metabolic' acidosis have been described separately, they not infrequently occur together in surgical patients. Under these circumstances pH rapidly falls and, if the patient is not treated promptly, the prognosis is poor.

Alkalosis

'Respiratory' alkalosis is associated with a fall in arterial carbon dioxide tension below 4.7 kPa (35 mmHg). Arterial pH tends to rise. This form of acid-base disturbance is unusual in clinical practice. It occurs in hysterical states

and at high altitudes. Renal compensation leads to the excretion of an alkaline urine, containing bicarbonate, less dihydrogen phosphate, and no ammonium salts.

'Metabolic' alkalosis is associated with a rise in base excess and a trend towards a higher pH. This condition may follow chronic ingestion of alkali, vomiting with loss of hydrogen ion, and potassium depletion. All three factors are involved in the acid-base disturbance of pyloric stenosis. The sequel of events in this condition has been divided into two stages (LeQuesne, 1968). In the anionic stage (Fig. 3.12), chloride is exchanged via the gastric mucosa for bicarbonate which accumulates in the plasma in higher than normal quantity. The urine is alkaline with an increased bicarbonate content. In the cationic stage, sodium continues to be lost both in the vomit and in urine until it requires to be preserved to retain the extracellular fluid volume. Hydrogen then replaces sodium in the urine which aggravates the extracellular alkalosis. Potassium is also lost in the vomit and urine (Fig. 3.13), and the urine loss increases as the alkalosis becomes more severe because of the normal competition between hydrogen and potassium for tubular excretion. Potassium eventually leaves the cells to make up for extracellular losses and is replaced

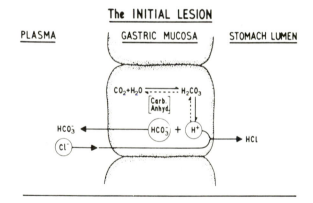

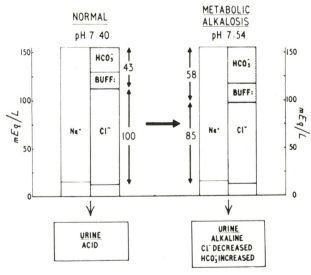

Fig. 3.12 Anionic stage of pyloric stenosis (After Le Quesne, 1968)

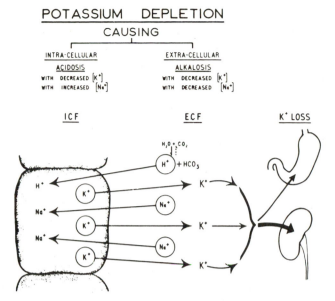

POTASSIUM DEPLETION
CAUSING

INTRA-CELLULAR	EXTRA-CELLULAR
ACIDOSIS	ALKALOSIS
WITH DECREASED [K⁺]	WITH DECREASED [K⁺]
WITH INCREASED [Na⁺]	WITH DECREASED [Na⁺]

Fig. 3.13 Early cationic stage of pyloric stenosis (After Le Quesne, 1968)

there by sodium and hydrogen. There is finally a combination of an extracellular alkalosis and an intracellular acidosis.

The importance of this complex story is that the acid-base disturbances in pyloric stenosis are closely inter-related with fluid and electrolyte disturbances (Clark &

Norman, 1964). Alkali normally has no part to play in treatment which consists essentially of rehydration with added sodium, potassium and chloride. The acid-base disequilibrium corrects itself spontaneously.

In a small number of patients in the post-operative period, particularly after open-heart surgery, it is not unusual to find a degree of extracellular alkalosis, maximal on the third day and persisting for 1–3 weeks. This alkalosis may result from the administration of base (ACD (acid-citrate-dextrose) blood and bicarbonate), increased urinary loss of hydrogen, extracellular to intracellular shifts of hydrogen, and chloride or potassium deficiency. The hydrogen ion changes are secondary to increased aldosterone secretion. The clinical importance of this type of acid-base disturbance is that there is an inability to excrete base in the post-operative period, digoxin may be dangerous to administer under these circumstances, a deficiency of ionic calcium may occur, and prognosis appears to be adversely affected. The administration of potassium is of value.

APPENDIX

The tables overleaf illustrate the relationship between the new SI units and older terminology. The hatched areas refer to the 'normal' range for adults.

REFERENCES

Baylis P H 1983 Chayen J, Bitensky L (eds) Measurement of antidiuretic hormone in cytochemical bioassays: techniques and clinical applications. Marcel Dekker, Bristol

Bates R G 1966 Acids, bases and buffers. Annals of New York Academy of Sciences 133:25

Black D A K, McCance R A, Young W F 1944 A study of dehydration by means of balance experiments. Journal of Physiology 102:406

Clark R G, Normal J N 1964 Metabolic alkalosis in pyloric stenosis. Lancet i:1244

Cohen R D 1974 Body fluids. In: Campbell E J M, Dickinson C J, Slater J D H (eds) Clinical Physiology 4th edn Blackwell, Oxford p 1

Davenport H W 1958 The ABC of acid-base chemistry 4th edn. University of Chicago Press, Chicago

Felig P, Baxter J D, Broadus A E, Frohman L A 1981 Endocrinology and metabolism. McGraw-Hill, New York

Frohlich E D (ed) 1976 Pathophysiology — altered regulatory mechanisms in disease, 2nd edn. Lippincott, Philadelphia

Kinney J M, Egdahl R H, Zuidema G D (eds) 1971 Manual of preoperative and postoperative care, 2nd edn. Saunders Philadelphia

Ledingham I McA, Norman J N 1962 Acid-base studies in circulatory arrest. Lancet ii:967

LeQuesne L P 1968 Pyloric stenosis in the adult. Journal of the Royal College of Surgeons of Edinburgh 13:59

Marriott H L 1947 Water and salt depletion. British Medical Journal 1: 245 285 328

Morgan H G 1969 Acid-base balance in blood. British Journal of Anaesthesia 41:196

Norman J N, Clark R G 1964 Metabolic acidosis in general surgery. Lancet i: 348–350

Prys-Roberts C, Smith W D A, Nunn J N 1967 Accidental severe hypercapnia during anaesthesia. British Journal of Anaesthesia 39:257

Severinghaus J W 1966 Blood gas calculator. Journal of Applied Physiology 21:1108

Shoemaker W C, Walker W F 1970 Fluid-electrolyte therapy in acute illness. Year Book Medical Publishers Inc, Chicago

Siggaard-Andersen O 1965 The acid-base status of the blood, 3rd edn. Munksgaard, Copenhagen

Siggaard-Andersen O 1974 The acid-base status of the blood, 4th end, Munksgaard, Copenhagen

Winters R W, Engel K, Dell R B, Berkson R P 1967 Acid-base physiology. Radiometer, Copenhagen

Wynn V 1965 Water and electrolyte metabolism. In: Irvine W T (ed) Scientific Basis of Surgery. Churchill, London p 340

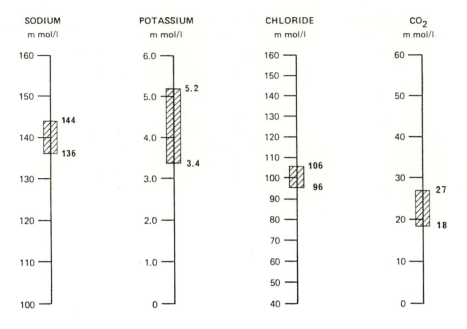

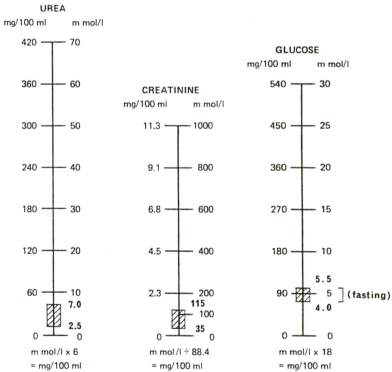

Appendix. The relationship between new SI units and older terminology.

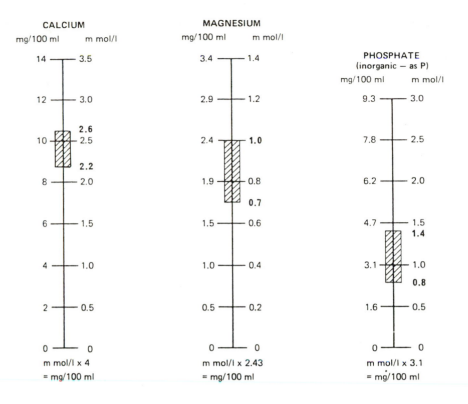

CALCIUM

mg/100 ml   m mol/l

14 — 3.5

12 — 3.0

2.6
10 — 2.5
2.2

8 — 2.0

6 — 1.5

4 — 1.0

2 — 0.5

0 — 0

m mol/l x 4
= mg/100 ml

MAGNESIUM

mg/100 ml   m mol/l

3.4 — 1.4

2.9 — 1.2

2.4 — **1.0**

1.9 — 0.8
0.7

1.5 — 0.6

1.0 — 0.4

0.5 — 0.2

0 — 0

m mol/l x 2.43
= mg/100 ml

PHOSPHATE
(inorganic — as P)

mg/100 ml   m mol/l

9.3 — 3.0

7.8 — 2.5

6.2 — 2.0

4.7 — 1.5
1.4
3.1 — 1.0
0.8

1.6 — 0.5

0 — 0

m mol/l x 3.1
= mg/100 ml

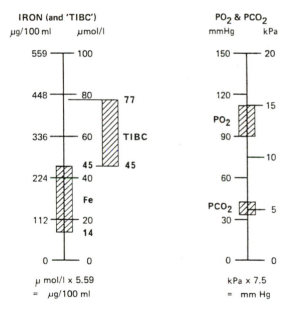

IRON (and 'TIBC')

µg/100 ml   µmol/l

559 — 100

448 — 80   **77**

336 — 60   **TIBC**

45 — **45**
224 — 40
Fe
112 — 20
14

0 — 0

µ mol/l x 5.59
=   µg/100 ml

PO$_2$ & PCO$_2$

mmHg   kPa

150 — 20

120 — 15

PO$_2$
90

— 10

60

PCO$_2$ — 5
30

0 — 0

kPa x 7.5
=   mm Hg

Metabolic response to injury

INTRODUCTION

Trauma is the commonest cause of death in males under 40 years of age. It is also the most common reason for admission to hospital, accounting for 10–15% of admissions.

The changes in metabolism which follow most elective surgery result in slight loss of body weight and do not require specific therapy, consequently they are usually ignored. In contrast, the metabolic problems of those resuscitated by modern intensive care therapy after severe injury or shock, clearly demonstrate the requirement for an understanding of the metabolic response to injury.

Intensive studies, stimulated by two world wars and subsequent hostilities, led to the general recognition of the necessity for active fluid therapy in shock and other measures of resuscitation (see Ch. 28). Progress in understanding the metabolic changes after injury has not been so dramatic. Studies of nitrogen metabolism were impossible until the introduction of the chemical estimation of nitrogen in the mid 19th century. Numerous quantitative studies of metabolism followed. An early example is Muller's demonstration in 1884 of the increased excretion of nitrogen in the urine during typhoid fever. Bernard's observation in 1877 of the hyperglycaemia provoked by haemorrhage is another example of a metabolic discovery made possible by a technical innovation. The studies of van Slyke in the early 20th century on acid base regulation preceded the observations of acidosis in shock mentioned by Cannon in 1918. In recent years, the development of methods for estimating hormones, especially radio-immuno-assay techniques, has contributed to our understanding of some of the metabolic interactions which occur after injury.

Although there were earlier studies of the effects of injury on metabolism, it was the publication of Cuthbertson's observations in 1932 (see Fig. 4.1) which led to wide acceptance of the concept that the predominant effect of injury is a net increase in catabolism which leads to a generalized loss of body protein. This concept, which has

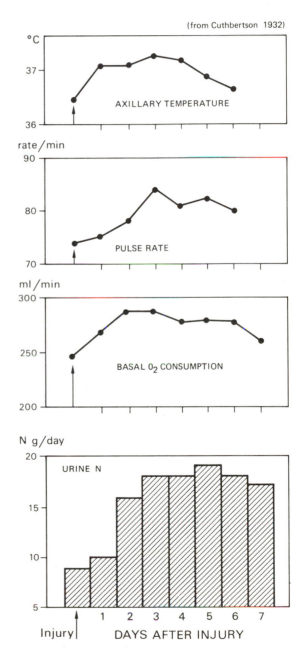

Fig. 4.1 Response to injury (from Cuthbertson, 1932).

been modified slightly in recent years will be discussed on page 58. Cuthbertson also demonstrated that there was an increase in oxygen consumption after injury. At this time the temporal and quantitative relationships of the increase in nitrogen excretion in urine after injury, the increase in oxygen consumption, the transient increase in pulse rate and in body temperature (Fig. 4.1) were summarized. The increase in excretion in the urine of phosphorus and sulphate which followed fracture of a long bone were described and these changes shown to be greater than after simple immobilization. Since nitrogen, potassium, phosphate and sulphate are major components of body tissue, an increase in their excretion in the urine has been taken as indicating a generalized net catabolism of body proteins following injury.

Almost 15 years after his initial observation, Cuthbertson suggested that the metabolic changes provoked by injury could be described in two phases: an early ebb phase, during which there is a depression of metabolic processes and a subsequent flow phase, during which metabolism is increased. When the ebb phase is manifested as severe clinical shock which progresses despite therapy and from which there is no recovery, the related metabolic processes have been referred to as the necrobiotic phase (Fig. 4.2). The ordinate in Figure 4.2 is generally taken as oxygen consumption, resting metabolic energy expenditure (RME) or heat production. The ebb or shock phase is characterized by decreased oxygen consumption and the flow phase by an increase to a value above normal followed by a gradual decline towards normal oxygen consumption. The necrobiotic phase is characterized by an initial gradual continuation of the metabolic changes of shock followed by a terminal rapid decrease in oxygen consumption.

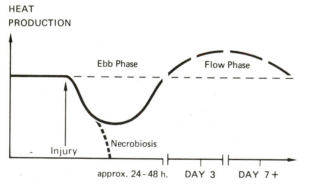

HEAT
PRODUCTION

Fig. 4.2 Phases of the response to injury.

METABOLIC CHANGES IN THE EBB PHASE AND SHOCK

From the above summary it is clear that the early concept of the ebb phase was that it is the period immediately after injury (including elective surgery) during which there is a depression of various metabolic processes, especially those of energy production, oxygen uptake and hence heat production. In recent years, mainly due to progress in anaesthesia and intensive care, many have come to question whether the ebb phase is an invariable concomitant of the controlled injury of elective surgery or severe burning injury when effective therapy is begun within a very short time after the injury.

The syndrome of clinical shock as described by Cannon in 1923 and summarized by Ledingham is still encountered. The clinical syndrome (see Ch. 28) consists of hypotension, tachycardia, pallor, sweating, peripheral cyanosis, hyperventilation, clouding of consciousness and oliguria.

For the present discussion we can regard shock as being roughly synonymous with the ebb phase provided it is remembered that in many cases of injury, shock does not develop and the ebb phase may be so transient that it is not detected.

Some of the metabolic changes in shock may be modified by the cause. For example, shock may be traumatic, cardiogenic, haemorrhagic, ischaemic, septic or due to burning injury (Ch. 28). The effects on metabolism of traumatic shock as seen in battle casualties are summarized in Table 4.1.

Table 4.1 Metabolic changes in shock

Plasma/Blood	Cells
Hyperglycaemia	Decrease in oxygen consumption
Acidosis	Decreased glucose oxidation
Lacticacidaemia	Glycogen depletion
Increase in free fatty acids (FFA) &	Mobilization of fat
Increase in glycerol	Depletion of ATP
Increase in non-protein nitrogen	Reduced membrane potential
	(Possible) stimulation of
	gluconeogenesis
Urine	
Increased excretion of ketones	
Increased excretion of nitrogen	

The hyperglycaemia was observed first by Claude Bernard in experimental haemorrhagic shock in 1877. The acidosis, the increased production and excretion of ketones, the increase in nitrogen excretion and the increase in non-protein nitrogen were all observed in First World War casualties in France. The lacticacidaemia and increased free fatty acids and glycerol are more recent observations. In severe shock, increase in free fatty acids (FFA) has on occasion not been observed, although the increase in plasma glycerol usually is. The explanation offered is that, in the absence of good tissue perfusion, the free fatty acids which are transported bound to albumin cannot leave the fat depot whereas glycerol is freely diffusible. Cellular effects include reduced membrane potential, a decrease in oxygen utilization, decreases in mitochondrial metabolism and glycolysis, glycogen depletion and mobilization of fat.

The different causes of shock may accentuate one aspect of these metabolic changes more than another. For example, the hyperglycaemia of haemorrhagic shock is well known although hyperglycaemia may not occur in some cases of septic shock. Lacticacidaemia tends to be more severe in haemorrhagic shock than in the others.

The changes in levels of metabolites in the blood, urine and cells after injury, which are summarized in Table 4.1, can be rationalized. Recent observations of changes in the endocrine system after injury, which will be discussed later, offer a basic explanation for the metabolic disturbance.

An early hypothesis was that in shock, reduced blood flow and peripheral vasoconstriction led to tissue hypoxia and consequently to a larger proportion of the energy requirement of the body being derived from anaerobic glycolysis. This, being much less efficient than aerobic carbohydrate metabolism (Fig. 4.3), leads to increased glycogenolysis and, when prolonged, to depletion of tissue glycogen. Anaerobic glycolysis leads to accumulation of lactic acid, lacticacidaemia, and the development of acidosis.

Although this mechanism may occur in haemorrhagic and traumatic shock, it has been shown that lactic acid production is increased in shock in tissues in which it has not been possible to demonstrate a reduced oxygen supply. This may be due to direct impairment of oxidative phosphorylation by a mechanism similar to that in endotoxic shock. The endocrine effects on carbohydrate metabolism would also tend to lead to an increase in lactic acid and all three mechanisms could be additive. Depletion of cellular ATP or 'available energy' could result from these changes in carbohydrate metabolism together with reduced oxygen consumption. The latter presumably would lead to a reduction in the amount of ATP produced by the

oxidation reactions of the cytochrome system of mitochondria. However, the total carbohydrate stores (glycogen) of the body are sufficient to supply only about one-half of one day's energy requirements. Therefore from the first day after injury, endogenous fat and protein will be the only sources of energy. It has been shown that after injury protein provides from 12–22% of the energy expenditure and fat the remainder.

Other metabolic observations on shocked individuals can be explained by an increase in gluconeogenesis. In gluconeogenesis, the source of glucose is three-carbon precursors derived mainly from amino acids and lactate and since the amino acid alanine has the same carbon skeleton as pyruvic acid, the observed increase in plasma alanine after injury could be consistent with increased gluconeogenesis. (see Fig. 4.4). The glucose-alanine cycle (Fig. 4.4) is likely to have a significant role in this process. Since muscle is a major site for metabolism of the branched-chain amino acids (BCAA), leucine, isoleucine and valine, a mechanism is required to transfer the amino groups removed in the first stage of metabolism to the liver for conversion to urea and subsequent excretion in the urine. The mechanism is to transfer the amino groups to oxaloacetate and to pyruvate to form the amino acids glutamate and alanine. The alanine is transferred to the liver, in which the pyruvate again produced can be converted to glucose. This is also consistent with early observations of increased blood non-protein nitrogen (NPN) in shock. Non-protein nitrogen is composed predominantly of urea (approximately 60%) and about half the remainder (residual NPN) is amino acid nitrogen. The increase in NPN in shock was shown to consist of increases in both urea nitrogen and residual nitrogen. The increase in residual nitrogen is compatible with increases in plasma amino acids, especially alanine. Unlike in renal failure, the ratio of urea-N to total NPN remains approximately normal in most patients in shock. The increase in urea at this early stage could be accentuated by 'dehydration' or by redistribution of fluid from the extracellular space to the intracellular fluid. This redistribution of body water, it has been suggested, may be due to osmotic changes caused by breakdown of some of the cell polymers. Examples include protein breakdown to amino acids (which in turn leads to increased gluconeogenesis) and glycogen breakdown to glucose. The breakdown of ATP to ADP and inorganic phosphate and other analogous reactions would also increase the osmotic load within the cell.

The reduced flux of available energy in the cell (ATP) influences fluid and electrolyte metabolism. There are two ways of describing this. Firstly and more simply, the reduced energy supply leads to failure of the sodium pump mechanism. Secondly, as the energy supply fails, the cell membrane potential must fall. Because the membrane potential determines the distribution of ions across the membrane, a fall in potential leads to increased intracellu-

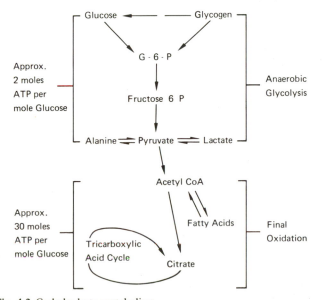

Fig. 4.3 Carbohydrate metabolism.

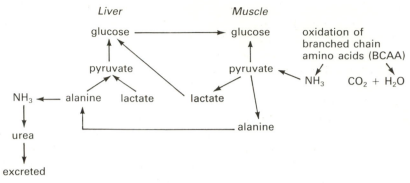

Fig. 4.4 The glucose-alanine cycle.

lar sodium and an increase in extracellular potassium. This, with fluid deprivation or hypovolaemia can explain the hyperkalaemia often observed in shock. It may also be one explanation for the hyponatraemia frequently encountered after shock.

The observation of ketonuria in war wounded in 1918 is supported by recent studies. The explanation is that fat is mobilized immediately after injury leading to increased plasma free fatty acid and glycerol levels. Consonant with these observations, there is an increase in the proportion of the energy production of the body from ketones from the normal 7% to about 15%. There is also a slight increase in the urinary excretion of ketones, which is observed very early after injury so that the metabolic effect is prompt and, in this respect, different from the ketosis of starvation which develops only slowly. However, the amount of ketones found in the urine after injury is generally much less than that found in diabetic ketoacidosis or after 3 or 4 days of starvation.

THE FLOW PHASE

The main metabolic changes which take place immediately after recovering from shock and which follow the ebb phase have been summarised in the introduction to this chapter and in Figure 4.1.

In addition to the increased urinary excretion and net losses (i.e. food or intake minus urine output) of nitrogen, potassium phosphate and sulphate, losses of creatine, magnesium and zinc have also been recorded. The increase in the net losses of these substances together with the commonly observed loss in body weight after injury, and the increase in resting metabolic expenditure (RME) have been taken as indicating an overall increase in protein catabolism. However, in a small number of cases in which carcase protein synthesis has been measured directly after elective surgery using isotopes, protein synthesis has been found to be decreased for the first 24–48 h.

From the early observations of nitrogen excretion and oxygen consumption in injured patients and experimental animals after injury, it was suggested that the increase in oxygen consumption was largely due to the increased breakdown of protein and subsequent oxidation of amino acids. Later studies on energy metabolism after injury using indirect calorimetry and isotopes have confirmed that the loss of lean tissue is the largest component of the body weight loss. Protein provides 12–22% of the resting metabolic expenditure after injury and fat oxidation provides the greater part of the remainder. In contrast, as shown in Table 4.2, if the catabolism of body protein contributes 20% of the energy requirement after injury, the consequent weight loss will be composed of 2/3 lean tissue and 1/3 depot fat.

Table 4.2 Source of body weight loss after injury

Energy source[a](%)	Corresponding mass[b]	Loss of tissue[c]	Tissue contribution to weight loss
Protein 20	20/4	$20/4 \times \dfrac{100}{25} = 20$	20/31 approx 2/3
Fat 80	80/9	$80/9 \times \dfrac{100}{80} = 11$	11/31 approx 1/3

[a] After injury, in the fasting patient, 20% of the energy is derived from protein and the remainder from fat.
[b] The energy content of protein is 4 cal/g and of fat, 9 cal/g.
[c] Assume depot fat is 80% anhydrous fat, and lean tissue contains 25% protein.

Recent studies of the excretion in the urine of the amino acid 3-methylhistidine have provided some additional evidence about muscle protein breakdown after injury. 3-methylhistidine is produced by methylation of histidine after it has been incorporated into the protein of the myofibrils and it is not re-incorporated into protein following protein degradation. Its excretion in the urine can therefore give a guide to the extent of protein breakdown. A recent study of 3-methylhistidine excretion in patients showed no change during a short period of starvation and a reduction in patients with myxoedema. There was an increase by a factor close to 2 in volunteers given prednisolone and also after injury. Thyrotoxicosis was also associated with an increase as was carcinomatosis. Obviously, meat eaters ingest 3-methylhistidine with their normal intake of meat and it is usual to give subjects a meat-free intake for at least 3 days before beginning to assess muscle protein breakdown by this approach.

It is not yet possible to present a clear picture of the changes in protein metabolism after injury. Summarizing the recent evidence, it would appear that immediately after a moderate injury, food intake is decreased and for a short time there is a decrease in carcase protein synthesis, while the catabolic rate may remain unchanged, resulting in net negative nitrogen balance. Later in the flow phase, the evidence suggests increased protein catabolism greater than synthesis to account for the negative N balance lasting for several days. Although carbohydrate oxidation is reduced in the shock phase, there is evidence from studies on patients, that glucose turnover is increased and its oxidation is doubled in the flow phase.

The magnitude of the response to injury corresponds roughly to the extent of the injury, although the nature of the injury also influences the response. Even minor surgical operations (e.g. herniorrhaphy) usually lead to a transient negative nitrogen balance and slight weight loss. Despite this, the alteration in RME is not usually detectable. In more serious injuries the loss of body nitrogen corresponds approximately to the increase in resting metabolic expenditure as illustrated in Figure 4.5. Fractures of the long bone or orthopaedic surgery lead to increases of 10–30% in RME and to a net loss of nitrogen in the first 4 days of approximately 8 g nitrogen per day in the urine. Sepsis, including peritonitis, may result in increases in RME of 30–50% and major burns, depending largely on the extent of the body surface affected, may increase the RME by 100%. Severe burns also lead to the greatest losses in body weight.

Weight loss is a common occurrence even after minor trauma. After moderate injury such as the operation of hip arthroplasty the loss of body bulk can be visibly evident.

Immediately after injury, weight may be gained and the increase reaches a maximum in 1–3 days depending on the severity of the injury and the extent to which attempts to replace the circulatory fluid volume have been successful, for example, in the severely burned. The cause of this initial weight gain is fluid retention which is due to two mechanisms. The first is the intracellular osmotic change which may lead to a relative increase in the intracellular fluid in relation to the extracellular fluid (see p. 57). The second possible reason is that the secretion of antidiuretic hormone is apparently increased after injury and this leads to both sodium and water retention.

During the flow phase this 'excess' water is gradually lost and by the end of the first week the patient's weight is usually less than before the injury or operation and gives a closer indication of the true loss of lean body mass and fat consequent on the injury. In the severely burned patient it may take somewhat longer before the weight loss becomes evident. In these patients the catabolic phase may be prolonged for several weeks so that these patients, unless given appropriately high energy and nitrogen intake, may become severely wasted. Severe burns and sepsis thus cause the most severe metabolic upsets which are encountered after injury and an understanding of the altered metabolism can be of considerable importance for the successful management of these cases.

ENDOCRINE CHANGES

It is now possible to link the metabolic changes of the ebb and flow phases of the injury response in a simple way with the known endocrine changes after injury.

The pattern of the main aspects of the endocrine response to injury is summarized in Figure 4.6. Immediately after injury there is a very rapid (within seconds) increase in the secretion of the catecholamines, adrenaline and noradrenaline. The increase is prolonged for several days and in cases of severe burns, for weeks. This is clearly demonstrated by the increase in excretion in the urine of the catecholamines. Because of the rapid disappearance of catecholamines from the blood, increased levels in peripheral blood are not so readily demonstrated after injury or following shock.

The main metabolic effects of the catecholamines are mediated via the 'cell messenger' or intermediate cyclic AMP (cAMP) and include: increased lipolysis with its consequent increase in plasma FFA and glycerol, promotion of gluconeogenesis, and glycogenolysis. These changes are compatible with the observed metabolic changes in shock.

It is interesting to note that the stimulation of adrenocortical secretions is also rapid. The elevation of plasma cortisol is transient and of short duration, 24–48 h. Increased levels of excretion of urinary hydroxycorticoids may, however, be found for several days after injury. Subsequent increases in plasma cortisol some days after the initial response to injury have been reported after secondary infection or additional stress such as dressing a large burned area. The gluconeogenic, protein-catabolic

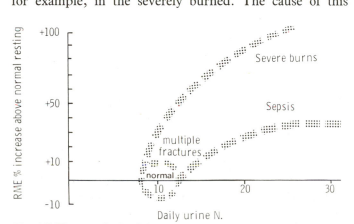

Fig. 4.5 The magnitude of the response to injury. Urine N is expressed as g/day.

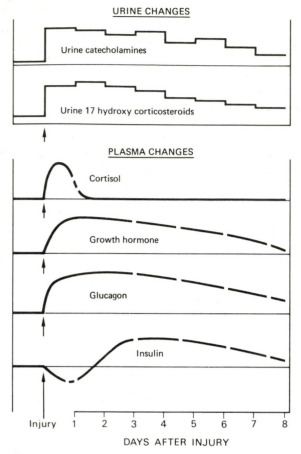

Fig. 4.6 Hormone changes after injury.

influence of cortisol is well known so that the increased levels of cortisol early in the ebb phase would tend to enhance the response to the catecholamines.

The response to cortisol after injury is said to be permissive in that adrenalectomized animals given constant maintenance therapy still show the metabolic response to injury while those without maintenance therapy do not show the usual response. A permissive effect related to cAMP is the stimulation of gluconeogenesis by glucagon which requires the presence of glucocorticoids.

Adrenalectomy without replacement therapy leads to a massive increase in mortality rate in experimental animals subjected to suitable injury. Adrenal medullectomy alone however, leads to a similar outcome.

The full role of growth hormone in the response to injury is difficult to comprehend. There is an initial very rapid rise and the elevation of blood levels may be prolonged for several days. One well-recognised effect of growth hormone is to mobilize fat. This leads to the commonly observed increase in FFA. High levels of growth hormone after injury might be expected therefore to accentuate this influence of the catecholamines. It is noteworthy that starvation is accompanied by increased growth hormone and increases in FFA; also that the

anabolic effects of growth hormone may require the presence of insulin.

The response of glucagon to injury is as rapid as the increase in catecholamines and high plasma levels have been observed for several days after injury. Among the main metabolic effects of glucagon are the stimulation of glycogenolysis, gluconeogenesis and lipolysis.

The changes and main metabolic effects of these hormones (i.e. catecholamines, cortisol, growth hormone and glucagon) are consistent with the observed metabolic changes in the ebb phase (i.e. hyperglycaemia and increased FFAs following the stimulation of gluconeogenesis, glycogenolysis and lipolysis). Lacticacidaemia and increased production and utilisation of ketones would follow.

The metabolic action of insulin is virtually the opposite of those hormones summarized above. Hypoglycaemia follows the increased uptake of glucose into cells and the stimulation of glycogen synthesis by insulin. Insulin also has a profound anabolic effect on protein metabolism. Cell amino acid uptake and protein synthesis are stimulated, and mucle protein breakdown inhibited. It is of considerable interest therefore that there are several reports of subnormal plasma insulin levels in the ebb phase after injury. Thus the humoral changes in the ebb phase tend to act together to result in the observed hyperglycaemia, increase in FFA, gluconeogenesis, glycogenolysis, etc. and increased net protein breakdown.

The interaction of these hormones and the changes in metabolism which ensue are much more complex than the above very simplified summary. There are several examples which illustrate the complexity of the metabolic response in injury. Glucagon is known to stimulate catecholamine secretion very rapidly. There could be a 'positive feed back' or potentiation effect in shock. In contrast, free fatty acids are potent inhibitors of glucagon secretion. Also, acidosis inhibits the metabolic effects of catecholamines such as lipolysis but stimulates catecholamine secretion. Finally, catecholamines inhibit insulin secretion but glucagon stimulates it. There is obviously enough scope in these apparently contradictory mechanisms to explain the differing observations in shock produced by different stimuli.

It is rather more difficult to relate satisfactorily the observed metabolic and endocrine changes in the flow phase. The levels of catecholamines, growth hormone and glucagon remain high for several days even following trauma or injury which could not be classified as severe. The increase in insulin observed early in the flow phase might effectively block lipolysis sufficiently to reduce the inhibitory effect of FFAs and other metabolites on the citric acid cycle and so promote aerobic metabolism. Also it is possible that the increase in insulin levels leads to the observed increase in glucose turnover which would also be consistent with an increase in oxygen uptake. The balance of decreasing catabolism and increasing anabolism must be presumed to be related to the gradual decline in levels of the predominantly catabolic hormones, the catecholamines, glucagon and cortisol.

The early and subsequently well established observations of increased oxygen consumption and energy production in the flow phase of the injury response naturally prompted investigations of a possible role of thyroid hormone. Some changes have been described in thyroid binding globulin (TBG), the level of which falls after injury in the same way as some other acute phase reactants (see below) and it has been suggested that this might lead to increases in the active circulatory thyroid hormones T3 and T4. There is evidence for the appearance of the inactive product 'reverse T3'. The mechanism and role of this substance in injury is unclear. There is therefore no consistent evidence which links alterations in thyroid function with the changes in energy expenditure in either the ebb or flow phases of the injury response. An early response in man in adapting to a cold environment is to increase both catecholamine and cortisol secretion, and it is possible that the considerable increases in the secretion of these hormones in patients who have suffered severe burns occurs due to the increased energy demand by the evaporation of water from the raw surface area.

A considerable reduction in 17-ketosteroid excretion has been described after injury. It is tempting to speculate that this might be related to the injury response being much less in women than men and that the return to normal levels would coincide with the anabolic phase of recovery.

SEPSIS

Although in many aspects the metabolic changes during infection are similar to those after trauma, it has been suggested that some of the metabolic accompaniments of sepsis differ from those following physical injury, surgery or haemorrhage.

Observed metabolic changes in sepsis may depend on whether the patient is stable with a high cardiac output and high oxygen consumption, or whether cardiac output is low and peripheral perfusion inadequate. During the latter, the metabolic changes might resemble those of the ebb phase (Fig. 4.2) whereas during the former, the changes would be anticipated to resemble those of the flow phase.

In patients with severe sepsis who are stable with high cardiac output and increased oxygen consumption, high levels of blood glucose and very high levels of insulin have been described. However, glucose uptake by skeletal muscle is reduced, and there is poor utilization of fat, implying tissue 'resistance' to insulin.

A possible explanation of the observed metabolic changes is different sensitivity of various metabolic processes to insulin. High levels of circulating insulin would be expected to inhibit lipolysis and ketone production, as has been noted in these patients. In contrast, the observed changes in glucose metabolism are those of insulin lack which, since this is not the case, implies tissue resistance to insulin.

Tissue energy requirements are met by proteolysis, with increased metabolism of branch chain amino acids (BCAA) and there is also a considerable increase in blood lactate. In the contrasting septic state with low cardiac output, septic shock, the levels of catecholamines are very high and insulin is low, giving a typical 'ebb phase'.

FACTORS INFLUENCING THE METABOLIC RESPONSE

Metabolism after injury may be influenced in numerous ways, summarized in Table 4.3.

Table 4.3 Factors influencing metabolism after injury

1. Nature and extent of injury	7. Age
2. Infection	8. The activity of patient
3. Stress	9. Environmental temperature
4. Pain	10. Therapy directed at minimising the metabolic response
5. Nutrition	
6. Gender	11. Pre-existing pathology

The most important determining influence is the nature and the extent of the injury. Infection is specifically mentioned because it may lead to serious complications and significant net catabolism, for example in patients who have suffered burning injury. There is evidence that stress with its concomitant increased secretion of catecholamines and cortisol can result in net protein catabolism. Pain may contribute to negative N balance because N balance has been improved by analgesia alone.

Several other influences might be classified as secondary, rather than those numbered 1–4 in Table 4.3, which could be regarded as primary. Protein depletion before injury results in a lesser degree of negative N balance after the injury than in controls. It is recognized that the metabolic and endocrine response in females is less than in males. The relative response to an injury in geriatric patients is likely to be less than in infants because of the considerable differences in metabolic rates in relation to body weight and surface area at these ages in man. The activity of the patient is another factor. Immobilization or bed rest alone induces negative N balance. Energy consumption is related to muscular activity and is obviously less if a patient is unconscious and requires mechanical ventilation than when alert, sitting in a chair, and occasionally exercising. The temperature of the environment can be an important influence on the metabolic response, and indeed survival, of patients who have suffered extensive burns. Those patients who are maintained after a burn in an environment at between 25 and 31°C have a much reduced catabolic response. In experimental animals wound healing is faster at such environmental temperatures.

There is only a small number of therapeutic agents with a direct effect on metabolism after injury. The most widely used is cortisol or prednisolone or similar analogues. These have been successfully used as an adjunct to other therapy in shock but the exact mechanism and indeed the direct metabolic effects are not clearly understood. In contrast there is no satisfactory evidence for beneficial effects of anabolic steroids given shortly after injury.

The administration to patients showing an extensive catabolic response of adequate protein or amino acids and energy (in the main as carbohydrate) may not reduce an extensive negative N balance; on the other hand, the addition of small doses of insulin may induce a prompt return to N balance. Pre-existing pathology such as cancer with cachexia or active rheumatoid arthritis may also influence the response to superimposed injury if the condition is associated with an increased metabolic rate.

IMMOBILIZATION

With the present policy of rapid mobilization and physiotherapy after surgical operations, injury or acute illness, the metabolic effects of immobilization are now seen only in patients who cannot move their limbs or are immobile.

Cuthbertson (1928) and later Deitrick et al (1948) studied the metabolic effects of immobilization in human volunteers. Although there was gradual loss of muscle bulk in immobilized limbs the net loss of nitrogen in the urine was small, about 1 g/day. The most significant observation was the loss of calcium, the urinary excretion of which approximately doubled. In general, immobilization leads to a gradual loss of calcium, phosphorus and muscle protein but not to the considerable and relatively rapid loss of protein, potassium, etc. which follows trauma. The metabolic changes which accompany immobilization are therefore qualitatively and quantitatively different from those following trauma and are generally of lesser significance.

PLASMA PROTEINS

Electrophoresis remains in wide use as a method of studying plasma proteins. The changes in the electrophoretic pattern of the serum proteins after injury have been reviewed by Owen (1967). In recent years, with the introduction of immunological methods of determining individual proteins, the immunological techniques have been applied increasingly to the study of plasma protein changes

after injury. Some of these changes have been summarized in Table 4.4 and Figure 4.7 which also give an indication of the position in which the specific protein is found on electrophoresis.

Table 4.4 Changes in plasma proteins after injury

Electrophoresis position	Increase	Decrease
Albumin	—	Albumin
α_1 Globulins	α_1 Antitrypsin α_1 Acid glycoprotein	α_1 Lipoprotein
α_2 Globulins	Ceruloplasmin Haptoglobin	
β Globulins	γ_1 region	Transferrin β Lipoprotein
γ Globulins	C-reactive protein Fibrinogen	

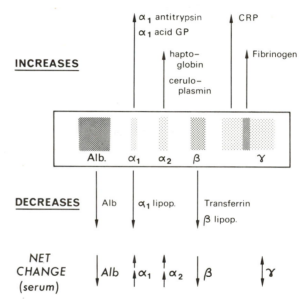

Fig. 4.7 Changes in plasma proteins after injury.

Albumin

Typically the albumin concentration in plasma decreases by 25–30% by the fourth or fifth day after a moderate injury and thereafter slowly returns towards normal. The time taken to return to normal depends on the injury but may be more than 14–20 days. After severe burns, the depression of albumin may last for many weeks.

α_1 Globulins

The α_1 globulin fraction is usually observed to increase after injury. This may be explained by increases in both α_1 antitrypsin and α_1 acid glycoprotein. These changes tend to reach a maximum about the third day after injury. After minor injury, however, the α_1 acid glycoprotein level may not increase above the normal range. The quantitatively less significant α_1 lipoprotein component decreases after injury.

α_2 Globulins

Both ceruloplasmin and haptoglobin, important components of this electrophoretic fraction, increase after injury by 50–100% and attain a maximum about the third day. These increases account for the commonly observed increase in the α_2 globulin fraction on electrophoresis of plasma or serum after injury.

β Globulins

This electrophoretic fraction has been reported as unchanged or decreased after injury. Two important components, transferrin and β lipoprotein, show a decline in concentration after injury of 25–50% to a minimum in from 3–9 days.

γ Globulins

After injury, the immunoglobulins do not alter significantly in concentration unless there is infection. A specific protein, C-reactive protein (CRP) which is scarcely detectable by simple immunological methods in serum from normal individuals appears very rapidly after injury and reaches a maximum usually within 48 hours then declines. The presence of significant amounts of this protein in serum therefore indicates a response to injury — trauma, infection, or some other source of tissue damage.

Fibrinogen is widely reported as increasing in concentration after injury. The increase occurs rapidly, approximately in proportion to the magnitude of the injury and levels of 100% or more above the upper limit of normal have been observed. The elevation may persist for several days or, in the case of severe burns, for weeks.

Because fibrinogen usually migrates to the γ region on electrophoresis, and thus would obscure any changes in the immunoglobulins, it is common practice to use serum to study electrophoretic changes rather than plasma. The proteins discussed above could be included in the group of 'acute phase reactants' because of the changes which take place in their concentration in plasma after injury.

The metabolism of albumin, immunoglobulin G (IgG) and fibrinogen after injury, has been studied using iodine (^{125}I or ^{131}I) labelled proteins. The results of such studies are usually expressed as fractional catabolic rate (FCR) or absolute catabolic rate (ACR). The FCR is the fraction of the intravascular pool which is broken down or catabolized per day and the ACR is the actual amount of protein (g) catabolized per day. Although it is possible to measure the synthesis of some plasma proteins directly using ^{14}C, the technique is complex and in man after injury, synthesis rates of proteins have been derived by calculation from the observed catabolic rates and changes in plasma pools. This is not entirely satisfactory because subjects after injury cannot be regarded as being in a 'steady state' and this complicates the interpretation of results. After severe burning injury, the FCR and ACR of albumin increase and it is concluded that the synthetic rate also increases. However, direct determination of albumin synthesis after the less severe injury of long bone fracture indicates that synthesis is decreased for the first few days following the injury.

There is a change in the distribution of albumin in the body after injury. This is usually expressed as the extravascular to intravascular ratio which is markedly increased especially after burns. After severe burns, gamma globulin catabolism has been shown to be increased for many days, and the calculated synthesis rate is increased by a factor of 2. Similarly, fibrinogen catabolism is increased after injury by from two to three times the upper limit of normal. In studies in patients after severe burning injury, the increases in albumin and IgG catabolism were found to be in proportion to the increase in resting metabolic energy expenditure.

The factors which determine the concentration of a plasma protein are: (a) changes in the amount and distribution of body fluids; (b) loss from the plasma to the extravascular spaces (e.g. by increased vascular permeability); (c) impaired lymphatic return; (d) direct loss from the intravascular space (e.g. haemorrhage, nephrosis, protein-losing enteropathy; (e) synthesis; and (f) catabolism. Some values for these factors are of interest. In man, somewhat more than 100% of the intravascular albumin exchanges with the extravascular spaces per day while only 10% of the intravascular albumin is broken down and replaced by synthesis each day. Changes in vascular permeability and lymphatic return are therefore likely to lead to greater and more rapid changes in plasma albumin concentration in man than changes in the rates of synthesis and catabolism. In normal individuals the most rapid changes are produced by altering the attitude of the body and by exercise. There is an increase of albumin concentration of 15%, within 15 minutes of a recumbant individual standing up.

For the less-rapidly synthesized proteins such as albumin and the immunoglobulins, the factors of greatest significance in determining their concentration after an injury are likely to be the amount of haemorrhage or direct losses (as in burns), the amount of non-protein fluid replaced and increased vascular permeability.

It is interesting to consider the proportion of the increase in urinary nitrogen excretion which occurs after injury which may be due to the increased catabolism of some of the plasma proteins. Table 4.5 summarizes approximate data for the three main plasma proteins which have been investigated after injury in man. Taking the upper limit

Table 4.5 Catabolism of plasma proteins after injury

	'Normal' ACR (70 kg man) g/d	Increase after injury (approximate) g/d
Albumin	14	4
Fibrinogen	2	2
IgG	22	
Total Increase	—	8
Increase in N output from plasma proteins (assuming protein contains 16% N)		1.3

of the normal absolute catabolic rate of albumin in man as 14 g per day, it might be expected that after moderate to severe injury the increase in catabolic rate would not exceed 4 g per day. Similarly, taking the 'normal' fibrinogen catabolic rate as approximately 2 g per day, in moderate to severe injury this might be anticipated to increase by 100% giving an additional 2 g per day catabolized. Approximately the same values might apply to immunoglobulin G. Summing these increases in catabolism gives a total increase of approximately 8 g per day catabolized. This is equivalent to an increase of approximately 1.3 g of nitrogen output in the urine per day. Referring to Figure 4.5, it can be seen that these increases might correspond to an increase in urinary nitrogen excretion in moderate to severe injury of approximately 10 g of urinary nitrogen per day. Thus the increase in plasma protein catabolism following injury could account for approximately one-eighth of the increase in urinary nitrogen excretion. This, of course, assumes that all the amino acids released by this increase in the breakdown of the protein are completely catabolised to CO_2, H_2O and ammonia, of which in turn, 80% appears as urea in the urine. There is no evidence that this assumption of complete catabolism of the additional amino acids is justified, so we must conclude that changes in plasma protein metabolism do not make an important contribution to the increased urinary N excretion after injury.

NUTRITION AND THE RESPONSE TO INJURY

It is not uncommon after an injury that a patient's nutritional requirements must be administered intravenously. Parenteral nutrition has been the topic of several books and symposia (see Ballinger et al, 1975; Johnston, 1978, 1983; Karran & Alberti, 1980) in recent years so that only a brief summary is given here.

Foodstuffs are usually classified as proteins, carbohydrates, fats, vitamins and minerals and preparations for parenteral nutrition can be discussed under these headings.

Protein

Because of the hazards of an immunological response or anaphylactic reaction, the only source of protein which can be usefully administered intravenously is a mixture of amino acids. Mixtures containing both the D- and L-forms of the amino acids have been used but the modern tendency is to restrict the administration to mixtures containing only L amino acids. Some of the special mixtures of amino acids have a composition which has been selected to mimic that of egg protein and so have a high biological value. The quantity of amino acid administered must be adjusted to suit each particular case and obviously in those in the flow phase after a severe injury must be much greater than those in whom there is a much smaller catabolic response. However, apart from patients with renal failure it is probably best to aim at a minimum protein intake not less than 1 g protein/kg body weight (i.e. 0.76 g N/kg) per day of 100% biological value protein and to adjust the input of the particular amino acid preparation selected accordingly.

Energy sources

Early in the metabolic response to injury there is a mobilization of free fatty acids and a reduction in plasma lipoproteins. Increased clearance of intravenously administered fat has been observed after injury so that the use of triglyceride intravenously as a source of energy would seem to be, and has proved in practice to be, satisfactory. Stable fat emulsions are expensive in relation to carbohydrate which for many years has been the main source of energy to be provided during intravenous feeding. For long term, especially home, parenteral nutrition, the requirement for essential fatty acids must be met. At least one source of fat emulsion available for intravenous use provides these.

Many carbohydrates have been administered over the years, the main ones being glucose, fructose and sorbitol. The modern trend is to use glucose and to avoid other carbohydrates.

Glucose is not utilized quite so rapidly as fructose and is usually metabolized at rates not exceeding 0.4 g/kg body weight per hour. If given at greater rates than this glucose has the effect of an osmotic load and glycosuria and polyuria result. However, it is a very simple matter to check the urine for the presence of glucose during its administration and alter rates of administration accordingly. Glucose also stimulates endogenous insulin production and its administration in large amounts should not be stopped suddenly or, if this is necessary, care should be taken to check on and prevent undue hypoglycaemia.

Fructose is metabolized by the liver and its utilization is more rapid than that of glucose (approximately 1 g/kg body weight per hour). It is, however, possible that too rapid fructose administration may lead to depletion of liver ATP and also to lactic acidosis.

Sorbitol is converted to fructose as the first stage in its metabolism.

At present the balance of the advantages probably rest

with glucose as the best source of carbohydrate and it may have the positive advantage of stimulating endogenous production of an important anabolic hormone — insulin — which fructose lacks.

There is evidence that in some patients, careful consideration should be given to the energy provided intravenously and that the administration of excess energy should be avoided. It is a simple matter to estimate a patient's basal energy requirement from tables knowing the body weight, age and sex. In the injured, especially those suffering burning injury, estimates of the additional energy requirement must be made if the energy consumption cannot be directly measured. The giving of excess energy leads to fat synthesis and if a large excess is given a respiratory quotient (RQ) greater than unity results. If the patient has respiratory insufficiency or is being artificially ventilated, problems may occur in the elimination of the consequent large excess of CO_2, and there is the hazard of the development of a respiratory acidaemia. Unfortunately, although the aim is to produce fit patients not fat ones, no simple formula exists to achieve this.

Vitamins

In short-term parenteral nutrition there is no clear evidence that administration of vitamins is beneficial. It is possible, however, that additional vitamin C may be beneficial since after injury there is a depletion or fall in leucocyte ascorbic acid levels. If, however, the patient shows signs of inadequate intake of vitamins or there is a dietary history of inadequate vitamin intake, then supplementation with both fat-soluble and water-soluble vitamins should be carried out. This, of course, becomes essential in long-term parenteral nutrition.

Minerals

In shock and early in the flow phase after injury, it is usual only to be concerned with the minerals sodium and potassium. However, phosphate and magnesium depletion are not uncommon and when parenteral nutrition is required for more than a few days, possible deficiency of these essential minerals should be carefully investigated and corrected.

After injury, zinc is lost in relatively large amounts from the urine and, especially in alimentary tract problems, zinc depletion may exist. Zinc is known to be an essential element with a role in both protein synthesis and nucleic acid metabolism. Correction of assessed zinc depletion does no harm and may assist in wound healing.

In long-term parenteral nutrition it is important to administer appropriate levels of all minerals and trace elements. Special attention should be given to iron and calcium, but manganese, copper and cobalt have also been administered.

REFERENCES

Ballinger W F, Collins J A, Drucker W R, Dudrick S J, Zeppo R 1975 Manual of surgical nutrition: American College of Surgeons, W B Saunders and Company, London

Black E A, Denning P A 1973 The study of injured patients — a trauma conference report: National Institute of General Medical Sciences, National Institute of Health Publication No (NIH): 74–603

Cannon W B 1918 A basis for discussion of traumatic shock. Comptes rend. Hebd des Seances et mem de la Societe de Biologie, Paris 81:850

Cuthbertson D P 1929 The influence of prolonged muscular rest on metabolism. Biochemical Journal 23: 1328–1344

Cutherbertson D P 1932 Observations on the disturbance of metabolism produced by injury to the limbs. Quarterly Journal of Medicine 25: (New Series 1), 233–246

Cuthbertson D P 1964 Physical injury and its effects on protein metabolism. In: Munro H N, Allison J B (eds) Mammalian Protein Metabolism Vol II, 19. Academic Press, New York

Cuthbertson D P, Tilstone W J 1969 Metabolism during the post-injury period. Advances in Clinical Chemistry 12:1

Cuthbertson D P, Wilkinson J H 1976 Metabolism and the response to injury. Pitman: Tunbridge Wells

Deitrick J E, Whedon G D, Shorr E 1948 Effects of immobilisation upon various metabolic and physiologic functions in normal men. American Journal of Medicine 4:3

Fleck A, Ledingham I. McA (ed) 1976 Shock: clinical and experimental aspects. Monographs in Anaesthesiology, Excerpta Medica, Amsterdam 4:57

Hinshaw L B, Cox B G 1972 The fundamental mechanisms of shock. Advances in Experimental Medicine and Biology, 23 Plenum Press, London

Hunt A C 1972 Report of a working party of the Royal College of Pathologists, Pathology of injury. Harvey Miller, Medcalf: London

Johnston I D A 1978 Advances in Clinical Nutrition, vol 1 and vol 2 1983 M T P Press Limited, Lancaster

Karran S J, Alberti K G M M 1980 Practical nutrition support, Pitman Medical, London

Kinney J M, Egdall R H, Zuidema G D 1971 Manual of pre-operative and post-operative care, 2nd edn. Saunders, Philadelphia

Kovach A G B, Stoner H B, Spitzer J J 1973 Neurohumoral and metabolic aspects of injury. Advances in Experimental Medicine and Biology 33 Plenum Press, London.

Lee H A 1974 Parenteral nutrition in acute metabolic illness, Academic Press, London

Lusk G 1928 The elements of the science of nutrition, 4th edn. Saunders, London

Moore F D 1959 Metabolic care of the surgical patient. Saunders, Philadelphia

Moore F D, Ball M R 1952 The metabolic response to surgery. Thomas Springfield, Illinois

Owen J A 1967 Effect of injury on plasma proteins. Advances in Clinical Chemistry 9:9

Porter R, Knight J 1970 Energy metabolism in trauma. A Ciba Foundation Symposium, Churchill, London

Selye H 1950 The physiology and pathology of exposure to stress. Acta Inc. Medical Publishers, Montreal, Canada

Sevitt S, Stoner H B 1970 The pathology of trauma. Journal of Clinical Pathology 23: supplement 4

Shoemaker W C, Walker W F 1970 Fluidelectrolyte therapy in acute illness. Year Book Medical Publications, Chicago

Wretlind A 1972 Complete intravenous nutrition. Nutrition and Metabolism 14

Adrenal

The adrenal glands each comprise two distinct endocrine organs, the adrenal cortex and the adrenal medulla, which differ in development, structure and function.

STRUCTURE

The adrenal glands lie on each side of the vertebral column. They lie immediately above the kidneys but are outside the perinephric fascia, and are in no danger of being accidentally removed during nephrectomy.

The adrenal cortex develops from mesoderm, and the medulla from neural ectoderm. Aggregations of cortical cells appear at an early stage of development on each side of the root of the mesentery, and at the 12 mm stage are invaded by the sympathochromaffin tissue which will eventually form the medulla.

The adrenal gland in the human fetus is 10–20 times larger in relation to body weight than in the adult. Its large size is due to a broad zone in the deepest layer of the cortex, containing large and sparsely distributed cells, and known as the 'fetal zone'. This fetal zone shrinks soon after birth, often with haemorrhagic necrosis, and the adrenal does not regain its birth-weight till after puberty (Lanman, 1962).

The mature cortex has three layers, but there is no break in cellular continuity: an outer zona glomerulosa, a middle zona fasciculata, and an inner zona reticularis (Fig. 5.1). The glomerulosa in man is inconspicuous, narrow and in places lacking, but in rats and other rodents is well developed and entire. The fasciculata is much the broadest layer, and the reticularis again narrower. The cells of the glomerulosa are small, with deeply staining nuclei, and with scanty cytoplasm containing abundant mitochondria and ribonucleic acid (RNA), but little lipid. The cells of the fasciculata are large and distended with lipid: the lipid gives the fresh cortex its golden colour, but is lost after fixation in alcohol leaving the cells 'clear' on routine staining. The cells of the reticularis have a scanty eosinophilic cytoplasm, again containing abundant mitochondria

and RNA. It is possible that the fasciculata is renewed from the reticularis, for it is only in the reticularis that mitotic figures can be found.

Symington (1962a) believes that the zona reticularis and zona fasciculata are functionally a single unit, the inner zone producing all steroids except aldosterone, while the fasciculata acts as a storehouse for steroid precursors. It should be noted that both androgens and oestrogens are found in the adrenal glands of both sexes.

The adrenal medulla is composed of large granular cells

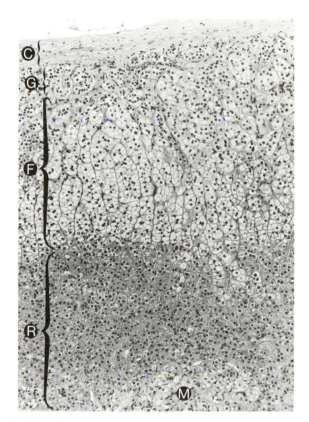

Fig. 5.1 Normal human adrenal cortex. C, capsule; G, glomerulosa; F; fasciculata; R, reticularis; M, medulla (By courtesy of Professor RNM MacSween, Western Infirmary, Glasgow).

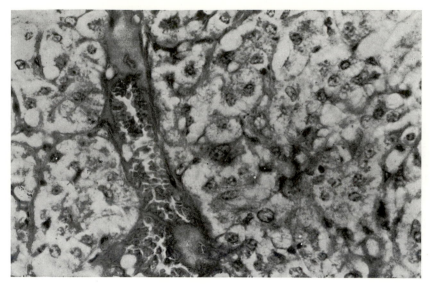

Fig. 5.2 Histology of adrenal medulla showing large granular 'chromaffin' cells disposed round a vascular sinusoid. ×310

termed 'chromaffin' from their affinity for potassium dichromate which stains them deep yellow. The cells are disposed in irregular columns forming a lattice-work around vascular sinusoids (Fig. 5.2). The medulla is known to produce adrenaline and noradrenaline. Noradrenaline is also a neurotransmitter, being secreted locally by sympathetic nerve endings.

Blood supply

The adrenal is very vascular and more blood passes through it than through any other endocrine gland except the thyroid. Its arteries are variable, but its venous drainage is relatively constant.

There are often three arteries, one from the phrenic, one from the aorta and one from the renal, and of these the branch from the phrenic is the least inconstant. The arteries, after penetrating the capsule, form a subcapsular plexus from which small arteries pass to the medulla, and capillaries pass to the cortex. The capillaries surround the cells of the glomerulosa, pass as columns between the cells of the fasciculata and open into the intercommunicating sinuses of the reticularis. Blood then passes into the central vein which runs through the medulla in the long axis of the gland. The wall of the central vein is characterised by thick longitudinal muscle bundles whose function has given rise to much speculation. According to Symington and his colleagues (1962b), the muscle bundles act as stop-cocks on the tributaries draining the cortex. Several small accessory veins connect the central vein with the surface of the gland, and the large principal vein empties on the left side into the renal vein, and on the right into the inferior vena cava.

Nerve supply

The adrenal gland receives many nerve filaments derived from the greater splanchnic nerve, the upper lumbar sympathetic ganglia, the vagus and the phrenic. These filaments form a plexus of medullated and non-medullated nerves in the fibrous capsule before entering the gland. Most of this rich supply is destined for the medulla and the innervation of the cortex is poor. It has been shown that stimulation of the nerve filaments entering the gland leads to an increased output of adrenaline.

Accessory adrenal tissue

The frequency of occurrence of accessory cortical tissue is debatable, but accessory medullary tissue occurs commonly at any of the sites illustrated in Figure 5.3.

ADRENAL CORTEX

Although more than 40 steroid compounds have been extracted from the adrenal cortex, most of them appear to be precursors or derivatives of the small number of active hormones secreted into the blood of the adrenal vein. These active hormones include cortisol and corticosterone, aldosterone, androgens, oestrogens and progesterone.

Therapeutic advances have made the operation of bilateral adrenalectomy safe. It is rarely resorted to in the treatment of advanced mammary cancer, but is an accepted treatment for Cushing's syndrome resulting from bilateral adrenocortical hyperplasia.

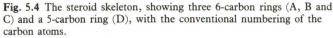

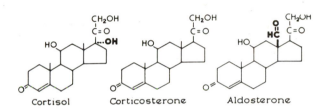

Fig. 5.4 The steroid skeleton, showing three 6-carbon rings (A, B and C) and a 5-carbon ring (D), with the conventional numbering of the carbon atoms.

mainly in the number and positions of various oxygen atoms and hydroxyl radicles attached to the basic skeleton and in the presence or absence of double bonds between ring-carbon atoms (Fig. 5.5). The simplest method of classifying natural steroids is by the number of carbon atoms in the molecule; it should be noted that C_{21} means a molecule with 21 carbon atoms, but C-3 refers to carbon atom number 3. Corticosteroids, a term which includes glucocorticoids (influencing carbohydrate metabolism) and mineralocorticoids (influencing electrolyte and water

Fig. 5.3 The distribution of chromaffin tissue in a 45-day-old child. (After Kohn, 1903).

The surgeon should know the basis of tests for assessing adrenal cortical function, and understand the pre-operative and postoperative management of patients requiring bilateral adrenalectomy.

THE ADRENAL CORTICAL HORMONES

Historical review

A hundred years ago Thomas Addison drew attention to the importance of the adrenal glands when he described the syndrome of adrenal insufficiency. At this time also, Brown-Sequard showed that bilateral adrenalectomy in animals invariably resulted in death. For the next 50 years the adrenals were generally believed to produce a single vital substance.

At the turn of the century a hormone of the adrenal medulla, adrenaline, was isolated. When it was found that adrenalectomized animals did not survive on substitution therapy with adrenaline it became evident that the adrenals must produce at least two hormones.

By 1930 extracts of whole adrenal cortex had been made and found beneficial in the treatment of Addison's disease. This was the first good evidence of the importance of the cortex as opposed to the medulla. During the next 30 years intensive research led to some 40 steroids being isolated from crude extracts of the adrenal cortex. Gradually the chemical structure of these compounds was elucidated and their interrelations clarified. All were found to have in common a basic structure consisting of three 6-carbon rings designated A, B and C attached to a 5-carbon ring designated D (Fig. 5.4). The substances differed

Fig. 5.5 Various corticosteroids.

Cortisol   Corticosterone   Aldosterone

Cortisone   11-deoxycorticosterone (DOC)

Dehydro-epi-androsterone

9-α-fludrocortisone   Prednisone

metabolism), are C_{21} compounds; androgens are C_{19} compounds and oestrogens C_{18} derivatives.

The discovery of cortisone and deoxycorticosterone acetate (DOCA) was a notable therapeutic advance. Cortisone was isolated in 1934, but DOCA, which was synthesized in 1937, was the first to become commercially available. Treatment with DOCA was a great step forward in the management of Addison's disease, for it allowed correction of the electrolyte disturbance and of hypotension. With the advent of cortisone the abnormal carbohydrate metabolism could be corrected also, and Addisonian crises became largely preventable. Treatment with cortisone was also a great advance in the management of sensitivity states, including especially rheumatoid arthritis and acquired haemolytic anaemia.

Within the last few years the refinement of analytical procedures and the development of chromatographic techniques have made possible the identification of the adrenal hormones present in the blood of the adrenal vein itself. It has become evident that the chief corticosteroids secreted into the bloodstream in man are cortisol (about 25 mg per day), corticosterone (about 2.5 mg per day), aldosterone (about 200 μg per day), dehydro-epiandrosterone (DHA) (about 25 mg per day), and small amounts of progesterone and oestrogens.

Apart from natural hormones, several hundred analogues of cortisol have been prepared. Synthetic glucocorticoids such as prednisone or dexamethasone are less suitable for long-term replacement therapy than cortisol itself because of their weak salt-retaining action. Fludrocortisone has the mineralocorticoid effect enhanced out of proportion to the glucocorticoid activity; its mineralocorticoid action is 50 times greater than that of cortisol, while its glucocorticoid effect is very much less. It should be noted that routine corticosteroid maintenance therapy does not reduce resistance to infection and it is important to remember that dosage should be increased where a patient on replacement therapy develops infection, or requires operation.

Metabolism of the corticosteroids

Most of the cortisol entering the bloodstream is bound to protein. Transcortin, an α globulin, has a much greater affinity for cortisol than has albumin; however, because of the greater amounts of albumin present, its total capacity for cortisol is greater. More than 95% of the cortisol present in the circulation is normally bound to protein, this fraction being in equilibrium with the unbound fraction that is able to enter cells and exert its physiological action. With a rising blood level of cortisol, the binding capacity of transcortin is exceeded and the unbound fraction may reach in excess of 25% of the total. The free or unbound hormone can alone be filtered by the glomerulus and so the amount of cortisol normally found in the urine is small. Pregnancy and administration of oestrogens result

in a rising level of circulating transcortin which increases the amount of bound cortisol but, as the level of free cortisol is normal, the clinical features of cortisol excess do not arise. In cirrhosis of the liver there is a decrease in cortisol binding power.

About 60% of aldosterone is bound to albumin in health but this fraction may be reduced when albumin levels fall, as in the nephrotic syndrome.

The main site of cortisol degradation is in the liver. Initially it is broken down to tetrahydrocortisol, cortisone and tetrahydrocortisone. The solubility of these compounds is increased by conjugation with glucuronic acid and, being poorly bound to protein, the glucuronides are readily excreted in the urine. A small proportion of cortisol is converted to 17-oxosteroids by removal of the side chain. Because of the high degree of protein binding, cortisol is removed from the circulation quite slowly, the half-life of injected labelled cortisol being of the order of 80–110 minutes.

Aldosterone is converted to its tetrahydro derivative and part of this is excreted unchanged and part conjugated and excreted as the glucuronide. About 5% of aldosterone secreted each day is in the form of a 3-oxo-conjugate and only 0.5% is in the free form.

DHA is converted in part to its sulphate and is also metabolized to aetiocholanolone and androsterone.

Excretion of steroids and their metabolites is by way of the kidney and the amount excreted depends on the protein binding and tubular reabsorption. Less than 150 μg of free cortisol are found in the urine each day and about 60 μg of cortisone.

Cortisol

The secretion of cortisol and of androgens by the adrenal cortex is largely controlled by pituitary adrenocorticotrophic hormone (ACTH) whereas the secretion of aldosterone is less dependent on pituitary control. ACTH regulates cortisol secretion by way of the circadian rhythm, the negative feedback mechanism and stress mechanisms.

In interpreting the results of cortisol measurements it is important to note that the older methods, particularly those using fluorimetry, are not specific. The results should then be more correctly recorded as plasma 'cortisol' or fluorigenic corticosteroids. Concentrations of cortisol in the plasma are not constant throughout the day. The highest concentrations are found just before awakening and thereafter, under restful conditions, fall gradually throughout the day to reach their lowest levels at about bedtime and begin to rise again a few hours before waking. This circadian rhythm is maintained by secretion of ACTH, is controlled by an intrinsic 'biological clock' mechanism within the mid-brain, and is presumably mediated by variations in the secretion of corticotrophin-releasing factor (CRF) from the median eminence of the

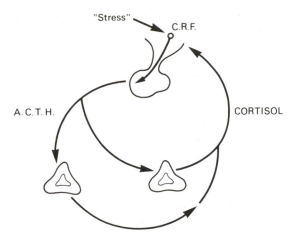

Fig. 5.6 The normal relationships between plasma cortisol, hypothalamic corticotrophin releasing factor (CRF) and ACTH release.

hypothalamus. CRF is carried to the anterior lobe of the pituitary by the portal venous system of the pituitary stalk where it acts on the basophil cells causing them to synthesize and release ACTH (Fig. 5.6).

Under basal conditions there is a negative feedback mechanism whereby CRF, ACTH and therefore cortisol secretion are inhibited when plasma cortisol levels are too high, and increased when the levels of cortisol are abnormally low. It should be noted that an excess of cortisol, by suppressing the output of ACTH, indirectly suppresses the output of adrenal androgens. This has important implications when we come to consider the mechanism of the adrenogenital syndrome. So far as is known, cortisol is the only naturally occurring suppressor of ACTH secretion in man.

The third controlling mechanism is that which operates during physical or psychological stress. Under these circumstances CRF, ACTH and cortisol secretion are increased with a promptness which overrules both the circadian rhythm and the negative feedback mechanism. In adrenal, pituitary or hypothalamic disease leading to adrenocortical insufficiency, the stress response fails and the patient is liable to collapse in circulatory failure.

ACTIONS OF CORTISOL

The main action of cortisol is on carbohydrate metabolism. It stimulates the formation of glucose from non-carbohydrate precursors and the laying down of glycogen in the liver. The precursors from which glucose is formed are chiefly amino acids, which are normally in plentiful supply, and to a lesser extent, fatty acids. This diversion of amino acids retards the synthesis of new protein throughout the body. Eventually, body protein and body fat may require to be broken down to supply the precursors needed for making glucose. Over-production of cortisol results in centripetal distribution of fat, hyperlipaemia and hypercholesterolaemia.

In excess, cortisol suppresses the normal inflammatory response to trauma or infection; wound healing is retarded and infective processes tend to spread. It has been shown that there is a decrease in all components of the inflammatory response with a reduced passage of fluid and cells out of capillaries and a reduction in the formation of fibrous tissue.

In large doses cortisol results in lysis of lymphocytes and plasma cells with the release of antibody; this is subsequently followed by a lowering of antibody levels.

Water diuresis is enhanced, the shift of water into cells prevented, and extracellular fluid volume maintained by the action of cortisol. In the absence of cortisol, diuresis does not occur and this may be due to its ability to antagonize the effect of vasopressin on the renal tubule and to increased destruction of vasopressin by the liver.

Cortisol and its analogues have an effect on haemopoiesis and haemostasis. Neutrophil polymorphs are increased, lymphocytes decreased and eosinophils greatly decreased or even absent. The polymorph leucocytosis is attributed to stimulation of the bone marrow, the lymphopenia to destruction of lymphocytes themselves and of lymphoid tissue, and the eosinopenia to increased destruction of the eosinophils and reduced formation in the bone marrow. In addition there is a tendency to increased clotting.

The skeletal system is also influenced by cortisol which impairs both the secretion of growth hormone from the pituitary and also its action on the tissues. Formation of cartilage is impaired and osteoporosis results from diminished absorption of calcium from the gut where cortisol antagonizes the action of vitamin D.

The gastrointestinal tract is not immune from the effects of an excess of cortisol and peptic ulceration, frequently heralded by major bleeding, may occur in patients on heavy steroid dosage. This has been attributed to increased gastric acid secretion combined with a reduction in the production of gastric mucus.

Finally, cortisol sensitizes the arterioles to the action of noradrenaline, thereby maintaining blood pressure.

As has been noted earlier, the administration of cortisol or its analogues suppresses the secretion of ACTH, and this in time may lead to atrophy of the adrenal glands. This atrophy makes it dangerous to stop the administration of cortisol abruptly and the alternatives are to reduce the dose gradually, or to give ACTH during the period of withdrawal.

CUSHING'S SYNDROME (excessive production of cortisol)

The term 'Cushing's syndrome' describes the clinical disorder that results from raised levels of cortisol in the circulation. A few patients may also present features of androgen excess, especially if the disorder is due to an

1. Bilateral Adrenocortical Hyperplasia

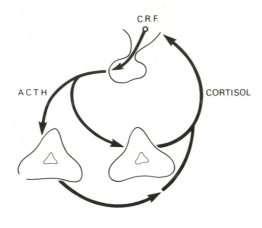

2. Ectopic A.C.T.H. Syndrome
(Extra pituitary "A C T H" producing tumour)

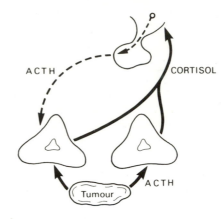

3. Adrenocortical Tumour

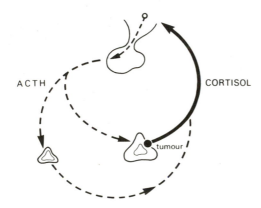

4. Bilateral Adrenocortical Nodular Hyperplasia

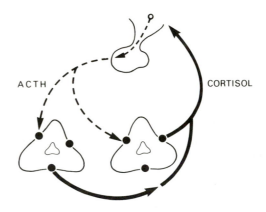

Fig. 5.7 Pathophysiology of Cushing's syndrome.

adrenal adenoma or carcinoma. The clinical picture may also result from prolonged treatment with ACTH or its synthetic analogues, or from heavy steroid dosage: this iatrogenic group is not discussed here.

The syndrome can be divided into two main groups depending on whether or not the condition results from excessive ACTH drive (Fig. 5.7). The first group includes pituitary-dependent bilateral adrenocortical hyperplasia due to increased pituitary ACTH secretion (Cushing's disease), and the ectopic ACTH syndrome where the secretion of ACTH arises in a tumour of non-endocrine origin. In the second group, which is not ACTH-dependent, the excess of corticosteroid arises in an adenoma or carcinoma of the adrenal cortex. The distinguishing feature between the two groups is that plasma ACTH levels are high in the first, whereas in the second group the negative feedback mechanism causes circulating ACTH levels to be very low or even undetectable. If iatrogenic and ectopic cases are excluded, pituitary-

dependent Cushing's disease comprises 80% of all adult cases, whereas adenomas and carcinomas each make up about 10%.

Whether the primary abnormality in Cushing's disease lies in the pituitary or the adrenals has been debated since the time of Harvey Cushing, who believed that the essential lesion was a basophil adenoma of the pituitary. It is now thought that the abnormality probably lies at the hypothalamic level resulting in excessive CRF secretion which in turn promotes increased secretion of ACTH. Instead of a normal circadian rhythm of ACTH and cortisol output, a continuous secretion is found. The continued ACTH drive on the adrenal cortex results in hyperplasia so that the adrenal glands weigh in excess of the normal maximal amount (6 g each). Approximately 20% of patients with Cushing's disease have enlargement of the pituitary fossa when they are first seen due to the presence of an expanding pituitary basophil adenoma, the remainder have tiny microadenomas which are again basophilic but are not large enough to interfere with the visual pathways.

Adenomas or carcinomas of the adrenal cortex may secrete very large amounts of cortisol, frequently with various androgens (especially DHA) and, occasionally, aldosterone. It is particularly to be noted that if one adrenal contains a tumour, the other is atrophic as a consequence of the suppression of ACTH secretion brought about by the outpouring of cortisol from the tumour itself. Consequently, the immediate effects of excising a cortisol-secreting tumour are about the same as the effects of removing both adrenals and so the same precautions must be taken to avoid a fatal Addisonian crisis. Carcinomas outwith the adrenal, especially of the lung, may secrete ACTH-like peptides in large quantity and thereby stimulate the adrenal glands to produce exceedingly high amounts of cortisol. Finally, the commonest cause of Cushing's syndrome in childhood is an adrenocortical carcinoma.

Clinical features

The main actions of cortisol have already been described and a consideration of these readily explains most of the signs and symptoms in Cushing's syndrome.

The anti-anabolic and catabolic effects of cortisol result in protein depletion, with muscular weakness, osteoporosis, thinning of the skin, and (if the syndrome develops in youth) cessation of growth.

The altered distribution of the body fat leads to obesity involving the face, neck, trunk and roots of the limbs. Rounding of the face is characteristic and is often referred to as 'moon face' (Fig. 5.8). The rapid deposition of fat, especially on the flanks and hips, stretches the dermis and gives rise to purple striae analogous to the striae gravidarum.

Hypertension may be the cause of death in patients with Cushing's syndrome. Salt retention, induced by cortisol and related corticosteroids, may be one factor causing the rise in blood pressure but there is some evidence that cortisol also has a direct action on the peripheral vessels in concert with the catecholamines: it has to be conceded that our knowledge of the causation of hypertension in this condition remains incomplete.

Osteoporosis of the spine leading to compression fractures, and spontaneous fractures typically in the ribs and feet, may be due to loss of the protein matrix of bone: healing is slow and often accompanied by an excess of callus formation.

Skin pigmentation of Addisonian type is found in patients where both ACTH and β melanocyte stimulating hormone (β-MSH) levels are high, and indicates that there is likely to be bilateral adrenal hyperplasia, probably due to a pituitary tumour. It occurs more commonly after total

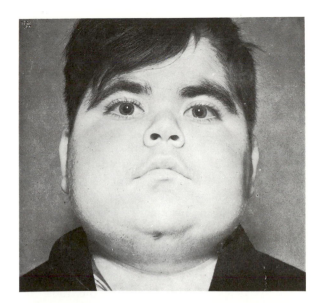

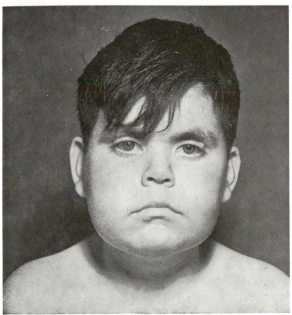

Fig. 5.8 Cushing's syndrome due to adrenal cortical hyperplasia in an 11-year-old boy. Photographs before and 3 months after bilateral adrenalectomy.

bilateral adrenalectomy for Cushing's disease and reflects the presence, probably from the beginning, of a primary pituitary lesion resulting in persistent high plasma ACTH and β-MSH levels.

The syndrome has some additional features which cannot readily be attributed to the actions of cortisol alone — polycythaemia, bruising tendency, hirsutism without other evidence of virilism, acne, psychoses and polyuria. Finally, hyperglycaemia and glycosuria develop in some patients because cortisol interferes with the action of insulin and lowers the renal threshold for glucose; frank diabetes occurs in 10–15% of patients.

Confirmation of diagnosis

The diagnosis of Cushing's syndrome is often obvious but investigations are required to demonstrate cortisol over-production and to determine its cause.

Direct evidence of raised cortisol production is best obtained by measuring the cortisol secretion rate. Where the facilities are not available for this estimation, other estimations can be of value. Thus plasma cortisol levels may reveal a loss of the normal circadian rhythm, and a raised midnight cortisol level is particularly helpful; withdrawal of blood demands care in order to avoid even slight stress as this stimulus alone may raise cortisol secretion in non-Cushing's subjects. Again, estimation of the urinary oxogenic steroids is useful in advanced cases of Cushing's syndrome but when the cortisol levels are only moderately raised, urinary tests may give values within the normal range. It is generally accepted that the most reliable urinary excretion test for routine use involves the measurement of the urinary free cortisol using the comparatively specific protein displacement method described by Beardwell, Burke and Cope (1968): most patients with Cushing's syndrome show a raised 24-hour excretion which correlates well with the cortisol production rate; values greater than 100 μg per 24-hour are usually obtained in Cushing's syndrome but because of the fluctuations in steroid output from day to day, several estimations should be performed.

A disadvantage of the tests so far described is that abnormal results may be due to stressful situations such as anxiety, pain or infection, and under these conditions the increased adrenocortical activity may not reflect a true Cushingoid state. To differentiate this situation from true Cushing's syndrome either of the following investigations is helpful.

The ACTH feedback control mechanism is set at an abnormally high level in Cushing's disease and adrenocorticoid production will not be suppressed by doses of dexamethasone which suppress the adrenal function in normal subjects. When 0.5 mg dexamethasone is given 4 times a day for 2 days adrenocorticoid output will be suppressed in normal subjects but not in patients with any cause of Cushing's syndrome. It is usual to measure plasma or urinary 17-hydroxycorticosteroids (17-OHCS) or oxogenic steroids (17-OGS) or, urinary free cortisol.

An insulin tolerance test is of at least equal reliability since the plasma cortisol levels do not rise in patients with Cushing's syndrome despite a fall in blood sugar to below 40 mg per 100 ml. This is due to the fact that the high cortisol levels have succeeded in suppressing the hypothalamic response to stress. Because of cortisol's antagonism to the actions of insulin, it is often necessary to give as much as 0.3–0.5 units of soluble insulin per kg body weight. A rise of plasma cortisol of at least 8 μg per 100 ml excludes Cushing's syndrome.

In summary, abolition of the circadian rhythm of plasma cortisol, raised urinary corticosteroids, resistance to suppression of blood or urine corticosteroids or dexamethasone, and failure of plasma cortisol to rise during severe hypoglycaemia are useful for establishing the existence of cortisol over-production. It is now necessary to determine which of the various causes of this over-production operates.

There can be no doubt that measurements of plasma ACTH by radioimmunoassay offer the best method of determining the cause of Cushing's syndrome (Fig. 5.9). If ACTH cannot be detected in the plasma, the patient will have an adenoma or carcinoma of the adrenal gland. The presence of high plasma ACTH levels shows that the excess cortisol production is ACTH-dependent and therefore that the patient has either Cushing's disease or an extra-adrenal tumour secreting ACTH.

Although other tests are less reliable, the best of these is the metyrapone test. This drug blocks 11-hydroxylation

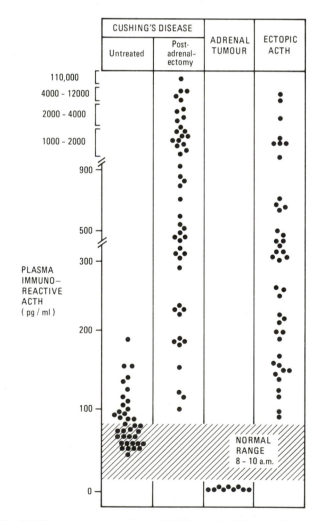

Fig. 5.9 Plasma immunoreactive ACTH levels in 137 cases of Cushing's syndrome. (From Besser & Edwards 1972 Clinics in Endocrinology and Metabolism, Vol. 1, No. 2.)

of corticosteroids so that plasma cortisol falls and the pre-cortisol metabolites accumulate and are excreted in the urine as 17-OHCS or 17-OGS. With the falling cortisol level, ACTH secretion increases in patients with Cushing's disease and there is therefore an exaggerated urinary output; this differentiates a lesion in the pituitary from adrenal tumour or the ectopic ACTH syndrome where pituitary ACTH output is already suppressed and so there will be little or no increase in ACTH or urinary 17-OGS (Hall et al, 1974). It is worthwhile noting that if the serum potassium in an untreated case of Cushing's syndrome is less than 3.0 mmol/l, the underlying lesion is usually a carcinoma with the ectopic ACTH syndrome.

Although attention has been directed so far towards laboratory investigations, helpful information can be obtained from radiological studies in these patients. Thus an X-ray of skull may reveal expansion of the sella tursica by a pituitary tumour; chest X-ray may reveal a carcinoma of the lung which could be the site of ACTH secretion; a urogram may show downward displacement of the kidney or distortion of the calyceal pattern by an adrenal tumour. Renal arteriography can render the adrenals visible when the presence of a tumour may be confirmed by alteration in the vascular pattern; however, this technique has been largely replaced by the increasing sophistication of CAT scanning which has the advantage of being non-invasive. In doubtful cases, selective catheterization of the adrenal veins may outline a tumour or show enlargement of the adrenal glands in bilateral hyperplasia; this technique has the additional advantage in that it is possible to obtain blood samples from each adrenal vein for subsequent corticosteroid assay.

Treatment

The commonest pathology in pituitary-dependent Cushing's syndrome is bilateral adrenal hyperplasia. This can be treated either at the pituitary or at the adrenal level.

Bilateral total adrenalectomy was regarded as the method of choice until a few years ago. This operation requires cortisol cover and thereafter permanent replacement therapy with cortisol and a mineralocorticoid. The earlier procedure of total adrenalectomy on one side together with a subtotal adrenalectomy on the other has been abandoned; in some patients the adrenal remnant failed to function, while in others it underwent hyperplasia and produced a recurrence of symptoms. As mentioned earlier, some 20% of patients having total bilateral adrenalectomy can be expected to develop pigmentation of the skin due to rising β-MSH levels and enlargement of the pituitary fossa (Nelson's syndrome). This situation is likely to respond to pituitary irradiation. However, there is an increasing tendency to use this form of treatment at the time of adrenalectomy to limit the development of the 'postadrenalectomy syndrome', especially if the plasma

ACTH level rises markedly in the immediate postoperative period.

Today, opinion is strengthening in favour of initial treatment of all mild or moderate cases of Cushing's disease by pituitary irradiation. Pituitary irradiation is most effectively provided using a proton beam and cure can be anticipated in about 40% of patients although some of these may require supplementary treatment with an adrenocortical inhibitor such as metyrapone or aminoglutethimide. If a satisfactory reduction in blood cortisol levels is not achieved over a period of up to 2 years, removal of the adrenal glands is advised. Surgical attack on the pituitary is less effective in Cushing's disease than the methods described and its main use is now confined to removal of an expanding pituitary tumour which is encroaching on the visual pathways.

Tumours of the adrenal gland are now usually localized before operation and the surgical treatment involves removal of the affected gland. If localization has not been achieved, the surgical approach is best made through an upper transverse abdominal incision which allows ready exposure and examination of both adrenal glands; one will be the site of the tumour and the other will exhibit atrophy. In view of this atrophy the patient will require cortisol cover during and immediately after the operation, but a course of ACTH will usually revive the remaining gland.

A secreting carcinoma outwith the adrenal glands, commonly a carcinoma of the lung, will be treated on its own merits. However, as the tumour will frequently have metastasized, full remission is not common and adrenal inhibitors have little to offer in these patients.

Aldosterone

Aldosterone is a very potent mineralocorticoid and is also a weak glucocorticoid. Its most striking action is to increase the amount of sodium in the body by increasing absorption of this ion from the distal renal tubule in exchange for potassium and hydrogen ions excreted by the tubular cells. The extent of this exchange depends on the relative availability of the ions concerned. Spironolactone, a synthetic steroid, blocks the action of aldosterone on the tubular reabsorption of sodium by competitive inhibition. It should be noted that the drug is effective only when there is an excess of aldosterone in the circulation, in the clinical conditions of primary or secondary aldosteronism.

Aldosterone also influences the exchange of electrolytes in other parts of the body. Thus it reduces the sodium content and increases the potassium content of sweat, saliva and small bowel secretions.

When aldosterone is given to a normal subject it will initially induce sodium and water retention. However, if the administration is continued for a longer period, this retention ceases through an escape mechanism, the nature of which remains unknown. This explains why most patients with primary aldosteronism do not develop oedema. Although plasma aldosterone levels are usually raised in the nephrotic syndrome and in congestive cardiac failure, the hyperaldosteronism is not the primary cause of the oedema although it may aggravate the situation in these conditions.

Control of aldosterone secretion

The secretion of aldosterone is influenced by a variety of stimuli predominantly by way of the renin-angiotensin system (Fig. 5.10). Sodium restriction, diminution of the blood volume, increased sodium loss by giving diuretics, a potassium load, and injection of angiotensin all increase the rate of aldosterone production. Potassium depletion, the administration of sodium, and any increase in the blood volume result in a decreased secretion rate.

ACTH has a minor influence on aldosterone secretion: a transient increase in aldosterone output follows ACTH infusion, but in most physiological situations levels of aldosterone are dissociated from cortisol levels. On the other hand, changes in the plasma aldosterone levels in normal subjects are almost always associated with corresponding changes in the concentration of renin or angiotensin II levels in the plasma. This provides confirmation of the central role of renin in the control of aldosterone secretion.

The precise mechanism by which the various stimuli to aldosterone secretion effect renin release has not been worked out in detail. One of the main stimuli is a reduction in blood volume; this is known to activate renin release, perhaps partly by stimulating an intrarenal sensing mechanism and partly indirectly through the sympathetic nervous system. Renin itself is produced by the cells of the juxtaglomerular apparatus in the afferent arteriole and on entering the circulation, it acts on angiotensinogen to form angiotensin I. 'Converting enzyme' converts angiotensin I to angiotensin II which, in addition to being the main substance to stimulate the secretion of aldosterone, is also a potent vasopressor agent.

Excessive production of aldosterone

An over-production of aldosterone may be primary or secondary. Primary aldosteronism, which is of particular surgical interest, results from an adrenal lesion and is considered in detail later.

In secondary aldosteronism the adrenal glands are normal but are stimulated excessively as a result of disease of other organs. Thus the nephrotic syndrome, sodium-losing nephritis and hepatic cirrhosis lead to a reduction in blood volume which is a major stimulus to the secretion of aldosterone; these patients frequently have oedema. Again, in renal artery stenosis, and in most cases of malignant hypertension, there is ischaemia of the kidney which leads to an increased production of renin which in turn stimulates aldosterone production; these patients are usually free from oedema. Measurements of plasma renin or angiotensin II allow differentiation between primary and secondary aldosteronism; in primary aldosteronism high levels of aldosterone are associated with low levels of renin or angiotensin II, in secondary aldosteronism the levels of both substances are raised.

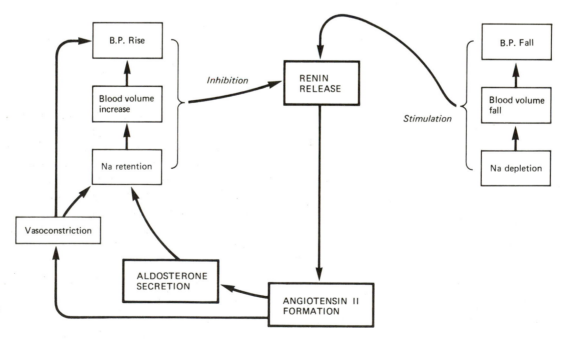

Fig. 5.10 Renin, angiotensin, and aldosterone relationships. (From Hall et al, 1974)

Primary aldosteronism (Conn's syndrome)

Primary aldosteronism was described by Conn in 1955. The incidence of this syndrome is probably less than 1% of hospitalized hypertensive patients (Brown et al, 1972). The lesion in the adrenal gland is usually an adenoma arising in the zona glomerulosa, it almost always is unilateral, and about 1–2 cm in diameter with a characteristic vivid yellow colouration on section. In a minority of patients there is bilateral adrenal hyperplasia often with multiple micro-adenomata. Rarely, more than one adenoma may be present either in the same gland or in both glands. Very rarely, the adenoma may occur in heterotopic adrenocortical tissue — one has been described in the kidney and another in the ovary.

The clinical picture in primary aldosteronism results in the main from an increased urinary loss of potassium and the consequent state of hypokalaemia. The symptoms can be grouped into three categories: renal (polyuria and consequent polydipsia); hypertensive (headaches and dyspnoea); and neuromuscular (paraesthesiae, muscular weakness, tetany and cramps). The hypertension is usually moderate and rarely malignant.

The diagnosis is suspected when a patient with raised blood pressure is found to have a low serum potassium. It should be noted however that hypokalaemia may be intermittent and that it may require several estimations to establish its presence. The significance of the potassium deficiency calls for the exclusion of such other causes as the imprudent use of diuretics, intestinal loss of potassium in chronic diarrhoea, and primary anomalies of renal tubular absorption. It is helpful to remember that these anomalies are accompanied by acidosis whereas primary aldosteronism is associated with alkalosis. Although several indirect investigations can be of assistance, the direct way of confirming that there is an over-production of aldosterone is to measure the plasma and urinary aldosterone levels. This done, the next step is to differentiate between primary and secondary aldosteronism and, as noted above, this can be done reliably by measurement of plasma renin levels: these are low in primary aldosteronism and elevated in secondary aldosteronism. It is recommended that these estimations should be made in all patients with a raised blood pressure associated with hypokalaemia which cannot be explained in other ways. In a review of 50 patients with primary aldosteronism we found that all patients had a raised plasma aldosterone concentration (> 18 ng/100 ml) on at least one occasion, while plasma renin concentration was below the normal mean (8.4 u/l) at least once in all cases and below the normal range (4–20 u/l) at least once in 38 patients. Further support to the diagnosis can be obtained in the majority of patients by demonstrating a satisfactory hypotensive response to spironolactone in adequate dosage (300–400 mg per day).

When the diagnosis of primary aldosteronism has been confirmed it is important to differentiate between tumour and non-tumour patients prior to a decision on management. In our experience, patients in whom hypertension, aldosterone excess and low plasma renin concentration are associated with an adenoma, and in whom the pre-operative administration of spironolactone has resulted in a fall of blood pressure to normal or near-normal levels, the removal of the gland bearing the adenoma has usually produced an excellent result. In those patients in whom an adenoma is not found, adrenal surgery is no longer recommended; prolonged treatment with spironolactone or amiloride is preferred. Clearly, total adrenalectomy will remove the site of aldosterone production and ensure the correction of the syndrome and its biochemical effects, but the patient will thereafter be dependent on replacement therapy. In five patients whom we have treated by removing one adrenal gland and most of its fellow, corticosteroid replacement therapy has not been necessary but we recognize the possibility of recurrence of hyperaldosteronism.

The investigation of choice to determine the presence of an adenoma is by adrenal vein catheterization, by way of the femoral vein. This technique not only permits demonstration of the adenoma itself but sampling of plasma from each adrenal vein allows differential aldosterone measurements to be made thus localizing the site of excessive aldosterone production. Stress has frequently been placed on the technical difficulties of adrenal venography but in expert hands both adrenal veins can be catheterized in over 90% of patients and in our experience the risk of adrenal infarction is low. Another technique of value is that of scintillation scanning of the adrenal glands (Conn et al, 1971). CAT scanning has been used and, being non-invasive, might well become the investigation of first choice. Finally, the computer-assisted technique of quadric analysis, described by Ferriss et all (1970) has proved valuable in making the distinction between tumour and non-tumour cases.

In summary, surgical treatment is advised in most patients with a confirmed adrenal adenoma: where surgery is refused or when the syndrome is the result of bilateral adrenal hyperplasia, spironolactone therapy is an acceptable alternative. However it should be noted that prolonged use of spironolactone may lead to impotence, gynaecomastia, amenorrhoea, menorrhagia and epigastric discomfort; if this occurs it may be preferable to switch to the use of the alternative potassium-sparing diuretic, amiloride (Kremer et al, 1973).

THE ADRENOGENITAL SYNDROME AND VIRILIZING ADRENAL TUMOURS

These diseases are rare. Their clinical presentation is similar, but they differ in mechanism and treatment.

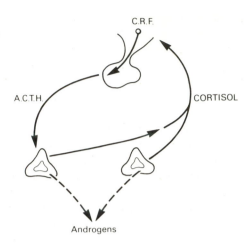

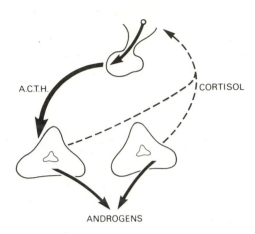

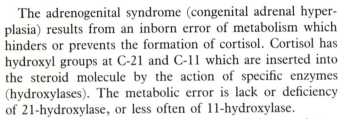

NORMAL   CONGENITAL ADRENAL HYPERPLASIA

Fig. 5.11 Pathophysiology of congenital adrenal hyperplasia.

The adrenogenital syndrome (congenital adrenal hyper-plasia) results from an inborn error of metabolism which hinders or prevents the formation of cortisol. Cortisol has hydroxyl groups at C-21 and C-11 which are inserted into the steroid molecule by the action of specific enzymes (hydroxylases). The metabolic error is lack or deficiency of 21-hydroxylase, or less often of 11-hydroxylase.

With cortisol output reduced, there is little restraint on the secretion of ACTH, leading to an accumulation of cortisol precursors. These are shunted into adrenal andro-genic pathways (which do not require 21- or 11-hydroxy-lation) and the resulting androgen excess leads to varying degrees of virilization in the female or precocious puberty in the male (Fig. 5.11).

Severe grades of the malady are apparent in infancy, and the milder grades in childhood or adolescence.

In infancy, females are pseudohermaphrodite and may be mistaken for males unless 'nuclear sexing' is carried out. Males may appear normal at birth, but within a few weeks develop macrogenitosomia praecox and become 'infant Hercules'.

In childhood, females develop pre-pubertal virilism, and males again become 'infant Hercules'. In both sexes the epiphyses appear early but close prematurely, with the result that the patients are tall for their age as children, but short as adults.

In adults, the syndrome may escape notice in males, but is more obvious in females. The clinical features are virilism, with deepening of the voice, hirsutism, and enlargement of the clitoris, and defeminization, with amenorrhoea and atrophy of the breasts. Androgenic inhi-bition of gonadotrophin release has been postulated to explain this phenomenon. Some cases (perhaps those with the more complete enzyme deficiency) are incapable of retaining sodium normally, and may die from this cause particularly during infancy. Cases with the rarer 11-hydroxylase deficiency are hypertensive.

At all ages the metabolic block to the formation of cortisol alters the pattern of steroids excreted in the urine, and in particular the output of 17-oxosteroids and of preg-nanediol and pregnanetriol is much increased.

The logical treatment is by giving cortisol, which suppresses the secretion of ACTH and the consequential secretion of androgens. The discovery that treatment with cortisol is effective is an important therapeutic advance.

Virilizing adrenal tumours give rise to much the same clinical syndrome. Here, however, the tumour continues to pour out androgens and cortisol when ACTH is suppressed by cortisol replacement. For this reason, cortisol therapy is without benefit in these cases.

Virilizing adrenal tumours are much rarer than the adrenogenital syndrome, especially in infancy. The possi-bility of a tumour comes more into consideration in chil-dren and especially in adults.

The treatment is surgical. During adrenalectomy, corti-sone cover is usually unnecessary. However, some viril-izing tumours by virtue of their cortisol secretion give rise to Cushing's syndrome, and cortisone cover is then essential.

Although the only enzymatic defects considered here have been interference with cortisol production at the C-21 and C-11 points in the steroid molecule, the number of defects described is increasing and deficiencies of almost all of the enzymes of the corticosteroid biosynthetic pathway have been described. The interested reader is referred to the work of Rimoin and Schimke (1971) and to the review by Hamilton (1972). The syndrome of congenital adrenal hyperplasia is one of the commonest inborn errors of metabolism, the gene frequency for the 21-hydroxylase defect being as high as 1 in 50 in some regions. The pattern of inheritance is generally accepted to be as an autosomal recessive.

ADRENOCORTICAL INSUFFICIENCY

Chronic adrenal insufficiency, first described by Thomas Addison in 1855 and thereafter called Addison's disease, and acute adrenal insufficiency are discussed here.

Chronic adrenal insufficiency

Hypoadrenalism is said to be primary when the adrenal glands are damaged or destroyed by disease, and secondary when the lesion is in the pituitary gland.

In Addison's disease the adrenal cortices may be congenitally hypoplastic, or partially destroyed by tuberculosis or other chronic inflammatory conditions, and by auto-immune processes. This last mentioned condition probably includes most of those patients who were formerly regarded as having idiopathic adrenal insufficiency; it is now known that they have antibodies to adrenal cortex which can be detected by immunofluorescence or by complement fixation in the majority of females but in only about 10% of males. A clinical and immunological overlap occurs between idiopathic Addison's disease and auto-immune thyroid, gastric, parathyroid and ovarian failure. The disease process affects almost solely the adrenal cortex, whereas tuberculous disease of the adrenals affects the entire gland.

The decreased production of cortisol, androgenic hormone and aldosterone in hypoadrenalism explains the clinical manifestations which include muscular weakness, low blood pressure, changes in fluid and water balance, pigmentation, insulin sensitivity, gastrointestinal symptoms attributable to loss of sodium, and eventual renal and circulatory failure. The reduced plasma cortisol levels result in an increase in the output of the pituitary hormones, particularly of ACTH but the latter is accompanied by a rise of β-MSH which produces the characteristic pigmentation, very often the first evidence of hypoadrenalism.

The diagnosis is confirmed by obtaining direct evidence of hormonal deficiencies: cortisol secretion rate is reduced but sometimes only marginally and it is advisable to demonstrate that it will not increase under stress, and this can be done by showing an impaired response to the administration of exogenous ACTH. If cortisol production rate measurements are not available, the Synacthen test may be used. In the short version of this test, 250 μg of tetracosactrin (Synacthen) is given by intramuscular injection and blood taken before, and at 30 and 60 minutes thereafter for measurements of plasma cortisol. This agent is a synthetic polypeptide with ACTH-like activity. If the plasma cortisol rises by more than 7 μg per 100 ml to a level of over 20 μg per 100 ml, a diagnosis of primary adrenal insufficiency can be excluded. A lesser rise indicates adrenocortical insufficiency but does not distinguish between Addison's disease and adrenal atrophy secondary

to a pituitary or hypothalamic lesion. The next step is to use the 'long' Synacthen test in which the agent is given in depot form in a dose of 1 mg intramuscularly daily over 3 days prior to repeating the short Synacthen test. In Addison's disease there will still be little or no response whereas, if the glands are atrophic from lack of ACTH stimulation, the plasma cortisol may rise above 20 μg per 100 ml. Aldosterone deficiency is reflected in reduced levels of plasma sodium and chloride associated with a high plasma concentration of potassium and urea.

All patients with chronic adrenal insufficiency require permanent maintenance therapy with a glucocorticoid and a suitable regime is 20 mg cortisol each morning and 10 mg each evening. As some deficiency of aldosterone production can be expected in primary hypoadrenalism it is customary to give fludrocortisone; most patients will be controlled on a dose of 0.1 mg per day.

In secondary hypoadrenalism there is a lack of the pituitary trophic hormones, including ACTH and thyrotropin and so there is a secondary depression of adrenocortical activity and secondary myxoedema. The adrenal atrophy is not always complete and the condition sometimes becomes apparent only when a patient collapses under conditions of stress. Although the secretion of cortisol and androgens is much reduced, the basal secretion of aldosterone (which is not primarily under ACTH control) remains normal, and there is usually little disturbance of electrolyte metabolism. The clinical picture is very much the same as that in Addison's disease except that pigmentation is not present (the blood ACTH and MSH levels are low and not elevated) and there will commonly be signs of deficiency of other pituitary hormones including the gonadotrophins, prolactin and growth hormone. The treatment is the same as for primary hypoadrenalism except that fludrocortisone is not required but thyroxine may be indicated.

General surgical operations performed on patients with adrenocortical insufficiency merit careful pre-operative management. Where there is fluid depletion, due to sodium and water loss from the kidneys and from the intestinal tract, saline and fludrocortisone (0.1–0.2 mg orally) should be given for 2 days before operation. Soluble hydrocortisone can be given in a dose of 50 mg intramuscularly every 6 hours for 2 days before and again on the day of surgery. With adequate restoration of the blood volume, the use of vasoconstrictors is rarely required.

Acute adrenal insufficiency

Acute insufficiency can arise in a variety of conditions: in the crises of untreated chronic insufficiency; in patients with chronic insufficiency under treatment with cortisol, but subjected to severe stress, such as an acute infection or emergency operation; after bilateral adrenalectomy; in Cushing's syndrome, after total adrenalectomy and after removal of an adrenal tumour; and as a complication of some serious infection, most often septicaemia. The last is considered in detail in Chapter 28; the discussion here is restricted to adrenalectomy.

The indications for bilateral adrenalectomy have widened in recent years, thanks to the reliability of modern substitution therapy. The operation is done for advanced cancer, especially of the breast, for Cushing's syndrome when there is bilateral hyperplasia of the adrenal cortices, and occasionally for primary aldosteronism in the absence of the usual solitary adenoma. The motive that prompts adrenalectomy is not always the same. In cancer, the motive is to remove sources of oestrogens; in Cushing's syndrome to prevent excessive secretion of glucocorticoids; and in Conn's syndrome to correct the over-production of aldosterone.

Now that adrenalectomy is performed frequently, the surgeon must understand the pre-operative and postoperative management, and be able to recognize symptoms of impending adrenal crisis. This takes the form of acute peripheral circulatory failure, the preliminary symptoms being apathy, lassitude, malaise and nausea followed later by vomiting. Collapse, hypotension and tachycardia may develop with dramatic suddenness, particularly in patients having total adrenalectomy for Cushing's syndrome. It is recommended that an intravenous saline infusion be in place, that pulse and blood pressure be monitored frequently, and that hydrocortisone be at hand for immediate infusion if required. Except in patients with Cushing's syndrome, the postoperative course is usually smooth provided 100 mg hydrocortisone is given intramuscularly each 6 hours, starting with premedication and continuing by this route, or intravenously, until the patient is able to take oral replacement therapy. Provided that the convalescence is smooth, the patient can usually be stabilized on the maintenance dose of cortisone within about 10 days. However, if convalescence is complicated by a respiratory or wound infection, careful watch must be kept for the signs of impending adrenal crisis, and it may be necessary to resort to parenteral hydrocortisone.

Before leaving hospital the patient must be told that maintenance doses of cortisone will be required permanently, and that in the event of any infection, injury, or further operation the dose will require to be increased temporarily. He should be issued with a 'steroid card' and carefully instructed to carry it at all times; this card gives details of the current corticosteroid replacement therapy.

ADRENAL MEDULLA

The structure of the adrenal medulla has already been described (p. 68) and the occurrence and situation of accessory nodules of chromaffin tissue has been mentioned.

The adrenal medullary hormones are discussed here.

Actions of adrenaline and noradrenaline

The biological activity of catecholamines in the circulation will depend upon the amount fixed in the tissue and also on the sensitivity of the binding sites of tissue receptors. These receptors have not been isolated and derive from a theoretical concept which is, however, of considerable value in clinical practice. Alpha and beta adrenergic receptors are described: the former cause smooth muscle contraction and the latter smooth muscle relaxation. Noradrenaline acts almost entirely on α receptors and has little action on β receptors except in the heart. Adrenaline is thought to act on both types of receptor and so may cause smooth muscle contraction in certain sites, and relaxation in others. The main actions of adrenaline and noradrenaline are given in Table 5.1. Receptor blocking drugs are available and these will be discussed in greater detail in relation to the diagnosis and treatment of phaeochromocytoma. Meantime it is sufficient to note that propranolol and practolol act mainly as blockers of the β receptors; phentolamine and phenoxybenzamine are α blockers.

Phaeochromocytoma

Three types of tumour, all rare, are found in the adrenal medulla, and of these only phaeochromocytoma regularly secretes adrenaline and noradrenaline. The highly malig-

Table 5.1 Actions of adrenaline and noradrenaline. (Modified from Goldberg et al, 1950, in Archives of Internal Medicine)

Action	Adrenaline	Nor-adrenaline
Cardiac:		
Heart rate	+	−*
Stroke volume	+ +	+ +
Cardiac output	+ + +	0, −
Arrhythmias	+ + + +	+ + + +
Coronary blood flow	+ +	+ + +
Blood pressure:		
Systolic arterial	+ + +	+ + +
Mean arterial	+	+ +
Diastolic arterial	+, 0, −	+ +
Mean pulmonary	+ +	+ +
Peripheral circulation:		
Total peripheral resistance	−	+ +
Cerebral blood flow	+	0, −
Muscle blood flow	+ +	0, −
Cutaneous blood flow	−	+, 0, −
Renal blood flow	−	−
Splanchnic blood flow	+ +	0, +
Metabolic effects		
Oxygen consumption	+ +	0, +
Blood sugar	+ + +	0, +
Blood lactic acid	+ + +	0, +
Eosinopenic response	+	0
CNS:		
Respiration	+	+
Subjective sensations	+	0, +

+ = increase   0 = no change
− = decrease   * = after atropine

nant neuroblastoma and the relatively benign ganglio-neuroma are usually non-secreting.

A phaeochromocytoma is most often a solitary benign tumour arising in an adrenal gland, but a few are multiple, or malignant, or arise in extra-adrenal chromaffin tissue. About 90% of tumours occur in the adrenal glands with the right gland the more commonly affected. The incidence of multiple tumours has been variously reported as being between 10–20%; in children the tumours are bilateral in about 25%, and multiple in about 40% of patients. As noted earlier, tumours may occur in chromaffin tissue anywhere along the sympathetic chain, the aorta and inferior vena cava from the diaphragm to the urinary bladder; only tumours localized in the bladder are likely to produce symptoms which enable the site to be predicted from the clinical features, in that patients may have an attack precipitated by micturition. Occasionally vigorous palpation of the loins may, by a sudden release of catecholamines, suggest that the tumour is on the side examined. Finally, the incidence of malignancy has been reported to be of the order of 10%.

The tumour may be as little as 1 cm or as much as 10 cm in diameter. Usually well encapsulated, the tumour is vascular and, on sectioning, shows areas of haemorrhage and necrosis in a greyish brown surface. Histologically the appearances resemble adrenal medullary tissue which, like normal adrenal medulla, stains brown with dichromate.

Assay of the tumour tissue shows it to contain adrenaline and noradrenaline in various proportions. Noradrenaline often preponderates, instead of constituting only 15% of the total as in the normal adrenal.

Clinical features in phaeochromocytoma

The clinical findings in patients with phaeochromocytoma can be explained by the known actions of noradrenaline and adrenaline. However patients may present in a variety of ways.

Some patients present with *paroxysmal hypertension* with vasomotor features and this is the easiest presentation to recognize. The factor precipitating a hypertensive attack is frequently physical movement and it commonly lasts for about 15 minutes, but attacks lasting for several hours and even days have been reported. They tend to occur with increasing frequency and it seems probable that paroxysmal hypertension may eventually give way to permanent hypertension. During an attack there is a sharp rise in arterial blood pressure, the face and extremities become pale, the skin is cold and sweating and there may be headache, nausea, vomiting and visual disturbance.

Persistent hypertension in the benign or malignant phase is a more common presentation. The arterial pressure is persistently elevated and may show further increments on close monitoring — presumably due to unrecognized paroxysms. In sustained hypertension there is (in addition to the usual symptoms of hypertension) a special tendency to sweating, to changes in skin colour from pallor to flushing, and there may be tremors and paraesthesiae in the limbs.

Hypotension has been described in some patients, usually after spells of raised blood pressure. The mechanism of the fall in blood pressure is not clearly understood; it is not due to adrenaline since hypotensive episodes have been reported in patients with purely noradrenaline secreting tumours.

Occasionally patients present with features suggesting *hyperthydroidism*. However, although the basal metabolic rate is often raised, thyroid function is normal and these patients do not respond to antithyroid drugs.

The diagnosis of *diabetes mellitus* has been made in patients with phaeochromocytoma and treatment instituted before the adrenal tumour was discovered. Hyperglycaemia and glycosuria occur in about 50% of patients with phaeochromocytoma, and these carbohydrate abnormalities usually return to normal after tumour removal. In this regard it should be remembered that adrenaline increases the concentration of glucose in the blood by bringing about the breakdown of liver glycogen, and probably also facilitates the breakdown of muscle glycogen.

It is of particular importance to the surgeon to consider the possibility of phaeochromocytoma when a patient has an unexpected reaction during induction of anaesthesia, following a minor surgical procedure, or after an invasive diagnostic test. The reaction may constitute hypertension, hypotension or arrhythmias.

Phaeochromocytoma has been described in families and in this situation the patient is liable to have multiple tumours. Again, adrenal medullary tumours occur in 10% of patients with the familial condition of von Recklinghausen's neurofibromatosis.

Finally, *thyroid carcinoma* occurs with about 15 times the expected incidence in patients with phaeochromocytoma; the tumour — so-called medullary type — contains the calcitonin secreting parafollicular cells and is sometimes associated with a parathyroid adenoma (Sipple syndrome).

Confirmatory diagnostic tests

When a patient with hypertension presents some or all of the features of phaeochromocytoma, the next step is to demonstrate an overproduction of catecholamines. Fluorometric and radio-enzymatic techniques are available for the direct estimation of catecholamines in the plasma, and more commonly of their metabolites in the urine. The total catecholamine level in the plasma is normally less than 1.0 μg per litre and much higher values are found in most patients with phaeochromocytoma: false positive results in patients with hypertension from other causes are exceedingly rare.

The most commonly used procedure is to estimate the

daily urine output of vanillyl mandelic acid (VMA). Values vary between different laboratories but it can be said that less than 8 mg of VMA are normally excreted daily. Certain precautions must be taken to prevent false positive results: catecholamine excretion is higher during the day, when the patient is standing, and during stress; excessive intake of coffee, tea, chocolate, bananas and ice cream should be avoided because they may result in an excessive level of catecholamines in the urine; drugs including phenothiazines, tetracycline and α-methyldopa interfere with the fluorometric estimation of catecholamines.

In addition to estimating urinary VMA output it is helpful to measure the excretion of metadrenaline and normetadrenaline in the urine as this helps to determine the type of catecholamine predominantly being produced by the tumour. In this last regard it has been suggested that an excess of adrenaline indicates the likelihood of the tumour being in the adrenal medulla, whereas a predominance of noradrenaline raises the possibility of an extra-adrenal phaeochromocytoma.

Less reliance is now placed on blocking tests such as the phentolamine test in which 5 mg of the drug is injected intravenously and the blood pressure measured every half minute for 10 minutes. A positive response is indicated by a fall in blood pressure of 35/25 mmHg below control values. The recognition that both false negative and false positive results can occur has greatly reduced the status of this test in clinical practice.

The final step in diagnosis is to attempt to locate the site of the tumour. It should be noted at this stage, however, that the successful location of a single tumour does not relieve the surgeon of the need to search the entire retroperitoneal space, for in about 10% of patients.there is more than one tumour. A large adrenal tumour may displace and distort the calyceal pattern after urography (Fig. 5.12). These tumours are usually large enough to be located readily either by ultrasonography or CAT scanning; these techniques are now preferred to invasive procedures, particularly as the latter can provoke potentially dangerous paroxysms. Even using these techniques it may not be possible to localize the tumour, and under these circumstances we frequently have been helped by the following procedure. The inferior vena cava is catheterized and serial samples of blood taken for catecholamine estimation during the gradual withdrawal of the venous catheter. Rarely today is it necessary for the surgeon to proceed to operation without some reasonably clear idea of the site of the phaeochromocytoma; even so, the need to perform a full exploratory operation has already been noted and for this it is our custom to use an adequate anterior approach.

Surgical management

Death during operation was formerly common, either from hypertension during the early stages of operation or from

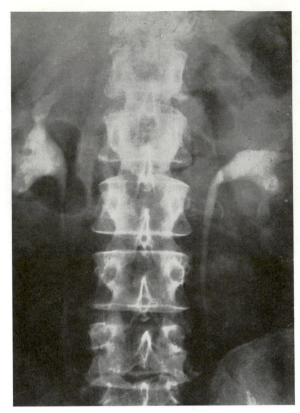

Fig. 5.12 Intravenous pyelogram showing downward displacement of kidney and distortion of upper calyces and renal pelvis by a tumour of the left adrenal.

profound hypotension after removal of the tumour. The hypertension was due to handling of the tumour and the consequent increase in release of catecholamines. The hypotension developing when the adrenal veins were ligated was due to the sudden withdrawal of noradrenaline, the consequent expansion of the vascular bed, and the inability of the blood volume to fill this expanded space. Prior to the introduction of effective blocking agents this hypotension was treated by infusion of plasma or by adding noradrenaline to the intravenous infusion; neither is usually required nowadays. These hazards together with the risk of arrhythmias arising from the effects of increased catecholamines upon a myocardium sensitized by anaesthetic agents are avoided by inhibiting the actions of noradrenaline and adrenaline with α and β blockers respectively.

It is customary to give the α-adrenergic blocker, phenoxybenzamine starting with a dose of 1 mg/kg/day for at least 3 days before operation, although it may be given for longer periods with safety and with effect. This abolishes the vasoconstriction and thereby controls the hypertension. As a result of the α-adrenergic blockade, catecholamines act upon β receptors in an unopposed way and this results in tachycardia. Very fast heart rates may occur during induction of anaesthesia or when the surgeon handles the tumour, but this situation can be controlled by β-adrenergic blockage using propranolol; for rapid effect the drug is given in a dose of 1–5 mg by slow intravenous injection. It is now customary to commence treatment with phenoxybenzamine and shortly thereafter to add propranolol and so obtain adequate double blockade for at least 3 days prior to operation.

The surgeon has the responsibility, not only of locating the phaeochromocytoma at its expected site, but of excluding more than one tumour. It is therefore necessary to examine the opposite adrenal gland and all likely areas of extra-adrenal chromaffin tissue. Each possible site is examined in turn and firm pressure will usually result in a sharp elevation of blood pressure despite α-adrenergic blockade with phenoxybenzamine. Careful monitoring of pulse, blood pressure, electrocardiogram and central venous pressure is mandatory. The development of arrhythmias may require additional administration of propranolol intravenously. Hypotension following removal of the tumour — now uncommon — should be treated by administration of blood or plasma until the central venous pressure and blood pressure are restored to normal.

Finally, about 1 week after operation the catecholamines and their metabolites should again be measured to ensure that all tumour tissue has been removed.

REFERENCES

Beardwell C G, Burke C W, Cope C L 1968 Urinary free cortisol measured by competitive protein binding. Journal of Endocrinology 42: 79–89

Brown J J, Chinn R H, Davies D L, Dusterdieck G, Fraser R, Lever A F, et al 1968 Plasma electrolytes, renin, and aldosterone in the diagnosis of primary hyperaldosteronism. Lancet ii: 55–59

Brown J J, Davies D L, Ferriss J B, Fraser R, Haywood E, Lever A F, Robertson J I S 1972 Comparison of surgery and prolonged spironolactone therapy in patients with hypertension, aldosterone excess, and low plasma renin. British Medical Journal 2: 729–734

Brown J J, Fraser R, Lever A F, Robertson J I S (1972) Aldosterone: Physiological and pathophysiological variations in man. In: Mason A S (ed) Clinics in Endocrinology and Metabolism Vol 1. Saunders, London p 397–449

Conn J W 1955 Primary aldosteronism: a new clinical syndrome. Journal of Laboratory and Clinical Medicine 45: 661–664

Conn J W, Beierwaltes W H, Lieberman L M, Ansari A N, Cohen E L, Bookstein J J, Herwig K R 1971 Primary aldosteronism: pre-operative tumour visualisation by scintillation scanning. Journal of Clinical Endocrinology 33: 713–716

Conn J W, Knopf R F, Nesbit R M 1964 Clinical characteristics of primary aldosteronism from an analysis of 145 cases. American Journal of Surgery 107: 159–172

Court Brown W M, Harnden D G, Jacobs A, Maclean N, Mantle D J 1964 Abnormalities of the sex chromosome complement in man. Medical Research Council, Special Report Series No 305–1–239 HMSO, London

Currie A R, Symington T, Grant J K (eds) 1962 The human adrenal cortex. Livingstone, Edinburgh

Ferriss J B, Brown J J, Fraser R, Kay A W, Neville A M, O'Muircheartaigh J G, Robertson J I S, Symington T, Lever A F 1970 Hypertension with aldosterone excess and low plasma-renin: pre-operative distinction between patients with and without adrenocortical tumour. Lancet ii: 995–1000

Ferriss J B, Brown J J, Fraser R, Haywood E, Davies D L, Kay A W, Lever A F, Robertson J I S, Owen K, Peart W S 1975 Results of adrenal surgery in patients with hypertension, aldosterone excess, and low plasma renin concentration. British Medical Journal 1: 135–138

Hall R, Anderson J, Smart G A, Besser M 1974 Fundamentals of clinical endocrinology 2nd edn. Pitman Medical, London

Hamilton W 1972 Congenital adrenal hyperplasia. In: Mason A S (ed) Clinics in Endocrinology and Metabolism. Disease of the Adrenal Cortex Vol 1, Saunders, London p 503–547

Irvine W J, Stewart A G, Scarth L 1967 A clinical and immunological study of adrenocortical insufficiency (Addison's disease). Clinical Experiments of Immunology 2: 31–69

Kaplan N N 1974 Adrenal causes of hypertension. Archives of Internal Medicine 133: 1001–1006

Kremer D, Beevers D G, Brown J J, Davies D L, Ferriss J B, Fraser R, et al 1973 Spironolactone and amiloride in the treatment of low renin hyperaldosteronism and related syndromes. Clinical Science and Molecular Medicine 45: 213–218

Lanman J T 1962 An interpretation of human foetal adrenal structure and function. In: Currie A R, Symington T, Grant J K (eds) Livingstone, Edinburgh p 547–558

Rimoin D L, Schimke R N 1971 Genetic disorders of the endocrine glands p 225. C V Mosby Co, Saint Louis

Symington T 1962a Morphology and secretory cytology of human adrenal cortex. British Medical Bulletin 18: 117–121

Symington T 1962b The morphology and zoning of the human adrenal cortex. In: Currie A R, Symington T, Grant J K (eds) The human adrenal cortex. Livingstone, Edinburgh p 3–20

Welbourn R B, Montgomery D A D, Kennedy T L 1971 The natural history of treated Cushing's syndrome. British Journal of Surgery 58: 1–16

Breast

INTRODUCTION

The breast is an exocrine gland. Its prime function is to secrete milk to nourish the neonate. Rudimentary in early life, it develops as a secondary sexual character at puberty but only becomes fully functional with pregnancy. Following pregnancy and at the menopause there is involution with atrophy of parenchymal breast tissue and a variable accumulation of fat. Thus, the breast is in a resting state for much of its life.

Development of the breast is brought about by the hormones secreted by the ovaries, adrenals and pituitary. This sensitivity of the breast to hormones may have a bearing on the susceptibility of the organ to disease, both benign and malignant. The breast is also the commonest site of cancer in Western women.

STRUCTURE

The breast is composed of fat, glandular tissue, ducts and fibrous stroma contained within an incomplete fascial envelope. These structures intertwine and there are no definable planes of dissection. The shape of the breast is maintained by fibrous 'ligaments' which are believed to form a supporting framework attached posteriorly and fusing with the overlying fascia.

The breast has a rich arterial blood supply derived from the lateral thoracic artery and perforating branches of the intercostal and internal mammary arteries (Fig. 6.1). Venous drainage is by veins accompanying the artery. The active breast of a young person is more vascular than the involuted breast of a postmenopausal woman; blood supply increases markedly during pregnancy.

A network of lymphatics runs centrifugally throughout the breast to lymph nodes in the axilla and medially to nodes alongside the internal mammary blood vessels. Lymph from any part of the breast may drain to both groups of nodes. This is of relevance to the spread of malignant disease (Fig. 6.2).

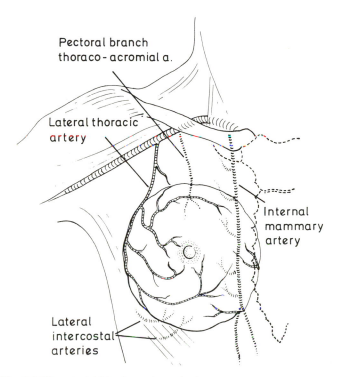

Fig. 6.1 The arterial blood supply to the breast.

The nerve supply to the breast is relatively unimportant except in the area of the nipple where there are profuse sensory nerve endings.

The secreting units of the breast are the breast lobules. These are composed of groups of acini lying within loose, fine connective tissue which contains vascular and lymphatic channels (Fig. 6.3). The lobules are separated by dense, inter-lobular fibrous tissue. The acini drain into ductules which join to form segmental ducts. These run towards the nipple and further join to form 6–10 main ducts which open onto the surface of the nipple. Each terminal duct dilates to form a 'lactiferous sinus', a dilated irregular sac-like reservoir lying beneath the nipple (Fig. 6.4).

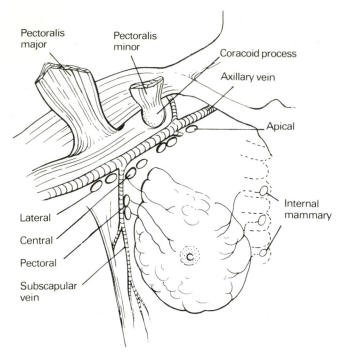

Fig. 6.2 The lymphatic supply to the breast.

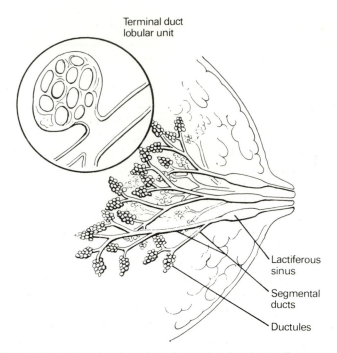

Fig. 6.4 Vertical section through the breast showing the lactiferous sinuses, ducts and terminal ductule-lobular units.

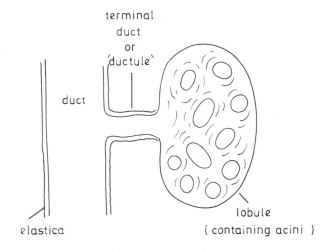

Fig. 6.3 The structure of the terminal ductule-lobular unit of the breast (from Azzopardi, 1979).

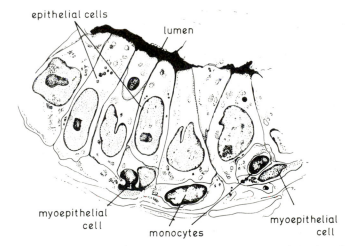

Fig. 6.5 Section through part of a breast ductule to show the main cell types (from Ferguson & Anderson, 1981).

The acini and ducts are lined by two types of cell (Fig. 6.5): (i) epithelial secreting cells which border on the lumen and, in the resting state, may form a double layer; and (ii) the myoepithelial cells which lie on the basement membrane and send out processes which intermingle with the epithelial cells. Myoepithelial cells are sparse in the acini but more plentiful within the ducts. The ducts of the breast, but not the acini, are surrounded by elastica. At the nipple the terminal ducts are lined by stratified squa-

mous epithelium and contain a plug of keratin.

The nipple is composed of connective tissue and smooth muscle. Cold, sexual excitement or physical stimulation cause the nipple to become hard and prominent. The surrounding areola is studded with a number of prominent sweat glands, the glands of Montgomery. The nipple is pink in the nulliparous woman but during pregnancy may become deeply pigmented with melanin, some of which is permanently retained.

DEVELOPMENT AND FUNCTION

The possession of 'mammary glands' is the prime characteristic of mammals. In primitive forms, lactation occurred as a result of 'weeping' of milk from diffusely scattered glands onto the skin or fur. This was licked off by the offspring. With evolution, these glands became conglomerated into well-developed structures provided with nipples for ease of suckling. These occur on a line between axilla and groin (the milk line or crest) and usually are paired, the number and site being determined by the likely number of offspring and convenience for suckling. In some animals, e.g. the cow, conglomeration has extended to the formation of a single large mammary gland provided with multiple nipples or teats.

The human mammary glands lie in the pectoral region. They develop during the sixth week of fetal life from ectodermal thickenings which appear on each mammary ridge. Epithelial downgrowth into the dermis follows to form 'mammary buds'. By the fifth month of intra-uterine life, these primary buds have proliferated to form 15–25 secondary buds which elongate into solid cellular cords from which the ducts are formed. These open onto the nipple which, at birth, is flush with the skin surface.

Apart from the production of a milky secretion in some newborn infants due to stimulation with maternal hormones ('witch's milk'), the breast remains rudimentary until puberty. Then, the onset of ovarian activity stimulates growth. Beginning several years before the onset of full menstruation, discs of stromal connective tissue develop beneath the nipple and areola within which the lactiferous ducts lengthen and branch. The nipple becomes everted. At this time, the primitive lobular components of the breast are formed but these contribute less to the size and shape of the pubertal breast than fat which is deposited between the lobular units.

As a result of this development, the adult breast consists of 5–10 anatomical lobes, each formed from many lobules which, as indicated above, are the functional units for secretion. The adult, non-lactating breast undergoes changes in cellular activity during the menstrual cycle. It produces a small amount of secretion (see below). After the third month of pregnancy, ductal and glandular elements proliferate greatly so that by the end of pregnancy, the breast is composed of a compact mass of lobules each containing multiple acini lined by secretory cells. These produce colostrum during the later months of pregnancy and milk during the post partum (lactational) period.

Following pregnancy, involution occurs rapidly and the breast returns to a resting state. Following the menopause, the lobules of the breast atrophy, secretions diminish and the gland becomes composed mainly of fat and fibrous tissue.

Hormonal factors

Large hormonal fluctuations occur at puberty, during pregnancy and at the menopause and these influence the development of the breast. It was believed that the ovarian hormones oestrogen and progesterone were mainly responsible for breast development, but work in animals whose ovaries, adrenals and pituitary were ablated, indicated that these ovarian hormones could stimulate breast development only in the presence of pituitary hormones. It is now recognized that the hormones of all three endocrine glands, supported by those of the placenta during pregnancy, act synergically to provide the necessary stimulus for full breast development (Fig. 6.6).

In the rat, the minimal requirements for the growth of ducts are oestrogens, corticosteroids and pituitary growth hormone (Fig. 6.7). Alveolar formation requires prolactin; for full lobular alveolar development, such as is seen in late pregnancy, oestrogen, progesterone, prolactin and growth hormone, the 'growth tetrad' are necessary. The placenta contributes to the supply of these hormones including the secretion of chorionic somatotrophin which has both prolactin-like and growth hormone-like effects.

Lactation in the fully developed breast is also hormone-dependent requiring the 'lactational triad' of prolactin, growth hormone and cortisol. Thyroid hormone and insulin may also be concerned. Several factors are involved in the initiation of lactation. The sudden reduction of placental oestrogens and progesterone which follows delivery sensitizes the breast epithelium to prolactin, the secretion of which is stimulated by the 'suckling reflex'.

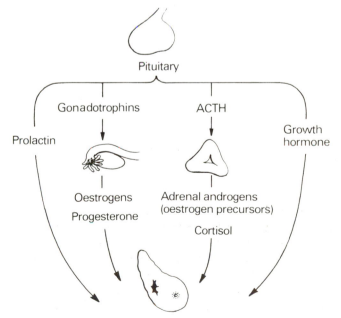

Fig. 6.6 The glandular sources of hormones essential to the development of the breast.

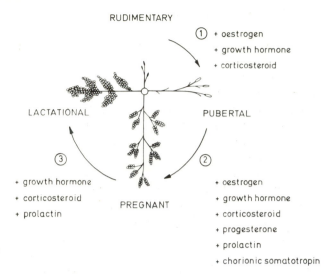

Fig. 6.7 The minimal requirements for the growth and full development of the breast in the rat (from Lyons et al, 1958).

Table 6.1 Comparative concentrations of some major constituents of human milk, plasma and breast secretions.

	Milk	Plasma	Secretions
Na$^+$	low	high	high
K$^+$	high	low	low[a]
casein	high	absent	low/absent
lactalbumin	high	absent	low
immunoglobulin A[b]	11S	7S	11S
GCDFP-15[c]	low	low	high
DHA-sulphate[d]	low	high	very high

[a] Although [K$^+$] are lower than [Na$^+$] in breast secretions the concentration of K$^+$ is still significantly higher than in plasma.
[b] Predominant class of IgA.
[c] GCDFP-15 = gross cystic disease fluid protein (molecular weight of monomer ~15 000).
[d] DHA-sulphate = dehydroepiandrosterone sulphate.

Liberation of the posterior pituitary hormone oxytocin promotes prolactin release and stimulates the myoepithelial cells to eject milk into the main duct system and lactiferous sinus. Provided there is suckling, milk will continue to be secreted.

Reversal of these influences occurs rapidly as a result of weaning.

BREAST SECRETIONS

As indicated above, the non-lactating breast secretes small amounts of fluid. The secretions, produced in the terminal duct lobular unit, do not normally appear at the nipple, but are reabsorbed as they pass along the ducts. Keratin plugs in the outlets of the major ducts are believed to prevent leakage onto the nipple. Little is known about the process of reabsorption of breast secretions; the lymphatic network which surrounds the mammary parenchyma is the likely route.

If the keratin plugs are dissolved by swabbing the nipple with an organic solvent, and the breast is massaged or suction is applied to the nipple, small amounts of secretion appear at the orifice of one or more ducts in approximately one-half of normal women. The likelihood of yielding secretions varies according to several factors including race, parity, menstrual status and genetic type. Thus, secretions are more commonly obtained from Caucasian rather than Oriental women, parous rather than nulliparous, premenopausal rather than postmenopausal and those with wet as opposed to dry cerumen (this representing distinct genetic types). The fluid which is aspirated varies in colour and consistency, but there are common biochemical characteristics which distinguish it from milk and from plasma (Table 6.1). These include excessively high concentrations of androgen conjugates and of the 11S secretory form of IgA. Breast secretions also contain a specific protein which is secreted only into breast cysts, saliva and sweat. The extent to which the concentrations of these components are altered during passage along the duct system is unknown.

Galactorrhoea

Milk secretion is a normal event in pregnancy and, in some circumstances, may persist for long periods following cessation of suckling. Pregnancy apart, the breast of both nulliparous and multiparous women may produce milk. This is termed galactorrhoea; it may be associated with elevated plasma levels of prolactin, 'hyperprolactinaemia', a condition which should be suspected if the patient also is amenorrhoeic.

Hyperprolactinaemia may be due to (i) treatment with psychotrophic or other prolactin-stimulating drugs; (ii) impaired thyroid function with excess secretion of thyrotrophin-stimulating hormone (TRH) which stimulates prolactin release; (iii) prolactin-secreting pituitary adenomas. In non-pregnant women, the latter are small (micro-adenomas) but, during pregnancy, they may rapidly enlarge and cause visual disturbance. For this reason, micro-adenomas should be removed surgically or treated by the suppressing drug, bromoergocryptine, should pregnancy occur.

Galactorrhoea should not be confused with nipple discharge associated with pathological conditions in the breast. Differentiation may require assay of the fluid for the milk proteins, lactalbumin or casein.

THE MALE BREAST

In the male, testicular androgens inhibit the development of the breast which remains rudimentary. Should there be a disturbance of hormonal relationships, however, the breast may enlarge from growth of the primitive duct system. Such 'gynaecomastia' may be unilateral or bilateral. Causes include alteration in the circulating oestrogen-to-androgen ratio; increased prolactin secretion; or the ingestion of drugs which, by binding to the oestrogen receptor, exert a weak oestrogenic effect. Most commonly, gynaecomastia occurs at three periods of life:

1. Late fetal life, when circulating levels of maternal hormones are high, a condition which may persist for a brief period after birth.

2. Puberty, when many boys experience a mild transient enlargement of the breast due to variations in the ratio of oestrogens to androgens.

3. Later life (the male menopause), when testosterone levels in the plasma fall due to testicular atrophy.

Gynaecomastia can occur at other times when it may be due to abnormal hormonal drive. Oestrogen excess occurs in a variety of conditions which include chronic liver disease, refeeding after a period of starvation, tumours of the endocrine glands or hormone-secreting tumours of ectopic (non-endocrine) type. More commonly, however, gynaecomastia is due to the ingestion of such medicines as digitalis, spironolactone, phenothiazines or cimetidine. Marihuana ('pot') is a cause of gynaecomastia in some young men.

Most cases of gynaecomastia require no treatment; however, should enlargement of the male breast persist or become painful or tender, surgical excision is indicated. Exclusion of an endocrine-secreting tumour may necessitate hormone studies.

ABNORMAL DEVELOPMENT OF THE BREAST

Failure of the development of the female breast may result from genetic, endocrine or traumatic causes.

Unilateral non-development may be due to an isolated genetic defect which may be associated with absence of the underlying pectoral muscles (Poland syndrome). Bilateral atrophy is a feature of ovarian agenesis (Turner's syndrome), castration in youth, or hypopituitarism in later life.

Trauma to the breast area in youth, e.g. by a burn, may result in failure of the breast to develop. More common is the surgical removal of an asymmetrically developing breast, this on the belief that it may contain a cyst or tumour. Such iatrogenic 'mastectomies' should not occur.

Breast hypertrophy may be troublesome. It is due to massive accumulation of fat. The cause is unknown. It can be treated by reduction mammoplasty.

BENIGN BREAST DISEASE

A variety of benign diseases of the breast are believed to result from abnormal hormonal stimulation. These are characterized by proliferation of glandular and/or stromal components of the breast and vary from the small solitary fibroadenoma of young women to the ill-defined areas of fibrosis and epithelial tissue which form the so-called dysplastic breast of older women and which may be associated with the formation of cysts.

Diffuse 'dysplastic disease' of the breast may become particularly prominent in the immediate premenstrual period and may cause cyclical breast discomfort or pain. It has been suggested that these conditions may be associated with a deficiency in progesterone during the luteal phase of the menstrual cycle so that the breasts are subject to unopposed oestrogen stimulation: however, to date the evidence for this deficiency has been conflicting. Women who take oral contraceptives are reported to have a lower incidence of benign breast disease. Other workers have suggested that excessive stimulation by gonadotrophins, prolactin or testosterone may be implicated.

On the basis of a suspected hormonal aetiology, the management of benign painful breast disease has included the administration of progesterone (both systemic and by local application), the antigonadotrophin, danazol, and the antiprolactin, bromoergocryptine. Some evidence has been presented for objective benefit from the latter two drugs.

Composition of cyst fluid

The fluid aspirated from breast cysts has been subjected to study. Two main types of cyst have been defined: one which contains fluid with high concentrations of potassium and low concentrations of sodium; the other with lower concentrations of potassium but high concentrations of sodium. It is believed that the former type of fluid is found in cysts lined by active secretory epithelium of apocrine type and this is supported by the finding of higher concentrations of the androgenic steroid conjugate, dehydro-epiandrosterone sulphate (DHA-sulphate), and of secretory immunoglobulin in cysts of high potassium type. There is evidence that women with cystic disease of the breast have an increased risk of breast cancer. The cause of this association is not known.

HORMONES AND BREAST CANCER

Traditionally, the process whereby a malignant cell is formed has been divided into two distinct phases: (i) initiation, (ii) promotion (Fig. 6.8).

Initiation is induction of neoplastic change in a cell, transforming it from one with normal growth characteristics to one with potential for uncontrolled growth and

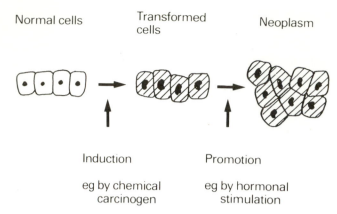

Normal cells   Transformed   Neoplasm
                 cells

Induction   Promotion

eg by chemical   eg by hormonal
carcinogen   stimulation

Fig. 6.8 The key steps in cancer formation.

invasion. Initiation is often caused by a single agent with an immediate biochemical effect on the sequence of the bases in the DNA. Once a malignant or transformed cell has been formed by initiation, its development into a tumour is enhanced by the subsequent action of other stimuli, i.e. the process of 'promotion'. Promoting factors may be chemical, hormonal or immunological.

Recent advances in molecular biology indicate that the separation of carcinogenesis into these two phases is an over-simplification. Neoplastic transformation is likely to involve a minimum of two events in which 'proto-oncogenes' (normal genes, but with a cancer-forming potential) are altered or activated. Strictly speaking, only the altered/activated genes are called 'oncogenes' (genes associated with cancer formation), but both the altered gene and its precursor are often loosely termed 'cellular oncogenes'. Promoters are thought likely to increase the rate of proliferation of cells at risk, either of normal cells or of 'intermediate cells', i.e. cells which have undergone one alteration and are now at risk of a second, critical event. The genes (proto-oncogenes) which may be the target of such alterations are considered to be critically involved in normal cell growth in at least two ways: their protein products may (i) within the nucleus, regulate the transcription of genes influencing proliferation and the finite life of the cell, or (ii) control the perception and transduction of growth stimuli from outside the cell, through the cytoplasm. Such proto-oncogenes may code, for example, for growth factors or their receptors and alteration or over-activation of these genes confers upon the cells an infinite life-span ('immortalization') and an apparent escape from the normal influence of factors controlling growth, including the influence of cells upon each other's growth.

Despite the oversimplification in dividing carcinogenesis into two phases, the approach is useful. Hormonal factors may act in both phases, but in the aetiology of breast cancer, their ability to act as promoters would appear to be the more important.

Evidence for this promoting effect of hormones in breast cancer comes from studies of experimental tumours in laboratory animals. Thus it was observed that (i) spontaneous breast cancer in mice was limited to females; (ii) their susceptibility was dependent on the secretions of the ovaries; (iii) this could be decreased by oophorectomy and enhanced by oestrogens and (iv) grafting of ovaries or the administration of oestrogens to male mice rendered them susceptible to tumour growth. Other studies have implicated progesterone and prolactin as also having a promoting role. Prolactin is particularly important in the dimethylbenz (a) anthracene-induced (DMBA) breast cancer of rats, though probably not in women.

Human breast cancer

There is every reason to suspect that cancer of the human breast is similarly promoted by hormonal influences. Evidence is as follows:

1. Hormones influence the risk of developing breast cancer. The disease occurs predominantly in females and is rare in males. Ovariectomy performed early in life reduces the incidence of the disease; in addition, the disease is rare in women with hypopituitarism. Women taking oestrogenic hormones are reported to have an increased incidence of the disease in later life.

Full-term pregnancies early in life protect against breast cancer. Nulliparous women and those whose first pregnancy occurs late in life have an increased risk. The duration of the menstrual life also is a risk factor, early menarche and late menopause being associated with an increased incidence of the disease.

2. Hormonal factors also affect the prognosis of established disease. Cancer of the breast arising during the later months of pregnancy carries a bad prognosis. Cyclical variations in endocrine activity during the menstrual cycle or the administration of oestrogens can enhance tumour growth. Conversely, spontaneous regression of established disease may occur during the menopause.

3. Hormonal deprivation can cause regression of established disease. Removal of ovarian oestrogen by oophorectomy or ovarian irradiation effects regression of tumour deposits in approximately 30% of young women with advanced breast cancer. In older women, adrenalectomy, hypophysectomy or pharmacological inhibition of adrenal or pituitary function can act similarly. Pharmaceutical agents which inhibit the uptake of oestrogen by the tumour cell (e.g. tamoxifen) are also beneficial.

It is important to appreciate that hormones are only one of several risk factors which influence the occurrence of breast cancer. The greatest is geographical. The incidence of the disease in the western world is very much higher than in the east or in developing countries. Although recent reports suggest that hormonal status may be implicated, this is likely to be a secondary effect to such environmental factors as diet. Female children of women from oriental countries who emigrate to the western world develop the western prevalence of the disease.

Hormone estimations in relation to breast cancer

Despite evidence that the endocrine environment markedly influences the behaviour of cancer of the human breast, numerous studies of circulating plasma and of urinary hormones have failed to reveal any consistent, major abnormality in women with breast cancer. There may be several reasons for this. Recent evidence suggests, for example, that the non-protein-bound ('free') fraction of plasma oestrogen is increased in women at risk. Probably, however, the most important reason is that circulating hormones reflect poorly the hormonal content of the breast and thus the environment of the tumour. The excessively high levels of conjugated androgenic hormones (dehydro-epiandrosterone sulphate) found in breast secretions and in breast cyst fluid compared to the levels in plasma support this statement.

Local synthesis of hormones

It is important to appreciate that the synthesis of hormones can occur peripherally. Fat, muscle and liver possess enzymes which can synthesize active hormones including oestrogens from such precursors as androstenedione, testosterone and dehydroepiandrosterone sulphate. In postmenopausal patients, such peripheral conversion of adrenal androgens represents the main source of oestrogens.

Breast tumours, in common with some tumours at other sites, also possess enzymes which can metabolize and synthesize steroid hormones. For example, breast cancer tissue, through the action of 5α-reductase can reduce testosterone to active androgenic metabolites; or through its possession of aromatase enzymes, convert testosterone to active oestrogen. Thus, provided precursor steroids of adrenal origin are available, breast cancer can produce its own supply of active oestrogen.

Oestrogen receptors

One of the most significant advances in endocrinology is the recognition that the selectivity of oestrogen action was explained by the presence, in target cells, of a specific receptor for that hormone. This is a protein with a high affinity for binding oestrogen, thought initially to be localized in the cytoplasm, but now believed to be nuclear. A two-step mechanism is involved (Fig. 6.9). Firstly, following diffusion into the cell, oestrogen binds to this oestrogen receptor (ER) protein to form a hormone-receptor complex; for the second stage, the hormone-receptor complex binds to nuclear chromatin and modifies

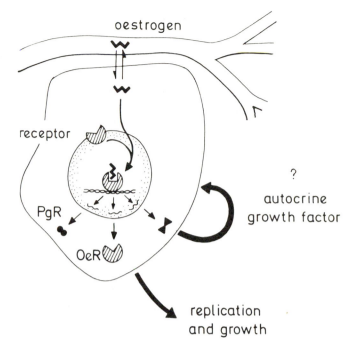

Fig. 6.9 The two step mechanism of oestrogen action: (1) binding of hormone to receptor; (2) stimulation of the genome by the hormone-receptor complex. The stimulation of DNA synthesis, however, may be mediated via production of an autocrine growth factor.

gene expression. Synthesis of RNA, DNA and proteins and the stimulation of cell growth and division result. It may well be that stimulation of DNA synthesis is mediated in an autocrine manner, by a glycopeptide growth factor, synthesized in response to oestrogen (Fig. 6.9). An important part of this action is to replenish the cell cyto-plasm with new ER and possibly also stimulation of the synthesis of a receptor protein for progesterone.

Method of assay

The standard method of assay of ER protein is by satu-ration analysis (Fig. 6.10). Preparations of tissue extract (cytosol) are incubated with varying concentrations of radioactive (tritiated) oestradiol in the presence or absence of unlabelled oestrogen. Separation of bound from unbound oestrogen is carried out by adsorption of the bound steroid on dextran-coated charcoal or other agent and the concentrations of free and bound hormone are determined by scintillation counting. By plotting the ratio of bound to unbound hormone against that which is bound for each concentration of steroid, a 'Scatchard plot' is obtained which allows calculation of the dissociation constant of the reaction (and therefore its specificity) and the concentration of receptor protein. Alternatively, the concentration of oestrogen receptor protein can be deter-mined by incubation with a high concentration of (^{3}H)-oestradiol followed by centrifugation of the incubation mixture through sucrose gradients. The ER sediments in

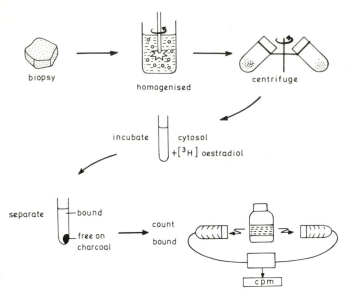

Fig. 6.10 The assay of oestrogen receptor activity by saturation analysis.

one or both of two molecular forms: large (8s) or small (4s). More recently the advent of monoclonal antibodies against the oestrogen receptor has permitted the development of newer methods, enzymimmunoassay (ER-EIA) and immunocytochemistry (ERICA). The former appears more sensitive and reproducible than steroid-binding assays and the latter permits localisation of receptor in tissue sections.

Receptor concentrations are normally expressed as fmol/mg cytosol protein. A better correction may be made for the degree of cellularity, either from microscopic examination or by expression of ER concentrations per milligram DNA.

Relevance of ER assays

ER protein has been demonstrated in both benign and malignant breast tissue. Some 70% of all breast cancers contain ER. The main value of ER assays is for the prediction of endocrine responsiveness. The 30% of tumours without ER activity are, in general, unresponsive to endocrine treatment. Unfortunately, the converse is not true; not all ER-positive tumours show benefit. The chance of remission of disease to endocrine therapy in an ER-positive tumour approximates 50%. Possible explanations for the lack of sensitivity of some tumours despite ER positivity are:

1. ER protein is present but defective so that the ER complex cannot bind to, or stimulate the nuclear genome

2. Heterogeneity within or between tumour deposits results in mixtures of ER-positive and ER-negative cells so that, although ER activity is present, remission is obscured by the number of insensitive cells

3. Factors other than oestrogens may be involved in endocrine responsiveness.

Several approaches have been used in an attempt to improve the accuracy of prediction of response to endocrine therapy. For example, the effectiveness of the ER complex to stimulate genomic activity can be assessed by study of an end point of oestrogen action, e.g. the synthesis of progesterone receptor (PR) protein. It has been stated that those tumours which possess both ER and PR, are more likely to respond to endocrine therapy than those with ER alone.

Compensation for heterogeneity has been attempted by defining ER activity in individual cells using fluorescein or peroxidase-labelled oestrogen-protein conjugates. However, more specific histochemical assays, involving the application of highly specific antibodies to ER protein are now available and being evaluated on tissue sections and fine needle aspirates.

Other parameters of endocrine responsiveness

Various other tissue parameters have been reported to relate to endocrine responsiveness. These include capacity to sulphate steroids, the presence or absence of periductal elastosis, the sensitivity of the tumour tissue to added hormones in vitro and its endogenous peroxidase activity. Their predictive value in the clinical situation has not been agreed.

Therapeutic considerations

The first demonstration that endocrine manipulation could affect the course of human breast cancer was in 1895. Beatson then treated a 31-year-old Glasgow woman with recurrent cancer by ovariectomy. With the discovery of cortisone, other surgical procedures (adrenalectomy, hypophysectomy, radioactive implantation of the pituitary) were used in older women to deprive the tumour of promoting hormones. Pharmacological agents also were introduced to treat advanced disease. Testosterone, synthetic oestrogens and progestagens were found to be effective in a proportion of women but, as side effects could be severe, many preferred a surgical attack. The situation has now changed. The availability of two new agents which are well tolerated, tamoxifen and aminoglutethimide, has largely led to the abandonment of surgical methods of achieving hormonal suppression other than in the young woman.

Tamoxifen

Tamoxifen is a triphenylethylene derivative which has marked anti-oestrogenic effects in the human female. This action is believed to be due to binding of the drug to the nuclear oestrogen receptor which, on binding to the

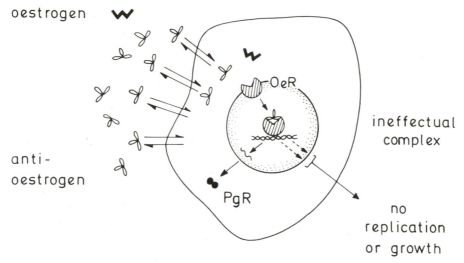

Fig. 6.11 The mechanism of action of tamoxifen: the drug competes for binding to the oestrogen receptor (OeR) and yields an ineffectual drug-receptor complex.

genome, is ineffective in stimulating protein synthesis or cell growth. Synthesis (replenishment) of new oestrogen receptor protein is depressed so that the cell is also starved of oestrogen receptor (Fig. 6.11).

The rate of response of advanced human breast cancer to tamoxifen is similar to that to other endocrine manipulations. Approximately 35% of tumours show evidence of remission; an additional 20% becoming static.

Tamoxifen is well tolerated and without side effects in 95% of patients. It is now also used as an adjuvant agent for the treatment of micrometastatic disease in patients with primary cancer of the breast.

Aminoglutethimide

Originally developed as an anti-convulsant, this synthetic drug inhibits the synthesis of adrenocortical steroids in the human adrenal cortex. As in older (postmenopausal) women, circulating oestrogen is derived from peripheral conversion of androgens secreted by the adrenal gland; aminoglutethimide, like adrenalectomy, directly lowers this source of precursors for oestrogen synthesis. Aminoglutethimide also inhibits the conversion of androgen to oestrogen by aromatising enzymes at peripheral sites such as fat and liver and within the tumour. This may compliment its central action (Fig. 6.12).

The initial side effects of the drug (nausea, a maculopapular rash and, occasionally, a flu-like illness) may be troublesome, but these usually do not persist and the drug can be tolerated well over long periods of time. Because the adrenal gland is suppressed, cortisone maintenance therapy is necessary.

It has been shown in controlled trials that the proportion of patients with advanced breast cancer who have a remission with aminoglutethimide, is similar to that with tamoxifen or surgical adrenalectomy.

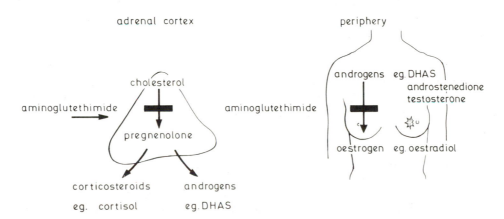

Fig. 6.12 The mechanism of action of aminoglutethimide: cytochrome p_{450}-mediated hydroxylations in the adrenal, tumour and peripheral tissues are inhibited.

PROGNOSIS OF BREAST CANCER

It is now recognized that breast cancer is a systemic disease. By the time a primary tumour is clinically obvious, micrometastases have developed in many sites. The outlook for the patient depends on the growth potential of these deposits of tumour. This in turn is related to various tumour factors. These include the histological type of the tumour, its cellular and nuclear grade, the degree of necrosis, the presence or absence of elastica and the concentration of ER protein. All of these are indices of differentiation. Lymphocytic infiltration and reactive change in the regional lymph nodes (immunological indices) are also regarded as having prognostic significance.

From a clinical standpoint, most of these factors are of little practical value. The best guide to the aggressiveness of a tumour is the degree of lymphatic and vascular invasion and the extent of metastatic spread to regional lymph nodes. The number of axillary lymph nodes which are involved by tumour is closely related to recurrence and survival rates.

Tumour markers

Like other tumours, breast cancer can secrete products which may be detected in the circulating blood. These include the alpha and beta subunits of chorionic gonadotrophin, α-fetoprotein, pregnancy-associated α_2-globulin, α-lactalbumin, casein and carcino-embryonic antigen. They have not yet proved to be of value in either diagnosis or detection of metastatic spread. The drawback with most of these tumour 'markers' is their lack of specificity for breast tissues. It is clear, however, that the breast may express more specific antigens and recently, two major classes of monoclonal antibodies reactive against breast cancer-associated antigens have been developed. These include (i) antibodies raised against breast cancer cell lines, which are highly directed against breast cancer and not expressed or normal breast cells, and (ii) antibodies raised against differentiation antigens of normal breast epithelium, which identify cell surface components of normal cells but are also expressed by the majority of breast cancers. Such antibodies may be useful in the diagnosis of breast cancer, the detection of micro-metastasis and the estimation of tumour burden.

REFERENCES

Azzopardi J G 1979 Problems in breast pathology. W B Saunders, London

Ferguson D J P, Anderson T J 1981 Ultrastructural observations on cell death by apoptosis in the resting human breast. Virchow's Archives (Pathology and Anatomy) 393: 193–203

Lyons W R, Li C H, Johnson R E 1958 The hormonal control of mammary growth and lactation. Recent Progress in Hormone Research. 14: 219–254

Thyroid

A short description of the embryology, anatomy and physiology of the thyroid is followed by an outline of the physiological disturbances and relevant investigations in the principal thyroid diseases.

EMBRYOLOGY AND ANATOMY

Thyroid tissue is found first in vertebrates and, although its location varies, in most mammals including man it is a single bi-lobed gland in front of the trachea. In man the isthmus connecting the two lobes crosses the front of the second and third tracheal rings. It is invested with a fibrous capsule connected with the pretracheal fascia.

The thyroid which is derived from the midline endoderm can be recognized in the developing embryo at the end of the first month. It develops as an outgrowth of the foregut at a point later marked by the foramen caecum of the tongue. The course of descent is indicated by the thyroglossal duct, which occasionally persists, and its mode of development accounts for ectopic tissue being occasionally found at any point between the dorsum of the tongue (lingual thyroid) and the pericardium, in or near the median plane. Such ectopic thyroid tissue may be the sole functioning thyroid tissue present, with hypothyroidism the sequelae of surgical removal. More commonly thyroglossal cysts may arise from remnants of the thyroglossal duct. The pyramidal lobe, an upward extension of the thyroid isthmus, is a residue of the thyroglossal duct. The 'lateral ectopic thyroid' of old accounts is now known not to be ectopic healthy tissue but metastatic thyroid carcinoma in the lower cervical lymph nodes.

The thyroid is the largest of the endocrine glands, weighing in adults approximately 25 g. The right lobe of the gland is normally slightly larger than the left lobe. A convenient clinical standard in assessing goitre size is that each lobe should not exceed the size of the terminal phalanx of the subject's thumb. Palpation from behind with both hands, from the side using the fingers to feel the trachea and retrosternal space or from the front, fixing the gland with the thumbs, may be required to define the gland accurately and exclude lymphadenopathy.

The structure of the thyroid is simple. It is built of colloid-containing acini 200–300 μm in diameter, lined by a single layer of epithelial cells. Both the amount of colloid and the shape of the cells vary with the gland's activity. The epithelial cells are flat in the resting state and tall when the gland is active. Colloid is largely made up of proteins, especially the iodinated glycoprotein, thyroglobulin, a large 19S protein to which tyrosine residues are bound and in which thyroid hormone synthesis and storage takes place. The follicles are bound together in groups to form lobules each supplied by an end artery. Calcitonin is secreted by the parafollicular or 'C-cells' which are distinct from the follicular cells of the thyroid being derived from neural crest rather than endoderm. This explains why medullary carcinomas are associated with phaeochromocytomas and other tumours with a common cell origin.

There are four main arteries, the paired superior and the paired inferior thyroid arteries. An inconstant fifth artery, the thyroidea ima, may occasionally be a large vessel. In addition, the tracheal and oesophageal arteries contribute many unnamed branches which are normally small, but which enlarge in thyrotoxicosis and may bleed briskly during thyroidectomy. The veins draining the thyroid collect into three paired channels, the superior, middle and inferior thyroid veins.

LYMPHATICS

The peri-acinar lymphatic plexus does not communicate with the lumen of the acini and indeed lies outside the peri-acinar plexuses of blood vessels. The lymphatic capillaries of the right and left lobes communicate freely by channels running across the thyroid isthmus. The main lymphatic vessels leave the gland in two groups, ascending and descending. Ascending lymphatics from the isthmus and from the medial part of the lateral lobes, pass upwards to lymph nodes in front of the larynx. Ascending lymphatics from the rest of the lateral lobes pass upwards and backwards to lymph nodes lying along the upper part of the internal jugular vein. Descending lymphatics from the isthmus and medial part of the lateral lobes pass down to the pretracheal and retrosternal lymph nodes, and descending lymphatics from the rest of the lateral lobes pass laterally to lymph nodes along the lower part of the internal jugular vein. Enlargement of the regional lymph nodes from metastases may be the first evidence of papillary adenocarcinoma of the thyroid.

INNERVATION

The thyroid receives both sympathetic and parasympathetic nerve fibres. Sympathetic fibres emerge from the middle cervical ganglion and pass into the substance of the gland in the peri-arterial plexus of the superior and inferior thyroid arteries. Parasympathetic fibres are derived from the superior and recurrent laryngeal branches of the vagus. Nerve fibres terminate in relation to both arterioles and follicular cells and thyroid function may be influenced indirectly through changes in blood flow (the delivery of thyroid stimulating hormone (TSH, thyrotropin) iodine and other substances) and by a direct effect on the follicular cell. The recurrent laryngeal branch of the vagus is not concerned in thyroid physiology, but is important in thyroid surgery. Destruction of the nerve, by the spread of thyroid carcinoma or accidental division during thyroidectomy, paralyses the vocal cord.

THYROID HORMONES

Although thyrotoxicosis was recorded by Parry as early as 1786 and Gull first described myxoedema in 1874 it was not until 1895 that iodine was shown by Kocher to play a part in thyroid function, until 1915 that Kendal isolated thyroxine and 1951 that the discoveries that led Gross and Pitt-Rivers to identify tri-iodothyronine were made.

Dietary iodine, principally from fish, milk, eggs and iodinated salt or bread, is absorbed from the stomach and upper small intestine as iodide ions and circulating iodide is trapped and concentrated by the thyroid up to 40 times the plasma level (Fig. 7.1). There is no homeostatic mechanism for conserving iodide and the plasma level depends on the balance between renal and faecal losses and dietary intake. Within the thyroid cell a peroxidase enzyme system rapidly oxidises iodide, covalently binds the active form with tyrosine or monoiodotyrosine (MIT) attached to thyroglobulin in colloid at the apical border to form MIT and di-iodotyrosine (DIT), and is involved in the coupling of these iodotyrosines to form thyroxine (tetraiodothyronine, T4) and tri-iodothyronine (T3).

Synthesized thyroid hormone attached to thyroglobulin is stored in colloid until required. Microvilli on the apical surface of the cell engulf colloid droplets (pinocytosis) which fuse with lysosomes whose proteolytic enzymes hydrolyse thyroglobulin to release thyroid hormones. It is mainly T4 that is released into the blood-stream but a small amount of T3 and thyroglobulin (used as tumour marker in the follow-up of the treatment of thyroid carci-

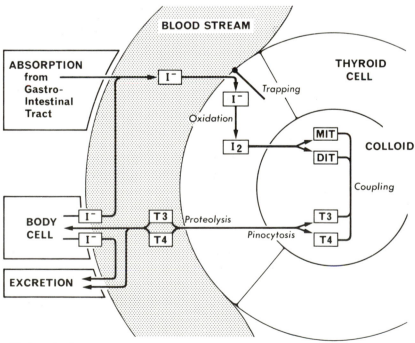

Fig. 7.1 Thyroid hormone synthesis and release

noma after ablative therapy) are also released. Most T3 (approximately 75%) and nearly all the other iodothyronines and their derivatives are derived by peripheral deiodination of thyroxine. The T3 and T4 content of the normal thyroid is about 200 μg/g and 15 μg/g respectively. In the normal adult male, on average, 80 μg of T4 and 30 μg of T3 are produced daily. T4 and T3 are the two major calorigenically active hormones.

The ratio of circulating T4 to T3 is about 70:1. T3 is, however, about four times more active than T4 by weight. The majority of circulating thyroid hormone is protein-bound but it is the free thyroid hormone that is assumed to be metabolically active (approximately 0.03% of total T4 and 0.3% of total T3 is 'free' or non-protein-bound). With decreasing affinity, thyroxine binding globulin (TBG), thyroxine binding prealbumin (TBPA) and albumin bind thyroid hormones. TBG has a low capacity and albumin a very high capacity for binding. T3 is much less firmly bound than T4 and this difference accounts for its lower serum levels and shorter half life. The functions of the binding proteins are regulation of the rate of delivery of free hormone, buffering of changes in secretion or degradation and prevention of loss by way of the liver or kidneys.

Although the concentration of T4 in the tissues is lower than the free level in serum, the reverse is true for T3. It is possible that T3 is the metabolically active thyroid hormone and that T4 is a prohormone.

There are several routes of T4 metabolism. The major route (85%) is deiodination to T3 (monodeiodination at the 5′ position) or to reverse-T3 (monodeiodination at the 5 position) in the liver, kidney and other sites. Reverse-T3 is calorigenically inactive. Other routes include conjugation to form glucuronides and sulphates and alteration of the alanine side chain to form acetic or proprionic acids.

A number of physiological and pathological states and medications influence T4 metabolism. In the fetus and newborn, T3 levels are low and reverse-T3 levels are high. With ageing there is a tendency for T3 levels to fall and reverse-T3 levels to rise. Some non-thyroidal diseases (e.g. acute medical or surgical stress, starvation, severe systemic disease, hepatic cirrhosis and renal failure) are associated with low T3 levels, the ' low T3 syndrome'. These patients are clinically euthyroid and usually have normal or low total and free T4, elevated reverse-T3, low protein binding and normal TSH. If the free T4 is low, the TSH and reverse-T3 levels help to exclude primary hypothyroidism. The exact significance of these changes remains to be elucidated but in nonthyroid illness it may be a beneficial adaptation to reduce the metabolic rate. Propylthiouracil (but not carbimazole), dexamethasone, radiocontrast dyes and amiodarone also influence the direction of T4 metabolism with decreased production of T3 and a reciprocal increase in reverse-T3.

Hypothalamic-pituitary-thyroid regulatory mechanisms

TSH, a glycoprotein, stimulates both synthesis and release of thyroid hormones (Fig. 7.2). TSH binds to a specific thyroid cell membrane receptor with activation of adenylate cyclase and subsequently cyclic AMP-dependent protein kinases but subsequent steps linking these changes to the metabolic and morphological effects of TSH are not well established and some work suggests that not all the effects of TSH are mediated by cAMP. TSH stimulates practically all the processes of thyroid function involved in thyroid hormone biosynthesis. Its secretion from basophilic cells of the anterior pituitary is in turn controlled by releasing (thyrotropin-releasing hormone, TRH), and perhaps release-inhibiting hormones (dopamine, somatostatin) from the hypothalamus and the level of circulating thyroid hormone. TRH also acts as a releasing factor for prolactin and under certain conditions it may affect secretion of other pituitary trophic hormones. TRH is a tripeptide, pyroglutamylhistidylprolineamide, widely distributed throughout neural tissue and is probably a neurotransmitter as well as a releasing hormone. The factors controlling the synthesis and secretion of TRH are not well established.

Competitive interaction exists at the pituitary level between TRH and thyroid hormones to determine TSH

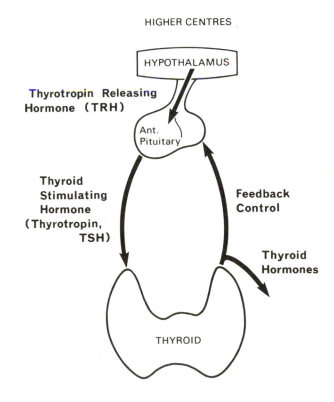

HIGHER CENTRES

HYPOTHALAMUS

Thyrotropin Releasing Hormone (TRH)

Ant. Pituitary

Thyroid Stimulating Hormone (Thyrotropin, TSH)

Feedback Control

Thyroid Hormones

THYROID

Fig. 7.2 The hypothalamic-pituitary-thyroid axis

secretion. Although both thyroid hormones antagonize the action of TRH it is likely that the action of T4 is via intracellular conversion to T3. If the blood concentration of free thyroid hormone falls, an increased secretion of TSH stimulates the production of thyroxine and tri-iodothyronine. On the other hand, increased levels of these hormones inhibit TSH release and consequently, thyroid hormone synthesis until the free hormone level has returned to normal (negative feedback). It is not established whether there is also feedback control through the hypothalamus as well as the pituitary, and whether there is a short feedback loop of TSH itself.

Intrinsic thyroid autoregulatory mechanisms are also important and come into action particularly when there are changes in the availability of iodine. Iodine deficiency leads to enhanced responsiveness to TSH and in areas of endemic iodine deficiency the T3:T4 ratio is increased.

Action of thyroid hormones

The biochemical mechanism at the cellular level is still uncertain despite extensive recent research. Present data indicate that both the cell nucleus and the mitochondria are sites of interaction with thyroid hormones. Interaction with the nuclear receptor results in an increase of messenger RNA and subsequently in protein synthesis and with the mitochondrial receptor, probably in the uncoupling of phosphorylation from respiration with increased oxygen consumption and heat production.

As well as the rate of tissue metabolism, thyroid hormones affect growth and differentiation, cardiac function and fat, sugar and protein metabolism. Their importance for normal growth and development is emphasized by the dwarfism associated with cretinism and the accelerated growth in childhood hyperthyroidism. They affect the activity of the nervous tissue and the nervousness and irritability of hyperthyroidism contrast with the apathy and mental retardation of hypothyroidism. In hyperthyroidism gastrointestinal motility is increased while in hypothyroidism it is sluggish and constipation occurs. Delayed relaxation of the tendon reflexes is one of the classical findings in hypothyroidism. Thyroid hormones increase the rate of absorption of glucose from the intestine, favour the conversion of liver glycogen to glucose and promote the formation of glucose from non-carbohydrate sources. In hyperthyroidism the oral glucose tolerance test may give a diabetic pattern whereas in hypothyroidism a flat curve may be found.

Some of the actions of thyroid hormones are compatible with augmentation of the sensitivity of beta receptors to catecholamines. These effects, e.g., the tachycardia of hyperthyroidism, are blocked by β-adrenergic blocking agents, such as propranolol, without affecting thyroid hormone levels.

INVESTIGATION OF THYROID DISEASE

Whilst an experienced clinician can often make the correct diagnosis on the basis of the history and physical examination alone, appropriate confirmatory investigations should always be performed. In hypothyroidism lifelong therapy with thyroid hormone will be necessary and in hyperthyroidism treatment with either radioiodine or surgery may be associated with significant morbidity.

Many different tests are available and this may pose problems of selection of the most appropriate and their interpretation. The serum free T4 (direct or indirect measurement) should be measured in all patients, the serum T3 in suspected hyperthyroidism and the serum TSH in suspected hypothyroidism.

Care is required in the interpretation of thyroid function tests in seriously ill patients. Ideally, if strong clinical evidence of thyroid dysfunction is absent, the tests should be performed when the patient is back to normal health.

Thyroid function may be investigated by tests of (i) primary thyroid function, (ii) hypothalamic-pituitary-thyroid relationships and (iii) peripheral metabolism.

As different values are obtained by different techniques each laboratory must establish its own normal range for each assay.

Tests of primary thyroid function

Circulating thyroid hormone levels

The concentration of free thyroid hormones determines the clinical thyroid status and can be measured directly or indirectly (by estimating free thyroid hormone from measurement of total thyroid hormone together with a test of residual protein binding capacity).

The half life of T4 is greater than T3 and if tests of thyroid function are required after treatment with thyroid hormone, a period of 6 weeks or 10 days respectively off medication is required.

Total serum thyroxine (T4) and triiodothyronine (T3)

The total serum T4 is measured by competitive protein binding or radioimmunoassay (RIA) and the total serum T3 by RIA.

Anomalous T4 or T3 values at variance with the clinical assessment are seen in patients with altered protein binding but values are not affected by other iodinated components unless thyroid function itself is affected. The normal concentration of T4 in plasma or serum ranges from approximately 50–150 nmol/l and of T3 from 1–3 nmol/l.

Assessment of protein binding and measurement of free thyroid hormone

Total thyroid hormone levels vary directly with the levels

of binding proteins. Homeostatic adjustment keeps the free hormone concentration stable. The common causes of increased thyroid hormone-binding proteins are pregnancy and treatment with oestrogens. Protein binding is decreased in the nephrotic syndrome, severe liver disease, androgen therapy and by drugs that compete for binding sites (salicylates, diphenylhydantoin and phenylbutazone). Changes in either direction may be familial.

There has been confusion in interpreting tests measuring binding (T3 resin uptake) as the results are expressed in different ways, depending on the test used, and because they are often referred to as 'T3 tests' (they neither directly nor indirectly measure serum T3). In some laboratories TBG levels are directly measured.

An indirect estimation of free thyroxine, free thyroxine index (FTI) or effective thyroxine ratio (ETR), can be derived from the total T4 level and a measurement of residual thyroid hormone binding capacity. These calculations give values corrected for alterations in binding proteins and a good correlation has been shown with the free T4 level measured directly. Similarly, an indirect estimation of free T3 can be calculated (free T3 index). These indirect estimations of free hormone reliably establish thyroid status when there are changes in TBG concentrations but are less accurate in accounting for the presence of circulating inhibitors of protein binding.

Direct measurements of both free T4 and free T3 by radio-immunoassay are now replacing indirect estimations in many laboratories and have similar diagnostic accuracy as the indirect methods in most patients. However, low free T4 values may be seen in nonthyroid illness with most of the available methods. Measurement of free hormone levels by equilibrium dialysis permits excellent differentiation of thyroid function but is cumbersome and in nonthyroid illness may give elevated free T4 levels.

Uptake studies

The proportion of a known tracer dose of iodine or technetium taken up by the thyroid at a standard time after administration reflects the level of thyroid function. Uptake studies have poor discrimination between hypothyroidism or mild hyperthyroidism and normality and have no place in the initial investigation of thyroid disease; they are useful however, in identifying those cases of hyperthyroidism due to thyroiditis, iodine-induced thyrotoxicosis and thyrotoxicosis factitia in which the thyroid uptake is suppressed. Recognition of these unusual conditions is important as they are transient and do not require definitive treatment.

Technetium is trapped but not organically bound by the thyroid. It is replacing radio-iodine because of its low radiation dose and short half-life. It is given by intravenous injection and the count and scan can be done 20 or 30 minutes later.

Thyroidal uptake may be reduced by iodine-containing mixtures and X-ray contrast media and by drugs that interfere with the trapping and retention of iodide.

The TSH stimulation test has been used to distinguish between primary (impaired response) and secondary (normal or stepwise response) hypothyroidism, but is not consistently abnormal in minor degrees of primary thyroid failure and has now been replaced by measurement of serum TSH.

Hypothalamic-pituitary-thyroid relationships

Serum TSH

Serum TSH is measured by radioimmunoassay. With most assays it is not possible to distinguish reliably between normal and low TSH values (e.g. in thyrotoxicosis), but any increase in TSH can be detected. An increase in serum TSH reflects reduction in thyroid hormone concentrations but does not necessarily imply clinical hypothyroidism. A normal TSH virtually excludes primary thyroid failure.

Approximate normal values range from below the limit of detection of the assay up to 10 mu/l.

Thyrotropin-releasing hormone (TRH) stimulation test

In the standard test TRH is administered as a 200 μg intravenous bolus with sampling for TSH prior to and 20 and 60 minutes after administration. In normal patients the peak TSH response is at 15–20 minutes, in primary hypothyroidism there is an exaggerated and prolonged response and patients with hyperthyroidism fail to show any rise in TSH (because of the negative feedback of increased levels of thyroid hormone). An abnormal TSH response may also be found in hypothalamic-pituitary disease.

Although a normal TSH response excludes hyperthyroidism, patients with ophthalmic Grave's disease, autonomous thyroid adenoma, multinodular goitre, in clinical remission after Grave's disease or receiving throxine or tri-iodothyronine may have an impaired response despite being clinically euthyroid. The majority of these patients have thyroid hormone levels that are high enough to inhibit TSH release but not high enough to cause clinical features of hypermetabolism. Some patients rendered euthyroid after treatment of hyperthyroidism have persistent suppression of the pituitary similar to that seen after corticosteroid therapy. Treatment with steroids, spontaneous Cushing's syndrome or treatment with L-dopa may also cause an impaired response. Side effects of intravenous TRH include transient nausea, flushing, dizziness, a peculiar taste and a desire to micturate.

T3-suppression test

Suppression tests are also used to demonstrate thyroid

autonomy in patients with possible hyperthyroidism in whom routine tests of thyroid function do not establish a definite diagnosis. The lack of suppression of thyroid uptake after administration of T3 indicates that the thyroid is functioning independent of pituitary control either due to an abnormal thyroid stimulator or autonomous functioning nodule(s). There is a close correlation between lack of suppressibility and impairment of TSH response to TRH in patients without previous thyroid disease. The TRH stimulation test is simpler to perform and should be used in the elderly patient or patients with cardiac disease where suppression tests are potentially dangerous in that they may precipitate atrial fibrillation, angina or heart failure.

Suppression of radio-iodine uptake by tri-iodothyronine is very strong evidence against hyperthyroidism but impairment of suppression may be found in some clinically euthyroid patients with Graves' disease, autonomous functioning adenomas, mutlinodular goitres or treated Graves' disease. The test is of greatest value in distinguishing between the high uptake of dyshormonogenesis (defects in thyroid hormone synthesis) or iodine deficiency and that of hyperthyroidism.

Peripheral metabolism

These tests are insensitive and non-specific and now have little place in the routine investigation of thyroid disease.

The relaxation phase of the Achilles tendon reflex is prolonged in overt thyroid failure but is not significantly delayed in the patient with mild hypothyroidism in whom there is diagnostic difficulty. Serum cholesterol and/or triglyceride concentrations are often increased in thyroid failure but there is a substantial overlap with the normal range. Electrocardiographic changes in hypothyroidism are non-specific (bradycardia, flattening or inversion of T waves and decreased amplitude of the R waves). Estimation of the basal metabolic rate requires meticulous supervision to obtain a valid result.

OTHER THYROID INVESTIGATIONS

Thyroid auto-antibodies

Auto-antibodies to thyroglobulin and a microsomal cell component reflect lymphocytic infiltration of the thyroid gland and high titres are indicative of Hashimoto's disease. Auto-antibodies which stimulate the thyroid membrane receptor and mimic the action of TSH may be detected in patients with Graves' disease but at present play no part in routine investigation. The different names (long-acting thyroid stimulator — LATS, LATS protector, thyroid stimulating antibodies or immunoglobulins) ascribed to

this heterogeneous group of immunoglobulins reflects the different assay procedures and the species specificity of antibodies. Several limited applications for these assays have been proposed. Persistently high titres in treated diffuse toxic goitre are predictive of relapse of hyperthyroidism following discontinuation of antithyroid drugs, demonstration in patients with exophthalmous supports the diagnosis of euthyroid Graves' disease and high concentrations in a pregnant woman may increase the likelihood of neonatal Graves' disease.

Thyroid scanning

Scanning of the thyroid gland is used (i) to define the extent of the thyroid (e.g. possible retrosternal extension) and its size; (ii) to define the function of the gland (diffuse uptake is found in Graves' disease and localised uptake in toxic adenomata) or of nodules (cold nodules have a significant incidence of malignancy); (iii) to identify ectopic thyroid tissue or to locate functioning metastases after ablation of normal thyroid tissue.

Radio-iodine kinetic studies

These may be useful in studying patients with dyshormonogenesis. The principal test available is the perchlorate discharge test which identifies subjects with an organification defect. Perchlorate competes with iodide for transport within the thyroid causing discharge of iodide not yet organifically bound.

Ultrasonic scanning

Ultrasonic scanning may be used in evaluating cold thyroid nodules, distinguishing between apparent and true single nodules (true single nodules have a greater risk of malignancy) and solid from cystic lesions (true cysts without solid components are rare but have a low incidence of malignancy) and in determining thyroid size.

Radiology

X-rays may be useful to define the extent of a goitre with retrosternal extension or to determine if tracheal compression is present.

Thyroid biopsy

Needle aspiration biopsy may identify the underlying disease process but the samples obtained may be non-representative (a negative biopsy does not exclude malignancy) and require special cytological expertise for proper interpretation. Benign and malignant follicular neoplasms cannot be separated preoperatively but papillary carcinomas, colloid adenomas and autoimmune thyroiditis can often be identified.

HYPERTHYROIDISM

Hyperthyroidism is commonly due to either autoimmune thyrotoxicosis or toxic adenomata.

Types of hyperthyroidism

Autoimmune thyrotoxicosis (Graves' disease)

Autoimmune thyrotoxicosis is the commonest type of hyperthyroidism. Females are affected six times more often than males with a maximum incidence in the third and fourth decades. It is part of a syndrome (Graves' disease) comprizing one or more of the following features: goitre, hyperthyroidism, eye signs and rarely, localized myxoedema (plaques of thickened subcutaneous tissue usually over the pretibial or calf areas) or thyroid acropachy (clubbing of the fingers and toes with subperiosteal new bone formation). Ophthalmic Graves' disease describes the occasional patient with ocular manifestations in the absence of hyperthyroidism. Neonatal Graves' disease describes the rare case of transient hyperthyroidism in children born to mothers who have or have had thyrotoxicosis.

The differentiation between autoimmune thyrotoxicosis and toxic adenomata may be difficult. Although in the former the goitre is typically diffuse and vascular at first, autoimmune thyrotoxicosis may occur in patients who have had a nodular goitre for some time (hyperactivity of internodular tissue) or nodularity may arise in the course of the disease. Diffuse hyperfunction as shown by scanning and the presence of thyroid-stimulating antibodies in the serum of some of these patients with nodular goitre supports a common aetiology with classical Graves' disease. Pretibial myxoedema, thickening of the skin and subcutaneous tissues, occurs in about 5% of patients with autoimmune thyrotoxicosis whereas thyroid acropachy is much rarer.

Observations on the natural history of hyperthyroidism show the variable course of the disease. The illness may be characterised by a single episode followed by prolonged remission (Fig. 7.3), by fluctuations in the activity of the disease with phases of remission and relapse (Fig. 7.4) or by persistent disease activity lasting many years despite control of thyroid function (Fig. 7.5). In these three figures whilst the patient is on triiodothyronine non-suppression of the thyroid uptake reflects persistent disease activity and non-suppression of the FTI whilst the patient is on triiodothyronine alone after cessation of carbimazole also reflects disease activity.

Apart from relapse there are no significant sequelae after spontaneous remission of thyrotoxicosis. In view of the close association of the disease with autoimmune thyroiditis, it is not surprising that the occasional patient, not treated with radioiodine or surgery, develops hypothyroidism.

The sera from patients with autoimmune thyrotoxicosis contain thyroid-stimulating auto-antibodies. They were first discovered by Adams and Purves in 1956 and termed long acting thyroid stimulator (LATS). Because of the species specificity of these antibodies it was only possible to detect activity in less than half the patients with Graves' disease with the original bioassays. Immunoglobulins in the serum of LATS-negative patients with autoimmune thyrotoxicosis stimulate the human but not the mouse thyroid. More recently radio-receptor assays which measure the effects of thyroid stimulating auto-antibodies on the binding of labelled TSH to human thyroid membranes and assays dependent on adenyl cyclase activation have been developed. With these assays, thyroid-binding or thyroid-stimulating auto-antibodies are detectable in nearly all patients with untreated autoimmune thyrotoxicosis. The role of abnormal stimulating immunoglobulins appears inescapable but the initial triggering event remains unexplained. One hypothesis is that there is an underlying defect of immune surveillance and the disease arises in susceptible individuals either randomly or in response to triggering factors.

The evidence for an autoimmune basis for this type of hyperthyroidism is considerable. The finding that the disease is more frequently associated with autoimmune thyroiditis and other autoimmune diseases, the enlargement and/or hyperplasia of lymphoid tissues, the lymphocytic and plasma cell infiltration of thyroid and retro-orbital tissues, the deposition of immunoglobulins in the thyroid and the finding that corticosteroids and immunosuppressive agents may cause remission of hyperthyroidism and eye signs all point to a disturbance of immune mechanisms.

Toxic multinodular goitre and toxic adenoma

Plummer's disease, or toxic adenomata, describes the case of thyrotoxicosis with one or more functioning nodules. It is not associated with thyroid stimulating auto-antibodies. In its natural history, an adenoma initially becomes independent of outside influences (autonomous functioning nodule) as demonstrated by a lack of suppressibility in contrast with the rest of the thyroid and in time produces excess thyroid hormone resulting in the clinical features of hyperthyroidism. Toxic adenomata, which account for 5–10% of cases of hyperthyroidism are more common in women and have their maximum prevalence between 40 and 60 years of age.

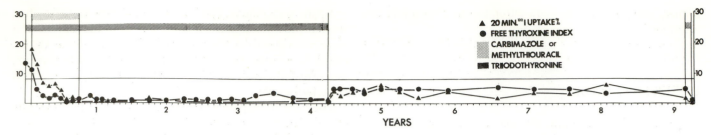

Fig. 7.3 Thyrotoxicosis characterized by a short-lived illness

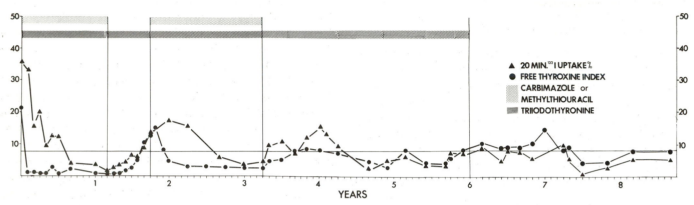

Fig. 7.4 Thyrotoxicosis characterized by fluctuating disease activity

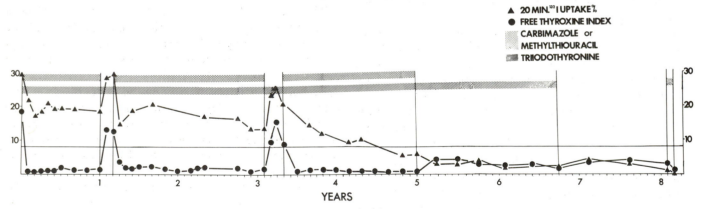

Fig. 7.5 Thyrotoxicosis characterized by persistent disease activity

Iodine-induced (Jod-Basedow)

Iodine administration may expose underlying thyroid dysfunction and cause hyperthyroidism presumably by providing more substrate for thyroid hormone production. This may be seen in the treatment of non-toxic goitre with iodine, when iodine prophylaxis is introduced for endemic goitre, when iodinated radiological contrast media are used or when iodinated medications (e.g. amiodarone) are prescribed.

Thyroiditis

Subacute thyroiditis, autoimmune thyroiditis or radiation-induced thyroiditis may cause hyperthyroidism due to release of thyroid hormone secondary to thyroid cell damage. Subacute thyroiditis may be 'silent' without the classical painful thyroid, recognized only by a suppressed thyroid uptake.

Factitious hyperthyroidism

Rarely, the patient who surreptitiously takes unprescribed thyroid hormone may present a diagnostic problem. The absence of goitre and a characteristic pattern of test results will alert the clinician to this possibility.

Malignancy

Clinical hyperthyroidism associated with secretion of TSH or TSH-like peptides from pituitary, trophoblastic or other malignant tumours or excess thyroid hormone from metastatic thyroid carcinoma or struma ovarie, is a rare occurrence.

Clinical features

The symptoms which most commonly suggest hyperthyroidism are recent heat intolerance, increased appetite with weight loss, excessive sweating, palpitations and nervousness. The presence of a goitre and a hyperkinetic circulatory and nervous system are the most helpful signs. These are classical features. It must be remembered that not infrequently there is an atypical presentation especially in elderly patients, 20% of whom will not have a tachycardia and/or goitre. The presence of myasthenia, proximal myopathy, atrial fibrillation, paroxysmal tachycardia, unexplained or resistant cardiac failure or diarrhoea, osteoporosis and unstable diabetes require the exclusion of hyperthyroidism. It should also be remembered that the different facets of Graves' disease can occur separately and exophthalmos may occur without hyperthyroidism.

Investigation

Confirmation of the diagnosis of hyperthyroidism is possible in most cases with measurement of free serum thyroxine directly or indirectly. In a small percentage of cases hyperthyroidism may be present with normal serum T4 but elevated T3 levels (T3 toxicosis). On rare occasions the diagnosis will still be in doubt and more complex tests (TRH stimulation or T3 suppression) will be required. The steps in diagnosis are:

1. Measurement of free T4 and free T3 (direct or indirectly)
   (a) High — establishes hyperthyroidism
   (b) Normal — thyrotoxicosis unlikely
   (c) Marginal or conflict with clinical impression — step 2
2. TRH stimulation test (or T3 suppression test)
   Normal — thyrotoxicosis excluded.
   Impaired or absent response — consistent with thyrotoxicosis

Treatment of thyrotoxicosis

Despite advances in our knowledge of the pathogenesis of Graves' disease, rational treatment of aetiological factors is not yet possible and treatment is directed towards controlling excess thyroid activity. The criteria for selection of the main therapeutic choices (radio-iodine treatment, subtotal thyroidectomy or antithyroid drugs) vary in the different leading centres and a detailed discussion of this subject is outside the scope of this text.

Antithyroid drugs

The thiouracil drugs (Carbimazole, its derivative methimazole and propylthiouracil) which act by blocking organification, are most widely used. Propylthiouracil blocks T4 and T3 conversion peripherally but has the disadvantage of a shorter half-life. The advantages of the thiouracils include efficacy of control, low incidence of side-effects and lack of damage to the thyroid. The chief disadvantage is a high relapse rate. Side-effects to both drugs seldom occur. The most serious side effect is agranulocytosis (0.05%) which can occur at any time in treatment and if the drug is not discontinued fatal infection can supervene. Initial doses are 30–60 mg/day of Carbimazole and 300–600 mg/day of propylthiouracil in divided doses. The patient usually becomes euthyroid in 6–8 weeks. With definite improvement the dose is reduced at intervals to maintenance dose of 5–15 mg/day of Carbimazole (100–200 mg/day of propylthiouracil) or thyroid hormone is added ('block-replace therapy' for easier control and prevention of hypothyroidism due to over-treatment). Treatment is usually maintained for 12–24 months.

β-adrenergic blockade, by blocking the peripheral effects of thyroid hormone (and less importantly by diverting peripheral T4 metabolism from T3 to reverse-T3), achieves rapid control of many clinical features of hyperthyroidism within 24–36 hours. Initial doses of propranolol are 80–160 mg/day in divided doses. On withdrawal of therapy hyperthyroidism may recur within 4–6 hours. Beta-blockade is valuable in severe hyperthyroidism, in conjunction with antithyroid drugs, to achieve rapid relief and although sometimes used alone in preparation for surgery, omission of a single dose may cause thyroid storm.

Surgery

Bilateral subtotal thyroidectomy effectively and decisively controls thyrotoxicosis with, in good hands and proper preparation, no mortality and little morbidity. Hypoparathyroidism and damage to the recurrent laryngeal nerves are rare in skilled hands. Thyroid storm should not occur with adequate prior control with antithyroid drugs. Propranolol, if used, should be continued for 72 hours postoperatively. The incidence of recurrence (up to 5%) is higher in patients whose radioiodine uptakes remain non-suppressible after surgery and in whom thyroid stimulating immunoglobulins are found. Thyroidectomy itself has a dramatic effect on circulating levels of thyroid stimulating auto-antibodies. The risk of hypothyroidism, though not as great as with radioiodine, is significant (20–35% in 10 years) and may be cumulative. The incidence is higher in patients with significant titres of microsomal antibodies. Transient hypothyroidism may occur in the first few months after thyroidectomy and a high TSH is not in itself an indication for replacement therapy.

Radio-iodine

Radio-iodine is simple to administer, usually on an outpatient basis. It is however, not possible to choose a dose that will accurately destroy the appropriate amount of thyroid tissue. With conventional doses (3–6 mCi) over 50% of patients are controlled within 3 or 4 months and over 90% within 12 months. Antithyroid drugs or propranolol cover is usually needed for several months. Repeated doses may have to be given and it is customary to give the second dose, if needed, 4–6 months after the first. An alternative is to give an ablative (15–20 mCi) dose of radio-iodine followed by thyroxine replacement. With conventional doses, about 20% of patients are hypothyroid in 2 years with a cumulative increase of about 3% per year thereafter. Radio-iodine therapy does not increase the risk of subsequent cancer or leukaemia and there is no evidence of gonadal damage. It is contraindicated in pregnancy.

Choice of therapy

Selection of the most appropriate therapy for a particular patient remains at the present time empirical. As there is a strong tendency to spontaneous remission and since sequelae, other than relapse, after antithyroid drugs are rare, it would appear rational to treat the great majority of patients with antithyroid drugs selecting out those patients with unfavourable prognostic factors for radio-iodine therapy or surgery. Surgery would be the more appropriate initial choice in patients with very large goitres or compression, radio-iodine in the elderly or thyrocardiac patient and the patient with recurrence after thyroidectomy, and either surgery or radioiodine in the patient with autonomous adenomata. During treatment with antithyroid drugs unfavourable prognostic features (e.g. persistence of high titres of thyroid-stimulating antibodies or of thyroid non-suppressibility and progressive increase in goitre size) may indicate that prolonged remission after drug therapy is unlikely and surgery or radio-iodine is more appropriate. In pregnancy either antithyroid drugs (minimal dose as these drugs cross the placenta and may cause fetal goitre and hypothyroidism whereas T4 and T3

do not significantly cross the placenta and do not protect the fetus) or surgery in the second trimester (when the risk of miscarriage is least) is appropriate.

Thyroid crisis

This is a rare complication of uncontrolled thyrotoxicosis occurring after surgery, radio-iodine therapy or in patients with an intercurrent infection or other illness.

The features are those of an exacerbation of thyrotoxicosis and are dominated by manifestations of severe hypermetabolism. There is fever, tachycardia, dehydration and often atrial fibrillation and heart failure.

The treatment is aimed at inhibiting hormone synthesis and release, and T4 conversion to T3 with iodine, antithyroid drugs (propylthiouracil) and dexamethasone and antagonizing the peripheral effect of thyroid hormones by β-adrenergic blockade. Supportive therapy (rehydration, oxygen, sedation, reduction of fever, treatment of cardiac failure) is also required.

Exophthalmos

Most patients with Graves' disease have relatively mild occular involvement. A small number of patients have more severe exophthalmos with chemosis, conjunctival infection, periorbital oedema, lacrimation, diplopia and ophthalmoplegia. Progressive or malignant exophthalmos may threaten vision. Exophthalmos may occur at onset of hyperthyroidism, after treatment or without evidence of thyroid disease. Treatment of mild ophthalmopathy involves artificial tears and tinted glasses. Treatment of severe disease is difficult requiring steroids and immunosuppressive agents and possibly surgical decompression. Cosmetic surgery may be indicated if complete resolution does not occur.

HYPOTHYROIDISM AND NON-TOXIC GOITRE

Hypothyroidism is the disease state that results from thyroid hormone deficiency and its synonym, myxoedema, is derived from the myxomatous thickening of the skin that is a characteristic, but not invariable, finding. 'Primary' hypothyroidism is due to a lack of functioning thyroid tissue. 'Secondary' hypothyroidism, due to thyroid failure that is the sequel of hypothalamic-pituitary disease, is usually associated with a loss of other pituitary hormones.

Apart from thyroid neoplasia most non-toxic goitres result from the action of TSH on a thyroid that has failed to produce sufficient thyroid hormone. The resultant hyperplasia is characterized by an increase in the height and number of thyroid cells with papillary outgrowth into the follicles which lose colloid. The hyperplasia and hypertrophy results in compensated thyroid function, which may be sufficient to prevent overt hypothyroidism. The gland is initially diffusely hyperplastic but with variation in activity hyperplastic nodules appear. Some nodules undergo haemorrhagic or cystic degeneration with resultant fibrosis or calcification and as these areas lose function new nodules appear. Early detection and correction of the thyroid hormone deficiency often results in reduction of goitre size but when the goitre is longstanding and nodular or cystic, thyroid hormone has little effect. If stimulation fails to effect a normal hormone output, goitrous hypothyroidism will ensue.

Aetiology

Iodine deficiency, autoimmune thyroiditis and less frequently, dyshormonogenesis, goitrogens or other types of thyroiditis may cause non-toxic goitre and/or hypothyroidism. Hypothyroidism may also occur as a result of dysgenesis, destructive treatments (surgery or radiation) and in hypothalamic-pituitary disease.

Iodine deficiency

Iodine deficiency usually presents as a goitre but hypothyroidism may occur. It is responsible for most endemic goitres and in highly endemic areas, e.g. New Guinea, the Himalayas, the Andes and the Congo, cretinism is found. The thyroid function is usually well compensated with preferential secretion of T3 and significant elevation of TSH level is not usually found unless the iodine deficiency is severe. Programmes of iodine supplementation have done much to eradicate the disorder.

Dyshormonogenesis

This is an uncommon cause of non-toxic goitre and six separate intrathyroidal disturbances have been incriminated in dyshormonogenesis: defects of the iodine trap, organification or coupling, dehalogenase or protease enzyme deficiencies and synthesis of abnormal iodoproteins. Of the various forms of dyshormonogenesis, an organification defect is most often found. The development of goitre and/or hypothyroidism depends on the severity of the defect; mild defects may only present if there is concurrent iodine deficiency or goitrogens. Sometimes because of their hyperplasia they may simulate malignancy. All these conditions respond to thyroxine while the iodine trapping and dehalogenase defects respond to a high iodine intake.

Goitrogens

Goitrogens, by blocking steps in thyroid hormone synthesis or inhibiting iodine uptake, usually cause a hyperplastic gland with compensated thyroid function or hypothyroidism. Natural goitrogens by themselves have not been shown to be significant in goitre production but some drugs, given for non-thyroidal disease, have a goitrogenic action. Phenylbutazone, para-aminosalicylates and resorcinol inhibit organification in a similar fashion to the thiouracils used to treat thyrotoxicosis. Sulphonylureas used as oral hypoglycaemic agents are also potential goitrogens and lithium used in the treatment of manic depressive disorders has an antithyroid action. Iodine in proprietary cough mixtures if taken in excess may cause goitre and either hypothyroidism or hyperthyroidism.

Autoimmune thyroiditis

The thyroiditis described by Hashimoto in 1912 is due to an autoimmune disturbance. There is an associated genetic predisposition to both this condition and Graves' disease and a familial history of one or other disorder is often obtained. 95% of cases occur in women, especially in the middle-aged, and its incidence is increasing. Thyroid tissue is gradually destroyed and as a result of diminished function and reduced thyroid hormone output, TSH stimulation of less severely affected areas takes place. This may result in goitre and/or hypothyroidism. It is characterized by a moderately enlarged firm diffuse or bosselated goitre, usually without discrete nodules which, if present, require exclusion of co-existent carcinoma. The incidence of carcinoma is about 3%, with the majority of cases coming to light as an occult finding on pathological examination. Usually the diagnosis is made on clinical grounds supported by laboratory investigation. Auto-antibodies to thyroglobulin or microsomal antigens, if present in high titres, are diagnostic; in some patients a biopsy may be required with the characteristic histological appearance of lymphocyte and plasma cell infiltration, lymphoid follicles and dense fibrous tissue being found.

Surgery is rarely necessary unless neoplasia is suspected. Even if myxoedema is absent, treatment with thyroxine (0.1–1.2 mg/day) is advocated to suppress TSH production, reduce goitre size and prevent further growth. Little if any decrease in size occurs in longstanding goitres with extensive fibrosis.

Spontaneous myxoedema may present without the presence of a goitre. The thyroid shows a variable degree of fibrosis and atrophy as well as changes of chronic thyroiditis resembling those of Hashimoto's disease. Titres of circulating antibodies are usually lower than in Hashimoto's thyroiditis.

Dysgenesis

Thyroid deficiency during fetal or early neonatal life causes neurological and skeletal retardation (cretinism). Mental development continues throughout the first year of life and delay in treatment in this period results in irreversible defects.

Secondary hypothyroidism

In secondary hypothyroidism the skin tends to be finer and paler and other endocrine deficiencies are often present.

Clinical features

Grades of hypothyroidism occur: overt hypothyroidism with major symptoms of thyroid hormone deficiency (mental and physical lethargy, cold intolerance, weight gain, hoarseness, coarse dry skin, typical facies, bradycardia and delayed relaxation of the tendon jerks), mild hypothyroidism with minor and non-specific symptoms that are common in elderly people, and subclinical hypothyroidism in which increased TSH output maintains thyroid function. Atypical presentations include faecal impaction, deafness, angina, anaemia, depression, dementia, paraesthesia, muscle or joint discomfort, neuropathies and coma. Goitre symptoms usually depend more on its position than its size. If retrosternal, effort dyspnoea, dyspnoea with certain postures and dysphagia may occur.

Investigation

A clinical diagnosis of hypothyroidism must be confirmed by investigation as lifelong therapy is required.

In overt hypothyroidism, measurement of free T4 levels will confirm the diagnosis and a high serum TSH will establish primary thyroid disease. In mild hypothyroidism routine tests may be borderline or normal. A normal TSH excludes primary hypothyroidism whereas a raised TSH level makes primary hypothyroidism the likely cause of the patient's symptoms and a trial of thyroxine justified. The TRH stimulation test is useful to clarify the thyroid status of the patient with borderline basal TSH levels. In subclinical hypothyroidism there is a low or low normal serum T4 but normal or slightly elevated serum T3 level maintaining euthyroidism in response to high TSH levels. If pituitary hypothyroidism is suspected other hypothalamic-pituitary functions should be tested.

The steps in investigation of suspected hypothyroidism are:

1. Measurement of free serum T4 level
   (a) Low — hypothyroidism established
   (b) Normal — hypothyroidism unlikely
   (c) Marginal, conflict with clinical impression or secondary hypothyroidism suspected — step 2
2. Measurement of serum TSH
   (a) High — establishes primary hypothyroidism
   (b) Normal — primary hypothyroidism excluded

   (c) Marginal, in conflict or normal with a low free T4 — step 3
3. TRH stimulation test
   (a) Exaggerated response — primary hypothyroidism
   (b) Delayed, impaired or normal response with a low free thyroxine level — consistent with a secondary hypothyroidism, exclude other endocrine deficiencies, X-ray pituitary fossa, visual field charting, etc.

Having assessed the state of metabolic function the cause of a goitre needs to be established. Country of origin, family history and drug history may provide useful clues. The presence of thyroid antibodies points to an autoimmune basis. The important question is whether the patient has thyroid cancer or not. Malignancy is suspected if one or more of the following features are present: a single thyroid nodule or asymmetrical enlargement; rapid increase in size; vocal cord paraesis; cervical lymphadenopathy, and/or a history of irradiation to the neck in childhood or adolescence. If malignancy is suspected, thyroid scanning (a hot nodule carries little risk whereas a cold thyroid nodule carries a 10–15% risk of malignancy), thyroid ultrasound (simple cysts are rarely malignant) and fine needle aspiration biopsy are useful.

Treatment

The treatment of choice for hypothyroidism is l-thyroxine. Thyroid extract has variable potency and T3 has no advantage over T4 apart from situations in which rapid correction of hypothyroidism is required. The optimal replacement dose for an individual patient is established by using gradual increments of T4 until the patient is asymptomatic and serum TSH and thyroid hormone levels are within the normal range. The daily maintenance dose usually lies between 0.1 mg and 0.2 mg. The elderly or patients with cardiac disease should be commenced on 0.05 mg or less daily.

Myxoedema coma (severe myxoedema with hypothermia and coma) is associated with a high mortality. Rewarming and correction of hypothyroidism must be gradual with careful monitoring to detect onset of arrythmias or cardiac failure. Hydrocortisone, intravenous fluids, oxygen, assisted respiration and treatment of infection may also be required.

Early diagnosis and treatment within 6 weeks of birth is essential in neonatal hypothyroidism to minimize mental retardation.

The treatment of non-toxic goitre without hypothyroidism depends on many factors. A small, soft, symmetrical goitre found incidentally does not usually require any therapy and it is wise to leave the patient unaware of its presence. If the patient has symptoms or if it is of significant size treatment with thyroxine is justified. There is usually a decrease in size in diffuse goitres within a few months but the more nodular the goitre the less chance there is of response. Surgery is indicated for cosmetic reasons, if there are pressure effects or if there is suspicion of malignancy.

THYROID CARCINOMA

Tumours of the thyroid arise mainly from three different groups of cells: (i) follicular cells give rise to papillary, follicular and anaplastic tumours, (ii) parafollicular cells give rise to medullary carcinoma and (iii) lymphocytes give rise to lymphomas. Papillary tumours are the commonest type followed by follicular, anaplastic, medullary and lymphoma. All, with the exception of medullary carcinoma, are more common in women. Papillary tumours usually present in late adolescence or early adult life, follicular tumours somewhat later, lymphomas in late middle age and anaplastic carcinomas in the elderly.

Differentiated carcinomas of follicular cell origin fall into two broadly different but overlapping types. 'Papillary' tumours are encapsulated, often multifocal, invade lymphatics and spread to lymph nodes. On histology they may have a pure papillary architecture or a mixture of follicules and papillae. 'Follicular' tumours are encapsulated, solitary, invade veins and spread characteristically to lung and bone. On histology they show a pure follicular pattern or a mixture of follicules and trabeculae. Both tumours are TSH dependent and may follow external neck irradiation. Anaplastic carcinomas of the spindle and giant cell type may arise from pre-existing differentiated carcinoma. Differentiated thyroid carcinomas have a very slow growth rate and can often be successfully treated even when disseminated. In addition to thyroidectomy, TSH-suppressive doses of thyroid hormone and radio-iodine (most differentiated tumours concentrate radio-iodine, although much less than normal thyroid tissue) may be appropriate and the choice will depend on the stage of the disease and other prognostic factors. If normal thyroid tissue has been ablated, the serum thyroglobulin can be used as a tumour marker. There is no significantly effective treatment for anaplastic thyroid cancer.

Medullary carcinoma is the only thyroid tumour where inheritance (20%) plays a major part and there are three disease patterns: medullary carcinoma alone, associated with phaeochromocytomas, or associated with phaeochromocytomas and mucosal neuromas. Calcitonin is secreted and is a useful tumour marker both in screening and in detecting recurrence. Histologically, the cells are distinctive with large nuclei and a characteristic finding is amyloid in the stroma. It is slow growing with early spread by lymphatics. Treatment is surgical with or without external radiotherapy but once it has spread beyond the thyroid, eradication is unlikely.

Thyroid lymphoma, which may be associated with chronic thyroiditis, has a similar presentation to undifferentiated carcinoma but responds to radiotherapy and/or chemotherapy.

REFERENCES AND FURTHER READING

Brennan M D 1980 Thyroid hormones. Mayo Clinic Proceedings 55: 33–44

Calder E A Irvine W J 1975 Cell-mediated immunity and immune complexes in thyroid disease. Clinics in Endocrinology and Metabolism 4:287–318

Enger D, Burger A J 1984 The deiodination of the iodothronines and of their derivatives in man. Endocrine Reviews 5: 151–184

Evered D, Hall R (eds) 1979 Hypothyroidism and goitre. Clinics in Endocrinology and Metabolism 8: 1–245

Hall R, Smith B R, Mukhtar E D 1975 Thyroid stimulators in health and disease. Clinical Endocrinology 4: 213–230

Hall R, Anderson J, Smart G A, Besser M (eds) 1980 Fundamentals of clinical endocrinology, 3rd edn. Pitman, London

Hamburger J I, Miller J M (eds) 1981 Controversies in clinical thyroidology. Springer-Verlag, New York

Ladenson P W 1985 Diseases of the thyroid gland. Clinics in Endocrinology and Metabolism 14: 145–174

Lever E G, Medeiros-neto G A, DeGroot L J 1983 Inherited disorders of thyroid metabolism. Endocrine Reviews 4: 213–239

Toft A D (ed) 1985 Hyperthyroidism. Clinics in Endocrinology and Metabolism 14: 249–511

Wartofsky L, Burman K D 1982 Alterations in thyroid function in patients with systemic illness: the 'euthyroid sick syndrome'. Endocrine Reviews 3: 184–217

Weetmen A P, McGregor A M 1984 Autoimmune thyroid disease: developments in our understanding. Endocrine Reviews 5: 309–355

Weiner S C, Ingbar S H (eds) 1978 The thyroid. A fundamental and clinical text, 4th edn. Harper & Row, London

Respiratory system

The preliminary paragraphs include a brief anatomical account, followed by a consideration of the mechanics of respiration, and the manner in which respiration is controlled. The main body of the chapter is devoted to those aspects of respiratory physiology which are of special importance in practical surgery. Successive sections deal with the assessment of respiratory function, the adjustments which take place after pneumonectomy, the effects of the various kinds of pneumothorax, the effects of injuries of the chest, the common postoperative chest complications, pulmonary embolism and the mechanism of pleural and tracheo-bronchial pain. Some non-respiratory functions of the lung are mentioned.

ANATOMY

A brief account of the structure of the air passages, the alveolo-capillary membrane and the pleura suffices as a preliminary to the discussion of respiratory function. For an account of the detailed arrangement of the bronchi the reader is referred to the standard monograph by Brock (1954). The smallest lung unit is the acinus, a pyramidal-shaped section of lung supplied by a single terminal bronchiole (Dilly, 1984) (Fig. 8.1).

The wall of the trachea and of the extra-pulmonary part of the bronchi is composed of a strong fibro-elastic membrane in which is embedded a series of C-shaped

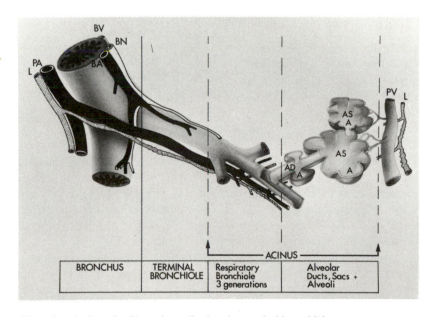

Fig. 8.1 Structure of the lung. The acinus is the unit of lung tissue distal to the terminal bronchiole.
PA, PV = Pulmonary Artery, Vein. BA, BV = Bronchial Artery, Vein. BN = bronchomotor nerve. L = Lymphatic. AD, AS = Alveolar Duct, Sac. A = Alveolus

cartilages. As the bronchi branch through 23 generations within the lung and become smaller, the cartilage is first reduced to irregular plates and nodules, and is finally lacking from the bronchioles. In the larger airways smooth muscle extends between the arms of the C-shaped cartilages and controls minor adjustments of bore, but in the smaller bronchi and bronchioles the muscle forms an investing lattice capable of almost obliterating the lumen when in spasm.

The submucosa of the conducting airways (trachea, bronchi and terminal bronchioles) which constitute the first 16 generations of passages contains lymphoid tissue, and both serous and mucous glands. It is surmounted by a ciliated columnar epithelium in which mucus-secreting goblet cells are interspersed. The cilia propel the surface mucus layer upwards. This important clearing action is inhibited by smoking, anticholinergic agents and general anaesthesia. In the final seven generations of passages (respiratory bronchioles, alveolar ducts and alveolar sacs) there is a transition to a predominantly squamous respiratory epithelium where gas exchange occurs. Two types of epithelial cell are seen here; Type I pneumocytes are flat cells which, with the pulmonary capillary endothelium and basement membrane constitute the alveolo-capillary membrane (Fig. 8.2). Type II pneumocytes are thicker and contain numerous osmophilic lamellar inclusion bodies. They play no part in gas exchange, but have a vital role in the production of surfactant. At the alveolar level collateral ventilation through pores of Kuhn exists. Other specialized cells found in the lungs include pulmonary alveolar macrophages, lymphocytes, plasma cells, amine precursor uptake and decarboxylation (APUD) cells and mast cells.

The alveolocapillary membrane is highly permeable to carbon dioxide and, to a lesser extent, to oxygen. In health, rapid diffusion of these gases across the membrane occurs along a partial pressure gradient. In disease processes involving the alveolocapillary membrane, such as fibrosing alveolitis, oxygen transport is more compromised than carbon dioxide transport.

The structural stability of the alveoli raises a problem in mechanics, for they might be expected to collapse under the influence of the surface tension of their walls (cf. the Law of Laplace which relates pressure in a bubble to its surface tension and radius; $P = 2T/R$). Their stability is due to the lining layer of surfactant, a complex 2-phase mixture of protein and lipid whose major constituent is the phospolipid dipalmatoylphosphatidylcholine. The surface tension of surfactant changes in a manner appropriate to the maintenance of stability as the alveoli expand and contract during inspiration and expiration, presumably as a result of changing intermolecular relationships in the surfactant layer. Surfactant appears in fetal lungs during the last trimester of pregnancy. Its relative deficiency in the premature neonate is responsible for the respiratory

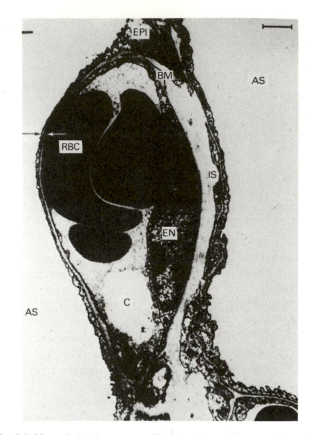

Fig. 8.2 Normal alveolar septum. The alveolar capillary membrane is composed of capillary endothelium, epithelium and interstitial space. Note thin portion (arrows) where fused basement membranes separate endothelium from epithelium and most of the gas exchange takes place. AS = alveolar space, EPI = Type I epithelial all, BM = basement membrane, IS = interstitial space, EN = endothelial cell, C = capillary. Horizontal bar represents 1 μm (After Fein A M, Goldberg S K, Lippmann M L, Fischer R & Morgan L, British Journal of Anaesthesia (1982), 54, 723)

distress syndrome (RDS), or hyaline membrane disease. Disruption of the surfactant layer may also be part of the pathophysiology of the adult respiratory distress syndrome (ARDS).

It is to be noted that the pulmonary arteries, like the bronchi, radiate from the hilum of the lung branching as they go (see Fig. 8.8c). Every bronchus is accompanied by a branch of the pulmonary artery (carrying deoxygenated blood) down to the alveolocapillary level. It is important to remember that the bronchial arteries, which are branches of the aorta, supply oxygenated blood to the bronchial tree as far as the terminal bronchioles. There is in health no anastomosis between the pulmonary and bronchial arteries though there may be some overspill of bronchial capillaries into the pulmonary capillaries. In certain inflammatory pulmonary diseases dilatation of this capillary anastomosis may lead to a physiologicallly significant shunt. The pulmonary veins are formed by tributaries which do not closely follow the bronchi, and drain into the left atrium. The bronchial veins drain into the azygos vein on the right, and into the accessory hemiazygos on the left.

The innervation of the lung is from the pulmonary plexus, formed at the hilum of the lung by the vagus, by branches from the upper four thoracic ganglia of the sympathetic chain, and by communications from the cardiac plexuses which are themselves formed by branches from the cervical portion of the vagus and branches from the cervical sympathetic ganglia. The cholinergic (parasympathetic) receptors of the lung cause bronchoconstriction. The β_2-adrenergic receptors are bronchodilator.

Sensory end organs, ovoid and unencapsulated, lie in the walls of the trachea and bronchi but not in the alveoli. Their nerve fibres pass centrally via the vagus nerve. Stretch receptors in the bronchial smooth muscle and J (juxtacapillary) receptors mediate the Hering Breuer inflation and deflation reflexes. Chemoreceptors mediating haemodynamic responses have been demonstrated in the pulmonary circulation but their physiological significance is uncertain.

The right and left pleurae are thin sero-elastic membranes lining each half of the thoracic cavity, and embryologically invaginated by the developing lung. The parietal pleura lining the chest wall and covering the diaphragm is exquisitely sensitive to pain, for nerve fibres derived from the intercostal nerves and the phrenic nerve ramify in the areolar tissue just outside the serous membrane. The visceral pleura is insensitive. In health the parietal and visceral layers of the pleura are separated only by a thin film of tissue fluid which serves as lubrication. if the pleura becomes inflamed it pours out an exudate of high specific gravity (over 1020) and rich in protein (more than 40 g/l). This exudate contains fibrin which coagulates on the pleura. The pleural transudate of cardiac failure and chronic nephritis has a lower specific gravity, a protein content less than 20 g/l, and lacks fibrin.

THE MECHANICS OF RESPIRATION

The mechanics of the respiratory system are dependent upon the interaction of its two fundamental constituents with elastic properties, the lungs and the 'chest wall', which includes the ribs, intercostal muscles and diaphragm. In the intact respiratory system the lung volume at the resting expiratory level is known as the functional residual capacity (FRC). At this point the elastic tendency of the chest wall to expand from the FRC is balanced by the tendency of the lung to retract (Fig. 8.3). The pleural cavity is the potential space which separates these two constituents, and as they tend to pull away from each other a subatmospheric intrapleural pressure of some $-2.5\,cmH_2O$ results. Though intrapleural pressure cannot easily be measured directly, it can be estimated by measurement of the pressure in the middle

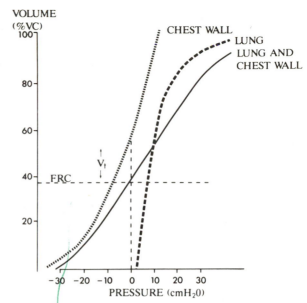

Fig. 8.3 Static pressure/volume relationships of the lungs and chest wall.

Note that the functional residual capacity (FRC) is the volume at which there is equilibrium between the expansile force of the chest wall and the retractile force of the lungs. The upper limit of inspiration (100% vital capacity–VC) is limited by the mechanical properties of the lungs, and the lower limit of expiration by the mechanical properties of the chest wall. The slope of the pressure/volume curve at any point represents the compliance at that volume, and is nearly linear in the mid-range.

of the oesophagus. To achieve inspiration by spontaneous respiration the inspiratory muscles must exert an expanding force upon the lungs up to the volume at which the isolated chest wall would come to rest. Beyond this point the muscles must also exert an expanding force upon the chest wall. During inspiration the intrapleural pressure becomes increasingly subatmospheric. Inspiration is limited by the mechanical properties of the lung.

Expiration occurs passively to the resting expiratory level beyond which the expiratory muscles must exert an elevating force on the diaphragm and a retracting force upon the chest wall. Forced expiration is limited by the mechanical properties of the chest wall, the isolated lung having a tendency to retract even further.

The static elastic properties of the lungs and the chest wall are described by their compliance, which is actually the reciprocal of elasticity. For the lung, volume can be plotted against the transpulmonary pressure gradient (pressure at the mouth-intrapleural pressure) and the compliance calculated as change in lung volume per unit change in pressure. Chest wall compliance may similarly be calculated by plotting volume against the transthoracic pressure gradient (intrapleural-atmospheric pressure). Over the middle range of lung volumes normal lung compliance is about $0.2\,l/cmH_2O$ and normal chest wall compliance about $0.1\,l/cmH_2O$.

Compliance, as we have seen, is a static property of the lung. Breathing is, however, a dynamic process and work must be done to overcome resistance to airflow within the lungs. Resistance is expressed as the pressure gradient necessary to move a unit volume of gas in unit time. Normal airway resistance at FRC is about 1 cmH$_2$O/l/s. The single most important factor responsible for airway resistance is the radius of the airway, and resistance is inversely proportional to a power of the radius, which can theoretically be anywhere between r^2 or r^5 depending upon the flow conditions. A reduction in airway radius (by bronchoconstriction or intraluminal obstruction) therefore causes a rise in resistance. In health about half the overall airway resistance is from the nasopharynx and larynx, and the remainder in the trachea and smaller airways. The very small airways contribute little to airway resistance as the sum of their cross-sectional areas is considerably greater than the sum of the cross-sectional areas of the larger airways.

Changes in the mechanical properties of the lungs and chest wall due to age, disease, surgery or even posture will result in changes in the FRC and work of breathing. For a more detailed treatise of the mechanics of respiration the reader is referred to Nunn (1977).

The expansion of the chest cavity during inspiration is brought about by contraction of the diaphragm and by rotation of the ribs. The axis of rotation of the ribs is oblique, so that when ribs are drawn upwards the thoracic cage expands both laterally and forwards. During this movement contraction of the external intercostals raises the lower ribs towards the first two ribs which are themselves prevented from descending by contraction of the scalenes. In forced inspiration added elevation of the chest wall is gained by contraction of accessory muscles — the sternomastoids, pectorals, trapezii, rhomboids and serratus anterior.

Quiet expiration is brought about by relaxation of the inspiratory muscles, aided by the elastic recoil of the lungs. In forced expiration the abdominal muscles contract and force the diaphragm up from below.

The total work of quiet breathing is very small. Even during exercise in health the energy cost of breathing represents only about 3% of the total expenditure. However, in the critically-ill patient with low pulmonary compliance, poor gas exchange and low cardiac output the high work of breathing may demand a high proportion of the total available oxygen and lead to metabolic acidosis and a rapid downward spiral which can only be helped by muscular paralysis and intermittent positive pressure ventilation (IPPV). Recent work has focused on the importance of respiratory muscle fatigue in respiratory failure (Cohen et al, 1982).

During manual or mechanical ventilation the transpulmonary pressure gradient required to inflate the lungs is achieved by applying a positive pressure at the mouth or airway; hence the term intermittent positive pressure ventilation. During the inspiratory phase of IPPV the intrapleural pressure becomes increasingly positive and this pressure is transmitted to the other intrathoracic structures, including the heart and great vessels. Decreased venous return accounts in part for the reduction in cardiac output which may occur during IPPV. Positive end-expiratory pressure (PEEP) is commonly used to improve arterial oxygenation in critically-ill ventilated patients. By maintaining a positive airway pressure during expiration the lung volume at the expiratory level (FRC) is increased.

REGULATION OF RESPIRATION

The muscles of respiration are innervated by lower motor neurones within the phrenic (C3, 4, 5), cervical and intercostal nerves; breathing stops if the cord is transected above the level of C3. Automatic rhythmic breathing is controlled by a respiratory centre in the brainstem; complete absence of respiratory effort is a feature of the clinical syndrome of brain death (Conference of the Medical Royal Colleges and their Faculties in the United Kingdom, 1976, 1979).

Breathing can also be controlled voluntarily by cortical activity via the corticospinal tracts. This fact is spectacularly demonstrated in the syndrome of Ondine's Curse in which the automatic pathways fail.

Reciprocal innervation of the respiratory muscles brings about relaxation of the expiratory muscles during inspiration and vice-versa. This phenomenon is not a spinal reflex, rather efferent impulses appear to simultaneously inhibit and excite the appropriate muscles, probably by exciting inhibitory interneurones.

The respiratory centre

The 'respiratory centre' (Fig. 8.4) is in the medulla oblongata, and consists of two anatomically distinct groups of neurones, the ventral (VRG) and dorsal (DRG) groups. Within both groups inspiratory (I) and expiratory (E) neurones can be identified by their pattern of discharge during the respiratory cycle. The DRG is in proximity to the tractus solitarius on each side and drives the diaphragm via the contralateral phrenic lower motor neurones. It possesses inherent rhythmicity and controls the VRG. The cranial division of the VRG is in the nucleus ambiguus and drives the accessory muscles of respiration via the ipsilateral lower cranial nerves, while the caudal division in the nucleus retroambigualis drives the intercostal muscles via the ipsilateral and contralateral intercostal nerves. The Botzinger complex is a group of expiratory neurones anatomically situated in the nucleus retroambigualis and therefore intimately associated with the VRG. These expiratory neurones discharge rhythmically, inhibiting the

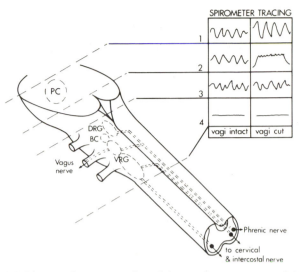

Fig. 8.4 Diagramatic representation of the respiratory neurons of the left side of the brainstem. Effects of transection at the level of 1 upper pons, 2 lower pons, 3 medulla and 4 spinal cord are shown. PC = pneumotaxic centre (nucleus parabrachialis); BC = Botzinger complex (nucleus retroambigualis). VRG = ventrolateral respiratory group (nucleus retroambigualis & nucleus ambiguus). DRG = dorsomedial respiratory group (nucleus tractus solitarius)

inspiratory neurones of both the VRG and DRG (Long & Duffin, 1984).

Two higher brainstem centres exert a modifying effect on the rhythmicity of the medullary respiratory centre but their precise physiological role is unclear. Lower pontine transection in vagotomized, anaesthetized animals results in the arrest of respiration in inspiration (apneusis), suggesting the presence of an 'apneustic centre' in the region of the floor of the fourth ventricle. However, respiratory neurones are rarely found here and the existence of such a centre is presently in doubt. Rhythmic respiration continues if the vagi are left intact. The pneumotaxic centre is in the nucleus parabrachialis within the upper part of the pons. It inhibits apneusis and facilitates rhythmic breathing (Mitchell & Berger, 1975).

Respiratory reflexes from the lung

Several reflexes can be elicited from the lungs, especially in anaesthetized animals, but their importance in man is uncertain.

Inflation and deflation reflexes, eponymously called the Hering-Breuer reflexes, are initiated by stimulation of the stretch receptors and J-receptors respectively and cause a vagally-mediated inhibition of inspiration or expiration. The J-receptors (deflation) are particularly sensitive to pulmonary congestion and embolisation and may contribute to the rapid shallow respiration seen in these conditions.

Irritation of receptors in the mucosa of the larger air passages leads to the expulsive reflex of coughing. The act of coughing involves irregular deep inspiration followed by

a series of forced expirations through the suddenly-opening glottis, preceding which the intrathoracic pressure may rise as high as 40 kPa. In addition, coughing is accompanied by reflex bronchoconstriction; both the afferent and efferent components of this reflex arc are contained in the vagi. It is a familiar and important observation that the cough reflex is attenuated by atropine and opiates, and abolished by anaesthesia. Until the cough reflex is regained, the unconscious patient must be safeguarded from the risk of inhaling vomitus.

Other respiratory reflexes

Apart from reflexes from receptors in the lungs, respiration is modified by many reflexes originating elsewhere. Sneezing is another expulsive reflex. Talking, swallowing, laughing and crying, pain and emotion are all associated with adjustment of the respiratory pattern. Exercise leads to increased ventilation of the lungs, mediated at least in part by stimulation of proprioceptors in muscles, tendons and joints. Important reflexes also originate from respiratory muscle spindles. The respiratory effects of baroreceptor reflexes are minor. Pulmonary and myocardial chemoreceptor reflexes demonstrated experimentally are probably insignificant.

Chemical control of respiration

The single most important factor in the control of respiration is the carbon dioxide tension (P_{CO_2}) of blood perfusing the medullary chemoreceptors which are anatomically distinct from the cells of the respiratory centre. Respiratory adjustments also occur to combat increases in blood hydrogen ion concentration (i.e. fall in pH) and dangerous falls in the oxygen tension (P_{O_2}) of arterial blood.

Carbon dioxide is a very soluble gas and readily crosses the blood/brain and blood/CSF barriers. Changes in arterial P_{CO_2} produce a rapid change in the P_{CO_2} of brain interstitial fluid and CSF, and consequently a change in brain and CSF pH as CO_2 combines with water and forms carbonic acid:

$$CO_2 + H_2O \rightleftharpoons H_2CO_3 \rightleftharpoons H^+ + HCO_3$$

A rising arterial P_{CO_2} produces a parallel rise in CSF and brain hydrogen ion concentration. The fall in pH stimulates the medullary chemoreceptors, increasing the rate and depth of respiration. CO_2 excretion is thereby increased, tending to restore the arterial P_{CO_2}. A fall in arterial P_{CO_2} has an opposite effect, leading to diminished respiration and even periods of apnoea. The peripheral chemoreceptors of the carotid and aortic bodies are innervated by the glossopharyngeal nerves and vagi; they are also sensitive to P_{CO_2} but play a very minor role in maintenance of normocapnia.

A fall in arterial pH stimulates the peripheral chemo-receptors, increasing respiratory centre activity and ventilation of the lungs. The consequent fall in $P\text{CO}_2$ tends to restore blood pH to normal. This is the mechanism of 'air hunger' or Kussmaul breathing seen in diabetic keto-acidosis. Conversely, metabolic alkalosis produces very little respiratory depression. The blood/brain barrier is relatively impermeable to the hydrogen ion, so that changes in arterial pH are only slowly transmitted to the medullary chemoreceptors.

A fall in the $P\text{O}_2$ of arterial blood perfusing the aortic and carotid bodies to about 8 kPa begins to cause stimulation of the chemoreceptors and to increase the rate and depth of respiration. Stagnant hypoxia of the chemoreceptors is in part responsible for the hyperventilation seen in circulatory shock. A rise in $P\text{O}_2$ does not depress respiration. The direct central effect of hypoxia is to depress the respiratory centre.

RESPIRATORY FUNCTION TESTS

The efficiency with which the lungs add oxygen to the blood and remove carbon dioxide depends upon three factors: the pulmonary ventilation, the pulmonary circulation and the rapidity of gaseous exchange. Respiratory function testing is a large and complex subject; the interested reader may refer to standard texts such as Cotes 1979. This discussion will be restricted to those tests of respiratory function which may be applicable in routine surgical practice. We shall begin by defining the terminology of lung volume measurements.

Terminology of lung volume measurements

A simplified scheme is shown in Figure 8.5. The total lung capacity (TLC) is the maximum volume of gas within the lungs during a powerful inspiration, and the residual volume (RV) is the smallest volume that must remain despite maximal expiration. The difference between these two volumes is the vital capacity (VC), and this denotes the greatest volume of gas that can be exhaled after a full inspiration: the vital capacity is measured without reference to the speed of expiration, and in this minor respect differs from the forced vital capacity (FVC). The functional residual capacity is the volume of gas remaining in the lungs after normal passive expiration. The resting tidal volume (V_t) is the volume of gas taken in from the exterior during any quiet single inspiration, but not all of this reaches the lungs. Thus the resting tidal volume in the adult is about 450 ml, but of this only some 300 ml reaches the alveoli (the alveolar ventilation), and the rest fills the conducting airways down to the respiratory bronchioles. The volume of these passages is known as the anatomical dead space.

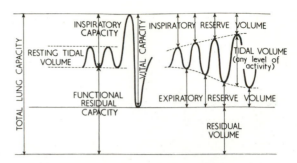

Fig. 8.5 Diagram illustrating the terminology of 'lung volume' measurements (after Papperheimer, 1950). In fact, increasing tidal volume encroaches mostly on inspiratory reserve volume; FRC reduced by only 15% at highest exercise tidal volumes.

Gases are exchanged partly by mass movement into the alveoli which dilate during inspiration, but more importantly by boundary diffusion between the respiratory bronchioles and the alveoli. In the normal subject at rest all alveoli are not equally ventilated; some receive more and others less than their share of inspired air. This has the effect of making the deadspace measured by physiological techniques larger than the anatomical deadspace. The total volume of the inspired air which does not take part in gaseous exchange is known as the physiological dead space. (V_D), and this averages about 150 ml for young men and about 100 ml for young women. It should be noted, however, that this varies with age, posture and depth of respiration; it rarely exceeds 250 ml.

The minute volume is the volume of air breathed in one minute and is therefore the product of the respiratory rate and the mean tidal volume. The alveolar ventilation is the volume of air participating in gas exchange each minute, i.e. $(V_t - V_D) \times$ respiratory rate. The alveolar ventilation is inversely proportional to the arterial CO_2 tension.

Spirometry

Spirometers are simple to use at the bedside and may provide valuable information in the clinical setting. The subject makes a maximal inspiration and then exhales forcibly and maximally into the spirometer. The healthy subject expels 80% of his FVC in 1 second, the forced expiratory volume 1 second (FEV_1), and the rest in a further 2 or 3 seconds (Fig. 8.6). Simple analysis of the data thus obtained from patients gives information about restrictive and obstructive patterns of ventilatory dysfunction. Tables of predicted normal values for age, weight and sex are available. Both obstructive and restrictive defects cause a reduction in the FVC, but the FEV_1/FVC ratio is reduced to less than 75% in patients with an obstructive defect. The reversibility of any detected airway obstruction may be tested by administering a bronchodilator such as nebulised salbutamol 200 μg and then repeating spirometry. In the assessment of patients for pneumonectomy

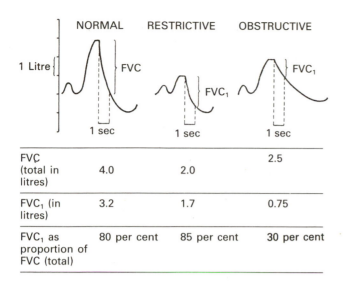

	NORMAL	RESTRICTIVE	OBSTRUCTIVE
FVC (total in litres)	4.0	2.0	2.5
FVC$_1$ (in litres)	3.2	1.7	0.75
FVC$_1$ as proportion of FVC (total)	80 per cent	85 per cent	30 per cent

Fig. 8.6 Spirograms during forced expiration. The tracing labelled 'restrictive' was from a patient with restricted rib movement owing to kyphoscoliosis, and the tracing labelled 'obstructive' from a patient with emphysema. FVC denotes total forced expiratory volume, and FVC$_1$ the forced expiratory volume in one second. Note that FVC is reduced in both restrictive and obstructive disease: the ratio of FVC$_1$ to FVC remains normal in restrictive disease but is reduced in obstructive disease. (Campbell E J M, Dickinson C J, Slater, J H D 1974 Clinical Physiology, 4th edition, p 142 Oxford: Blackwell.)

FEV$_1$ less than 1 l, or FVC less than 2 l is considered adverse.

The peak expiratory flow rate (PEFR) can be simply measured with a peak flow meter. Changes in PEFR tend to parallel changes in FEV$_1$/FVC in patients with obstructive airways disease.

The maximum breathing capacity (MBC), otherwise known as the maximum ventilatory volume (MVV), is sometimes used in the assessment of patients considered for pulmonary resection. The maximum volume of air which can be voluntarily hyperventilated through a low resistance circuit in 15 seconds is determined, multiplied by four and expressed as MBC in l/min. A value of less than 48 l/min is widely regarded as a contraindication to pulmonary resection.

Lung volume

Measurement of the total lung capacity by whole body plethysmography or inert gas dilution is a specialized technique which rarely gives more clinically useful information than simpler measurements such as FVC. FRC may also be measured by these methods. Closing volume is the volume at which airway closure begins, and may be measured by the special technique of nitrogen wash-out. The proximity of closing volume to FRC in the very young and elderly may be important in the tendency of these patient to develop more severe postoperative hypoxaemia when the FRC falls.

Pulmonary circulation

The pulmonary circulation is a low pressure system. The mean pulmonary arterial pressure is about one-sixth the systemic arterial pressure, yet this suffices to maintain the same volume flow rate through the lungs as through the systemic circuit. It is evident that the arteriolar resistance of the lungs must be low. Large increases in cardiac output (for example, during exercise) produce only a small rise in pulmonary arterial pressure, indicating that the arteriolar resistance in the lungs, already low, can be reduced still further in high output states. This is attributable to the distensibility of the pulmonary vessels, to dilatation of open arterioles, and to the recruitment of previously collapsed arterioles. Consequently pulmonary hypertension does not result from localized disease in the lungs, or even from resection of a whole lung. Hypertension does, however, result from generalized pulmonary disease such as emphysema or pulmonary fibrosis, and it can also result from mitral stenosis or patent ductus arteriosus. Pulmonary arterial pressure can be monitored with a pulmonary arterial balloon flotation catheter which is advanced from a central vein through the right heart to the pulmonary artery. When the inflated balloon wedges in a branch of the pulmonary artery the pressure distal to it approximates to the left atrial pressure (Fig. 8.8b). As the balloon obstructs a branch of the pulmonary artery it must always be deflated after determination of the pulmonary artery wedge pressure (PAWP). Normal pulmonary arterial systolic pressure is 18–30 mmHg, diastolic 7–12 mmHg, wedge pressure 4–12 mmHg. Pulmonary hypertension may be said to be present when the mean pulmonary arterial pressure exceeds 20 mmHg. High PAWP is associated with a high microvascular hydrostatic pressure which tends to increase the fluid filtration rate across the pulmonary capillary endothelium to the interstitial space and thereby predispose to accumulation of extravascular lung water, as seen in the pulmonary oedema of fluid overload or heart failure. Other determinants of the fluid filtration rate are the oncotic pressure gradient between the blood and pulmonary interstitium and the permeability of the capillary endothelium. Pulmonary oedema without raised PAWP is a feature of the adult respiratory distress syndrome, in which a pulmonary capillary permeability defect has been demonstrated. Measurement of extravascular lung water volume at the bedside is possible in clinical practice. The application of pulmonary arterial pressure monitoring the respiratory function testing to the monitoring of critically-ill patients is discussed by Weidemann et al (1984).

Gas exchange in the lungs

The transfer of oxygen to the tissues depends upon a series of partial pressure gradients known as the oxygen cascade

Table 8.1

Partial pressure kPa (mmHg)	Atmospheric air	Alveolar air	Arterial blood	Tissues	Venous blood
(PO_2)	20.30 (152)	14.00 (105)	13.33 (100)	2.67 to 0 (20 to 0)	About 5.33 (40)
(PCO_2)	0.03 (0.2)	5.33 (40)	5.33 (40)	8.00 (60)	6.13 (46)

(Table 8.1). Mixed venous blood in the pulmonary artery has an oxygen tension of about 5.3 kPa. Most of this blood is exposed to a PO_2 of 13.7 kPa at the alveolo-capillary membrane but an inevitable degree of venous admixture means that the PO_2 of arterial blood does not normally exceed 13.3 kPa. Venous admixture even in normal subjects occurs via Thebesian veins, the broncho-pulmonary capillary anastomosis and a degree of ventilation/perfusion mismatch. In the systemic capillaries oxygen diffuses from red cells down a pressure gradient to tissue cell mitochondria where it is utilised. The important mechanisms of oxygen transport are discussed elsewhere (p. 481).

A similar series of pressure gradients facilitates the excretion of carbon dioxide produced by the energy-producing metabolic oxidation of fats and carbohydrates. The high solubility of carbon dioxide is illustrated by the very small mixed venous blood/alveolar gas pressure gradient (0.9 kPa) required for the excretion of some 200 ml CO_2 per minute into alveolar gas from the pulmonary capillaries. In contrast, the transfer of some 250 ml O_2 per minute in the reverse direction requires a partial pressure gradient of some 8.4 kPa.

Neither ventilation nor perfusion are uniformly distributed throughout the normal lung. Perfusion of under-ventilated alveoli is wasted, contributing to the venous admixture which tends to lower the arterial PO_2. Also, ventilation of underperfused alveoli is wasted, contributing to the difference between physiological and anatomical deadspace and increasing the arterial PCO_2 at any given minute volume. The minute volume is some 5 l/min in the fit adult male, and the pulmonary blood flow (or cardiac output) 6 l/min, which gives an overall ventilation/perfusion ratio (V/Q) of 0.85. Both ventilation and perfusion tend to increase in the more dependent part of the lungs but the change is more striking in the case of perfusion with the result that the V/Q ratio tends to decrease from apex to base in the upright position (Fig. 8.7). The scatter of ratios throughout the lung determines the efficiency of gas exchange. Diffuse pulmonary disease, such as chronic bronchitis and emphysema, results in a gross increase in the scatter of ratios and is the commonest cause of hypoxaemia in these disorders. Similar disturbances occur during anaesthesia even in patients with normal lungs. For a full and lucid discussion of ventilation/perfusion relationships the reader is recommended to the work of West (1979, 1982).

The permeability of the alveolocapillary membrane to gas transfer can be assessed by measuring the gas transfer and transfer coefficient of carbon monoxide in the laboratory. As has previously been stated, reduced gas transfer has a more pronounced effect on oxygen than the more soluble carbon dioxide.

Facilities for blood gas analysis are widely available in modern hospitals. Determination of arterial blood gases in the patient with serious postoperative and traumatic respiratory complications is essential to the proper management of these disorders. While a mild degree of hypoxaemia can be treated with added inspired oxygen, refractory hypercapnia and severe hypoxaemia demand the institution of IPPV before cardiorespiratory arrest ensues. Care should be exercised in giving added oxygen to certain patients with emphysema, the 'blue bloaters', who may be dependent upon hypoxaemia to provide respiratory drive via the peripheral chemoreceptors.

CARDIORESPIRATORY ADJUSTMENTS TO PNEUMONECTOMY

The immediate effects of exclusion of a lung, uncomplicated by an open chest incision, have been studied in experimental animals. The late effects of pneumonectomy are known from clinical experience.

Immediate effects of exclusion of one lung

Exclusion of one lung by tightening a slip knot round the lung root of a spontaneously-breathing animal (Long et al, 1949) causes a temporary increase in pulmonary arterial pressure, which returns to baseline values within an hour. Effects on cardiac output are inconstant but, in the healthy lung, overall pulmonary arteriolar resistance is reduced. Ventilation of the remaining lung is increased in rate and depth to maintain normocapnia, and the total uptake of oxygen is not reduced.

Effects of pneumonectomy in man

Following pneumonectomy the chest is closed, often without a drain, and the air within the empty hemithorax is slowly absorbed to be replaced by a serosanguinous fluid. In the first few hours after pneumonectomy the midline position of the mediastinum can be maintained by ensuring a small negative end-expiratory pressure within the empty hemithorax (about -5 cmH$_2$O). The Maxwell

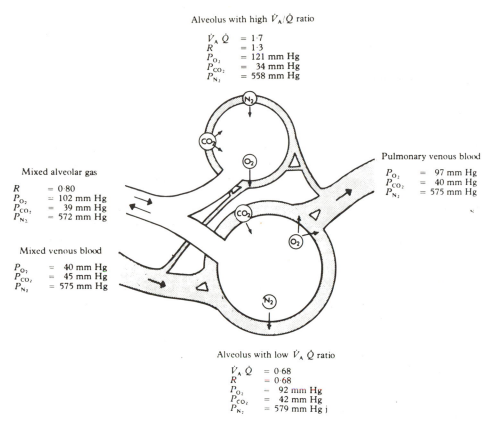

Alveolus with high $\dot{V}_A/\dot{Q}$ ratio

$$
\begin{array}{ll}
\dot{V}_A \dot{Q} & = 1\cdot7 \\
R & = 1\cdot3 \\
P_{O_2} & = 121 \text{ mm Hg} \\
P_{CO_2} & = 34 \text{ mm Hg} \\
P_{N_2} & = 558 \text{ mm Hg}
\end{array}
$$

Pulmonary venous blood

$$
\begin{array}{ll}
P_{O_2} & = 97 \text{ mm Hg} \\
P_{CO_2} & = 40 \text{ mm Hg} \\
P_{N_2} & = 575 \text{ mm Hg}
\end{array}
$$

Mixed alveolar gas

$$
\begin{array}{ll}
R & = 0\cdot80 \\
P_{O_2} & = 102 \text{ mm Hg} \\
P_{CO_2} & = 39 \text{ mm Hg} \\
P_{N_2} & = 572 \text{ mm Hg}
\end{array}
$$

Mixed venous blood

$$
\begin{array}{ll}
P_{O_2} & = 40 \text{ mm Hg} \\
P_{CO_2} & = 45 \text{ mm Hg} \\
P_{N_2} & = 575 \text{ mm Hg}
\end{array}
$$

Alveolus with low $\dot{V}_A \dot{Q}$ ratio

$$
\begin{array}{ll}
\dot{V}_A \dot{Q} & = 0\cdot68 \\
R & = 0\cdot68 \\
P_{O_2} & = 92 \text{ mm Hg} \\
P_{CO_2} & = 42 \text{ mm Hg} \\
P_{N_2} & = 579 \text{ mm Hg j}
\end{array}
$$

Fig. 8.7 Variation in ventilation and perfusion in different areas of the lungs (after Cotes J E, 1965, Lung Function — Assessment and Application in Medicine, Oxford: Blackwell).

box is a device which enables the pressure within the pneumonectomy space to be measured and adjusted by aspiration or injection of air.

In patients who have undergone pneumonectomy a normal cardiac output can be maintained through the remaining lung without pulmonary arterial hypertension because of dilatation and recruitment of pulmonary capillaries. There is, however, an inevitable reduction in the maximum cardiac output which can be accommodated (for example, during exercise) without a rise in pulmonary arterial pressure.

After pneumonectomy displacement of the mediastinum during deep inspiration allows increased expansion of the remaining lung. Provided that the lung does not become overdistended, the maximum breathing capacity remains good. Mediastinal shift during deep inspiration can, however, have the effect of stimulating the trachea and causing troublesome cough. In patients with initially impaired respiratory reserve, pneumonectomy may result in post-operative respiratory failure. Selection of patients with generalised pulmonary disease for pneumonectomy is aided by a number of tests, some of which have been mentioned. It is impossible to predict the prognosis for pneumonectomy in any individual patient, but the

following findings would generally be considered adverse signs (Gothard & Branthwaite, 1982):

1. MBC < 50% predicted, or less than about 40 l/min
2. $FEV_1 < 1$ l
3. FVC < 2 l
4. FEV_1/FVC < 50%
5. Pulmonary hypertension at rest or following balloon occlusion of the relevant pulmonary artery
6. Gas transfer of carbon monoxide < 50% predicted
7. Hypercapnia at rest, $P_a CO_2 > 6$ kPa

The cardiorespiratory response to exercise provides a rough guide to fitness for surgery in uncomplicated cases.

PNEUMOTHORAX

The term pneumothorax denotes the presence of air in the pleural cavity. In an open pneumothorax, as in surgical thoracotomy, air can pass freely in and out of the pleural cavity. In a closed pneumothorax, which may result from disease or injury of the lung, the air which has entered the pleural cavity is not free to escape. In tension pneumothorax, which most often results from injury to the lung, there is a valvular leak which allows air to enter but not leave the pleural space thereby causing progressive respiratory distress. All forms of pneumothorax interfere with lung expansion by disturbing the normal intrapleural pressure.

Open pneumothorax

When the pleural space is laid open the intrapleural pressure becomes atmospheric and, in the spontaneously breathing subject, the transpulmonary pressure gradient disappears allowing the lung to collapse by elastic recoil. Negative intrapleural pressure in the opposite intact hemithorax produces mediastinal shift in that direction, and inspiratory effort by increasing the negative pressure increases the shift. The resulting to-and-fro movement reduces the efficiency with which the lung can be ventilated. 'Paradoxical respiration', by which air discharged from the collapsing lung is inhaled into the good lung further reducing the efficiency of ventilation, is probably unimportant in clinical practice.

The loss of negative intrapleural pressure, particularly of the right hemithorax, would theoretically hamper venous return to the heart, but in practice simple open pneumothorax does not have detrimental effects on the circulation unless it produces respiratory failure.

Management during thoracotomy

When the chest is to be opened deliberately, steps are taken to prevent respiratory embarrassment. After induction of anaesthesia the trachea is intubated and IPPV instituted. The transpulmonary pressure gradient is then not affected by opening the chest, and the lung does not collapse. Inflation of the opposite lung supports the mediastinum and prevents shift.

A 'double-lumen tube' may be used to isolate the good lung and protect it from pus or secretions or, more commonly in modern practice, to allow deflation of the lung to be operated on. There are many varieties of such tubes, but the Robertshaw is perhaps the most widely used. The left Robertshaw tube has a left bronchial lumen with a bronchial cuff to isolate the left lung, and a tracheal lumen with tracheal cuff which ventilates the right lung. When the right hemithorax is opened the ventilation may be directed solely to the left lung and the right lung allowed to deflate by opening the tracheal lumen to atmosphere. During one-lung anaesthesia there is significant venous admixture through the collapsing, unventilated lung and the anaesthetist must take steps to minimise hypoxaemia. The right Robertshaw tube has a right bronchial lumen with a hole in the upper surface through the bronchial balloon to allow ventilation of the right upper lobe bronchus, which opens within 2 cm of the carina,

during surgery on the left lung. It is therefore technically more difficult to position a right-side endobronchial tube correctly. 'Bronchial blockers', with a narrow suction catheter to aspirate distal secretions, can be selectively placed within the bronchial tree to facilitate surgery but are rarely used today. High frequency ventilation of the lung has been used very recently during anaesthesia for thoracic surgery, and may be the technique of choice in the presence of bronchopleural fistula (Sjostrand, 1983). Before closure of the chest, the collapsed lung must be thoroughly re-expanded usually by controlled manual ventilation. The surgeon may aid this process by manually restraining the inflation of already-expanded segments thereby directing gas to the collapsed segments. A chest drain is often, but not always, inserted and connected to an underwater drainage bottle which does not allow air to enter the pleural space.

It is routine practice to X-ray the chest several hours after thoracotomy in order to verify that the lung is fully expanded.

Closed pneumothorax

A closed pneumothorax can result from laceration of the lung in crushing injuries, or from rupture of an emphysematous bulla.

In crushing injuries the lung is lacerated by the sharp end of a fractured rib; as the rib at once springs back into alignment, X-ray films give little indication of the initial displacement of the fracture. Air escapes from the lung into the pleural space, but the laceration becomes sealed as the lung collapses. The ill-effects of a closed pneumothorax are virtually limited to the partial or total collapse of one lung, and in contrast to open pneumothorax there is little disturbance of the opposite lung. Displacement of the mediastinum is slight, for the pressure in the pneumothorax remains negative. Also, what little mediastinal shift occurs during respiration is helpful to the good lung; there is increased negative pressure in the pneumothorax during inspiration, pulling the mediastinum and helping the good lung to inflate. Also, during expiration the mediastinum shifts slightly in the opposite direction, aiding deflation. The air trapped in the pleural space is gradually absorbed in about 10–14 days, and the lung usually re-expands. However, this delayed re-expansion cannot be relied upon in traumatic pneumothorax, for if the initial injury gives rise to haemorrhage or an intrapleural effusion the lung may become covered with an unyielding coagulum of fibrin. Further, institution of IPPV may convert a closed pneumothorax into a tension pneumothorax. In order to secure early re-expansion of the lung and protection against development of tension pneumothorax, the air within the pneumothorax should routinely be removed by insertion of a chest drain.

Tension pneumothorax

The valvular tear of the lung, which allows progressively more and more air to enter the pleural cavity, results most often from crushing injuries without any penetration wound of the chest wall, less often from disease of the lung, and less often still from penetrating injuries whose tract through the chest wall becomes sealed. A tension pneumothorax is often accompanied by haemothorax.

The mounting pressure in the pleural cavity leads to collapse of the lung, to progressive displacement of the mediastinum, and to compression of the opposite lung. Venous return to the heart is impeded and circulatory shock with asphyxiation ensues. IPPV only accelerates the process (cf IPPV and open pneumothorax during thoracotomy.) The emergency treatment is to allow the air in the pleural space to flow off through a wide-bore needle thrust through an intercostal space, but this cannot be relied upon and no time must be lost in placing a large chest drain, which is connected to an underwater seal. The usual site of insertion is in the second interspace in the mid-clavicular line anteriorly.

INJURIES OF THE CHEST

The mechanism, the effects, and the broad principles of treatment of the various kinds of chest injury merit brief discussion. These injuries may be classified as blunt or penetrating. Blunt injuries fall conveniently into three main categories:

1. Direct trauma to the chest wall
2. Compression of the thoracic contents
3. Sudden deceleration injuries

In clinical practice these injuries commonly occur in combination.

1. Direct injuries to the chest wall may be associated with simple fracture of the ribs, the pain of which leads to restriction of the depth of respiration, tachypnoea and suppression of cough.

Strapping the chest is almost certainly of no value. Provision of adequate analgesia immediately improves respiration and coughing; the form of analgesia used will depend upon the individual patient's requirements and the resources available. Intramuscular or intravenous administration of opiates such as morphine or pethidine is often necessary. The newer opioid buprenorphine may be given sublingually, and may be effective in some cases. When coughing is being encouraged by the physiotherapist a few breaths of Entonox (50% oxygen, 50% nitrous oxide) will dull the worst of the pain. In unilateral injuries intercostal or paravertebral nerve blocks with bupivicaine give several hours pain relief, following which, the returning pain is often less severe. Recently, thoracic epidural analgesia has been used in more severe chest injuries, and may reduce the requirement for IPPV. Local anaesthetics at this level cause sympathetic blockade with a risk of hypotension and so should only be used in the intensive care unit. Epidural opiates, particularly morphine and diamorphine, give good analgesia without autonomic or motor blockade or respiratory depression in many patients.

The possibility of underlying pulmonary contusions must never be overlooked even in a case of a simple fracture of the ribs (Figs 8.8a, b, c,). Repeated blood gas analysis and chest radiography will confirm the presence or absence of progressive deterioration in lung function.

2. Compression of the thoracic contents occurs most commonly when there is a sudden and often sustained squeezing of the chest wall, for instance when an individual is trapped beneath fallen masonry or in a collapsed trench. The condition is characterized by a diffuse ecchymosis of the skin of the face, neck and upper chest (Fig. 8.9). The surge of blood, driven out of the thorax, over-distends the veins and ruptures many of the small venules, giving rise to multiple tiny haemorrhages in the skin and conjunctivae. Dusky blue discolouration of the skin disappears over the course of 2 or 3 weeks.

In the condition known as blast lung, waves of high pressure may damage the lung without causing rib fractures or an open wound. The sudden concussion of the chest leads to multiple haemorrhages in the lungs, often to lacerations of the lung tissues, and occasionally even to the tearing of large vessels. Oedema of the injured lungs increases during the first few hours, and because of this the victim's condition usually deteriorates during the early period after rescue. Similar high pressure waves are generated by high-velocity penetrating missile injuries (e.g. rifle bullets).

3. The third type of blunt chest injury most often results from sudden deceleration such as that occurring in road traffic accidents. The injuries to the chest represent a combination of the effects of initial impact on the thoracic wall and the continuing momentum of the thoracic organs. The impact may lead to a 'stove-in' chest in which several ribs may be fractured in two places, most often at the sites of maximum curvature which lie posteriorly at the outer edge of erector spinae and anterolaterally (Fig. 8.10). The affected segment of chest wall, the 'flail' segment, is loose and moves paradoxically with respiration, sinking in with inspiration and floating outwards on expiration. If the flail segment is large, this paradoxical movement gives rise to the same difficulties as an open pneumothorax. The impact and momentum forces together produce damage of the thoracic contents to a greater or lesser degree. Bleeding may occur from torn intercostal vessels or from damage to the lung or mediastinum. Occasionally the forces are so great as to cause

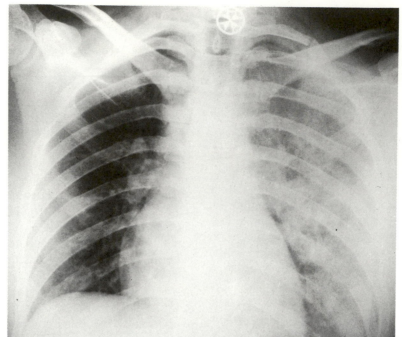

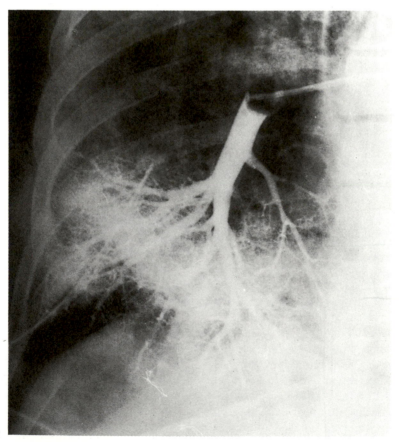

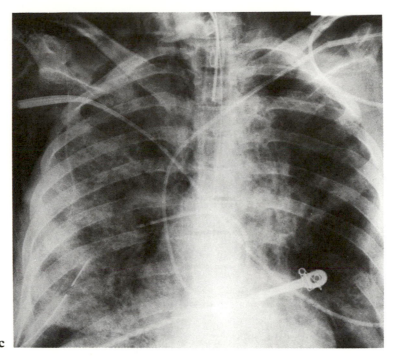

c

Fig. 8.8 (a) Chest radiograph of young patient after blunt chest injury showing left-sided haemopneumothorax. (b) Subsequent bilateral changes consistent with ARDS: Pulmonary artery balloon flotation catheter tip in right main pulmonary artery. Gross disturbance of pulmonary gas exchange was present (Pa_{O_2}–5 kPa; Pa_{CO_2}–6 kPa) in spite of mechanism ventilation, 100% inspired oxygen, positive end-expiratory pressure and a minute volume of 15 litres. (c) Pulmonary angiogram in above patient showing non-obstructive microvascular pattern.

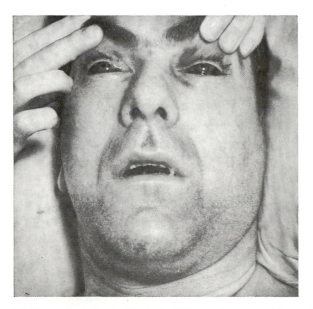

Fig. 8.9 Traumatic asphyxia. Note the diffuse ecchymoses of face and neck, and subconjunctival haemorrhage. These changes disappeared within 3 weeks.

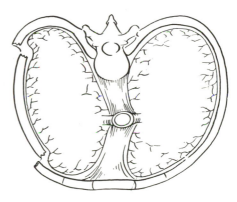

Fig. 8.10 Paradoxical movement of the loose fragment in 'stove-in' injury of the chest. On inspiration the loose fragment sinks inwards and the mediastinum shifts in the same direction.

sheering of the aorta, trachea or bronchi. Injury to the heart or great vessels is frequently and rapidly fatal. While anatomical considerations are important in all major blunt chest injuries, a clearer understanding of the underlying disturbances of lung function has led to more rational methods of treatment during the past few years. Respiratory distress may be severe, demanding urgent treatment. An initial chest radiograph is taken to determine the extent of bony injury to the chest wall and underlying injury to the lungs, heart and great vessels. At the same time arterial blood is taken for blood gas analysis. Characteristically the initial anatomical and functional assessment of the severity of injury may be misleading since haemorrhage, oedema and alveolar collapse continue to progress for several hours. Chest radiography and blood gas analysis must,

Table 8.2 Changes in blood-gas levels during treatment of class 3 chest injury (courtesy of Dr J. G. Mone, Western Infirmary, Glasgow). Woman aged 37: Flail Chest (left) and Multiple Injuries.

Time	SaO_2	PaO_2 (kPa)	pH	$PaCO_2$ (kPa)	Base excess	Remarks
Admission	78	5.73 (43)	7.36	4.13 (31.2)	−6.5	On air
+24 hours	94	9.60 (72)	7.52	3.73 (28.4)	+1.0	On 100% oxygen + IPPV + 120 mmol $NaHCo_3$
+2 days	95	10.40 (78)	7.35	5.20 (39.0)	−4.0	On 100% oxygen + IPPV
+7 days	96	10.67 (80)	7.43	4.26 (32.4)	−1.0	On 30% oxygen, spontaneous breathing. Tracheostomy
+13 days	100	42.00 (315)	7.43	6.00 (45.1)	+4.5	On oxygen 10 l/min Polymask. Tracheostomy closed.

therefore, be repeated as often as necessary until the full extent of injury is appreciated.

Blood gas analysis reveals a fall in arterial oxygen tension (Table 8.2). The underlying disturbance of pulmonary function is attributed to pulmonary parenchymal haemorrhage, oedema, alveolar collapse and increased scatter of V/Q ratios. A degree of hypocapnia is usual as pain and anxiety lead to hyperventilation. An elevation of carbon dioxide tension is found in association with pre-existing lung disease or as a result of over-enthusiastic administration of drugs with a sedative action. Hypercapnia occurring with chest injury alone is an indication of ventilatory failure and respiratory arrest is imminent. Hypoxaemia, particularly in association with hypotension, may lead to severe metabolic acidosis and a fall in arterial pH.

Concomitant head injury, hypercapnia, or hypoxaemia ($P_{aO_2} < 8$ kPa) refractory to added inspired oxygen administration are indications for the early institution of IPPV and, because this procedure carries the risk of producing a tension pneumothorax, the prior insertion of a chest drain is normal practice. The drain is introduced in the sixth or seventh intercostal space in the mid-axillary line and passed superiorly for a variable distance. It may be necessary to insert more than one drain, and on both sides of the chest if the injury is bilateral. The catheters are connected to chest drainage bottles in the normal fashion. As soon as possible thereafter a PVC endotracheal tube with low-pressure tracheal cuff is passed and IPPV commenced. The chest X-ray should then be repeated. Occasionally IPPV may be required for only 1 or 2 days if the chest wall injury is slight. More often IPPV is required until parenchymal contusions resolve or large flail segments acquire some stability, which may take up to 4 weeks. Under these conditions, to avoid the risk of laryngeal oedema, infection and subsequent stenosis, tracheostomy is performed at 10–14 days and extreme care taken to minimise superadded respiratory infection. In some units prolonged nasotracheal intubation is preferred to tracheostomy. After the first 24 hours the patient with adequate analgesia may tolerate the ventilator without excessive sedation or muscle relaxation; in the favourable

case the blood gas figures return towards normal over the next few days, but failure to improve may be associated with systemic sepsis, bronchopneumonia or the development of the adult respiratory distress syndrome (Fig. 8.8/b). The patient with a large flail segment may improve rapidly with IPPV, and it is tempting to remove the patient from the ventilator at this stage, but all too often the flail segment recurs and there is deterioration of pulmonary function.

In some centres operative stabilisation of flail chest is performed as an adjunct to IPPV in selected cases and may reduce the length of stay in hospital. However, the need for thoracotomy to insert wires used to stabilise the fractured ribs is a major factor in limiting the popularity of this mode of treatment.

While prompt intravenous fluid resuscitation is essential in all forms of trauma, care must be taken not to prescribe excessive volumes of fluid in patients with chest trauma as fluid overload may lead to accumulation of extravascular lung water. Indeed, some authorities advocate the use of diuretics and fluid restriction in such patients (Trinkle et al, 1975) though this may increase the risk of hypovolaemia and renal impairment. There is considerable controversy about the merits of colloid or crystalloid fluid therapy in trauma and sepsis patients (Lucas & Ledgerwood 1983); it is our practice to use colloidal solutions (e.g. gelatine plasma expanders, HPPF and blood) in the initial correction of intravascular hypovolaemia, and to use predominantly crystalloid solutions for maintenance, taking care to avoid excessive sodium loads.

THE ADULT RESPIRATORY DISTRESS SYNDROME (ARDS)

ARDS is characterized by clinical respiratory distress, hypoxaemia and radiological evidence of pulmonary oedema developing in a previously healthy adult patient after a major systemic or pulmonary insult (Petty & Fowler, 1982; Demling 1980). Of its many synonyms, 'shock lung' is perhaps the most familiar. Criteria for the

Table 8.3 Criteria for diagnosis of ARDS

1. Exclude pre-existing chronic pulmonary disease or left ventricular failure.
2. Clear history of a catastrophic pulmonary or systemic insult.
3. Clinical respiratory distress, defined as a respiratory rate of ≥ 20 breaths/min, with laboured breathing.
4. Diffuse pulmonay infiltrates on chest radiograph — interstitial in the early stages, alveolar later.
5. Hypoxaemia ($Pa_{CO_2} < 6.67$ kPa (50 mmHg), $F_{IO_2} > 0.6$), reduced total thoracic compliance (< 50 ml/cm H_2O), increased shunt fraction and increased dead space ventilation.

Table 8.4 Risk conditions commonly involving insult to the lung

Sepsis
Aspiratin of gastric contents or near-drowning
Multiple blood transfusions
Lung contusion
Disseminated intravascular coagulapathy
Long bone or pelvic fractures
Prolonged hypotension
Atypical pneumonia
Burns
Pancreatitis

diagnosis of ARDS, and a list of initiating insults are shown in Tables 8.3 & 8.4. It appears to be the pulmonary manifestation of intravascular neutrophil activation and aggregation (Lancet, 1984) which may occur in association with run-away complement activation. The result is a capillary permeability defect which predisposes to accumulation of extravascular lung water in the presence of low or normal left atrial pressure. Extensive damage to the alveolocapillary membrane leads to multiplication of Type II pneumocytes and repair by fibrosis which may progress to irreversible respiratory failure. Despite extensive research efforts to elucidate the underlying pathophysiology of ARDS in the past 15 years (Rinaldo & Rogers, 1982) no real advances in the basic principles of management have been made and mortality remains high at 40–90%, depending upon the number of organ systems involved. The cornerstones of treatment are:

1. Elimination of the shock state which often initiates or sustains ARDS
2. Eradication of sepsis and prevention of secondary infection which may eventually lead to death in multiple organ failure.
3. Intensive supportive therapy. IPPV with PEEP is virtually always necessary. Care must be taken to keep the inspired oxygen concentration as low as is needed to achieve a P_{aO_2} of 10 kPa

Controversy concerning the value of high-dose steroids in ARDS continues, but there is still no good evidence that this treatment improves the outcome from ARDS, while the side-effects of steroids may well be detrimental (Flick & Murray 1984).

Haemothorax and haemopneumothorax

Since wounds of the heart and great vessels are often rapidly fatal, bleeding into the pleural cavity in patients reaching hospital is most often from torn intercostal vessels. Bleeding from a pulmonary laceration is usually slight and soon ceases. It follows that a simple haemothorax commonly signifies a tear of intercostal vessels and that a haemopneumothorax (Fig. 8.8a) signifies a tear of intercostal vessels accompanied by a laceration of the lung. The mechanical effects of blood (or blood and air) in the pleural cavity are the same as air alone, but the presence of the blood increases the risk of intrapleural infection, and the blood also coagulates on the pleural membranes. Finally, the presence of blood leads to the out-pouring of an exudate which increases the volume of fluid present. In order to minimize these effects the blood and serum require to be removed at an early stage. The insertion of an inferior chest drain is the conventional treatment (Fig. 8.11a, b).

Mediastinal and subcutaneous emphysema

A laceration of the lung sometimes allows the escape of air under the visceral pleura, and the air may then pass by way of the lung root to the mediastinum, the fascial plains of the neck, and to the subcutaneous tissues of the face, neck and trunk. In extreme cases the subcutaneous emphysema may extend to the arms and genitalia. The laceration of the lung usually seals spontaneously, and the extravasated air is absorbed within about a week. Occasionally rupture of the pleura allows some of the air to escape into the pleural cavity, giving rise to a tension pneumothorax which must be decompressed. Also the tension developed by air in the mediastinum occasionally compresses the great veins, impeding venous return to the heart. This is particularly liable to happen postoperatively, if a ligature on a bronchus slips, or if the oesophagus is accidently torn during endoscopy. Emphysema which arises as a postoperative complication usually calls for surgical closure of the defect which has allowed the escape of air.

Penetrating injuries of the chest

Stab wounds of the chest are probably the commonest form of penetrating injury in British practice though missile injuries may be common in other parts of the world. Injuries which are known to be superficial by inspection of the weapon involved may be treated by surgical toilet and suture followed by careful observation, but in doubtful cases radiological assessment, close clinical

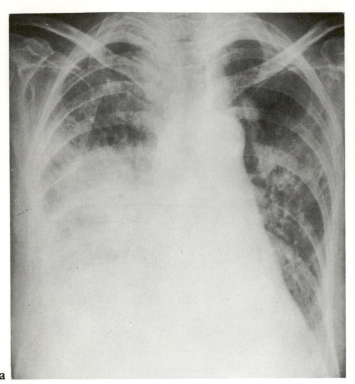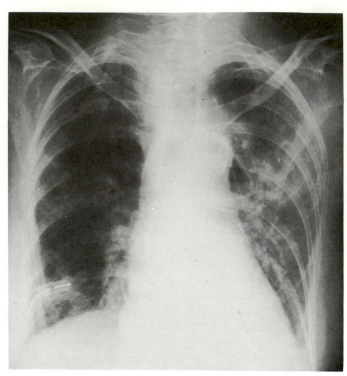

a   b

Fig. 8.11 (a) Direct injury to right chestwall with haemothorax and elevation of right hemi-diaphragm. (b) Same patient after insertion of lower chest drain (courtesy of Prof. W B Jennett, Institute of Neurological Sciences, Glasgow).

observation and early basal drainage of haemothorax must be performed (Muckart et al, 1984). In penetrating injuries of the mediastinum, haemodynamically unstable patients must be explored at urgent thoracotomy. In all patients blood loss in excess of 1 l, continued bleeding exceeding 200 ml/hour for 2 hours, or inadequate drainage of a large haemothorax are indications for thoracotomy (Richardson et al, 1981). An appreciation of the surface markings of the lungs and pleurae is clearly important in assessing penetrating injuries. In particular it should be noted that the dome of the pleura rises above the clavicle, and that the dome of the diaphragm rises to the level of the nipple. The chances of a penetrating injury to the lower chest having entered the abdomen are therefore high.

Diaphragmatic herniae

Occasionally sudden compression injuries of the chest or abdomen may rupture the diaphragm with subsequent herniation of abdominal viscera into the thoracic cavity. Since 98% of these injuries occur on the left side the liver would appear to be protective. Diagnosis of this condition may be difficult when many other causes of respiratory distress are present. Suspicion should be aroused by the finding on auscultation of bowel sounds in the chest; the diagnosis is confirmed by chest radiography. Surgical treatment is required immediately if strangulation of bowel is to be avoided.

POSTOPERATIVE CHEST COMPLICATIONS

Anaesthesia and surgery are often responsible for some degree of postoperative pulmonary dysfunction which may or may not be clinically significant. The well-known 'post-op chest' has many possible causes which will be mentioned here though it must be emphasized that the fundamental pathophysiology is still not fully resolved. The term 'postoperative pneumonia' is commonly used to describe the picture of pyrexia and pulmonary atelectasis commonly seen after surgery, but this description is not strictly correct and might obscure a proper understanding of the condition and its rational treatment. We shall discuss here the factors that predispose to post-operative pulmonary complications, the factors leading to pulmonary dysfunction even in the 'uncomplicated' case, and then discuss the diagnosis and management of atelectasis and pulmonary infections seen in postsurgical patients. We shall also consider the effects of pulmonary aspiration of oropharyngeal or gastric contents, massive collapse of lung and postoperative pleural effusion.

Factors predisposing to postoperative pulmonary complications

For any particular operative procedure the risk of post-operative pulmonary complications is primarily dependent upon the presence of pre-existing pulmonary disease, and most of the other associations are probably secondary to this single fact (Garribaldi et al, 1981). The type of surgery undertaken has an important impact on the risk of complications. Respiratory complications are very common after surgery of the thorax and upper abdomen, less common after lower abdominal surgery, and rare after minor surgery in ambulatory patients.

The normal arterial oxygen tension falls progressively with age as the closing volume rises and approximates to, or even exceeds, the FRC. In children, the closing volume may exceed FRC in the supine position up to the age of 6 years. Hypoxaemia due to a fall in FRC is therefore more pronounced in the very young and in the elderly. Postoperative respiratory complications are seen more frequently in the older age groups. The incidence of pre-existing lung disease is higher in the obese, and conditions peculiar to the obese patients include the Pickwickian syndrome, with sleep apnoea and pulmonary hypertension (Fisher et al, 1975). There may be a case for the use of regional analgesia or elective intermittent positive pressure ventilation in selected patients. In the western world malnutrition is a less common problem than obesity. An association between malnutrition and postoperative pneumonia has been demonstrated. Impaired immunocompetence is a possible factor in the susceptibility of these patients to pneumonia. The association between smoking and chronic bronchitis is irrefutable. In cigarette smokers, mucus is thick and tenacious, the normal ciliary clearance is impaired and defects in alveolocapillary permeability have been demonstrated.

Anaesthetic, analgesic and anticholinergic agents all tend to suppress ciliary activity in the respiratory tract and thereby reduce the clearance of secretions. This problem is compounded by the use of unwarmed, unhumidified anaesthetic gases. Nitrous oxide is a more soluble gas than nitrogen and pulmonary collapse distal to a bronchial obstruction will occur more readily when it is used. However, the conduct of the anaesthetic procedure is more important than the specific effects of any one anaesthetic agent. The anaesthetist must take steps to avoid provoking bronchospasm by the injudicious use of histamine-releasing anaesthetic agents, and ensure adequate depth of anaesthesia. Pulmonary ventilation, whether controlled or spontaneous, must be adequate during and after the procedure. The airway should be protected from infected foreign material, especially pus and vomit. Postoperative analgesia must be adequate without unduly obtunding the cough reflex or depressing respiration. In this respect the use of regional analgesia is advocated by some, though the incidence of post-operative pulmonary complications is not convincingly reduced thereby.

Postoperative pulmonary dysfunction

Derangements of pulmonary function are not infrequently seen following anaesthesia and surgery. The most commonly performed tests (arterial blood gases, forced expiratory volume and forced vital capacity) will not reveal clinically important changes in the respiratory pattern but are simple to perform at the bedside.

Postoperative respiratory changes may be considered to occur in two phases, early and late. They may also be broadly divided into two categories of hypoxaemia and respiratory depression.

Early hypoxaemia

Early hypoxaemia is a continuation of the disordered gas exchange which occurs during anaesthesia. While the causes are not entirely clear, changes in FRC and pulmonary vascular autoregulation leading to ventilation/perfusion abnormalities have been implicated. Derangements of chest wall tone and movement may adversely affect regional ventilation. Diffusion hypoxaemia, due to nitrous oxide washout, can be prevented by giving 100% oxygen for a few minutes after discontinuation of nitrous oxide. Hypoxaemia is exacerbated by respiratory depression.

Early respiratory depression

Early respiratory depression is a consequence of the anaesthetic technique and may be due to several factors including depletion of total body carbon dioxide stores, together with the central depressant effects of inhalational and systemically administered anaesthetic and analgesic agents. Inadequate reversal of neuromuscular block should always be considered as a potential cause of postoperative respiratory insufficiency in the early phase. It should be remembered that certain antibiotics, in particular the aminoglycosides, may potentiate neuromuscular blockade. For obvious reasons respiratory obstruction must be differentiated from respiratory depression.

Hypoxaemia in the late phase

Hypoxaemia in the late phase is more commonly seen in older patients and in patients who have undergone thoracic or upper abdominal surgery. It is associated with a reduced FRC which may be due to chest wall and diaphragmatic changes or pulmonary changes or a combination of both (Spence & Alexander, 1972) (Fig. 8.12). Attempts at ameliorating late phase hypoxaemia have concentrated on provision of adequate systemic or regional analgesia and the use of physiotherapy, breathing exercises and intermittent positive pressure breathing. Though none of these measures has yet been demonstrated to prevent late phase hypoxaemia, their implementation should not be neglected. Judicious use of added inspired oxygen may be necessary if hypoxaemia is severe. Late phase hypoxaemia may last for several days after anaesthesia and surgery.

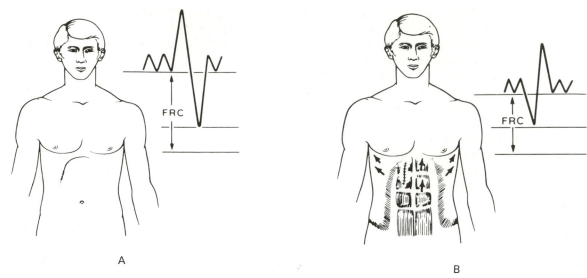

Fig. 8.12 Reduction in functional residual capacity following abdominal surgery (after Spence and Alexander 1972).

Respiratory depression in the late phase

Respiratory depression in the late phase is usually an expression of the depressant effects of the analgesic agents used and must be distinguished from ventilatory failure due to other pulmonary and extrapulmonary complications. Recently, the use of continuous respiratory monitoring techniques has revealed some alarming disturbances of the respiratory pattern, particularly during sleep, in patients receiving opiate analgesics (Jones, 1984).

Atelectasis

Whether the collapse of lung units in postoperative patients is a primary event in the reduction of the FRC or a result of FRC changes is not known. Partial or complete obstruction of the airway may be caused by accumulation of viscous secretions, and will lead to collapse of the distal airways. If atelectasis is extensive enough to produce clinical features, then a degree of tachypnoea, tachycardia and pyrexia will be seen. The chest radiograph may show patchy atelectasis. If atelectatic areas become confluent or larger airway obstruction leads to segmental or lobar collapse, the classic signs of pulmonary collapse will be evident on clinical examination. Treatment at this stage is primarily aimed at re-expanding the collapsed airways by physiotherapy and controlled breathing exercises. Fibreoptic bronchoscopy may sometimes be necessary.

Secondary infection of atelectatic areas may mimic pneumonia; the differentiation is probably not important.

Bronchitis

Exacerbation of chronic bronchitis is not infrequently seen postoperatively, and the responsible organisms will commonly be *Haemophilus influenzae* or *Streptococcus pneu-*

moniae. In the postoperative patient sputum samples must be sent to the laboratory though it would be reasonable to start treatment with cotrimoxazole or ampicillin without awaiting bacteriological confirmation. Physiotherapy and bronchodilators should also be prescribed.

Pneumonia

Postoperative bronchitis may progress to pneumonia, with malaise, pyrexia and tachypnoea. Examination of the chest usually reveals scattered coarse crepitations and sometimes bronchial breathing and dullness to percussion associated with pulmonary consolidation. Hypoxaemia often necessitates supplementation of the inspired oxygen concentration. Organisms are again likely to be *H. influenzae* and *S. pneumoniae*. Sputum samples and blood cultures must be sent to the laboratory, and treatment started with parenteral cotrimoxazole or ampicillin. Frequent physiotherapy is essential. Potential complications include lung abscess, pleural effusion and empyema.

Classic lobar pneumonia and the 'atypical' pneumonias are rare in the post surgical patient. In the severely immunocompromised patient (e.g. after transplant surgery) opportunistic infections may be life-threatening (Briggs 1981). Isolation of the pathogenic organism may be difficult. Potential causative agents include gram-negative bacilli, fungi, viruses and Pneumocystis carinii (Tobin and Grenvik 1984).

Aspiration

Inhalation of oropharyngeal or gastric contents may lead to pneumonia, atelectasis and lung abscess. In fit patients aspiration is only likely to occur when the laryngeal reflexes are obtunded by heavy sedation, anaesthesia or local anaesthetics but in debilitated patients aspiration may occur pre-operatively, most notably in conditions such as achalasia of the oesophagus.

The most florid pulmonary sequela of aspiration of gastric contents is aspiration pneumonitis, a form of ARDS which is known by the eponym Mendelson's syndrome when seen in obstetric practice. The damaging agent is the acidity of the stomach contents and it is routine practice to increase the intragastric pH in obstetric patients prior to anaesthesia by the use of antacids with or without histamine (H_2) antagonists. Application of cricoid pressure at induction of anaesthesia, prior to intubation of the trachea, is effective in preventing regurgitation in patients with a full stomach or hiatus hernia. Treatment of the established condition is as for ARDS. There is a case for the use of ampicillin and metronidazole to prevent pulmonary infection with upper gastrointestinal tract flora. Steroids have not been shown to be effective in clinical practice.

Massive collapse

This term is applied to collapse of the whole lung or one of its lobes from absorption of air trapped beyond an obstruction of one of the larger bronchi.

The common causes of bronchial obstruction are tumours and inflammatory oedema round an impacted foreign body. Postoperative massive collapse may result from obstruction by inhaled vomitus, blood clot or even a mucus plug. The air trapped beyond the obstruction is rapidly absorbed, the lung collapses and becomes radio-opaque, and the mediastinum is drawn over to the affected side (Figs. 8.13a, b, c). The rapidity of the process of collapse is worth noting. It is known, for example, that artificial blockage of an upper lobe bronchus leads to collapse of the upper lobe, with displacement of the superior mediastinum and trachea, within a few minutes.

The dyspnoea and hypoxaemia that result from collapse of a large volume of lung is initially severe, but later improves even though collapse persists. At first the pulmonary perfusion through the collapsing non-ventilating lung continues, causing venous admixture or shunting, and consequently arterial hypoxaemia. Later, more complete collapse of the lung and contained pulmonary vessels plus the reflex effect of hypoxic pulmonary vasoconstriction act to minimize blood flow through the area, leading to reduced shunt and improved arterial oxygenation.

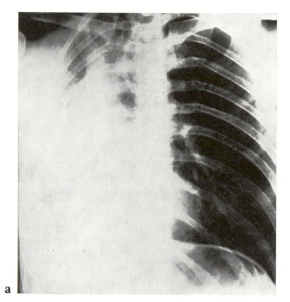

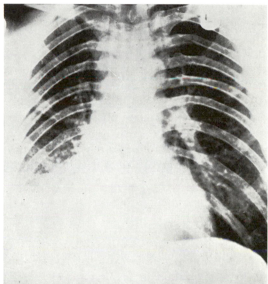

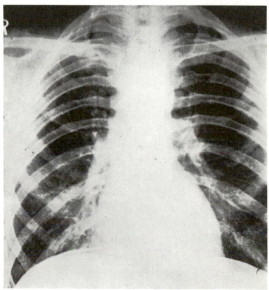

Fig. 8.13 (a) Post-operative massive collapse of the lung. The day after operation, before treatment by aspiration. (b) Massive collapse of the lung, treated by bronchial aspiration. The next day — the lung is clearing. (c) Massive collapse of the lung, treated by bronchial aspiration. The third day — the lung is clear.

In addition to the purely mechanical effects, the collapsed lung soon becomes infected and fever increases the patient's distress.

Treatment consists of bronchoscopic assessment and, where possible, removal of the obstruction. Physiotherapy and antibiotics are of secondary value.

Postoperative pleural effusion

After thoracotomy a serosanguinous effusion is a common complication. It results from inflammation of the pleura consequent upon exposure and handling, and from the unavoidable oozing of blood from the intercostal incision. The development of a small effusion is indeed so common that it is routine practice to provide intercostal drainage for the first 24–48 hours.

The purely mechanical effects of an effusion are here unimportant, for only a very large effusion embarrasses respiration. Even a moderate effusion, however, prevents full re-expansion of the lung and the portions of the lung which remain collapsed are liable to become infected. The pleural effusion may itself become infected, giving rise to a troublesome and even dangerous empyema. Finally, even in the absence of infection, the fibrin present in the exudate may coagulate on the pleurae giving rise to a thick clot which later becomes organised and forms dense fibrous adhesions.

To avoid these risks any pleural effusion which develops requires to be aspirated, and if it recurs it must be aspirated repeatedly.

PULMONARY EMBOLISM

Rarely, the lungs may be affected by fat embolism or amniotic fluid embolism leading to ARDS. Even more rarely tumour fragments or parasites may cause clinical evidence of pulmonary embolisation, but far and away the commonest cause of pulmonary embolism is the impaction in the pulmonary circulation of blood clot dislodged from a venous thrombus which was in the process of dissolution or organisation and canalisation.

In general terms there are three factors which predispose to thrombosis (Virchow's triad); the relative importance of one against another is impossible to assess. These factors are stasis or stagnation of blood, vascular endothelial damage and alteration of the coagulability of blood. It follows that venous thrombosis is most often seen in debilitated older patients who may be on prolonged bedrest. Surgery and trauma (particularly of the lower limbs and pelvis), pregnancy and the oral contraceptive pill all predispose to venous thrombosis. As one might expect, these patients are also at risk of pulmonary embolism. It is interesting to note that only some 50% of patients who suffer pulmonary embolism have clinical evidence of

venous thrombosis, but hardly surprising when one considers that the thrombus most likely to fragment or dislodge is one that does not occlude its vessel and has a good blood flow past it. The common sites of venous thrombosis are the veins of the calves and the iliofemoral veins.

Recognition of risk factors for venous thrombosis enables the practising surgeon to apply prophylactic therapy, such as low-dose heparin or dextran, in a rational manner. It has been suggested that the protective effects of thrombo-embolic deterrent stockings or epidural anaesthesia are due to enhanced fibrinolytic activity in the blood.

The clinical effects of pulmonary embolism vary widely and are dependent upon the size and number of embolic particles and the time course of the illness. Four clinical syndromes may usefully be recognised.

Actue minor pulmonary embolism

Impaction of a small embolus occurs in the smaller, more distal branches of the pulmonary artery causing pleuritic pain and sometimes haemoptysis. The mechanism is obscure, for the dual supply of blood to the lungs prevents infarction occurring in most cases. On examination a pleural rub or crepitations may be detected over the affected area and radiological examination may reveal one or more areas of opacification which are known as infarct shadows. In fact, they are due to exudation of fluid into the alveolar space which occurs rapidly but usually resolves within a few days. Necrosis of lung tissue is relatively unusual, and perhaps only occurs when there are complicating factors such as pre-existing cardiorespiratory disease. Pleural effusion or diaphragmatic elevation may also be seen. Pulmonary artery pressure is normal in such cases and there are no haemodynamic sequelae of acute minor pulmonary embolism. Perfusion lung scan will reveal the extent of embolisation. Treatment of the embolism is unnecessary, but as in all cases of pulmonary embolism anticoagulants should be considered for the treatment of venous thrombosis and prophylaxis of further embolism.

Acute massive pulmonary embolism

Larger emboli will lodge in the larger more proximal branches of the pulmonary artery where obstruction of the circulation causes haemodynamic disturbances and even sudden death. The presentation of acute massive pulmonary embolism is dramatic, with sudden onset of central chest pain, dyspnoea and cardiovascular collapse. Clinical examination reveals signs of right ventricular failure; the jugular venous pressure is raised, the pulse rate is raised, and an added heart sound is heard in diastole at the left sternal edge (gallop rhythm). The blood pressure is low due to reduced cardiac output, but the pulmonary artery pressure is raised by the dramatic increase in pulmonary vascular resistance. In about half the cases an S wave in Lead I, Q wave in Lead III and T wave inversion in Lead III are seen ('S1 Q3 T3' pattern). These represent right heart strain. Blood gas analysis typically shows hypocapnia due to hyperventilation and a degree of hypoxaemia due to ventilation/perfusion mismatch. The chest X-ray may show asymmetric oligaemia of the lung fields. Bedside pulmonary angiography confirms the diagnosis when this facility is available.

Occlusion of a major branch of a pulmonary artery alone does not lead to shock and hypoxaemia as seen in pulmonary embolism, and it seems likely that neuro-humoral responses complicate the clinical picture. Humoral mediators of pulmonary hypertension have been demonstrated in the plasma of animals with artificially-induced pulmonary embolism. Prostaglandins and thromboxane, histamine and serotonin may all play a role and may derive from pulmonary tissue or from leucocytes and platelets within the embolus.

Treatment is initially supportive. If the patient survives the early phase of acute massive pulmonary embolism and no further episodes occur the embolus will eventually dissolve or organise and canalise. Dissolution of the embolus is hastened by the use of fibrinolytic agents such as streptokinase or urokinase, but these agents have some important side-effects including increased bleeding diathesis and anaphylaxis. In specialist centres embolectomy may be undertaken in the acute phase, or if the patient relapses after the acute phase. In all cases anticoagulants should be considered for prophylaxis of further thrombus formation.

Sub-acute massive pulmonary embolism

In some patients the onset of symptoms related to massive pulmonary embolism is insidious. There is a gradual onset of dyspnoea over several days or even weeks. Haemoptysis and pleuritic chest pain may be features and evidence of deep vein thrombosis should be sought. Cardiac output and blood pressure may be maintained but signs of right ventricular failure will be detectable. Pulmonary artery pressure is high. Blood gas analysis shows evidence of ventilation/perfusion mismatch. The chest X-ray shows asymmetric oligaemia, and the diagnosis is confirmed by demonstrating defects on perfusion scan or pulmonary angiography. Treatment is as for acute massive embolism.

Chronic thrombo-embolic pulmonary hypertension

The pathophysiology of this condition is poorly understood. It could represent unresolved acute or sub-acute embolism or could conceivably be due to an abnormality of the pulmonary vascular endothelium or fibrinolytic processes. Onset of dyspnoea with effort syncope is insidi-

ous. Pulmonary artery pressure is markedly elevated to 80–90 mmHg systolic. Death occurs from progressive right heart failure. Treatment is ineffective, but anticoagulants are often prescribed.

PAIN IN PULMONARY DISEASE

Pleural pain

The visceral pleura is devoid of nerve end-organs and is insensitive. There is a plentiful supply of nerve end-organs immediately outside the parietal pleura, which is exquisitely sensitive. In patients with a pleural effusion, Capps and Coleman (1932) inserted a wide intercostal cannula through which they could stimulate the pleura mechanically with a piece of wire. They verified that the visceral pleura and indeed the lung parenchyma were insensitive. Stimulation of the parietal pleura gave rise to pain, described as sharp and knife-like, which was located over the area stimulated, but seemed to originate not deeply but superficially. Stimulation of the lowest part of the parietal pleura gave rise to pain which was located at the coastal margin and over the upper part of the abdominal wall. Stimulation of the pleura covering the marginal part of the diaphragm caused pain located round the costal margin in the distribution of the fifth and sixth intercostal nerves. Stimulation of the pleura covering the central part of the diaphragm caused pain over the top of the shoulder in the distribution of the supraclavicular nerves which, in common with the phrenic nerve, are derived from cervical segments 3, 4 and 5 (Fig. 8.14). The end organs lying outside the parietal pleura are segmentally supplied by branches of the intercostal nerves and, in the case of the central part of the diaphragm, by the phrenic nerve. Stimulation of the end-organs gives rise to pain in the cutaneous distribution of the corresponding spinal segment, and it is said that the pain can be abolished by infiltrating this area of skin with local anaesthetic solution. The abdominal reference of pain from the lower part of the parietal pleura has to be remembered if diagnostic errors are to be avoided.

In pleurisy the exact mechanism of pain is in some doubt. The pain is attributed most commonly to friction between the inflamed visceral and parietal pleurae. It is attributed by some to stretching of the inflamed parietal pleura by movements of the chest wall during respiration. Yet again it is attributed to tugging on the inflamed parietal pleura by intrapleural adhesions. This last suggestion gains support from the observation that the induction of artificial pneumothorax rarely caused pain if adhesions were not present, and that once these adhesions had been divided subsequent injection of air was painless. Similarly a spontaneous pneumothorax does not usually give rise to pleural pain unless adhesions are present.

Pleural pain may also occur in cases of pulmonary

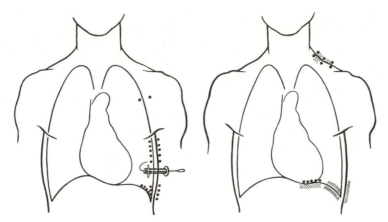

Fig. 8.14 Mechanical stimulation of the parietal pleura gives rise to pain experienced in nearby skin, but stimulation of the pleura (or peritoneum) covering the central part of the diaphragm gives rise to pain on the top of the shoulder.

'infarction' or of lung tumour which extends to the surface of the lung.

Tracheobronchial pain

The searing pain of tracheitis is a matter of common experience. It is usually located behind the upper sternum, but it may extend to one or other side when there is inflammation of the corresponding major bronchus.

Direct mechanical stimulation of the trachea and major bronchi during bronchoscopy gives rise to pain which is located over the throat or upper chest at a site overlying the area stimulated.

The impulses subserving tracheo-bronchial pain pass entirely in the vagal trunks, and the pain is thus abolished by cutting the vagi above the pulmonary plexus but below the origin of the recurrent laryngeal nerve.

The smaller bronchi and the parenchyma of the lung are insensitive, and can be cauterized painlessly in the conscious patient. Extensive disease in the periphery of the lung causes pain only when it spreads to involve the parietal pleura.

NON-RESPIRATORY FUNCTIONS OF THE LUNG

This chapter would not be complete without recognition of the fact that the lungs are now known to have important non-respiratory functions. As well as surfactant, the lungs are able to synthesize a wide range of prostaglandins and leukotrienes, histamine and kallikrein which may have systemic as well as local effects. Angiotensin I is converted to angiotensin II in the lung; this conversion is blocked by anti-hypertensive agents like captopril. A number of vaso-active substances are taken up by the lung, such as nor-adrenaline, serotonin, bradykinin and some prostaglandins.

REFERENCES

Brock R L 1954 The Anatomy of the Bronchial Tree, 2nd edn. Oxford University Press, London

Capps J A, Coleman G H 1932 An experimental and clinical study of pain in the pleura, pericardium and peritoneum MacMillan New York

Cohen C A, Zagelbaum G, Gross D, Roussos C H, Macklem P T 1982 Clinical manifestations of inspiratory muscle fatigue. American Journal of Medicine 73: 308–316

Conference of the Medical Royal Colleges and their Faculties in the United Kingdom 1976 British Medical Journal ii: 1187–8

Cotes J E 1979 Lung Function. Blackwell Scientific, Oxford

Demling R H 1980 The pathogenesis of respiratory failure after trauma and sepsis. Surgical Clinics of North America 60: 1373–1390

Dilly S H 1984 Scanning electron microscope study of the development of the human respiratory acinus. Thorax 39: 733–742

Fisher A, Waterhouse T D, Adams A P 1975 Obesity: its relation to anaesthesia. Anaesthesia 30:633

Flick M R, Murray J F 1984 High-dose corticosteroid therapy in the adult respiratory distress syndrome. Journal of the American Medical Association 251: 1054–1056

Garribaldi R A, Britt M R, Coleman M L, Reading J C, Pace N L 1981 Risk factors for post-operative pneumonia. American Journal of Medicine 70: 677–680

Gothard J W W, Branthwaite M A 1982 In: Anaesthesia for Thoracic Surgery. Blackwell Scientific, Oxford

Jones J G 1984 Pulmonary complications following general anaesthesia. In: Kaufman L (ed) Anaesthesia Review 2 Churchill Livingstone, Edinburgh p 21–38

Lancet 1984 Neutrophils and the Adult Respiratory Distress Syndrome. Lancet ii: 790–791

Long J H, Wester M R and Oppenheimer M J 1949 Immediate cardiovascular and respiratory adjustments to pneumonectomy. Journal of Thoracic Surgery 18:629

Long S E, Duffin J 1984 The medullary respiratory neurons: a review. Canadian Journal of Physiology and Pharmacology, 62, 161–82

Lucas C E, Ledgerwood A M 1983 The fluid problem in the critically ill. Surgical Clinics of North America 63, 439–454

Marshall B E, Wyche M Q Jr 1972 Hypoxaemia during and after anaesthesia. Anesthesiology 37:178

Mitchell R A, Berger A 1975 State of the Art: review of neural regulation of respiration. American Review of Respiratory Diseases 111:206

Muckart D J J, Luvuno F M, Baker L W 1984 Penetrating injuries of the pleural cavity. Thorax 39: 789–793

Nunn J 1977 Applied respiratory physiology Butterworths, London

Petty T L, Fowler A A 1982 Another look at ARDS. Chest 82: 98–104

Richardson J D, Flint L M, Snow N J, Gray L A, Trinkle J K 1981 Management of transmediastinal gunshot wounds. Surgery 90: 671–676

Rinaldo J E, Rogers R M 1982 Adult Respiratory Distress Syndrome: changing concepts of lung injury and repair. New England Journal of Medicine 306: 900–909

Sjostrand U H 1983 High frequency positive pressure ventilation. International Anaesthesia Clinics 21, 2: 59–81

Spence A A, Alexander J I 1972 Mechanisms of post-operative hypoxaemia. Proceedings of the Royal Society of Medicine 65:12

Tobin M J, Grenvik A 1984 Nosocomial lung infection and its diagnosis. Critical Care Medicine 12: 191–199

Trinkle J K, Richardson J D, Franz J L, Grover F L et al 1975 Management of flail chest without mechanical ventilation. Annals of Thoracic Surgery 19:355

Weidemann H P, Matthay M A, Matthay R A 1984 Cardiovascular-pulmonary monitoring in the Intensive Care Unit. Part 1 — Chest 85:537. Part 2 — Chest 85:656

West J B 1979 Respiratory Physiology — the essentials. Baltimore: Williams and Wilkins

West J B 1982 Pulmonary Pathophysiology — the essentials. Baltimore: Williams and Wilkins

Heart

An account of the fetal circulation and of the changes which normally take place at birth is followed by an outline of the manner in which the heart and circulation adapt to acquired and congenital lesions.

Because heart-lung bypass is an essential part of most cardiac surgery, recent developments in extracorporeal circulatory support are described.

Disease of the heart valves, congenital heart disease, coronary artery disease and heart block account for most of the work in a cardiac surgical unit. The common conditions in these groups are identified, their haemodynamic effects discussed and the appropriate surgery outlined.

All patients who undergo cardiac surgery require a period of intensive care. The common patterns of change in the vital functions in the early postoperative period are explained.

FETAL CIRCULATION

In the fetus, the lungs are not functional and so both ventricles feed the systemic circulation. The output from the right ventricle passes up the pulmonary artery and through the ductus arteriosus to join the left ventricular output in the aorta.

The fetal circulation is shown in Figure 9.1. Gas exchange occurs in the placenta and oxygenated blood flows to the fetus along the umbilical vein. This vein is functionally continuous with the ductus venosus and hepatic veins which empty into the inferior vena cava just below the right atrium. This stream of oxygenated blood from the inferior vena cava is largely directed through the foramen ovale into the left atrium. From here it flows into the left ventricle to be pumped into the aorta and distributed in the main to the vessels of the head and upper limbs. Blood entering the right atrium from the superior vena cava is joined by some blood from the inferior vena cava and flows through the tricuspid valve to the right ventricle. Since the fetal pulmonary circulation offers a

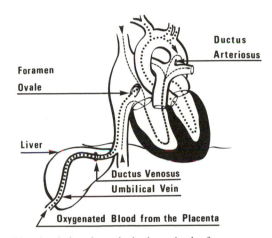

Fig. 9.1 The circulation through the heart in the fetus

high resistance to blood flow, blood from the right ventricle, which is largely venous, passes through the ductus arteriosus to the descending thoracic aorta. Some of this blood serves the trunk and lower extremities, the rest of it reaches the umbilical arteries and is carried to the placenta to gain oxygen and release carbon dioxide.

CHANGES IN THE CIRCULATION AT BIRTH
(Rudolph, 1970)

The principal anatomical events are closure of the ductus arteriosus and the foramen ovale. As the infant draws his first few breaths and expands his lungs, the pulmonary vascular resistance reduces by 90%, actively under the influence of the increased oxygen tension (P_{O_2}) in the pulmonary precapillary vessels, and passively by mechanical unfolding of the vasculature. Blood from the right ventricle flows freely through the pulmonary circulation and flow through the ductus arteriosus virtually ceases. During the subsequent 24 hours the ductus closes by contraction of its muscular wall and in the next 6 weeks obliterative fibrosis converts it into a fibrous cord. The stimulus which initiates closure of the ductus arteriosus is not yet known but the rise in oxygen tension of arterial blood probably plays a part. Arterial hypoxaemia in the neonatal period has been implicated as a cause of continued patency of the ductus (Hornblad, 1970). Recent studies on the circulatory effects of prostaglandins suggest that circulating prostaglandin E maintains patency of the ductus during fetal life and that prostaglandin F_2 alpha may constrict the ductus in a high Po_2 environment. Prostaglandin E infusion is used to maintain patency of the ductus in the management of some neonates with cyanotic congenital heart disease.

The foramen ovale closes when the increased flow through the pulmonary circulation causes the pressure in the left atrium to exceed that in the right. The foramen is closed by a flap of the original septum primum, which covers the left atrial side of the foramen. The flap can be pushed open by a catheter from the right atrium in 20% of adults, although the pressure differential between the left and right atria normally keeps it closed.

HAEMODYNAMIC PRINCIPLES

When the heart is diseased or congenitally abnormal, compensatory changes occur in order to maintain function. These compensatory changes can be recognized clinically and provide diagnostic clues to the nature of the causal lesion. A knowledge of the development of these adaptive changes is necessary for the correct interpretation of cardiac catheterization findings and for the correct choice and timing of surgical intervention.

Valvular stenosis

In common with other organs and muscles of the body, the heart responds to an increase in work load by hypertrophy and to a decrease by atrophy. A cardiac chamber may be called upon to perform extra work in order to force blood through a stenosed valve, or, in the case of an incompetent valve and an intracardiac shunt, in order to handle an increased stroke volume.

In aortic stenosis, the left ventricle becomes markedly hypertrophied and commonly generates an intra-ventricular pressure in excess of 200 mmHg in order to deliver a near normal stroke volume into the aorta. The apex beat becomes thrusting and sustained, the electrocardiogram (ECG) pattern alters in a characteristic manner (Fig. 9.2) and the X-ray silhouette of the heart may show a bulge corresponding to the enlarged left ventricle.

In mitral stenosis, the left atrium first shows enlargement and hypertrophy. It is the right ventricle, however, which propels blood through the mitral valve, having first pumped it through the pulmonary circulation (Fig. 9.3). The consequent right ventricular hypertrophy can be felt as a left parasternal heave with each systole. The left ventricle, which is 'down-stream' from the stenosis, becomes smaller and less muscular so that the apex beat is aptly described as being tapping in character. The ECG (Fig. 9.4) and X-ray both reflect the abnormal muscular dominance of the right ventricle.

Extreme degrees of ventricular hypertrophy are seen in patients who have survived into adult life with congenital stenosis of the aortic or pulmonary valves. Following correction of the valvular stenosis in these patients the excessively muscular walls of the ventricle approximate

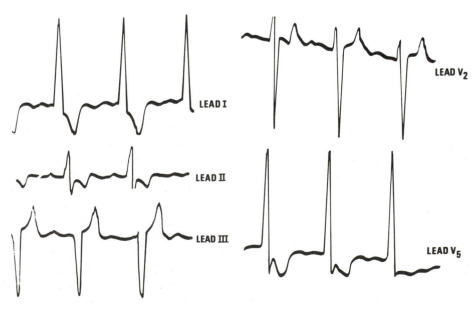

Fig. 9.2 Left ventricular hypertrophy — an electrocardiogram from a patient with aortic stenosis showing an abnormally high R wave in Leads 1 and V_5 and an abnormally deep S wave in Leads III and V_2. The ST segment is depressed in V_5

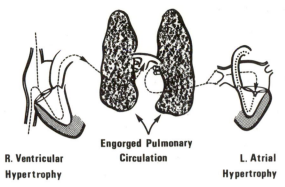

R. Ventricular
Hypertrophy

Engorged Pulmonary
Circulation

L. Atrial
Hypertrophy

Fig. 9.3 The consequences of mitral stenosis

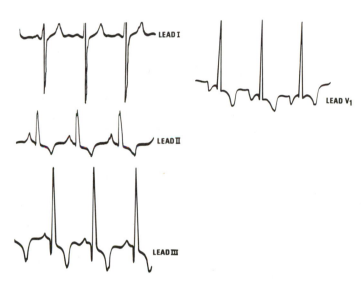

Fig. 9.4 Right ventricular hypertrophy. The tracing is from a patient with an atrial septal defect and pulmonary stenosis. It shows a deep S and a small R wave in Lead I with a tall R wave in Lead III. The T waves are inverted, the ST segments depressed in Leads II and III. The R wave is tall in V_1 and the S wave is absent.

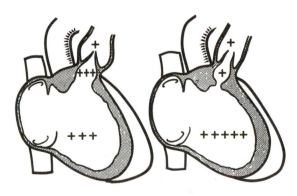

Fig. 9.5 'Suicidal Right Ventricle'. The drawing demonstrates how the excessively hypertrophied outflow tract of the right ventricle may obstruct blood flow after relief of pulmonary valvular stenosis (After Brock, 1957)

during systole and may constitute a continuing obstruction in the region of the outflow tract (Fig. 9.5). The post-operative course in these cases is dominated by evidence of a low cardiac output (viz. peripheral vasoconstriction, a narrow pulse pressure, a high central venous pressure and oliguria). Fortunately, involution of the muscle mass occurs with the passage of time after relief of the valvular obstruction.

Valvular incompetence

When one of the heart valves does not close properly a proportion of each stroke volume forwarded during systole leaks back during distole. This results in a net loss of output and the heart compensates by enlarging the capacity of the appropriate chamber. The normal left ventricle ejects about 70 ml (in an adult) into the aorta during each systole and none leaks back in diastole. In significant degrees of aortic incompetence, almost half the stroke volume leaks back during diastole, so that if 70 ml are ejected only 40 ml goes forward to the systemic circulation and 30 ml return to the ventricle in diastole. To compensate for this the left ventricle enlarges so that it can eject 110 ml during systole, and although 40 ml may leak back a normal output of 70 ml per beat has been regained.

In mitral incompetence, the left ventricle becomes more capacious for analogous reasons and in addition the left atrium becomes enlarged to accommodate the regurgitant stream and the right ventricle hypertrophies in order to forward blood through the pulmonary circulation against the back-flow from the left atrium. Thus, valvular incompetence results in cardiac enlargement, in which the affected chambers are both more capacious and have thicker walls than normal.

Septal defects

The principal consequence of a defect in either the atrial or ventricular septum or patency of the ductus arteriosus is an abnormal shunt of blood from one side of the heart to the other (Fig. 9.6). The direction of flow through the defect depends on the difference in pressure between the two chambers connected by the hole. Since pressures are higher in the left heart and aorta than in the right heart and pulmonary artery, blood flows from left-to-right through an atrial septal defect, a ventricular septal defect and a patent ductus arteriosus. Anomalous drainage of pulmonary veins into right atrium has a similar haemodynamic effect in that blood destined for the left atrium flows instead into the right atrium.

Left-to-right shunts increase the volume of blood flowing through the pulmonary circulation, because the right heart and pulmonary artery have to accept the additional arterial blood flowing through the shunt in addition to coping with the normal venous return from the

Shunts in C.H.D.

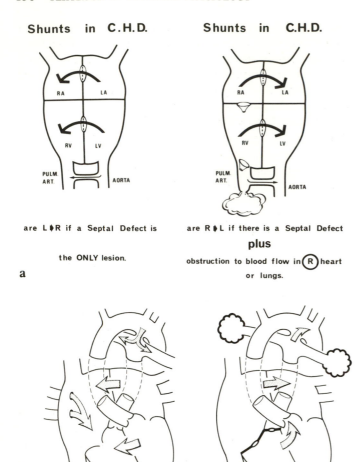

are L→R if a Septal Defect is

the ONLY lesion.

a

Shunts in C.H.D.

are R→L if there is a Septal Defect

plus

obstruction to blood flow in (R) heart

or lungs.

b   Left to Right   Right to Left

Fig. 9.6 The figure shows the direction of shunt in congenital heart disease in diagramatic form (a) and in anatomical form (b)

venae cavae and coronary sinus. In a patient with an atrial septal defect of moderate size (3 cm), the ratio of pulmonary blood flow to systemic blood flow is commonly 2.5:1. Adaptive changes take place in the pulmonary circulation in response to left to right shunts and these are described below (cf. pulmonary hypertension). In a proportion of infants with ventricular septal defects the shunt may represent such a large proportion of the stroke volume of the left ventricle that the output to the systemic circulation is insufficient to maintain life. In these infants an emergency operation is necessary to prevent flooding of the lungs (p. 145).

When, in addition to a septal defect, there is an obstructive lesion in the heart or pulmonary vasculature, the shunt may be right-to-left. Right-to-left shunts will occur through septal defects when the pressure in the right-sided chamber exceeds that in the left. Right-to-left shunts add venous blood to the systemic circulation and they cause cyanosis. The commonest defect in this group is Fallot's tetralogy. In this condition a ventricular septal defect is accompanied by stenosis of the outflow tract of the right

ventricle and of the pulmonary valve. The pressure in the greatly hypertrophied right ventricle exceeds that in the left and so venous blood is ejected into the systemic circulation through the defect.

The volume of a left-to-right shunt depends mainly on the size of the defect, and is expressed in terms of the pulmonary/systemic flow ratio. Measurement of this ratio is important in assessing the need for operation in a case of septal defect and it is calculated as follows. (The method used is an extension of the Fick principle for calculating cardiac output, using blood samples obtained during catheterization of the right heart.)

$$\frac{\text{pulmonary blood flow}}{\text{systemic blood flow}} =$$

$$\frac{\text{O}_2 \text{ consumption/pulmonary arteriovenous oxygen difference (A-VO}_2 \text{ diff.)}}{\text{O}_2 \text{ consumption/systemic arteriovenous oxygen difference}}$$

$$= \frac{\text{systemic A-VO}_2 \text{ diff.}}{\text{pulmonary A-VO}_2 \text{ diff.}}$$

The volume of a right-to-left shunt depends more on the severity of the obstructive lesion than on the size of the defect. An estimate of the volume of a right to left shunt can be made by measuring the $P\text{O}_2$ of an arterial blood sample. More precise quantitation of a right-to-left shunt can be derived from the extended Fick principle as follows:

right to left shunt = systemic blood flow minus pulmonary blood flow

$$= \frac{(\text{O}_2 \text{ consumption})}{(\text{arterial} - \text{right atrial O}_2 \text{ content})}$$

minus

$$\frac{(\text{O}_2 \text{ consumption})}{(\text{pulmonary venous} - \text{pulmonary arterial O}_2 \text{ content})}$$

Pulmonary hypertension

Elevation of the pulmonary arterial pressure results from the pulmonary vascular changes associated with left-to-right shunts; from obstructive lesions in the left heart such as mitral stenosis; from blockage of the pulmonary vessels in thromboembolic disease; as a late sequel of extensive fibrotic lung disease; and rarely, as a result of congenital vascular anomalies in the lungs.

The blood pressure in the main pulmonary arteries is normally low (20/10 mmHg) and such is the distensibility of the pulmonary vascular bed that it can accept a three-fold increase in flow without a significant rise in pressure. Thus, children with large atrial septal defects usually have a normal pulmonary arterial pressure despite a pulmonary blood flow which is commonly two or three times the systemic flow. Sooner or later however, an excessive pulmonary blood flow causes obliterative changes in the small pulmonary vessels which are progressive and which by raising the pulmonary vascular resistance lead to pulmonary hypertension.

The time of appearance of these changes and their rate of development is related to the site and size of the shunt and also varies from patient to patient. However, certain common patterns can be delineated (Wagenvoort, 1964). Before considering the pathogenesis of these, it would be appropriate to describe the normal maturation of the pulmonary vessels from fetus to childhood.

In the normal fetus at term the pulmonary vascular resistance is very high (about 40 000 dyn/sec/cm^{-5}), blood flow through the lungs is about 10% of the systemic flow and the pressure in the pulmonary artery equals that in the aorta.* Within a few hours or days of birth the pulmonary vascular resistance falls to a 10th of that in the fetus; flow increases five-fold and the pulmonary vascular resistance falls still further and flow increases; this process continues until the child is 5 or 6 years old, at which time 'normal' adult levels are attained. That is, the pulmonary flow equals the systemic flow; the pulmonary arterial pressure is one-sixth of the systemic pressure; and the pulmonary vascular resistance is one sixth of the systemic resistance (200 and 1200 dyn/sec/cm^{-5} respectively). Thus the normal fall in pulmonary vascular resistance occurs in two periods. A 90% reduction occurs at birth when the lungs expand and the ductus arteriosus closes. The second fall is spread over the next few years.

In about 15% of children born with a large left-to-right shunt, the pulmonary vascular resistance does not fall during the first year of life. It remains elevated, thickening of the media of the small pulmonary arteries persists or recurs, intimal hyperplasia follows and progressive obliteration of the pulmonary vascular bed ensues. Eventually the pulmonary vascular resistance becomes higher than the systemic, and the pressures in the right heart and pulmonary circulation exceed those in the left heart. When this stage is reached the shunt reverses, becomes from right to left and the patient becomes cyanosed. Eisenmenger described the end stage of this process first in 1897, and on the basis of post-mortem findings pointed out the association of a ventricular septal defect and narrowing of the pulmonary arteries. Further elucidation awaited the development of cardiac catheter techniques and the data were reviewed and brought together by Paul Wood in 1958. In particular he emphasised the diversity of lesions

*The relationship between flow, pressure and resistance is expressed by the hydraulic equivalent of Ohm's Law:

$$Pressure = Flow \times Resistance$$

In the mature circulation the systemic vascular resistance is 6 × the pulmonary vascular resistance. Since the output of both ventricles is identical this explains why pulmonary artery pressure = 20 and the aortic pressure = 120 mmHg.

which could result in the Eisenmenger syndrome. These include all the causes of increased pulmonary flow: ventricular septal defect, atrial septal defect, patent ductus arteriosus, truncus arteriosus, transposition of great vessels with ventricular septal defect, anomalous pulmonary venous drainage, A-V communis, and others.

Fortunately, in a majority of children with left-to-right shunts, these progressive obliterative changes in the pulmonary vasculature are of much slower onset and progression and do not cause pulmonary hypertension until the third or fourth decade.

The initial response of the pulmonary vasculature to an increase in flow is somewhat different if the shunt is at atrial level (e.g. atrial septal defect or anomalous drainage of pulmonary veins).

The first vessels to be affected in the presence of these defects are the pulmonary veins, which are the seat of intimal fibrosis. Subsequent changes occur in the pulmonary arteries, and these are identical to those described above. The changes take longer to develop, however, and it is rare to find pulmonary hypertension in association with an atrial septal defect in childhood.

Obstructive lesions in the left heart such as mitral stenosis (or incompetence) cause pulmonary venous hypertension in the first instance, followed with the passage of time by obliterative vascular changes which in turn lead to pulmonary (arterial) hypertension. These vascular changes are usually reversible following removal of the cause (Likoff, 1959).

The cause of the pulmonary hypertension which complicates thrombo-embolic disease is not yet clearly defined and controversy continues concerning the relative importance of mechanical blockage and vascular spasm in the aetiology. Long-term anti-coagulant therapy may halt the progress of this form of pulmonary hypertension but does not cure it.

HEART-LUNG BYPASS

The development of pump-oxygenators which maintain the systemic circulation while the heart and lungs are temporarily excluded has allowed operations to be carried out on an electively arrested, still and bloodless heart.

Although many heart-lung machines are now available, they differ only in detail of design and all consist of four basic parts: (i) cannulae and tubing which connect the patient to the machine; (ii) an oxygenator; (iii) a pump; and (iv) a heat exchanger to control blood temperature. Figure 9.7 shows a typical extra-corporeal circuit in more detail. Two cannulae are introduced into the superior and inferior venae cavae to collect the venous blood on its way to the heart and divert it through the venous line to the oxygenator. This lies about 18 inches below the patient so that venous blood will run into it by gravity-siphonage.

HEART-LUNG BY-PASS CIRCUIT

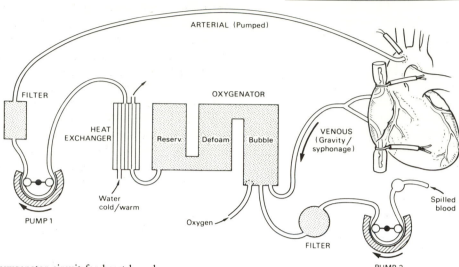

Fig. 9.7 A basic pump oxygenator circuit for heart-lung bypass.

There are several types of oxygenator but the most widely used type is a specially designed plastic bag divided into three compartments. The venous blood passes into the first compartment where oxygen is bubbled into the blood so as to oxygenate it. The second compartment is filled with a fine mesh, coated with a silicone anti-foam preparation so that the bubbles will burst and the oxygenated blood will leave this compartment free from bubbles. The third compartment is a reservoir to collect the blood from which the pump forces the oxygenated blood along the tubing to the arterial cannula. The pump consists of electrically-driven rollers which compress the tubing leading from the reservoir to the patient, so that the blood is 'milked' through the tubing to the arterial cannula and into the systemic arterial circulation. The pumping rate can be varied so as to maintain an adequate blood pressure in the patient's arteries. The arterial blood is usually returned to the ascending aorta through an arterial cannula introduced through a purse string suture. At some point in the circuit, depending on the type of machine used, the blood passes through a heat exchanger so that its temperature can be controlled.

Before connection is made between the patient's circulation and the machine, the latter is filled with fluid and the patient is heparinised (4.5 mg/kg body wt). The extra-corporeal circuit has a capacity of about 2.5 litres and is filled with Ringer's solution. When bypass is connected this clear fluid mixes with the patient's blood volume and reduces his haematocrit to about 25%. This degree of haemodilution has been shown to aid tissue perfusion, and by provoking a diuresis may offer some protection against renal tubular damage. It has the further major advantage that it reduces the usage of donor blood and so avoids the undesirable effects of large blood transfusions (Gadboys et al 1962).

Bypass is instituted by starting the pump and releasing the clamp on the venous line. The venous return to the heart flows out to the oxygenator, the heart quickly empties and the patient's blood pressure and arterial flow are maintained by the blood pumped back into the aorta by the machine. The intra-aortic pressure closes the aortic valve, and the heart remains empty except for some blood which passes through the coronary circulation to the right atrium via the coronary sinus. This blood is aspirated when the heart is opened and returned to the circuit through an additional entry to the oxygenator.

Pulsatile cardiopulmonary bypass

It has been appreciated from the outset that the vital organs of the body are accustomed to receiving pulsatile arterial blood flow from the heart. Though the early workers in the field of cardiopulmonary bypass pumps attempted to produce pulsatile systems, the technological complexity and high haemolysis ratings of these systems proved an insurmountable problem at the time. It was found that the substitution of steady flow non-pulsatile roller pumps were compatible with patient survival for up to 2 hours of total cardiopulmonary bypass. Thus non-pulsatile flow has over the years become accepted as the routine mode of perfusion despite its inherent unphysiological nature.

Over the past 15 years increasing attention has been paid to the possibility of developing reliable and relatively simple pulsatile perfusion systems and in the past 5 to 6 years at least two such systems have become available. Numerous studies of both haemodynamics and metabolism have emphasized, and continue to emphasize, the physiological superiority of pulsatile perfusion over conventional non-pulsatile flow. In particular, the use of pulsatile

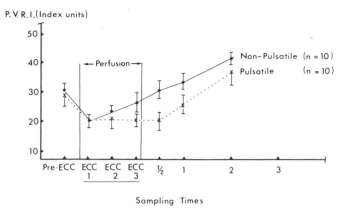

Fig. 9.8 The graph shows the change in peripheral vascular resistance in 20 cases during and after cardiopulmonary bypass (ECC). It can be seen that the resistance rises throughout bypass in the non pulsatile group but the rise in resistance is delayed until half an hour after bypass in those in whom flow was pulsatile

perfusion prevents the progressive rise in peripheral vascular resistance associated with non-pulsatile flow (Fig. 9.8). This is clearly advantageous, particularly in those patients with compromized left ventricular function in whom an excessive rise in peripheral resistance may precipitate left ventricular failure due to the necessary increase in left ventricular work. In addition, numerous studies have indicated that cellular metabolism in general and the specific organ metabolism in brain, kidney and pancreas, are significantly protected during periods of pulsatile perfusion as opposed to conventional non-pulsatile flow. Fears regarding the possible increase in haemolysis with pulsatile pump systems have proved unjustified, and the past 5 years have seen the increasing adoption of pulsatile perfusion as its clinical reliability and simplicity in use gains acceptance. At present pulsatile pump systems are of two major types:

1. Modified roller pump systems with pump heads which can accelerate and decelerate, generating pulsatile flow
2. Intermittent occlusive devices based on intra-aortic balloon pump. These systems incorporate an inflation/deflation chamber in the arterial return line and are inherently more invasive than modified roller pump systems.

Oxygenator design

As previously mentioned, bubble oxygenators are in widespread use in cardiac surgical practice. Modern oxygenators have high efficiency in terms of gas-to-blood flow ratios and are relatively atraumatic to the formed elements of the blood. There is, however, evidence indicating a small degree of blood cell trauma and of activation of platelet aggregation during bubble oxygenation which has

led to the search for alternative oxygenation techniques. In recent years membrane oxygenators have been developed in which a semi-permeable membrane (usually of silicone rubber or teflon) is interposed between the gas and blood films. This form of blood oxygenation has been shown experimentally to be less traumatic to blood-formed elements than bubble oxygenation though at present clinical studies suggest that the benefit may be marginal. Membrane oxygenation has also been introduced where long-term artificial oxygenation is required. Patients with severe but reversible pulmonary failure, for example, shock lung or extreme pulmonary oedema, may have such severe degrees of hypoxia that full intermittent positive pressure ventilation and the use of positive end expiratory pressure, may prove insufficient to provide adequate oxygenation. In such circumstances, partial circulatory bypass from femoral vein to femoral artery via a membrane oxygenation unit, may supplement oxygenation and allow patient survival until there is improvement in the underlying pulmonary condition. Extracorporeal membrane oxygenation (ECMO) is also used in conjunction with partial circulatory support in patients with severe cardiac failure though it must be said that at present this relatively new technique is associated with high mortality and morbidity figures.

MYOCARDIAL PROTECTION

During open-heart surgical procedures it is frequently necessary to stop cardiac action completely and to shut off the heart's own blood supply through the coronary arteries by cross-clamping the ascending aorta proximal to the arterial return cannula. During such periods the heart is clearly ischaemic and myocardial cellular damage will inevitably occur if this period of myocardial ischaemia is prolonged. Studies have indicated that the heart may be left ischaemic at normal temperatures for up to 20–30 minutes without there being significant evidence of myocardial cell injury. It is, however, frequently necessary to cross-clamp the aorta for longer periods than this during complex open-heart procedures and accordingly techniques of myocardial protection assume great importance. The earlier techniques of selective coronary artery perfusion have now largely been replaced by the widespread use of cold cardioplegic arrest techniques. A 4°C solution of cardioplegic agents is instilled under pressure into the aortic root after the aortic cross-clamp has been applied. The coronary arteries become perfused with the cardioplegic solution and cardiac arrest quickly ensues. The heart becomes totally arrested and flaccid and operating conditions are excellent for the cardiac surgeon. When the surgical procedure has been completed, the aortic cross-clamp is removed and re-perfusion of the coronary arteries restores ventricular action with the spontaneous return of the pre-operative cardiac rhythm. Current cardioplegic techniques provide the surgeon with a safe period of aortic cross-clamping up to and even exceeding two hours.

There are constituents in any cardioplegic solution which are directed towards three principal biochemical effects:

1. *Energy conservation.* Substances such as potassium and procaine induce rapid and complete cardiac asystole. This prevents the progressive depletion of intramyocardial cell energy compounds, for example, ATP.

2. *Hypothermia.* The introduction of cardioplegic solutions at around 4°C provides even and rapid myocardial cooling. When the myocardial temperature is reduced to less than 20°C there is a significant reduction in myocardial metabolism and this obviously reduces energy supply/demand inequality.

3. *Protection from ischaemic metabolites.* Some cardioplegic solutions include agents such as histidine buffer which are designed to protect the myocardial cells from the harmful effects of those substances produced during the period of myocardial ischaemia and also from the electrolyte and cell volume imbalance which tend to occur.

The present controversies regarding specific formulations should not detract from the fact that there is a consensus over the fundamental principles of myocardial protection.

Micro-aggregate formation and blood filtration

The compatibility of prosthetic materials with blood in extracorporeal circuits has prompted many studies which have indicated that aggregation of formed elements of blood, particularly the platelets, occurs to a considerable extent in the extracorporeal circuit. It is now generally recognized that blood trauma occurs mainly at the air/blood interface of high powered suction during the operative procedure, but in addition to this, bubble oxygenation and the pumping process are associated with the aggregation of platelets, the further deposition of blood cells and the formation of micro-aggregates which may pass down the arterial return line and into the patient's arterial circulation. Studies have demonstrated that micro-embolic pathology may be detected microscopically in numerous organs, particularly kidneys and brain, and at present there is considerable interest in possible prevention methods. Among these are:
(i) the use of small-pore blood filters and (ii) the inhibition of platelet aggregation.

The incorporation of small-pore ($<40 \ \mu m$) blood filters in the arterial return line distal to the perfusion pump, has been shown to retain significant amounts of blood cell microaggregates and particulate matter from the extracorporeal circuit. In addition, the oxygenation process may produce vast showers of micro-bubbles which may also be retained on suitably designed filters thus avoiding the pos-

sible occurrence of significant cerebral air embolism. Controversy exists as to the optimal design and site of incorporation of blood filters and further studies require to be carried out in order to evaluate the effects of arterial line filtration and end-organ morbidity.

Inhibition of platelet aggregation is presently the subject of many research studies. It must be stressed that full heparinization should be achieved in every patient on the heart-lung machine and that weight-related heparin dosage is not sufficient to ensure an adequate prolongation of blood clotting times. One of the several semi-automated blood clotting time systems allows the monitoring of each patient's coagulation status during the period of cardiopulmonary bypass and this has undoubtedly contributed to better control of both haemostasis and micro-aggregate accumulation during extracorporeal circulation. Recent studies using the prostaglandin substance prostacyclin appear encouraging. Such substances interfere with platelet aggregation and may prove to be of considerable benefit.

Circulatory assist devices

In patients with particularly severe left ventricular failure associated clinically with cardiogenic shock, inotropic drug therapy and manipulation of physiological parameters may prove insufficient to maintain an adequate peripheral circulation. The requirement for circulatory assist devices has been a stimulus to the appearance of such mechanical devices over the past few years. The use of such devices is at present linked to pathology in which spontaneous improvement is anticipated or where definitive surgical correction of an associated abnormality is likely to produce permanent improvement. Devices in use currently are:

1. *The intra-aortic balloon pump.* This system involves insertion of an inflation/deflation balloon chamber in the first part of the descending thoracic aorta. The inflation/deflation of the chamber is synchronised with the patient's ECG to allow augmentation of diastolic coronary blood flow and reduction in the presystolic left ventricular after-load. A typical trace of a patient on the intra-aortic balloon pump is shown (Fig. 9.9). When the patient's own cardiac function has improved sufficiently, the patient may be weaned from the balloon circulatory support. The balloon can then be removed and the defect in the femoral artery repaired.

2. *Left ventricular assist devices.* (*LVAD*) These devices are largely experimental at the present time and they usually consist of a valved pumping chamber which can be synchronized to the patient's own cardiac action providing partial circulatory support. Some devices are totally intracorporeal while others have cannulae or connections to the external pumping chamber. The development of a totally artificial heart continues experimentally but clinical feasibility still seems a long way off.

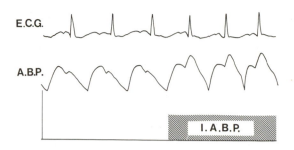

Fig. 9.9 The arterial blood pressure trace (ABP) before and during intra-aortic balloon counter pulsation (IABP). The diastolic augmentation of pressure can be clearly seen.

The principal areas of application of left ventricular assist devices and intra-aortic balloon counter-pulsation lie in the field of coronary artery surgery. In addition to patients who, because of left ventricular dysfunction have difficulty in being weaned from total cardiopulmonary bypass in the immediate postcardiac surgical situation, intra-aortic balloon pumps may be inserted in patients who have severe crescendo angina (the so-called pre-infarction angina) or in patients who have some postmyocardial infarction haemodynamic problem, e.g. postinfarct mitral valve incompetence or postinfarction ventricular septal defect. In these latter two conditions, a balloon pump may be inserted in the pre-operative phase in order to improve peripheral circulation and off-load the failing left ventricle until such time as definitive operation is undertaken.

DISEASE OF THE HEART VALVES

About two-thirds of those who have had rheumatic fever in childhood develop permanent valve damage and in two-thirds of these it is severe enough to warrant surgery. The mitral and aortic valves are most commonly affected. Tricuspid valve lesions are less common and the pulmonary valve is very rarely involved.

Because haemodynamically significant valvular changes are slow to develop and because the myocardium and pulmonary circulation can compensate for many years, symptoms do not usually become severe until the patients are in their thirties. Symptoms become clamant when the myocardium can no longer compensate for the narrowed or leaking valve(s), and eventually symptoms and signs of cardiac failure appear.

Mitral stenosis

This is the commonest form of rheumatic valvular disease, and it affects women more often than men in the ratio 4:1.

Haemodynamics

The stenosed valve impedes blood flow from the left atrium to the left ventricle. The left atrial wall thickens in an effort to maintain a normal throughput, but since there are no valves in the pulmonary veins, back-pressure into the pulmonary circulation is inevitable. The right ventricle therefore becomes hypertrophied and the pulmonary circulation is constantly over-filled with blood. The pulmonary blood vessels react and progressive changes occur first in the veins and then in the small arteries to produce a rise in pulmonary vascular resistance and the development of pulmonary hypertension.

The magnitude of the pressure changes in the pulmonary circulation and measurement of the gradient across the valve in diastole are an index of the severity of the stenosis, and the rise in these pressures in response to exercise are a valuable aid in the selection of patients for surgery.

Surgery

In most patients with mitral valve disease, the valve mechanism is so deformed once symptoms appear that replacement of the valve using heart-lung bypass is necessary. Less commonly, where the valve leaflets are still mobile, a valvotomy or valvuloplasty under direct vision can be performed.

In selected patients, with pure mitral stenosis with pliable, membranous valve cusps a blind mitral valvotomy without heart-lung bypass may be indicated. Mitral valvotomy is a 'closed heart' operation, i.e. separation of the adherent valve leaflets is achieved with a finger or instrumentally while the heart continues to maintain the circulation (Fig. 9.10). The operative mortality rate is low (3%), as is the incidence of postoperative complications. The two chief hazards are systemic embolism and the production of mitral incompetence. The latter may be produced if a valve leaflet is torn during valvotomy and replacement of the damaged valve with a prosthesis is necessary. Systemic embolism is a risk in the 15% of patients who are found to have thrombus in the left atrium at the time of operation.

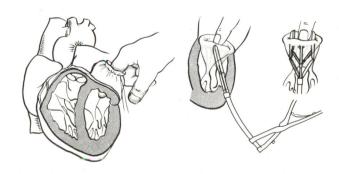

Fig. 9.10 Digital and instrumental splitting of the fused mitral valve leaflets: mitral valvotomy.

Re-stenosis

It has been found that in 65% of the patients who had a mitral valvotomy more than 10 years previously, symptoms have reappeared because the valve has re-stenosed. Because further scarring and deformation of the leaflets have occurred, these patients are candidates for replacement of the valve.

Mitral incompetence

This is less common than stenosis and affects men and women equally.

Haemodynamics

Mitral incompetence affects not only the left atrium and the pulmonary circulation and its pump (i.e. the right ventricle), it is also followed by left ventricular enlargement and hypertrophy. Left ventricular volume increases to compensate for the portion of each stroke volume lost back into the atrium. At the same time, the left atrium stretches to accommodate the leak-back.

As with mitral stenosis, mitral incompetence leads to overfilling of the pulmonary circulation with consequent obliterative vascular changes and right ventricular hypertrophy.

Surgery

When the mitral valve is incompetent, the operation of choice is replacement with a prosthesis. In the few cases where the valve cusps are still membranous and annular dilatation is the main lesion, some form of valvuloplasty is an alternative.

The operation is performed through the left atrium and requires heart-lung bypass (Fig. 9.11).

Aortic valve disease

The aortic valve is involved in about one-third of cases of rheumatic valve disease. It is rarely involved alone; concomitant mitral valve disease should be suspected. Isolated aortic stenosis is usually congenital in origin.

Haemodynamics

Stenosis or incompetence of the aortic valve overloads the main pumping chamber of the heart, the left ventricle.

This chamber has extraordinary powers of compensation, and by hypertrophying can maintain an adequate cardiac output for many years, in spite of a malfunctioning aortic valve. Extreme secondary changes in the left ventricle are seen in cases of severe aortic stenosis. Its myocardium enlarges concentrically at the expense of the cavity which becomes progressively smaller (Fig. 9.12). In time, the muscle mass outgrows the available coronary blood supply, which itself has been impaired by two factors: the reduced cardiac output and an increased resistance to blood flow in the intramural part of the coronary vascular bed. Consequently, the symptom of angina of effort appears as the overworked myocardium suffers hypoxia. Within months of the appearance of angina, signs of left ventricular failure follow, usually in the form of paroxysmal nocturnal dyspnoea. These arise because the failing ventricle does not relax completely in diastole and so impedes the inflow of blood from the left atrium and pulmonary veins. The consequent hold-up of blood in the pulmonary circulation leads to pulmonary oedema.

Surgery

Replacement of the damaged aortic valve is almost always necessary, because by the time symptoms appear and surgery is indicated, the architecture of the valve is so destroyed as to make any form of valvuloplasty impossible.

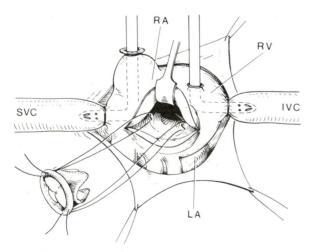

Fig. 9.11 Mitral valve replacement: The heart is cannulated for bypass; the left atrium has been opened from the right side in front of the pulmonary veins. A bioprosthesis is being sewn in place.

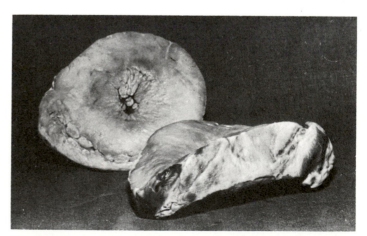

Fig. 9.12 Concentric hypertrophy of the left ventricle: Two slices taken at autopsy from the ventricles of a patient who had severe aortic stenosis. The cavity of the left ventricle would only admit a pencil.

Replacement may be with a prosthesis or with a biological valve, and the operation involves heart-lung bypass with cardioplegia.

Tricuspid stenosis and incompetence

This valve is diseased in about 15% of cases of rheumatic valve disease, and involvement of this valve is always associated with mitral and/or aortic valve pathology. In addition to this small group of patients in whom the tricuspid valve is damaged by rheumatic endocarditis, there is a larger group in whom chronic heart failure due to mitral valve disease leads to tricuspid incompetence induced by dilatation of the right ventricle and tricuspid annulus.

Haemodynamics

The most obvious feature of tricuspid valve dysfunction is elevation of the systemic and hepatic venous pressures, with consequent prominence of the visible veins such as the external jugular and enlargement of the liver. Peripheral oedema and ascites follow, and hepatocellular damage is progressive.

Tricuspid stenosis is characterized by the presence of an exaggerated 'a' wave in the jugular venous pulse. The 'a' pressure wave accompanies atrial contraction but if the neck veins are watched while the heart sounds are auscultated, it appears to accompany the first heart sound. This is because the wave takes about a sixth of a second to travel to the neck from the atrium. This sign is lost when atrial fibrillation occurs and co-ordinated atrial systole ceases.

In tricuspid incompetence, the prominent pressure wave (a 'v' wave) is due to ventricular contraction, as blood regurgitates back into the right atrium and great veins from the right ventricle.

Surgery

The valve is approached through the right atrium using heart-lung bypass and replacement or valvuloplasty are employed, depending on the extent to which the valve is damaged. When the valve is incompetent as part of the secondary pathology in long-standing mitral valve disease, simple plication of the annulus along with replacement of the mitral valve may suffice. When the valve is stenosed or significantly fibrosed, replacement is necessary.

Prostheses — heart valves

Some 5000 heart valves are replaced each year in the United Kingdom, with excellent and lasting results in 80% of patients.

The desirable attributes of the 'ideal' artificial valve are as follows:

1. It should function as well as the natural valve
2. It should last for the patient's life-time
3. It should be non-thrombogenic, non-haemolytic, and non-antigenic
4. It should not be readily colonized by circulating bacteria
5. It should be available in a wide range of sizes

All these ideals have not yet been achieved, but valve replacements are available which will function for many years with only a small risk of malfunction. The choice lies between the 'tilting-disc' or bi-leaflet mechanical prostheses and the gluteraldehyde-treated bioprostheses. Both have a woven fabric sewing ring surrounding the valve mechanism, to take the sutures which secure it to the host annulus. This sewing ring is invaded by fibroblasts and covered with endothelium within three months of implantation.

In mechanical prostheses, a disc or leaflets made of pyrolytic carbon open and shut with a tilting or hinged action within a rigid annulus with grooves or struts which guide and retain the disc or leaflets.

Bioprostheses are made by sewing porcine aortic valve leaflets, or leaflets made from bovine pericardium onto a plastic stent. The xenograft tissue is treated with gluteraldehyde which crosslinks the protein molecules (tanning) to give added strength and greatly reduce the antigenicity of the tissue.

The haemodynamic performance of an artificial valve is measured in terms of the pressure drop across it, throughout a range of blood flows.

The smaller sizes of all prosthetic valves offer varying degrees of obstruction to flow, and this factor influences the choice of replacement in children and small adults (Table 9.1).

The durability of an artificial valve is obviously important since it has to withstand the stresses of opening and closing with each heart beat (i.e. 38 million cycles per year with an average heart rate of 72 per minute). The gluteraldehyde-treated xenografts give cause for concern in this context. Early calcification and stiffening of the leaflets occurs in such implants in children and there is a significant incidence of leaflet disruption in adults several years

Table 9.1 Gradient across commonly used artificial valves in the aortic (A) and mitral (M) position

		Annulus (mm)	Pressure drop at mean flow of 5 l/min (mmHg)
Mechanical (Bjork-Shiley)	A	21	22
	A	27	10
	M	31	2→0
Xenograft (Carpentier-Edwards)	A	21	32
	A	27	16
	M	31	6→4

after implantation. It seems likely that many bioprostheses will require replacement within 10–12 years after implantation.

Thrombo-embolism was the most frequent complication of the valve replacements used in the l960s (e.g. the Starr-Edwards ball-in-cage valve). The use of highly polished, non-thrombogenic materials has greatly lessened the incidence of this problem. Nevertheless, the patient with a mechanical valve replacement must remain on anticoagulant therapy for life.

The thrombogenicity of bioprostheses is less and herein lies their chief advantage. Most centres do not require all patients who have bioprostheses to take anticoagulants in the long-term. Patients with atrial fibrillation or a large left atrium are maintained an anti-coagulants. This attribute makes the 'tissue valve' the first choice for valve replacement in young women who may become pregnant. (Long-term anticoagulant therapy is teratogenic and increases risk to mother and child at birth.)

Endocarditis due to bacterial colonization of the fabric sewing ring of a prosthesis or the leaflets of a xenograft, occurs in about 1% of patients receiving valve replacements. It is a serious complication. The infection is usually resistant to antibiotic therapy, and causes dehiscence of the prosthesis from the host annulus. Re-operation with replacement of the prosthesis is usually necessary.

Prostheses — patches and conduits

Congenital atrial or ventricular septal defects of more than a few millimetres in diameter are closed by sewing a fabric patch to the edges of the defect. Patches are also used as intracardiac baffles and as gussets to enlarge ventricular outflow tracts in other congenital cardiac malformations.

These patches are woven or knitted from synthetic polyester fibre which is chemically and biologically inert and very durable. The favoured material is terylene (Dacron) and various weaves of fabric are available with different degrees of porosity and elasticity for different applications.

CONGENITAL HEART DISEASE

About 7 of every 1000 babies born alive have a defect of the heart or great vessels. The defect may take the form of an abnormal communication between the right and left sides of the heart (e.g. atrial septal defect, ventricular septal defect, patent ductus arteriosus and anomalous drainage of the pulmonary veins); stenosis or occlusion of the inflow or outflow tracts of the ventricles at the valvular or sub-valvular area (e.g. aortic stenosis, pulmonary stenosis, infundibular stenosis, tricuspid atresia) or defects in the unfolding and rotation processes by which the primitive tubular heart of the embryo becomes the four-

chambered heart of the fetus (e.g. transposition of the great arteries). Not infrequently, more than one defect is found in the same heart.

The effects of left-to-right shunts are to cause an excessive pulmonary blood flow and a diminished systemic blood flow, so that children with such defects tend to be undersized and slender (poor systemic blood flow) and are subject to frequent respiratory infections (pulmonary plethora). With the passage of time, the excessive pulmonary flow may lead to pulmonary hypertension and fixed vascular changes (see p. 136).

The effect of right-to-left shunts is to cause systemic hypoxia and a diminished pulmonary blood flow. Children with these defects are also undersized for their age, but the main consequences of the systemic hypoxia are fatiguability and exertional dyspnoea. A compensatory polycythaemia develops as a result of the systemic arterial hypoxia and this may lead to spontaneous intravascular thrombosis.

Operations for congenital heart disease

These can be conveniently grouped under two headings: corrective and palliative.

CORRECTIVE OPERATIONS

The corrective operations are those in which a defect is closed, a stenosis relieved or a transposition corrected. These operations restore normal circulatory pathways and are usually followed by regression of the compensatory changes which accompanied the defect.

PALLIATIVE PROCEDURES

These are operations designed to improve the efficiency of the circulation for a number of years; to avert heart failure; and to allow the child to thrive and grow until he is large enough for a definitive corrective operation to be performed safely.

Banding the pulmonary artery

In this procedure the main pulmonary artery is constricted by a band of dacron tape in order to limit the volume of shunt through a large ventricular septal defect. The operation improves systemic blood flow and protects the pulmonary vasculature from the harmful effects of an excessive flow and pressure (Fig. 9.13).

Systemic to pulmonary anastomoses

This is indicated in some children with severe cyanotic congenital heart disease associated with a reduced pulmonary blood flow and a normal pulmonary vascular

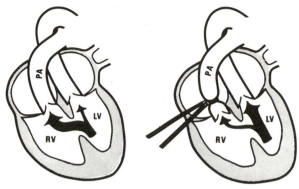

Fig. 9.13 Banding the pulmonary artery to protect the pulmonary vasculature in cases of excessive pulmonary blood flow associated with a large ventricular septal defect.

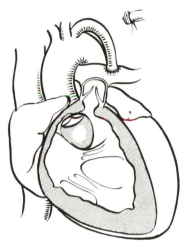

Fig. 9.14 The diagram shows the defects of Fallot's tetralogy, viz. pulmonary valvular stenosis, right ventricular infundibular stenosis, a ventricular septal defect with overriding of the aorta. The drawing also shows a left subclavian to pulmonary artery shunt (Blalock's operation)

resistance, e.g. Fallot's tetralogy. The operation increases blood flow through the pulmonary vasculature by making a communication between the left subclavian and pulmonary artery (Blalock-Taussig operation) (see Fig. 9.14).

Creation of an atrial septal defect

This is done in infants with transposition of the great vessels to allow some mixing of blood between pulmonary and systemic circuits.

The interatrial communication is made in the cardiac catheter room by passing a balloon-tipped catheter through the foramen ovale; inflating the balloon, then pulling the catheter back forcibly to enlarge the foramen and allow a shunt of oxygenated blood.

The relative frequency of the commoner congenital cardiac defects is shown in Table 9.2 and the altered physiology of each is described in the following paragraphs, with an outline of the choice and timing of operative treatment.

Table 9.2 A list of the congenital defects of the heart which are most commonly found in children who survive the first year of life.

Defect	Main effects	Percentage incidence
Ventricular septal defect (VSD)	Left-to-right shunt	25
Patent ductus arteriosus (PDA)	Excessive pulmonary blood flow	12
Atrial septal defect (ASD)	Reduced systemic blood flow	12
Fallot's tetralogy	Right-to-left shunt	12
Transposition of great vessels	Usually reduced pulmonary blood flow	5
Tricuspid atresia	Cyanosis	2
Pulmonary stenosis	Obstructive lesions Hypertrophy of left (coarctation and aortic stenosis) or right ventricle (pulmonary stenosis)	9
Coarctation of aorta		6
Aortic stenosis	—	5
Various uncommon defects		12

Ventricular septal defect

The usual site for this defect is in the membranous part of the interventricular septum, under the septal cusp of the tricuspid valve, and the defect commonly measures about 1.5 cm in diameter.

Haemodynamics

The consequences of a ventricular septal defect depend on the size of the defect and on the response of the pulmonary vascular bed to the increased flow. Three patterns can be defined:

1. A small defect allowing a pulmonary-systemic flow ratio of less than 1.5:1.0, with a normal pulmonary arterial pressure. These children are asymptomatic and do not require surgery.

2. A larger defect with a greater left-to-right shunt, but still having a normal pulmonary arterial pressure. These patients are followed carefully, many such defects close spontaneously. If the defect persists beyond the teens, most surgeons advocate closure to remove risk of endocarditis.

3. A defect with a high shunt flow and a high pulmonary arterial pressure. These children should be operated upon early (during the first year of life) to prevent the development of fixed pulmonary vascular changes.

Corrective surgery

In common with all surgery for congenital heart disease, the trend is to offer corrective surgery as early as possible. Cardiopulmonary bypass in neonates and infants is now commonplace and carries a low risk.

Operation to close defects of moderate size is best

undertaken before 5 years of age, using heart-lung bypass. The defect is closed with a fabric patch and the operative mortality is about 3%. The chief hazard of the operation is heart block, because the Bundle of His runs along the lower edge of the defect and may be caught by the stitches.

Patent ductus arteriosus

In about one infant in 1500 the ductus arteriosus fails to close after birth. A continuous flow of blood from the aorta to the pulmonary artery results, producing the classical systolic-diastolic murmur in the left infra-clavicular region called a 'machinery' murmur.

Haemodynamics

In common with the other causes of left-to-right shunt, a patent ductus arteriosus reduces blood flow to the systemic circulation and causes overfilling of the pulmonary circulation. The volume of the shunt is usually less than that due to a ventricular septal defect and much less than with an atrial septal defect. However, pulmonary vascular changes may develop with the passage of time and significant pulmonary hypertension is usual in cases who reach 30–40 years without treatment. Subacute bacterial endocarditis is a not infrequent complication of a patent ductus.

X-ray screening shows systolic expansile pulsation of the main pulmonary arteries and their first branches ('hilar dance'). A cardiac catheter with its tip in the main pulmonary artery will measure a rise in pulmonary pressure and a blood sample from this site will have a higher Po_2 than samples taken from the right ventricle.

Surgery

Operation is usually performed on diagnosis, after 1 year of age but may be indicated earlier in the case of a wide ductus with a large shunt. At operation the ductus is ligated, or if it is wider than 5 mm, divided between clamps and the cut ends oversewn. The operative mortality is less than 1%.

Atrial Septal Defect

The three common types of this defect are shown in Figure 9.15. In about 10% of secundum type defects, some or all of the right pulmonary veins join the right atrium instead of the left (anomalous drainage of pulmonary veins). In most cases of primum defects, there is an associated defect of the mitral valve. This takes the form of a cleft in the septal leaflet which usually renders the valve incompetent.

Haemodynamics

The principal effect of an atrial septal defect is an

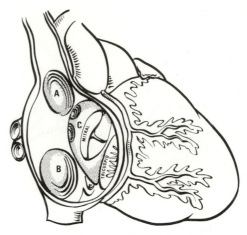

Fig. 9.15 Atrial septal defects: (a) a high defect, (b) a foramen ovale type defect and (c) an ostium primum defect associated with a cleft septal leaflet of the mitral valve.

abnormal flow of blood from the left atrium into the right atrium. This occurs because the pressure in the left atrium is normally 12 mmHg, whereas the normal right atrial pressure is only 5 mmHg. Blood flowing through the defect joins the normal venous return from the superior and inferior venae cavae. The right ventricle has to cope with this extra blood and it hypertrophies. The pulmonary artery becomes dilated and the pulmonary circulation is overfilled with blood. The excessive pulmonary blood flow leads in time (25–35 years) to the development of obliterative changes in the pulmonary vascular bed and ultimately to pulmonary hypertension.

The diagnosis is suggested by the finding of a systolic murmur over the pulmonary artery, with a fixed delay in the closing sound of the pulmonary valve. The EGG usually shows the pattern of a right bundle branch block. X-ray screening shows an engorged pulmonary circulation, a dilated pulmonary artery with excessive pulsation and an enlarged right ventricle. The diagnosis is confirmed by right heart catheterisation which reveals that blood samples from the right atrium have an increased oxygen content.

Surgery

Operative treatment involves closure of the defect using heart-lung bypass. A small defect less than 2 cm in diameter can usually be closed with sutures; if the defect is larger, a patch of pericardium is sewn over the hole. The operative mortality is less than 2%.

Fallot's tetralogy

This is the commonest cause of 'blue babies' who survive the first year of life. In infants, transposition of great vessels is commonest, but many babies with transposition die during the first weeks or months after birth.

Haemodynamics

The four defects are (Fig. 9.14):

1. Pulmonary stenosis,
2. Ventricular septal defect (VSD),
3. Gross hypertrophy of the right ventricle,
4. The root of the aorta straddling the VSD.

The first two abnormalities are the important ones from a functional point of view. The pulmonary stenosis is usually valvular with, invariably, narrowing of the outflow tract of the right ventricle. Because of this stenosis, the right ventricle hypertrophies until it becomes more powerful than the left. Venous blood is pumped into the systemic circulation and cyanosis results. The degree of cyanosis depends on the severity of the obstruction in the right ventricular outflow tract. In the most severe examples, the pulmonary valve is atretic, the pulmonary artery is represented by a thin cord and survival depends on patency of the ductus arteriosus and the development of a collateral circulation between the systemic and pulmonary circulation via the bronchial arteries. One-third of children with Fallot's tetralogy die during the first year of life. The survivors suffer from 'cyanotic attacks' in which they become very cyanosed and may lose consciousness. These attacks are due to excessive systolic contraction of the abnormally thick muscle in the outflow tract of the right ventricle. Blood flow to the lungs from the right ventricle virtually ceases and the right to left shunt through the ventricular septal defect becomes total.

A secondary polycythaemia is an invariable accompaniment of central cyanosis and children with cyanotic congenital heart disease have packed cell volumes and haemoglobin levels in excess of normal. Consequently, cerebral thrombosis is a common complication in children with Fallot's tetralogy.

Surgery

In most cases, corrective surgery involving remodelling of the outflow tract of the right ventricle and closure of the ventricular septal defect, is carried out as soon as the diagnosis is confirmed. Some very ill infants may require a temporizing operation to keep them alive and thriving until operation to correct the defects is done (p. 144).

Where the pulmonary valve is atretic and the pulmonary artery very small, the operation restores continuity between the right ventricle and the pulmonary arteries with a valved conduit of biological or prosthetic material.

Transposition of the great vessels

Although this complex defect is one of the commonest defects found in new-born babies, it is usually incompatible with life and few children survive untreated beyond the age of 1 year. In effect, the aorta arises from the right ventricle and the pulmonary artery from the left. The systemic and pulmonary circulations are circuits in parallel rather than in series and unless there is a septal defect or patent ductus arteriosus, through which mixing can occur, death is inevitable (Nadas & Fyler, 1972).

Babies born with these defects present an urgent diagnostic problem, since the mortality rate, untreated, in the first few months of life is about 60%. Where mixing between the systemic and pulmonary circuits is minimal, hypoxia is extreme. Where a large ventricular septal defect co-exists with lesser degrees of subaortic stenosis, the pulmonary circulation is exposed to high pressure and obliterative vascular changes progress rapidly to a point where corrective or palliative surgery is of no value.

Treatment

In those babies with inadequate mixing of the systemic and pulmonary circulations, the temporizing procedure, applicable in most cases, consists of creating a large interatrial septal defect. This can be done with a special cardiac catheter under fluoroscopy (balloon septostomy; Rashkind & Miller, 1966). The standard operation for simple transposition is inflow correction, which redirects the systemic venous return through the mitral valve to the left ventricle and pulmonary artery, and the pulmonary venous return through the tricuspid valve, right ventricle and aorta. Thus, it provides physiological but not anatomical correction.

If the transposition is accompanied by a large ventricular septal defect or patent ductus, the left ventricle may be accustomed to a higher pressure and this will allow anatomical repair by surgically transposing the aorta and pulmonary artery.

Tricuspid atresia

In this rare condition the tricuspid valve has not formed, the right ventricle is usually vestigial and the only exit for blood from the right atrium is through the foramen ovale into the left atrium. Children with this defect are darkly cyanosed and rarely survive the first few years of life.

Surgery

Complete correction is not yet possible, but a significant degree of palliation has been achieved by the Blalock-Taussig procedure. More recently, Fontan's operation, in which the right atrium is anastomosed to the pulmonary artery, has been followed by even greater palliation.

Pulmonary stenosis

This may be valvular or infundibular. The former commonly occurs as an isolated lesion, the latter is rarely seen alone but occurs as part of a defect such as Fallot's tetralogy.

A few cases of pulmonary stenosis are so severe as to cause right heart failure in infancy, but in most patients symptoms are few until late childhood or adolescence when dyspnoea and occasionally angina of effort and syncopal attacks occur.

Diagnosis is suspected from the findings of a harsh systolic murmur over the pulmonary area and a palpable right ventricular heave. X-ray screening shows an enlarged right ventricle, poststenotic dilatation of the pulmonary artery, and translucent (oligaemic) lung fields. Right heart catheterisation reveals an elevation of pressure in the right ventricle with a gradient in systole across the pulmonary valve.

Surgery

Operation is performed with heart-lung bypass. The stenosis is relieved by cutting the fused or rudimentary commissures of the valve, or by excising the abnormally thickened muscle on the outflow tract of the right ventricle. Because a patent foramen ovale frequently accompanies pulmonary stenosis, it is necessary to inspect the atrial septum and close the foramen with stitches.

Coarctation of the aorta

This is a constriction in the arch or descending part of the thoracic aorta. The most common type (postductal) is shown in Figure 9.16(b). The rarer pre-ductal coarctation is shown in Figure 9.16(a).

Haemodynamics

Post-ductal coarctation. This condition is characterized by hypertension in the head and arms, with hypotension and impalpable pulses in the lower half of the body. An extensive collateral circulation develops to feed the descending aorta, through the internal mammary, scapular and intercostal arteries. Notching of the ribs, seen on X-ray, is a manifestation of these greatly enlarged arteries. Untreated patients are at risk from cerebral haemorrhage and bacterial endocarditis and aneurysm formation at the site of the coarctation.

Preductal coarctation. Children born with this type usually suffer severe cardiac failure in infancy and other intracardiac defects usually accompany the aortic anomaly. The descending aorta is fed by unoxygenated blood from the pulmonary artery through the ductus which is usually wide.

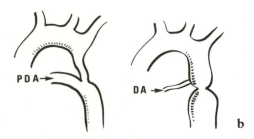

Fig. 9.16 Coarctation of the aorta: (a) preductal or infantile type (b) postductal or adult type

In either type of coarctation, the hypertension in the upper extremities may persist after successful resection of the narrowed segment. The cause of this has not been fully elucidated but it is unusual if operation is performed early enough.

Surgery

Cases of preductal coarctation usually present in infancy and the results of surgery depend largely on the complexity of coexisting defects and whether or not they can be corrected.

In the commoner type of postductal coarctation, the narrowed segment can be resected with end-to-end reconstruction of the aorta. Alternatively, if the narrowing involves some length of the aorta or where aneurysm formation has occurred, replacement of a segment of aorta by a tubular or patch prosthesis may be necessary.

Subclavian artery patch angioplasty is a relatively new but most successful technique for coarctation repair (Hamilton et al, 1978).

At operation, every effort must be made to leave some of the circumference of the aorta in situ so that the reconstructed segment can grow with the child.

An occasional complication of coarctation surgery is an acute intestinal crisis, characterized by ileus and distension and due to submucosal bleeding in the small bowel. It appears that in these cases release of the aortic obstruction is followed by disruption of arterioles in the gut wall and mesentery.

Congenital aortic stenosis

Three types are recognized: valvular (87%), subvalvular (10%) or supravalvular (3%). The latter is rare and is a coarctation of the aorta just above the aortic valve. Subvalvular stenosis may take the form of an abnormal ridge of myocardium protruding into the outflow tract of the left ventricle or a fibrous diaphragm just under the valve. In the commoner valvular stenosis, one or more commissures of the valve are absent and the valve is bicuspid or represented by a perforated diaphragm.

Haemodynamics

Congenital aortic stenosis is an insidious disease and secondary pathology tends to be advanced before symptoms become apparent. The left ventricle undergoes massive concentric hypertrophy in an effort to maintain a normal output though the obstruction and symptoms appear only when the myocardium begins to fail. Exertional dyspnoea occurs when the left ventricle fails to forward blood from the pulmonary circulation to the systemic. Angina occurs when the hypertrophied myocardium has outstripped the available coronary blood supply. When the failing ventricle cannot meet the demand for an increased cardiac output on exertion, episodes of syncope from cerebral ischaemia result. When angina and syncopal attacks occur in a patient with aortic stenosis, death is probable within 18 months.

Because a severe degree of aortic stenosis may exist in a patient who is symptom-free, the pressure gradient across the obstruction should be measured whenever the diagnosis of aortic stenosis is suspected clinically.

Surgery

Valvular stenosis. In children, it is usually possible to cut one of the rudimentary commissures to yield a functioning bicuspid valve. In adults, excision and replacement of the valve is always necessary because destruction of the architecture of the valve is invariable and calcification of the cusps is common. This progressive damage results from the turbulence set up by the jet-stream of blood forced through the stenosed valve.

Subvalvular stenosis. The obstruction is relieved by dividing the fibromuscular ridge which bulges into the outflow tract. Care must be taken to avoid damage to the conduction pathway.

Supravalvular stenosis. This form of coarctation is relieved by making a vertical incision across the narrowed segment, and then reconstructing a normal lumen by sewing in a lozenge-shaped patch.

These operations all require heart-lung bypass, with intermittent cold perfusion of the coronary arteries. In older patients the successful outcome of aortic valve surgery depends largely on maintaining the integrity of the left ventricle by adequate cardioplegia and selective cardiac cooling.

CORONARY HEART DISEASE

Arteriosclerotic narrowing of the coronary arteries is the principal cause of unexpected death in males between 35 and 65 years of age in Western societies.

Pathophysiology

The coronary circulation is unique and paradoxical in a number of respects. It supplies an organ which is continuously active, which cannot sustain an oxygen debt and which is very intolerant of hypoxia. The coronary vascular bed is squeezed during systole by the muscle which it supplies. Coronary flow occurs principally in diastole, yet during tachycardia, when myocardial oxygen demand is increased, the duration of diastole is reduced.

The myocardium extracts a relatively large proportion (50–60%) of the oxygen in the blood delivered to it. The oxygen tension in coronary venous blood is normally <20 mmHg. An increase of ventricular work requires a corresponding increase in coronary blood flow since oxygen extraction is already near maximal at rest.

Coronary flow in an adult, at rest, with a cardiac output of 5.0 litres represents 70 ml/min/100 g myocardium. (The normal myocardial weight is 300 g.) During maximal exercise this flow increases five- or six-fold to 300–400 ml/min/100 g. The coronary vasodilation which permits this increase in flow is largely mediated by metabolites, e.g. adenosine (Berne, 1964).

In the patient with coronary arteriosclerosis, where coronary flow is limited by obstructing lesions, the small vessels distal to the block display compensatory vasodilation to supply the myocardial oxygen needs. By so doing, however, the autoregulatory reserve is reduced. Sudden increases in ventricular oxygen demand such as accompanies exercise or strong emotions may then lead to a dangerous decrease in the ratio of coronary blood flow to tissue metabolism. A decrease in the supply/demand ratio can precipitate an attack of angina or even produce areas of hypoxia which can trigger ventricular fibrillation and sudden death.

Treatment

Pending discovery of the factors which lead to the formation of atheroma in blood vessels, treatment at present is designed to improve the vital ratio, coronary blood supply/myocardial demands.

Drug treatment aims at decreasing myocardial needs. Thus glyceryl trinitrate, by its dilator action on systemic veins, reduces venous return, cardiac output and hence ventricular work. Selective β-receptor blockade shields the heart from the sympathetic driving stimuli which normally accompany emotion and exercise.

Surgical treatment aims at improving the supply of blood to the myocardium. In 1969 Favoloro applied to the coronary circulation an operation which had been used in the amelioration of peripheral vascular disease for some 20 years. The autogenous vein bypass graft procedure (Fig. 9.17) has been shown to relieve angina in 75–80% of

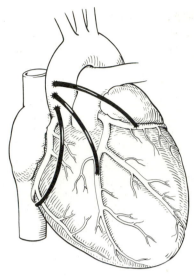

Fig. 9.17 Saphenous vein bypass grafts for the relief of coronary artery stenosis or blocks.

the cases operated on, and in a high proportion of these, improvement in myocardial function and exercise tolerance can also be demonstrated. Each vein graft delivers, on average, at rest, 50 ml/min blood flow to the distal coronary vascular bed.

The patient's own internal mammary artery divided as it leaves the chest and anastomosed end-to-side to the obstructed coronary artery, appears to function better than a vein graft. Prospective randomised trials designed to assess the effect of the operation on long-term survival are incomplete at the time of writing but evidence is now available to show that the 5-year survival rate of patients with critical stenoses of two or three main coronary arteries is significantly improved by the operation.

The criteria governing the selection of patients for the operation are still evolving. At present, the principle group for whom surgery is considered are those with angina of a degree which alters the life pattern of the patient and which has been unresponsive to drug therapy. Such patients should be investigated by coronary angiography and left ventriculography. Among those studied in this way, a small proportion are found to have extensive peripheral occlusions which imply a poor run-off for a graft, or a diffusely dyskinetic (poorly contracting) left ventricle. In these patients the risks of surgery are higher and the results poor. On the other hand, the demonstration, by ventriculography, of a localized area of poor contraction or an aneurysm is a further indication for surgery. Excision of an aneurysmal area improves ventricular function and improves the patient's exercise tolerance.

There is a group of patients in whom early surgery is mandatory. Several studies attest to the very poor prognosis in patients who have a block in their left main coronary artery, or at its bifurcation into the circumflex and left anterior descending arteries. The presence of these lesions on coronary arteriography calls for early surgery.

Surgery after an acute heart attack

There are three 'surgical' complications of acute myocardial infarction, viz. ventricular septal defect, mitral incompetence and ventricular aneurysm.

Postinfarction ventricular septal defect

This occurs in 1 or 2% of those who survive infarction. It is due to occlusion or critical stenosis of the left anterior descending coronary artery. The apical part of the interventricular septum softens and gives way some 7–10 days after the heart attack. The resultant defect permits a torrential left-to-right intracardiac shunt with pulmonary oedema and peripheral circulatory failure. Intensive medical management may save the patient's life in the short term, but unless the defect is closed at operation, heart failure and death within months is inevitable.

Mitral incompetence

A soft apical systolic murmur can be heard in 20–25% of patients who survive acute myocardial infarction. It is probably due to mitral incompetence but is of little haemodynamic significance and disappears in a few days. The mitral incompetence which develops suddenly 2 or 3 weeks after infarction is less common, but is life-threatening. Signs of left heart failure follow quickly and a steady downhill course is the rule. The underlying lesion is infarction of a papillary muscle with subsequent rupture of the muscle or its chordae tendinae. The correct management in most cases is replacement of the mitral valve with a prosthesis.

Myocardial aneurysm

In about 16% of patients who are recovering from an acute heart attack, a ventricular aneurysm forms (Mourdijinis et al, 1968). This sequel is most likely to complicate a large transmural infarct in the lateral wall of the left ventricle. A bulge can be seen in the cardiac silhouette on X-ray and in many cases paradoxical pulsation is obvious. It is a late complication, developing insidiously 6–8 weeks after infarction. The loss of contractile myocardium and the fact that it yields during systole results in a reduction in stroke volume. About half such aneurysms are lined by 'mural' thrombus which may fragment and release systemic emboli. Excision of the aneurysm with remodelling of the ventricle is indicated for all but the smallest myocardial aneurysms. Occasionally the aneurysm compromises the mitral valve mechanism, in which case, mitral valve replacement is also indicated.

Immediate postinfarct revascularisation

This relatively new concept in coronary artery surgery is based on the assumption that revascularization within the first 6 hours of an acute infarct may provide an adequate circulation to the peri-infarction zone which at that time is ischaemic and not frankly infarcted and may, therefore, in the long run reduce the infarct size. This technique is being used in some centres in North America and its value at present remains rather controversial. To undertake surgery of this nature requires rapid transit of the patient to the hospital and similar rapidity of coronary arteriography and transfer to surgery. A parallel approach at the present time involves intraluminal coronary artery dilatation techniques using suitable catheter and dilator and also the installation of thrombolytic agents, for example, streptokinase, into the coronary artery in an attempt to lyse recent thrombus. These techniques are currently under evaluation. The success of such techniques clearly depends upon accurate selection of suitable patients. If streptokinase therapy or intraluminal coronary dilatation are to be undertaken immediate open-heart surgical facilities must be available for cases of imperfect or even failed intervention.

BRADYCARDIA SYNDROMES ('HEART BLOCK')

Under this heading we are considering a group of patients in whom the heart rate is abnormally low. The conditions are due to a malfunction of the conducting system of the heart at atrial or ventricular level or both. In the most widely recognized type, conduction is blocked through the Bundle of His, consequently the ventricles are cut off from the impulse from the sino-atrial node and beat at their own intrinsic rate, which is usually between 30–40 times per minute. Less commonly, the malfunction is in the sino-atrial node or in the atrial conduction pathways. In both conditions, the ventricles are liable to periods of asystole or extreme bradycardia. They are also prone to dangerous tachyrhythmias such as ventricular tachycardia or frequent ventricular extrasystoles — both conditions can be life-threatening. The cause or causes of the various types of heart block are not fully elucidated. The conditions are commonest in elderly patients and an association with coronary artery disease has been described (Davies, 1967). Conduction defects may be a sequel of myocarditis (diphtheritic, viral), and in another small group are associated with calcific aortic valve disease. In a few cases it accompanies a congenital septal defect and it is occasionally a sequel of a congenital septal defect and it is occasionally a sequel of intracardiac surgery. Heart block develops acutely after coronary thrombosis in 5–10% of cases, but in this group recovery is the rule provided further arrhythmias are prevented.

Pathological bradycardia affects the circulation in two ways: (i) there is a reduction in cardiac output so that the patient experiences lassitude, exertional intolerance and dyspnoea and, occasionally, angina; (ii) the heart is liable to periods of asystole whereupon the patient loses consciousness and falls to the ground (Stokes-Adams attack); convulsions, coma and death may follow if ventricular action does not resume. In heart block of long standing, the heart undergoes considerable enlargement because the ventricles increase their capacity to achieve a larger stroke volume. This compensates to some extent for the reduction in rate (cardiac output = stroke volume × heart rate). The large stroke volume and slow heart rate combine to produce a wide pulse pressure with a higher than normal systolic pressure and a low diastolic pressure. The occurrence of heart block for the first time within a few days of coronary artery thrombosis calls for urgent management. The fall in cardiac output results in a further reduction in coronary blood flow and dangerous ventricular arrhythmias commonly supervene. At the same time, reduced tissue perfusion induces a metabolic acidosis which further impairs heart action.

Treatment

The aim of treatment is to restore a heart rate which will provide an adequate cardiac output.

In 1952, Zoll demonstrated that the ventricular rate could be controlled by electrical impulses applied externally. The artificial pacemaker has been developed from this work and is now the standard treatment for most cases of heart block. The pacemaker has three components: (i) the generator which consists of batteries and electronics capable of generating about 5 volts; (ii) wires, usually encased in a catheter, to convey the impulses to the heart; (iii) electrodes (of platinum) which transfer the current to the myocardium. The commonly used pacemaker systems are shown in Figure 9.18.

As a general rule, as soon as the diagnosis of heart block is made, a temporary pacing system should be introduced. In the emergency situation, where heart block has occurred acutely after a coronary thrombosis and is associated with ventricular arrhythmias, an electrode wire can be passed into the heart through a needle introduced percutaneously at the apex. A second electrode is applied to the chest wall and both are connected to the pacemaker generator.

In less urgent situations, a temporary pacing catheter is passed from an arm vein to the heart and the electrodes at its tip are wedged at the apex of the right ventricle under fluoroscopic control. The butt end of this catheter is connected to a generator unit, which stands on the bedside locker.

In patients with chronic established heart block, the treatment is the implantation of a miniaturised pacing

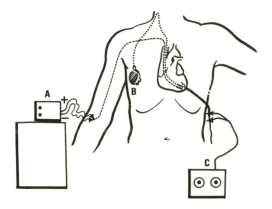

Fig. 9.18 Pacemakers. A: temporary pacing, the pacemaker generator at the bedside is connected to a pervenous electrode catheter. B: for permanent pacing, the entire unit is implanted. C: for emergency pacing, an external unit is connected to the electrode wires which are introduced through a needle into the apex of the heart ('Elecath')

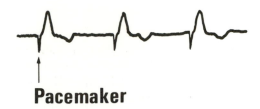

Pacemaker

Fig. 9.19 The electrocardiogram from an artificially paced heart. The sharp downward wave is the pacemaker impulse. It is followed by a widened QRST complex.

system. This requires general anaethesia, and because this can induce asystole in a patient with heart block, it is necessary first to introduce a temporary system under local anaesthesia, to gain control of the heart rate.

The implanted electrode catheter is usually introduced via the internal jugular vein, and manipulated under fluoroscopic control until the tip lodges in the apex of the right ventricle. The generator is implanted beneath the pectoral muscle and the catheter joined to it through a tunnel behind the clavicle.

The temporary pacing system is kept in position for a week, as a stand-by in case the permanent catheter should move and lose contact with the myocardium.

The ECG pattern during artificial pacing is shown in Figure 9.19.

The batteries in implantable pacemakers last for 8–10 years.

Battery exhaustion leads to pacing failure and is potentially life-threatening. This should be anticipated by measurements of pacemaker function made at a follow-up clinic, so that when early signs of battery depletion appear, elective replacement of the generator can be arranged. Normally, the ventricle will respond to an impulse of less than 2 volts and a current of 2 milliamperes.

The sympatheticomimetic drugs, isoprenaline and ephedrine, increase the rate and force of contraction of the ventricles and are used in the medical management of some cases of heart block, where pacing facilities are not immediately available.

In all patients, the 'pacing threshold', i.e. the lowest voltage which will consistently evoke ventricular contraction, rises during the first 3 weeks after commencement of artificial pacing.

In a few patients, a secondary rise in threshold occurs months or years after implantation and causes loss of pacing. The condition is termed 'exit block' and is thought to be due to fibrosis at the site of contact of the electrodes in the heart. When 'exit block' occurs acutely shortly after institution of pacing, the use of steroids may reduce the threshold. Where the threshold is found to be unacceptably high in a patient with a long standing endocardial pacing catheter, replacement of the catheter is necessary.

PHYSIOLOGICAL CHANGES AFTER HEART SURGERY: VITAL FUNCTION MONITORING

In the beginning of this chapter, attention was drawn to the adaptive changes which take place in the heart and circulation in the presence of a congenital or acquired defect. After surgical correction of the defect, these compensatory changes are redundant and may in some instances be harmful. Most of them undergo regression with the passage of time, and the circulatory system returns to normal. Others, however, are irreversible and their persistence may be associated with a continuing haemodynamic deficit. During the first few days after open heart surgery when circulatory re-adjustments are occurring most rapidly, the body's homoeostatic mechanisms are unstable, and careful monitoring of certain indices of circulatory efficiency is necessary in order to detect potentially harmful situations as soon as they develop. To this end, it is usual to nurse patients who have undergone major heart surgery in an intensive therapy area and to measure and record certain vital functions continuously or frequently. The significance of common patterns of changes in these functions is outlined here.

Arterial blood pressure

This measurement has gained acceptance as one of the more useful indices of circulatory well-being, and it is usually measured through an intra-arterial cannula connected to an electromanometer. It should be recognized, however, that while an adequate intra-arterial pressure is important, it is rather the volume and distribution of blood flow which determine the integrity of the various organs in the body.

Cardiac output

Maintenance of an adequate cardiac output is the principal objective in the management of the patient after cardiac surgery. This factor can be measured by indicator dilution techniques, of which, thermodilution with a Swan-Ganz catheter is most widely applicable (Swan et al, 1970). The signs of an inadequate output are restlessness, anxiety and drowsiness, coldness and pallor of the hands and feet, with empty superficial veins, a progressive reduction in urine output and the development of a metabolic acidosis.

The three common causes of a low output in the cardiac surgical patients are hypovolaemia, myocardial failure and tamponade.

Hypovolaemia

There is good evidence that early and rapid replacement of blood volume in the early post-operative period will augment the cardiac output (Fig. 9.20). The volume of blood lost at operation and subsequent losses through the chest drains are replaced as they occur. Direct measurement of the circulating blood volume in the early postoperative period has shown, however, that blood replacement must exceed the measured losses by about 20% in order to maintain normovolaemia. This is partly accounted for by the unmeasured blood losses into the mediastinum and pleural cavities and there is also evidence that some volume is lost to the circulation by 'pooling' in the splanchnic vascular bed. In the absence of direct measurements of the blood volume, the best guide to adequacy of replacement is the appearance of the superficial veins on the dorsum of the foot. If these veins are collapsed and empty the patient probably requires more blood. The central venous pressure, in contrast, is of little value as an index of blood volume in patients who have undergone cardiac surgery. Of the several factors which affect the central venous pressure in these patients, right ventricular function and peripheral vascular resistance override the influence of blood volume.

The following case is cited as an illustrative example. A patient aged 35 years has returned from theatre after the operation of mitral valve replacement. Shortly after arrival in the intensive therapy area, arterial blood pressure is 150/70, central venous pressure is 19 cm of water and rectal temperature is normal but the peripheral veins are empty and the extremities are cold and pale. The blood volume is 800 ml less than it was pre-operatively. 3 hours later, after infusion of 1000 ml of blood, the peripheral veins are full, arterial blood pressure is 115/80 and central venous pressure has fallen to 15 cm of water. In this case the initially high central venous pressure resulted from peripheral vasoconstriction which shifted blood from the periphery to the central great veins, and a poorly-acting

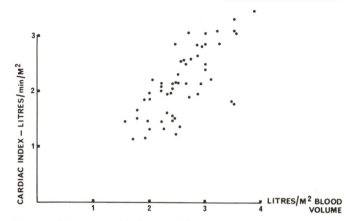

Fig. 9.20 The relationship between blood volume and the cardiac output (both related to surface area) in 55 patients studied 6–8 hours after major cardiac surgery

right ventricle which for a time failed to forward venous blood through the pulmonary circulation.

Myocardial failure

A low cardiac output due to pump failure is characterized by an elevated central venous pressure (which rises further in response to transfusion), a narrow pulse pressure, oliguria in the presence of adequate water intake, peripheral vasoconstriction, a falling arterial oxygen tension with a rising inflation pressure in patients who are maintained on intermittent positive pressure ventilation, or with increasing tachypnoea in patients who are breathing spontaneously. The patient will show evidence of impaired cerebral function and may be anxious and restless or drowsy and disorientated.

This low output state will be followed, within hours, by progressive renal and hepatic damage.

Treatment aims at improving cardiac output by manipulating the four principal determinants of ventricular function, viz. heart rate, ventricular filling pressure, ventricular after-load (systemic vascular resistance) and ventricular contractility. This is achieved by using artificial cardiac pacing, inotropic and chronotropic drugs such as isoprenaline or dopamine, peripheral vasodilator agents, such as sodium nitroprusside and nitroglycerin, and blood volume expansion.

Tamponade

Continuing bleeding from cardiotomy wounds may result in the collection of blood and clot under pressure in the pericardial sac. By compressing the atria and great veins, this leads to a progressive fall in cardiac output.

It is difficult to distinguish this cause of low output from myocardial failure. In both, the systolic blood pressure and pulse pressure are low and the venous pressure is high. Patency of the mediastinal and pericardial drains should be checked but if doubt remains the only recourse is to re-open the chest.

Blood Gases

Thoracotomy, intermittent positive pressure ventilation for some hours and heart-lung bypass cause multiple small areas of pulmonary atelectasis (Osborn, 1962). Perfusion of these unventilated alveoli allows venous blood to reach the systemic circulation with a consequent reduction in arterial P_{O_2}.

It is usually necessary to increase the inspired oxygen concentration to 50–60% in order to achieve a normal arterial P_{O_2} of 80–100 mmHg.

Carbon dioxide retention after thoracotomy is rarely due to intrinsic pulmonary pathology. It is due to hypoventilation and is seen in patients whose respiratory minute volume is subnormal because they are too drowsy, too weak or in too much pain to make adequate respiratory movements.

It is common practice during the first 6–8 hours after major heart surgery to keep the patients well sedated and maintain a correct respiratory minute volume with intermittent positive pressure ventilation. This practice has the added advantage of relieving the patient of the work of breathing.

Acid-base balance

A fall in the pH of the blood impairs myocardial contractility and in addition, induces ionic shifts which further weaken heart action and render arrhythmias likely. Three aberrations in acid-base balance may be seen after major cardiac surgery.

Respiratory Acidosis

This is due to hypoventilation and an arterial blood sample will yield the following figures: pH 7.20 units; P_{CO_2} 80 mmHg; standard bicarbonate 24 mmol. Bedside appraisal of the patient with a high P_{CO_2} can be misleading. He has warm flushed extremities, full peripheral veins, a bounding pulse and a raised blood pressure. Within a short time, however, 'carbon dioxide narcosis' occurs, the patient becomes drowsy, respiratory efforts become more inadequate, cardiac arrhythmias appear, and life is endangered.

Metabolic acidosis

This disorder develops when the systemic circulation is insufficient to meet the oxygen demands of the tissues. Typical figures are: pH 7.20 units; P_{CO_2} 40 mmHg; standard bicarbonate 18 mmol/l.

It is a sequel of a low cardiac output, and may be due to myocardial failure, hypovolaemia, peripheral vasoconstriction or cardiac tamponade. The immediate treatment is the intravenous administration of sodium bicarbonate, but at the same time steps must be taken to remove the cause, i.e. to improve the tissue perfusion.

Metabolic alkalosis

A metabolic alkalosis, characterized by a rise in pH and standard bicarbonate, results, amongst other causes, from the transfusion of relatively large volumes of donor blood. The acid-citrate-dextrose preservative in donor blood is metabolized in the body to produce sodium bicarbonate, with the production of a mild alkalosis. Typical figures are pH 7.55 units; P_{CO_2} 40 mmHg; standard bicarbonate 30 mmol/l. No treatment is necessary but a watch should be kept on serum potassium levels because these fall in the presence of an alkalosis.

The sick cell syndrome (Flear, 1971)

Some patients who have been in cardiac failure for months or years prior to surgery exhibit manifestations of this syndrome on the third or fourth day postoperatively.

Plasma sodium levels fall, urinary sodium levels fall and urinary potassium levels rise. Typical figures would be plasma Na 125 mmol/l; urine Na <20 mmol/l; urine K > 80 mmol/l.

The patient becomes weak and apathetic, with a reduced cardiac output, a poor peripheral circulation, bradycardia and a reduced digoxin tolerance.

The underlying mechanism is failure of the 'sodium pump' at cell membranes throughout the body, with the result that sodium leaks into the intracellular space and potassium leaks out.

In many patients spontaneous recovery takes place as the low cardiac output state improves after operation. In a few cases, active treatment is required. The sodium pump uses glucose as its energy source, and the administration of 50% glucose intravenously with insulin to allow its utilization has been shown to bring about improvement in the sick cell syndrome. Potassium supplements must be given to replace the urinary losses.

The glucose-insulin-potassium regimen consists of 50 ml of 50% glucose plus 20 units soluble insulin plus 10 mmol potassium every 2 hours.

REFERENCES

Berne R M 1964 Regulation of coronary blood flow. Physiology Review, 44:1

Brock R 1957 Anatomy of congenital pulmonary stenosis. Cassell, London

Davies M T 1967 A histological study of the conduction system in complete heart block. Journal of Pathology and Bacteriology 94:351

Favoloro R G 1969 Saphenous vein graft in the surgical treatment of coronary artery disease: operative technique. Journal of Thoracic and Cardiovascular Surgery 58:178

Flear C T G 1971 Electrolyte and body water changes after trauma Journal of Clinical Pathology, 23 (Supplement):4, 16

Gadboys H L, Slonim R & Litwak R S (1962) Homologous blood syndrome. I Preliminary observations on its relationship to clinical cardio-pulmonary bypass. Annals of Surgery 156:793

Hamilton D I, Di Eusanio G, Sandrasagra F A, Donnelly R J 1978 Early and late results of left subclavian flap aortoplasty for coarctation of the aorta in infancy. Journal of Thoracic and Cardiovascular Surgery 75: 699–704

Hearse D J, Stewart D A, Braimbridge M V 1976 Cellular protection during myocardial ischaemia. The development and characterization of a procedure for the induction of reversible ischaemic arrest. Circulation 54: 193–202

Hornblad P Y (1970). Ductus arteriosus and the mechanism of closure (Editorial) New England Journal of Medicine 282:566

Likoff W 1959 The change in pulmonary vascular resistance after relief of mitral obstruction. In: Adams W R, Veith I (eds) Pulmonary Circulation, Grune and Stratton, New York

Mourdjinis A, Olsen E, Raphael M T & Mounsey J P D 1968 The clinical diagnosis and prognosis of ventricular aneurysm. British Heart Journal 30:497

Mustard W T, Keith J D, Trusler G A, Fowler R & Kidd B S L 1964 The surgical management of transposition of the great vessels. Journal of Thoracic and Cardiovascular Surgery 48:953

Nadas A S & Fyler D C 1972 The transpositions. In: Pediatric Cardiology Saunders, London p 608

Osborn J J, Popper R W, Kerth W J & Gerbode F 1962 Respiratory insufficiency following open hert surgery. Annals of Surgery 156: 638

Rashkind W J & Miller W W 1966 Creation of an atrial septal defect without thoracotomy: A palliative approach to complete transposition of the great vessels. Journal of the American Medical Association 196:991

Rudolph A M 1970 The changes in the circulation after birth. Circulation 41:343

Swan H J C, Ganz W, Forester J, Marcus H, Diamond G, Chonette D 1970 Catheterisation of the heart in man with use of a flow-directed balloon-tipped catheter. New England Journal of Medicine 283:447

Taylor K M 1981 Pulsatile cardiopulmonary bypass. A review. Journal of Cardiovascular Surgery 22(6): 561–568

Taylor K M, Wright G S, Bain W H, Caves P K, Beastall G H 1978 Comparative studies of pulsatile and non-pulsatile flow during cardiopulmonary bypass. III Anterior pituitary response to thyrotrophin-releasing hormone. Journal of Thoracic and Cardiovascular Surgery 75:579

Wagenvoort C A, Heath D & Edwards J E 1964 The Pathology of the Pulmonary Vasculature. Charles C Thomas, Springfield USA p 146

Wood P 1958 The Eisenmenger syndrome or pulmonary hypertension with reversed shunt. British Medical Journal ii:701, 755

Zoll P M 1952 Resuscitation of the heart in ventricular standstill by external electric stimulation. New England Journal of Medicine 247: 768

Systemic circulation

This chapter gives a brief description of the anatomy of the blood vessels and the lymphatics. The circulation of blood through the peripheral vessels is discussed, along with methods of blood flow measurement. The factors which control blood pressure and abnormalities of it are described with reference to the role of the kidney in hypertension. The circulation through various specialized areas is briefly discussed, and the chapter ends with a description of the various pathological states which affect the peripheral vascular system.

ANATOMY

Arteries

The three tunics which form the wall of an artery have different functions in health and are subject to different diseases.

The *tunica intima* is relatively acellular, and is lined by a delicate endothelium marked off from the tunica media by the internal elastic lamina. The intima in health receives its nutrients by diffusion, but if it becomes thickened by atheroma, is liable to ulcerate. The function of the intima is to provide a non-wettable lining upon which the circulating blood does not clot.

Damage to the endothelium is followed by the deposition of platelets which may become the starting point for intravascular thrombosis. Such a thrombus may be overgrown by the endothelial layer, become incorporated in the substance of the intima, undergo fatty degeneration, and so give origin to a plaque of atheroma. In large arteries, atheromatous plaques do not materially encroach on the lumen of the artery, but by their tendency to ulcerate, are liable to lead to vascular thrombosis. In small arteries, the atheromatous plaques reduce the size of the lumen, and even without superadded thrombosis interfere with the flow of blood.

Finally, in prolonged hypertension, the intima of small arteries and arterioles becomes greatly thickened, by concentrically arranged cellular fibrous tissue. This end-arteritis reduces the lumen of the artery, and may eventually obliterate it.

The *tunica media* provides the mechanical strength of the arterial wall and is composed of fibro-elastic tissue and muscle in varying proportions. In large arteries, fibro-elastic tissue preponderates, but in smaller arteries, and especially in arterioles, the media is chiefly muscular. As age advances, the elastic tissue and muscle tend to be replaced by fibrous material so that large vessels become less elastic and the smaller ones less able to adjust the size of their lumen. The tunica media is thick and depends for nourishment on the vasa vasorum which enter it from the tunica adventitia.

The commonest disease of the tunica media is fibrosis in excess of the normal fibrotic change with advancing years, and the fibrous tissue may become calcified. Arteriosclerotic vessels are usually increased, not only in diameter but in length and are therefore often tortuous. Loss of elasticity of the arteries leads to an increased pulse pressure but does not in itself impede the transport of blood. However, plaques of atheroma are liable to develop in the intima which underlies areas of existing fibrosis or calcification of the media and these plaques may narrow the lumen. Finally, endarteritis of the vasa vasorum, especially in syphilis, may lead to the atrophy of the elastic and muscular tissue, and the weakened artery may stretch and form an aneurysm.

The *tunica adventitia* consists of areolar tissue, and serves to carry the vasa vasorum and the plexus of nerves destined for the tunica media.

The smaller arteries or arterioles contain smooth muscle which is innervated by adrenergic fibres. These vessels are the major site of resistance to flow and changes in their diameter lead to alterations of blood pressure.

Capillaries

Capillaries are the narrow vessels which link the arteriole to the venule. The capillary wall consists of a single layer of flattened endothelial cells cemented together edge-to-edge and is devoid of a muscular sheath. The capillaries are the area where most exchange of oxygen and nutrients occurs, and their exact structure varies from organ to organ. In some capillary beds, including those in cardiac muscle, the junctions between endothelial cells allows the passage of molecules 10 μm in diameter. In endocrine glands and the small intestine, the cytoplasm of endothelial cells contains gaps called fenestrations which allow the passage of very large molecules, and in the liver the endothelium is not continuous, allowing large gaps between individual cells.

The ability of the capillaries to open and close has been confirmed by many observers. How this is achieved in the absence of a muscular sheath is uncertain. One suggestion, so far only confirmed in the mesentery of the abdomen of the rat by Chambers and Zweifach (1944), is the existence of small, muscle-walled vessels called meta-arterioles. These are said to run from arteriole to venule with actual capillaries branching off them at intervals. The entrance to each capillary is thought to be guarded by a minute smooth muscle termed the pre-capillary sphincter. When these sphincters are opened, the vessels are about 6 μm in diameter.

Veins

The veins are wider channels than the arteries, have thinner walls and can adjust the size of their lumen to suit regional variations in blood flow. The large veins have walls composed mainly of fibro-elastic tissue, whereas small veins are muscular and can change their size. Valves are present in the veins of the limbs, which in longitudinal vessels permit only centripetal flow. In communicating veins between deep and superficial systems, flow is only allowed from superficial to deep. Veins of the abdomen, thorax, skull and spinal chord do not contain any valves.

Venous blood flow in the limbs depends on the veins being intermittently squeezed by the tissues in which they lie and this depends upon the limbs being moved. If a limb is held dependent and motionless, the venous return is arrested. It is, for example, impossible to stand quite still for longer than a few minutes, because sequestration of blood from veins of the legs leads to fainting. In varicose veins, the valves of the superficial system are incompetent and the direction of blood flow is centrifugal when the patient is erect.

Venous blood flow in the body cavities depends in part upon the great veins being subject to changes of pressure within the chest and abdomen caused by respiration. Centripetal flow is greatest during inspiration, when the descent of the diaphragm reduces the pressure within the thorax and increases it within the abdomen.

Arteriovenous anastomoses

In a number of areas, particularly in the skin, the hands and feet, and also in the gastrointestinal tract, there are short muscular channels which connect artery to vein, bypassing the capillary bed. These structures have muscular walls and are innervated by vasoconstrictor nerves. Opening and closing these shunts allows blood to bypass various capillary beds which is useful in situations where heat loss is required, for example, in the skin or in the gastrointestinal tract to allow arterialized blood to enter the portal system.

Lymphatic system

The lymphatic system drains fluids in the lungs and the body through a large number of narrow vessels which eventually coalesce to form large trunks which end in the blood stream at the junction of the right and left subclavian and internal jugular veins. Lymph vessels differ from capillaries in that the endothelial cells are not cemented together, leaving openings between individual cells. In addition, vessels contain valves and, in the course of their journey to the blood stream, pass through a number of lymph nodes.

CIRCULATION OF THE BLOOD

In the peripheral circulation, blood leaves the left ventricle at each systolic contraction and passes down the main arteries and then to the arterioles. From here it either bypasses or flows through the capillary bed to the venules and then returns to the heart by the great veins.

Haemodynamic changes

When every particle of a solution is moving with constant velocity in a tube parallel to the axis of the tube, the flow is described as undisturbed. In a steady state, undisturbed flow in a cylindrical tube results in laminar flow in which concentric laminae of flow occur because of the interface between wall and fluid, and the central laminae have a higher velocity than the peripheral laminae; the flow profile is parabolic. The law which governs steady flow in a cylindrical tube is Poiseuille's law:

$$Q = \frac{P\pi r^4}{8\,\mu L}$$

where Q = volume flow; P = pressure drop; r = radius of tube; L = length of tube; μ = viscosity.

This law describes the conditions present when the flow is undisturbed. At higher flow rates, the flow becomes disturbed and ultimately turbulent, in which, as well as the mass movement of the fluid along the tube, the particles of the fluid move randomly, some at right angles to the axis of flow. The equation describing the probability that flow in a certain situation is turbulent is Reynold's equation:

$$Re = \frac{\bar{V}r\rho}{\mu}$$

where Re = Reynold's number; V = mean velocity; ρ = fluid density; μ = viscosity.

When Reynold's number is greater than 2000 it is likely that flow is turbulent. When less than 2000, flow may be disturbed with peripheral eddies and local turbulence.

The importance of the change from laminar to turbulent flow is that there is a disproportionate increase in pressure drop from one point in the vascular system to another for higher flows, i.e. there is a dissipation of energy which constitutes energy loss.

Flow through an organ or limb can be simplified by considering mean flow and pressure drop across the organ, and the concept of peripheral resistance or the resistance in an organ can be expressed by analogy with Ohm's Law:

$$P_1 - P_2 = QR$$

where $P_1 - P_2$ = pressure drop; Q = volume flow; R = resistance to flow.

All these equations are oversimplifications and disregard the effect of the pulsatility of blood flow but nevertheless are useful when considering flow in a stenosed artery or through an organ or limb.

Arterial blood flow

In normal undiseased arteries, there is a pressure drop of about 10 mmHg between the aorta and the arterioles (Fig. 10.1).

In considering the total peripheral resistance, the various components are:

1. Arteries   25%
   (a) Aorta   4%
   (b) Large arteries   5%
   (c) Main arterial branches   10%
   (d) Terminal arterial branches   6%
2. Arterioles   41%
3. Capillaries   27%
4. Veins   7%

Blood flow in the normal arterial system is probably not truly turbulent, but disturbed, with the ascending aorta being the site of maximum disturbance.

In diseased arteries, where atheroma encroaches on the lumen and produces a stenosis, the result is a change in the type of flow, a dissipation of energy and a resultant drop in pressure. As classically described, a stenosis had

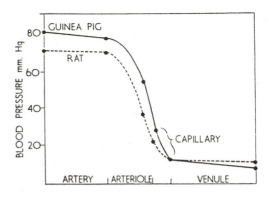

Fig. 10.1 The pressure gradient of the circulation. Note that the arterial pressure is mainly expanded in forcing blood through arterioles. Capillary pressure is lower in small rodents than in mammals. (After Landis, E. M. (1930). *Amer. J. Physiol.* **932**, 352.)

to reduce the luminal area to 20% of the normal area before there was a reduction in flow and before there was a significant pressure drop. This concept did not, however, take into account the possibility that blood flow might increase, e.g. in exercise, and that the patient's symptoms might only be experienced at higher flow rates. Under these circumstances, stenoses producing an area reduction to 60% of the unstenosed area might be haemodynamically significant (a stenosis reducing area to 60% constitutes a reduction in diameter by about 20%).

Pulsatile flow, although associated with a higher energy loss than steady state flow, has been shown to be more effective at achieving perfusion of organs or limbs. In one experimental situation, pulsatile flow produced an increase in perfusion pressure of more than 15%, compared with a comparable steady flow. This factor must also be considered when the effect of a stenosis is considered since flow profile will be damped at a stenosis and the effective distal flow will be reduced.

Capillary exchange

The exchange of fluid between the intravascular and extravascular compartments takes place in the fenestrated capillaries. The fluid exchange is described in Starling's hypothesis where the pressures promoting fluid loss from the intravascular compartment are the hydrostatic pressure in the capillaries and the osmotic pressure in the tissue fluid external to the capillaries; the pressures promoting absorption of fluid from the extravascular to the intravascular compartment are tissue pressure and intravascular osmotic pressure (oncotic pressure). The balance between these hydrostatic and osmotic pressures determines the net gain or loss of fluid in a capillary bed. The intravascular hydrostatic pressure may be raised in venous obstructive disease or congestive cardiac failure in which case fluid tends to accumulate in the extravascular compartment causing oedema. In early shock, the intravascular hydrostatic pressure can be reduced and there may be a net gain into the intravascular compartment helping to reduce the severity of the shock process. In hypoproteinaemic states, intravascular oncotic pressure is reduced and oedema may form.

Capillary pathology may affect the permeability of capillaries and thereby influence the effective plasma oncotic pressure. In thermal injuries, or after revascularisation of an ischaemic area, there may be a net loss of fluid from the capillaries because of a change in porosity.

Venous blood flow

Venous return from the lower limb is effected by two systems, superficial and deep, each of which contains bicuspid valves to direct flow to the heart. At the knee and the groin the superficial system anastomoses with the deep system at junctions containing valves permitting flow only from superficial to deep systems. At other sites in the leg, communicating veins (perforators) interconnect the superficial and deep venous systems. Valves on these communicating veins direct blood only from superficial to deep systems. Valves are not present in the inferior vena cava or in the common iliac veins and only infrequently in the external iliac veins.

The hydrostatic pressure from the heart to the leg would be in excess of 100 mmHg were it not for the presence of valves which interrupt the column of blood. In the muscle compartments of the leg, muscle contraction raises venous pressure and encourages venous return (the muscle pump). In the abdomen there is a pressure differential with reference to the thorax which is produced by respiration. With descent of the diaphragm in inspiration, abdominal pressure rises and thoracic pressure falls; the net effect is a pressure gradient from abdomen to thorax which encourages venous return to the heart.

In the normal situation, venous return is directed by the presence of valves and is produced by the muscle pump and the pressure effects of the respiratory cycle.

Where previous venous disease has occurred or valves have been damaged and become incompetent, the efficiency of venous return is impaired and there is back pressure on the distal capillary beds producing oedema. Because higher hydrostatic pressure may be transmitted retrogradely in the venous system when one or a few valves become incompetent, there may be progressive damage to valves as each one becomes subject to increasing hydrostatic pressure before becoming incompetent in turn. The rationale of compression sclerotherapy is to prevent this cascading effect and protect distal valves before they are damaged by hydrostatic pressure.

The circulation of lymph

The movement of fluid through the capillary walls normally exceeds the return. The function of the lymphatics is to allow the extra fluid to return to the circulation. The normal 24 hour lymph flow is between 2 and 4 litres. The factors producing lymphatic return are very similar to those helping venous return to the heart and include the contraction of muscles, the pulsation of adjacent arteries and the level of intrathoracic pressure, all helped by the valves within the lymphatic vessels. However, recent evidence suggest that lymphatics are able to contract rhythmically, which may account for the majority of centripetal movement. Lymph also carries protein, particularly in special areas such as the intestine, liver and kidney, in addition to long chain fatty acid such as cholesterol.

MEASUREMENT OF BLOOD FLOW

A variety of methods exist for measuring blood flow. They can be subdivided according to whether the method is invasive or non-invasive. Each method has its own applications and limitations.

Plethysmography

This is one of the earliest methods of measurement of blood flow, introduced in the early 1900s. The aim of the method is to occlude the venous return from a limb and measure the change in volume of the limb as arterial flow continues. Venous return is interrupted by application of a pneumatic cuff at a proximal point on the limb. The change in volume of the leg can be measured directly from air or fluid displacement from an air or fluid filled container applied around the limb, or it can be measured indirectly by weighing the suspended limb or detecting change in circumference with a strain gauge.

Air-filled plethysmographs are subject to errors since an observed change in volume may be related to a change in temperature rather than a true change of the volume of the leg. Fluid-filled plethysmographs exert a hydrostatic pressure on the enclosed limb and this may affect blood flow. Strain gauges, e.g. mercury-in-Silastic, are simple to use and are sufficiently accurate for most routine purposes.

Indicator-dilution

This invasive method is based on the Fick principle which enables blood flow to be calculated if a known amount of indicator is injected into the flowing stream and the arterial and venous concentrations of the diluted indicator can be measured. When applied to cardiac output measurements, the circulation through the pulmonary vascular system can be calculated by knowing the oxygen consumption of the patient, and the arterial and venous oxygen concentration. In this situation, oxygen is the 'indicator'.

In the peripheral circulation, indicator dyes or radioisotopic tracers can be utilized so long as there is no loss of the indicator into the peripheral tissues. This method can be used with limited accuracy to measure mean flow through an organ or limb or at a site in the arterial or venous systems, but the method is subject to errors inherent in the assumptions made before the calculations.

Local clearance

With increasing availability of radioisotopic tracers, this method has become applicable to measurements of the effectiveness of blood flow through an organ or tissue. In the peripheral circulation, radioisotopes of sodium, krypton or xenon can be used and the clearance of the isotope calculated mathematically from the reduction in the radiation counts over the injection site. This method is usually invasive, i.e. the isotope is injected, though it is possible to arrange that the isotope is either inhaled or applied to skin and absorbed by diffusion. Errors in the method are related to assumptions about the lack of tissue damage by the injection, or the lack of tissue binding of the isotope.

Electromagnetic flowmeters

Electromagnetic flowmeters are based on Faraday's laws of electromagnetic induction. When a mass moves through a magnetic field, a voltage difference is generated which is proportional to the size of the mass. In practice the appropriate vessel is surgically exposed and a flow probe is applied to encircle the vessel. A known magnetic field is generated electromagnetically and the potential difference produced by the blood flow is measured by two electrodes incorporated into the probe. A variety of methods of electrically producing the magnetic field are available — square wave, sine wave, modified square wave — each with its own advantages and disadvantages. All the methods are subject to assumptions that the probe closely fits the artery, that the vessel wall and the magnetic field are uniform, and that the flow is symmetrical and axial. Within the limitations of these assumptions, the method enables blood flow to be measured peroperatively and is often used in reconstructive arterial surgery.

A recent modification of the method uses an intravascular catheter-mounted probe which obviates the need for operative exposure of the vessel. The method, however, has its own errors, in particular that the flow is assumed to be even and that the dimensions of the vessel must be known.

Ultrasonic flowmeters

Ultrasonic flowmeters are a more recent and non-invasive type of flowmeter: strictly speaking, they should be described as velocity meters. They utilize low energy ultrasound of very high frequency, e.g. 10 MHz, which penetrates tissues for a few centimetres. They make use of the Doppler effect to measure the movement of reflecting particles through the ultrasound beam. The Doppler effect states that when a sound wave is transmitted from or reflected from a moving object, the transmitted frequency is altered by the movement. In practice with the velocity of flow in most peripheral arteries, the red cells in the blood produce a change in the incident ultrasound frequency which may be up to 10 kHz. The ultrasonic flowmeter compares the generated and received frequency and detects the difference due to the movement. This difference lies in the audible frequency spectrum so that commercial 'Dopplers' generate a flow noise which is audible with earphones or loudspeaker.

In order to measure flow, the dimensions of the vessel have to be known as has the angle between the ultrasound beam and the axis of blood flow. The noise can be analysed electronically for all its component frequencies and a measurement of mean or instantaneous flow derived.

This method has been of particular use in the diagnosis and management of peripheral vascular disease where artheromatous disease changes the flow profile of blood flow in arteries. Sophisticated machines which incorporate real time imaging and Doppler frequency analysis are now available. These 'Duplex' machines can measure volume flow and are particularly useful in the diagnosis of carotid arterial disease.

MEASUREMENT OF BLOOD PRESSURE

The methods of measurement of blood pressure are subdivided according to whether the measurement is made directly or indirectly. Both methods are applicable to measurement of arterial blood pressure while venous pressure is usually only measurable directly.

Direct measurement of blood pressure

In general, systems for direct measurement of blood pressure comprise a manometer and a hydraulic system for transmitting the intravascular pressure from the lumen of the vessel to the transducer.

For measurement of venous pressure the manometer can be a fluid filled column which is hydraulically connected to the required recording site by a narrow fluid or blood-filled tube, e.g. a central venous pressure catheter. Pressure is recorded from a predetermined zero by noting the height of the saline column which balances the venous pressure at the end of the catheter. The predetermined zero is important in venous pressure measurements because of the low venous pressures encountered relative to the errors associated with different arbitrary zeros. Pressure is notionally referred to the same hydrostatic level as the right atrium, the surface marking of which is the mid-axillary line when the patient is recumbent. To confirm the exact postion of the measuring catheter, it is recommended that radio-opaque catheters are used and the position of the catheter can then be determined radiologically. If required, the venous pressure can be recorded with a transducer in which the venous pressure distorts a sensitive electromechanical device and gives rise to an electrical signal which is proportional to the pressure. The magnitude of this signal can be displayed on a meter or on a pen recorder.

For measurement of arterial pressure it is not possible to use saline manometers to balance the arterial pressure because the column of saline corresponding to normal arterial pressure would be approximately 4 feet. Another problem associated with a fluid-filled column is the inertia of the fluid which results in a slow response to changing pressure. Both of these problems are overcome by using electrical transducers which have a high frequency response. Pressure is generally transmitted via a needle which punctures the artery and then via a manometer connecting tube — a narrow saline filled tube which is free of air bubbles.

For both venous and arterial measurements, a new intravascular transducer has been developed which is small enough to be passed into the lumen of a vessel and therefore dispenses with the need for manometer connecting tubes which may introduce errors into the measurements. This is, however, expensive and not available for routine use.

Because arterial pressures are high relative to the error associated with variation in the hydrostatic level of the transducer relative to the patient, no account need be taken of a predetermined zero pressure level when arterial measurements are to be made.

Direct pressure recording is used in low flow states, e.g. shock, when indirect measurement may be inaccurate or indeed impossible.

Indirect measurement of blood pressure

Arterial pressure may be measured by applying indirectly to the artery a known pressure which occludes the artery and then measuring the pressure at which flow occurs. This method of sphygmomanometry has been in universal clinical use since first introduced by Korotkoff in 1905. The pressure applied to the occlusive pneumatic cuff is usually measured either on a mercury column or on an aneroid meter. As originally described, the onset of flow was determined by auscultation over the artery distal to the cuff and when flow recommences, Korotkoff's sounds are clearly audible. The origin of these sounds has not yet been adequately explained. The method is, however, accurate in children and adults provided care is taken to use a cuff which is the appropriate size relative to the dimension of the arm.

A variety of other methods have been developed to signify the onset of flow and dispense with auscultation. Capacitance pulse pick-ups, ultrasonic flow detectors, strain gauge transducers, photo-electric and radio-isotopic methods will all signify the onset of flow and permit more objective measurement of systolic pressure; none of these methods can, however, be used to measure diastolic pressure.

In low pressure states, e.g. in peripheral vascular disease affecting the lower limb, and in infants, the auscultatory method may not be possible since the signals are inaudible and then one of the above methods may have to be employed.

A variation in the method using ultrasonic flow detectors is now available whereby systolic and diastolic pressures can be measured. In this method the ultrasound signal is filtered to select the signals from blood vessel wall motion and not from blood movement. This method has a high degree of correlation with systolic and diastolic pressures measured directly.

CONTROL OF THE PERIPHERAL CIRCULATION

Blood pressure is maintained by rhythmic cardiac contractions working against the peripheral resistance generated mainly by the arterioles in the peripheral vascular tree. Variations in the diameter of arterioles, or other factors such as the viscosity of blood can alter blood pressure and flow, as already described. In addition, the peripheral circulation is controlled by a number of local factors such as the autonomic nervous system, the endocrine system, or external pharmacological agents which act directly on arterioles or capillaries to produce particular changes in those areas. Furthermore, blood pressure and flow in peripheral vessels is dependent upon the mechanical properties of the vessel wall. Each of these factors will be discussed in turn.

Control of blood pressure

The normal control of blood pressure is achieved by the carotid and aortic baroreceptors and by variations in heart rate, stroke volume and arterial tone under the control of the autonomic nervous system. The diameter of these arterioles is altered by a central control mechanism situated in the medulla oblongata called the vasomotor centre which integrates various incoming impulses and produces

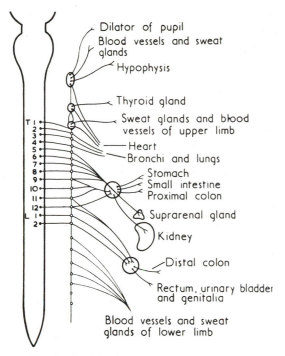

Fig. 10.2A The distribution of the sympathetic nerves.

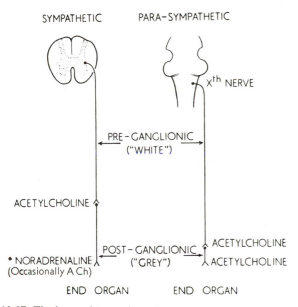

Fig. 10.2B The humoral transmitters in autonomic nerves.

The baroreceptors are stretch receptors in the carotid arteries and aortic arch. They are stimulated by distension of the structures in which they are located and discharged when blood pressure rises, thereby reducing the discharge of the vasometer centre and producing a reduction in the peripheral resistance. The reverse occurs during decreased distension, such as in hypotension.

The chemoreceptors are stimulated during hypoxia and cause peripheral vasoconstriction and tachycardia. The effects of the vasomotor centre on cardiac output and heart rate are discussed elsewhere.

Blood pressure can fall rapidly when the upright posture is suddenly assumed. Blood tends to pool in the legs, diminishing venous return which, in turn, reduces the discharge from the aortic and carotid baroreceptors. This leads to a reflex adjustment of the arteriolar diameter and an increase in peripheral resistance. The small and medium-sized veins also contract in response to sympathetic stimulation restoring venous return towards normal levels, which in conjunction with the increased peripheral resistance, restores blood pressure.

Sympathetic nervous system

Two types of sympathetic fibres innervate arterioles: cholinergic and adrenergic (Figure 10.2A and B). Cholinergic efferent fibres innervate resistance vessels in muscle, and are also sudomotor to sweat glands. The effect of acetylcholine injected into the main artery of the limb is to produce a peripheral vasodilation and an increase in blood flow through the limb.

Adrenergic efferent fibres innervate skin resistance and capacity vessels. The net effect of noradrenaline injected into the main artery of the limb is to produce profound peripheral vasoconstriction with a marked reduction in blood flow through the limb. This effect is mainly due to decreased muscle blood flow, although there is an accompanying reduction in skin blood flow which may be so severe that local ischaemic changes can occur.

Adrenaline administered intra-arterially initially increases blood flow, which soon returns to normal despite the continuation of the infusion (Figure 10.3). When the infusion is stopped, flow briefly increases. This effect is due to the presence of both α and β-adrenotrophic receptors in muscle arterioles with a difference in time of onset of effect.

Parasympathetic nervous system

Cranial nerves and sacral nerves contain the parasympathetic outflow which innervates the viscera. Stimulation of these nerves leads to vasodilatation and increased visceral flow necessary for lachrymal, salivary, bronchial, gastric and intestinal gland secretion. At some sites, bradykinin or prostaglandin may be mediators of the response.

a continuous vasoconstrictor discharge via the autonomic nervous system which controls the arteriolar diameter via the sympathetic outflow (Figure 10.2A). Information coming to the vasomotor centre arrives from the aortic baroreceptors, the carotid and aortic chemoreceptors, and other parts of the nervous system. In addition, the vasomotor centre can be directly stimulated by hypoxia and hypocapnia causing vasoconstriction.

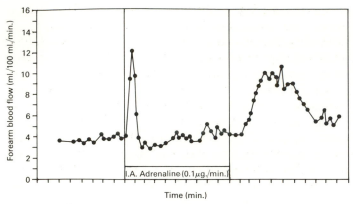

Fig. 10.3 Effect of infusing adrenaline into the brachial artery on forearm blood flow. Note the sharp but brief increase in blood flow when the infusion begins, the resumption of normal flow while the infusion continues, and the prolonged secondary increase in flow after the infusion is stopped. (Whelan & de la Lande, 1963.)

Endocrine system

Adrenaline from the adrenal medulla acts at different sites in different ways depending on the predominance of α or β receptors on the arterioles. Noradrenalin generally causes vasoconstriction of peripheral arterioles with an increase in peripheral resistance. Angiotension II (see p. 478) also causes peripheral vasoconstriction.

The circulatory effect of thyroxine is mediated predominantly via the sympathetic nervous system, although there is a general vasodilatory effect related to increased tissue metabolic activity.

Vasopressin has a visceral vasoconstrictor effect which is utilized in the management and control of gastrointestinal haemorrhage due to portal hypertension.

Pharmacological effects

Histamine

Histamine is concerned in pathological processes such as tissue injury and anaphylactic shock. It is present in most tissues in mast cells, smooth muscle, lung and skin. The effect of histamine is to produce general vasodilatation which affects arteries, arterioles, capillaries and veins. The release of histamine following skin trauma produces central redness due to vasodilatation, and a wheal due to increased capillary permeability, two of the components of Lewis' 'triple response'.

Histamine receptors are classified as H_1, which are responsible for the smooth muscle effect, and H_2, which are responsible for the stimulatory effect on gastric mucosa. Conventional 'anti-histamines' block the action of histamine H_1, but not H_2 receptors.

Prostaglandins

These were originally extracted from seminal fluid and the prostate gland, but now are identified in various tissues. These compounds are derived from unsaturated fatty acids and are extremely potent vasoactive agents. Their mode of action may be direct or indirect via a local effect on the sympathetic nerve endings. The metabolic effects are related to their action on adenylcyclase activity. At least four classes of these compounds have been described, a, b, e, and f and their effect varies for different compounds at different sites. For example, the recently synthesized prostacyclin is a very potent vasodilator acting directly on the arterial wall, and may be useful in treating either vasospastic conditions or patients with ischaemia due to peripheral vascular disease and occlusion of small vessels.

Kinins

These are formed from a number of circulating globulins called kininogens by the action of proteolytic enzymes called kallikreins. Their effect is similar to that of histamine: they cause relaxation of vascular smooth muscle and increased capillary permeability.

MECHANICAL PROPERTIES OF THE BLOOD VESSEL WALL

Blood vessels are viscoelastic tubes. Their diameter is determined by the equilibrium between the elastic filaments in the wall and the transmural pressure. This equilibrium is determined passively in the large vessels, both arteries and veins, whereas in arterioles, active control of the diameter is achieved because of the muscular elements in their walls.

Composition of vascular wall

Vessel walls consist of elastin, collagen and smooth muscle.

Elastin

Elastin fibres are present in all vessel walls except capillaries. The largest amounts are present in the thoracic aorta, decreasing progressively towards the capillaries. Veins have only small amounts in their walls. Elastin fibres are 5–10 times more easily stretched than rubber, and follow Hooke's law, i.e., when stretched, the increase in length is proportional to the applied stress. Elastin tolerates stretching by more than 60% from resting length before distortion occurs.

Collagen

Collagen is found in all blood vessels except capillaries.

Passing from the aorta, peripherally, the collagen content of arteries increases relatively to elastin and exceeds the elastin content of veins. The fibres are much less extensible than elastin and do not obey Hooke's law. Collagen does, however, have considerable tensile strength which is approximately 5×10^8 dyn/cm^2.

Smooth muscle

Smooth muscle becomes progressively more important the more peripheral the artery is located. In the arterioles, it is the predominant component where it is arranged in a helical fashion and responsible by contraction and relaxation for the peripheral resistance and hence blood pressure.

Vein wall characteristics

One function of the venous system is to accommodate large changes in blood volume with little change in transmural pressure. This occurs because of the tendency of veins to change shape and distort when at low pressure. The elastic modulus of vein wall may in fact be similar to arterial wall, but the ability to distort reduces the pressure volume change. The distensibility pattern of veins is also affected by the degree of smooth muscle contraction in the walls, so that a particular vein wall will exhibit stress relaxation in which sudden distension causes a sudden increase in pressure. This falls quickly at first, and then more slowly as the volume changes are accommodated with, in the end, little change in pressure.

Function of various vessels in health, age and disease

In the aorta, where elastin predominates, the main function is to act as a compliance reservoir where energy is stored in systole and dissipated in diastole. In this way the blood pressure is maintained between heart beats. With advancing age, the arterial wall becomes less distensible as the modulus of elasticity increases linearly with age; for the same change in volume there is a greater rise in pressure within the vessels. Degenerative disease, e.g. syphilis, may affect the elastin in the thoracic aorta, disrupting it and predisposing to aneurysm formation.

In peripheral arteries, the increase in content of collagen helps to protect the vessel wall from the effects of the intramural pressure. Ageing has a variable effect on the modulus of the elasticity of the peripheral arteries. There is a general increase in the pressure strain modulus, although some elderly patients have vessels with qualities similar to younger patients. With age, there is an increase in wall thickness which consists of additional amounts of both elastin and collagen in the same relative proportions. Disease processes may cause a great increase in rigidity in the vessel wall, particularly if calcification occurs.

This increasing tendency to rigidity can be assessed using two ultrasonic Doppler probes (see p. 161) to measure the pulse wave velocity between two points. Pulse wave velocity is enhanced as the vessels become less distensible as in ageing or when atherosclerosis occurs.

The problems seen with veins are discussed later. Capillaries can become more permeable in hypoxic situations, such as cardiac failure. This leads to oedema in dependent parts. Details of special circulations will already have been covered in other areas in this book. However, some relevant features of particular areas will be discussed briefly.

Cerebral circulation

The important point to remember about blood flow through the brain is that cerebral blood flow is generally maintained despite extensive changes in systemic blood pressure. This property is referred to as autoregulation. One important effect of this is that in hypovolemic states, the cerebral circulation is maintained even at very low systemic pressures. One of the important regulatory factors is the level of the arterial $P\text{CO}_2$ and this effect has recently been exploited in the treatment of brain oedema which commonly follows trauma. By hyperventilation of such a patient, arterial $P\text{CO}_2$ is reduced and this results in vasoconstriction of the cerebral blood vessels, which in turn provides more space within the skull to allow for increases in brain volume. In contrast, hypoventilation with an increase in arterial $P\text{CO}_2$ causes dilatation of the vessels in the brain.

Coronary circulation

The coronary circulation differs from others mainly by virtue of the fact that the blood vessels within the heart are compressed when it contracts, particularly in the left ventricle whose pressure exceeds that in the coronary arteries during systole. Consequently, most of the flow supplying the ventricles in particular, occurs during diastole. A number of factors affect coronary blood flow, and these can broadly be divided into neural and chemical factors.

The *neural control* is via the sympathetic nervous system, ending in both alpha adrenergic and beta adrenergic receptors. The net effect of stimulation of the sympathetic fibres is to produce vasodilatation. This, however, is almost certainly due to an increase in heart rate and accumulation of local metabolites. If β-adrenergic blocking drugs are used, then the effect of norepinephrine or α-adrenergic stimulation is vasoconstriction. Vagal stimulation causes dilatation of the coronary blood vessels.

As in the brain there is a certain amount of autoregulation of the coronary circulation; during hypertension, increased adrenergic discharge causes an increase in coronary blood flow due to an increase in heart rate and an accumulation of local metabolites. This occurs at a time when circulation to other areas, except the brain, is reduced.

The *chemical factors* which influence the coronary blood flow include P_{CO_2}, pH, lactic acid and prostaglandin. All of these substances are produced locally in ischaemic conditions, or when the work of the heart is increased. They are probably extremely important in maintaining the coronary circulation.

Coronary artery ischaemia is a very common problem and is covered in detail elsewhere in this book. Suffice to say that a reduction in coronary blood flow due to atheroma is common, and can be improved by coronary bypass surgery where a saphenous vein graft is placed from the aorta to distal coronary vessels.

Splanchnic circulation

The blood flow through the splanchnic area represents a large part of the peripheral vascular bed. The circulation to the liver is described in detail in Chapter 19. It is sufficient to point out here that the splanchnic circulation acts as an important reservoir for blood which allows rapid adjustments to take place in the event of an emergency such as bleeding. The intestinal circulation is one of the areas to suffer from vasoconstriction in order to maintain the circulating volume and divert blood to other important areas such as brain and heart.

Skin circulation

Alterations in blood flow to the skin allow heat to be lost or conserved depending upon the circumstances. As a result, the vessels in the skin are linked to the temperature control centre. Adrenergic nerve stimulation generally produces vasoconstriction in the blood vessels of the skin, but there are no known vasodilator fibres, increased flow being brought about by a decrease in vasoconstrictor activity. In shock states the circulation to the skin, as to other areas, is reduced by vasoconstrictor over-activity, leading to the pale, clammy, cold features commonly observed in such patients.

Local changes in capillary circulation occur due to the presence of substances such as the 'H' substance, which may or may not be histamine. These substances are released in relation to tissue damage and produce what is known as the triple response, which consists of a reddening around the injury, a weal and a flare. The red reaction is thought to be due to capillary dilatation, the weal due to increased capillary permeability, and the flare due to arteriolar dilatation, which is thought to be caused by a local axon reflex.

HYPERTENSION

By considering a simplified circulation in terms of cardiac output and peripheral resistance it follows that either an increased cardiac output or an increased peripheral resistance can cause an increased systemic pressure. In addition, disease processes which reduce the compliance of the blood vessel walls can increase systolic pressure and this is a part of the normal ageing process due to arteriosclerosis.

It seems likely that only in thyrotoxicosis is there an increased cardiac output contributing to hypertension and this reverts to normal when the thyroid overactivity is controlled medically, surgically or by radio-iodine treatment.

An increased peripheral resistance seems to be the commonest cause of hypertension. While treatment directed at the sympathetic nervous system may reduce the severity of the hypertension, there is no evidence that, per se, overactivity of the sympathetic nervous system is the primary cause of the hypertension. A number of disease states have been defined in which the mechanism of the hypertension is partly understood. These include phaeochromocytoma with increased output of adrenaline and noradrenaline, Conn's syndrome with increased output of aldosterone, Cushing's syndrome with increased cortisol secretion, and toxaemia of pregnancy. In some renal diseases, ischaemia of part of the renal cortex may cause increased renin secretion with subsequent hypertension.

The surgical importance of these endocrine causes of hypertension is that excision or ablation of the diseased endocrine gland usually allows the blood pressure to revert to normal. Diagnostic effort is at present directed towards defining the site of the particular endocrine abnormality since in some cases there is a diffuse overactivity of the gland or in some cases focal overactivity due to an adenoma. Radiological and biochemical tests are required before surgical excision is contemplated.

These surgically remediable causes of hypertension constitute only a small proportion of the group of patients with hypertension. In the majority the disease is labelled 'essential' and is related to age, obesity, and environmental and genetic factors. For these patients, control of the hypertension with drugs may reduce the cerebrovascular, coronary artery and peripheral vascular complications of the hypertension.

The various drugs available for the control of hypertension may be classified by their mode of action when it is known.

The ganglion blocking drugs, e.g. hexamethonium, were previously used in the control of hypertension but have now been superseded because of their side-effects due to wide-spread autonomic blockade. They act by producing sympathetic blockage at the sympathetic ganglia. Peripheral arteriolar tone is reduced and the antihypertensive effect is most marked when the patient is erect.

Some drugs affect the peripheral production of noradrenaline, e.g. methyldopa. By competitive inhibition of a step in the biochemical synthesis of noradrenaline, a less active analogue is produced, and the rate of production of noradrenaline is reduced. By this mechanism, peripheral arteriolar tone is reduced. Methyldopa may also have a central effect and part of the benefit of it may be due to reduced central sympathetic activity.

A further group of compounds affect the release and subsequent uptake of noradrenaline at the postganglionic sympathetic nerve endings. They include guanethidine and the shorter-acting bethanidine and debrisoquine. One of their side-effects is impotence and this may limit their clinical usefulness.

The β blockers are a newer group of compounds which are commonly used in association with a vasodilator. β blockers have a central mechanism of action as well as a peripheral action in suppressing renin release. They have a variable degree of selectivity for receptor site; unwanted effects include a cardiac effect which may seriously limit exercise tolerance and a pulmonary effect in which bronchospasm may be aggravated.

A group of compounds which act as vasodilators are available. Their mechanism of action is local, on the arterioles, and arteriolar tone is reduced. They include hydralazine, diazoxide and minoxidil. The principal side-effect of these drugs is tachycardia and increased cardiac output but this is off-set in the common therapeutic combination of a β blocker and vasodilator when the β blocker limits the tachycardia due to the vasodilator.

Thiazide diuretics are commonly used in the control of hypertension. Their mechanism of action may be partly via Na+ excretion, though more potent diuretics are in fact less efficient antihypertensive agents. They also have a local vasodilating effect. Dosage insufficient to achieve satisfactory diuresis may be sufficient for the control of hypertension.

Renovascular hypertension

The relationship between renal disease and hypertension was first described in 1827 by Richard Bright. In 1898 Tigerstedt and Bergman noted that a saline extract of renal cortex but not renal medulla could produce hypertension in dogs; they named this extract renin. Subsequently, in 1934 Goldblatt produced hypertension in dogs by partial occlusion of one renal artery after contralateral nephrectomy. In man, however, and in other animals including the rat, hypertension ensues after unilateral renal artery stenosis without contralateral nephrectomy. The first surgical application of these observations was in 1937 when Butler cured a hypertensive patient by removing a diseased, shrunken, chronically pyelonephritic kidney.

The mechanism of renovascular hypertension has recently been explained by clarification of the renin-angiotensin biochemical pathway. Renin is an enzyme secreted by the juxtaglomerular apparatus of the kidney. Renin acts on a circulating protein angiotensinogen-renin substrate converting it to the decapeptide angiotensin I. Converting enzyme present in plasma, the lung and vessel walls converts angiotensin I to the octapeptide angiotensin II.

Angiotensin II is a potent vasoconstrictor and is thus a pressor substance. It also stimulates the release of aldosterone from the adrenal cortex and this effect constitutes the feed-back which controls renin release. Aldosterone increases Na+ retention which in turn causes water retention. The resultant expansion of the plasma volume and extracellular fluid volume reduces the rate of release of renin from the juxtaglomerular cells. The feed-back control circuit is thus complete:

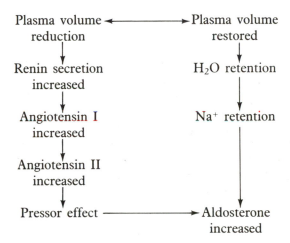

A number of disease states may affect the rate of secretion of renin and may give rise to renovascular hypertension. These diseases may be classified by whether they affect the renal artery or the renal parenchyma. Renal artery diseases include congenital fibromuscular hyperplasia and acquired atheromatous disease, embolism and thrombosis. Renal parenchymal diseases which may be unilateral and surgically important are chronic pyelonephritis, renal tuberculosis, hydronephrosis, and hypernephroma. Chronic glomerulonephritis affects the renal microvasculature and may cause renovascular hypertension though this will be bilateral and not amenable to surgical correction.

Investigation of a patient with hypertension should include intravenous pyelography in the first instance. This may indicate unilateral renal disease in which case retrograde pyelography, split function renal studies, isotope renography and renal angiography may be indicated singly or in combination. Confirmation of unilateral renovascular hypertension will, however, require renal vein sampling and measurement of renal vein renin levels.

In carefully controlled conditions, demonstration of renal vein renin levels of a ratio greater than 2:1 may indicate that significant unilateral renovascular hypertension is present. Surgery comprising nephrectomy for a kidney with diseased parenchyma or renal artery reconstruction or bypass for a kidney shown to have renal artery stenosis may be expected to relieve the hypertension provided that the contralateral kidney is not diseased primarily or has not become damaged secondarily to the hypertension.

The incidence of surgically correctable renovascular hypertension is approximately 0.5–2.0% of a population of hypertensive patients. Surgery may initially improve hypertension in 70–80% and may render 50–60% normotensive. At 5 years, however, only 30% are still normotensive though this percentage should improve with improvement in the diagnostic criteria and selection of patients for surgical procedures. The recently introduced dilatation of renal artery stenosis by balloon catheters introduced via the femoral artery has produced promising results in suitable cases.

Preliminary experiments with renin antagonists have, however, shown promise that medical control of renovascular hypertension may soon be achieved.

PATHOPHYSIOLOGY OF THE PERIPHERAL CIRCULATION

Acute ischaemia

Symptoms and signs

The symptoms and signs of acute ischaemia of a limb vary with the duration of the ischaemia and the site and nature of the arterial obstruction. The classically described symptoms and signs, referred to by their initial letter 'P', are:

1. Pain
2. Paraesthesia
3. Paralysis
4. Pallor
5. Pulseless
6. 'Perishing' cold

and to these may be added:

7. Tenderness of muscles
8. Rigidity of muscles
9. Guttering of veins

Diagnosis of the presence of arterial obstruction and prompt treatment to relieve the obstruction may permit complete recovery of the limb, though if paralysis and muscle rigidity are present, this is less likely.

Failure to relieve the obstruction leads to gangrene of the limb with irrecoverable loss of tissue. Skin pallor is replaced by mottling which does not blanche in response to local pressure and the muscles become hard, the state comparable to rigor mortis. The level of the demarcation between viable and non-viable tissue is determined by the site of the arterial obstruction, the presence of pre-existing arterial disease, and other general factors.

The development of dry gangrene in general only occurs when individual digits or the forefoot are affected and where there is pre-existing arterial disease. In dry gangrene, the tissues contract and mummify and eventually give rise to auto-amputation of the gangrenous part.

Where the ischaemia involves the lower leg or the whole leg, the gangrene usually progresses as moist gangrene in which there is purplish mottling of the limb with skin blistering, oedema and softening of the muscles from their previously tonic state. The surgical operation for this is amputation, either below the knee, through knee, or above knee, as determined by the level of viable tissue.

Moist gangrene should be differentiated from gas gangrene in which ischaemic tissues are invaded by gas-forming organisms, usually *Clostridium welchii*, where clinically there is profound general toxaemia, local muscle tenderness, and crepitus. Moist gangrene is a distinct entity and while it may, it need not, be followed by gas gangrene.

Aetiology

Local and systemic factors may singly or in combination give rise to acute ischaemia of a limb:

1. Thrombosis in peripheral arterial disease. Atheromatous plaques may be a focus for thrombus formation because of ulceration of their surface or they may produce a critical stenosis which causes stasis and thrombosis particulary when other general factors give rise to a low cardiac output, e.g. shock, myocardial infarction, congestive cardiac failure.

Aneurysmal dilatations may be the cause of acute ischaemia; aneurysms frequently contain lamellated clot which may encroach on the lumen remaining within the cavity of the aneurysm and cause obstruction. This rarely affects aortic aneurysms but often affects popliteal aneurysms and may be the mode of presentation of such an aneurysm.

2. Arterial embolism (q.v.).

3. Trauma. Penetrating wounds may cause local damage to the wall of an artery and give rise to acute ischaemia. In closed injuries of the limbs arterial trauma may be caused by sharp fragments of fractured or dislocated bones; the common sites for such injuries which result in significant acute ischaemia are in the thigh when a fractured shaft of femur may damage the superficial femoral artery or in the arm when the brachial artery is damaged by supracondylar fractures of the humerus or by dislocation of the elbow.

Inadvertent intra-arterial injection of irritant drugs can cause arterial thrombosis and acute ischaemia.

Operative trauma may damage arteries because of thrombosis on damaged endothelium, or by the inappropriate application of a ligature.

4. Dissection of the arterial wall. In this condition blood enters the media of the main vessels creating a false, blind-ending passage which compresses the true lumen and causes acute ischaemia. This is most commonly associated with systemic hypertension, but may occur in vessels weakened pathologically by an inherent collagen defect, e.g. Marfan's syndrome, or vessels weakened physiologically, e.g. pregnancy.

5. Raynaud's phenomenon and disease.

6. Frostbite.

7. Ergot poisoning.

Arterial embolism

Arterial embolism is the commonest cause of acute ischaemia which may be completely reversible if diagnosed and treated promptly. The commoner sites of origin of arterial embolus are:

1. Left atrium. In atrial fibrillation due to rheumatic heart disease or ischaemic heart disease, stasis in the atrium and the auricular appendage predisposes to thrombosis and a clot which may embolize to any of the systemic arteries.

2. Mitral or aortic valves. Acute or subacute bacterial endocarditis may result in vegetations on valve cusps which can be dislodged and embolize.

3. Left ventricle. A mural thrombus at the endocardial site of a myocardial infarction may give rise to arterial embolism, classically 7–10 days after the infarction.

4. Aorta and great vessels. Atheromatous plaques may disrupt and embolize or thrombus formed on their ulcerated surface may similarly embolize. Lamellated clot may form in aneurysms and be detached and embolize.

5. Paradoxical embolus. Where a foramen ovale remains patent, the rare event of 'paradoxical' embolus may occur. A thrombus on the venous side of the circulation, destined to be a pulmonary embolus, may be diverted from right atrium to left atrium and manifest as a systemic embolus.

Diagnosis

The diagnosis of acute ischaemia of a limb is made initially clinically by recognizing the symptoms and signs. The more marked the sensory loss and the more advanced the paralysis, the more likely it is that the limb has been ischaemic for some time and irrecoverably damaged. The site of arterial obstruction may be localized by knowledge of the site of an injury, or by inference from the pattern of presence and absence of pulses. Additional information may be obtained by measuring arterial pressure indirectly with occlusive cuffs (q.v.), or merely by auscultating over the vessels with an ultrasonic flow detector which may indicate the site of the obstruction. In cases of doubt, arteriography will demonstrate an obstruction in an artery and the aetiology can be determined, e.g. a narrow, tapered, diseased artery may suggest thrombosis related to pre-existing atheromatous disease or a sharp, transverse cut-off in an otherwise normal artery may suggest an arterial embolus.

Treatment

Treatment is directed generally and specifically, according to the aetiology, to remove the obstruction and prevent intravascular thrombosis which occurs distal to the obstruction due to stasis.

Systemic anticoagulation with heparin should be commenced as soon as the diagnosis is made. This reduces the tendency for distal thrombosis and may be crucial in preventing irreversible obstruction of the microvasculature. If delay is anticipated before surgical treatment can be instituted, the affected limb should be exposed and cooled to reduce the metabolic rate of the tissues.

Treatment of arterial embolism has been revolutionized by the development of the Fogarty catheter, a balloon catheter which is passed down an artery, past the embolus which is then removed by inflation of the balloon and removal of the catheter from the artery.

Treatment of thrombosis associated with atheromatous disease or trauma to the artery is usually performed surgically by bypassing the damaged area with a segment of one of the patient's own veins, or more rarely a synthetic Dacron prosthesis.

In some cases considered unsuitable for surgical treatment because of the peripheral nature of the embolism, treatment may be directed at promoting clot lysis by use of streptokinase or urokinase. These proteases obtained from Streptococci and human urine respectively enhance the natural fibrinolytic mechanism by plasmin and help reduce further clot formation and promote clot lysis. Both preparations have to be given parenterally by infusion. Previous streptococcal infection may have given rise to an antibody response and there may be an allergic reaction to streptokinase which precludes further infusion. Urokinase, which is even more expensive than streptokinase, is a human protease and allergic reactions are uncommon. Recently, direct infusion of small doses into the affected artery has produced promising results.

Where ischaemia is due to intra-arterial injection of irritant drugs, use of papaverine may eliminate arterial spasm and may help to reduce thrombosis.

Pathological dissection of the aortic wall is treated surgically by excision and grafting with a Dacron prosthesis or by performing fenestration where a re-entry for the false blind-ending track is made into the lumen of the aorta so that compression of the true lumen is relieved.

Following successful removal of an embolus or relief of one of the other aetiological factors, there is return of pulses and gradual recovery of sensation and muscle power. As a result of ischaemia of the muscles, the venous return from the re-vascularized limb may produce systemic hyperkalaemia and metabolic acidosis, both of which may have an adverse effect on cardiac rhythm and contractility. It may thus be necessary to measure and correct any metabolic acidosis by parenteral sodium bicarbonate and to attempt to correct hyperkalaemia by the use of insulin and dextrose.

In the first 24–48 hours after successful relief of acute ischaemia the limb will show sustained hyperaemia with increased temperature and heightened skin colour. In some cases, there develops an oedema usually involving the foot and ankle which may last 4–6 weeks. This is probably due to ischaemia of the skin and subcutaneous tissue capillary beds with increase in capillary permeability (q.v.).

In some cases, where the period of ischaemia was protracted, the muscles of the leg may become tense and tender indicating damage to the muscle capillary beds. Because the muscles are contained in compartments comprising bone and inelastic fascia, there is a limit to the degree of swelling of these muscles. When the limit is reached muscle ischaemia may occur because of the rising pressure in the muscle compartment. In the lower leg, the most commonly affected compartment is that of the ankle dorsiflexors, the syndrome is described as the anterior tibial compartment syndrome and the late effect may be a 'drop foot'. If appreciated sufficiently early, fasciotomy of the overlying deep fascia may relieve the muscle compartment tension and prevent ischaemic damage to the muscles.

Chronic occlusive arterial disease

The haemodynamic effect of arteriosclerosis is due to stenoses or occlusions related to atheroma. An increased resistance to blood flow occurs in the presence of a stenotic segment or of collaterals circumventing an occlusion. For the same blood flow as was present before a stenosis occurred, there is a drop in pressure due to dissipation of energy in passage of the blood through the stenosis. The resultant drop in pressure may become important when increased blood flow is required for exercising muscle.

Patients with occlusive arterial disease can be categorized according to whether their symptoms only occur with exercise, i.e. intermittent claudication, or whether their symptoms are present at rest, i.e. rest pain, pregangrene or gangrene.

Investigation

Investigation of a patient presenting with symptoms suggestive of peripheral arterial disease is directed towards defining the arterial segments which are affected.

Palpation of pulses at the aorta, common femoral, popliteal and pedal vessels will help to localize the disease though palpation may be subject to errors particularly in obese patients.

Pressure may be measured indirectly with occlusive cuffs and a flow detector, e.g. Doppler, placed over a vessel distal to the cuff. Systolic pressure gradients measured by this method may be useful in defining arterial segments across which there is a large pressure drop.

Pulse wave velocity may be measured using two flow detectors and the delay in the expected rate of transmission of the pulse wave through a particular segment may indicate that an occlusion is present and that a longer pathway via collaterals has been taken.

Mathematical analysis of the shape of the velocity profile can be performed non-invasively by spectral analysis of the 'noise' produced by a Doppler ultrasound flow detector. This method detects damping of the velocity profile such as may occur in passage through a stenosis.

Pressure may be measured directly by needle puncture of the common femoral artery at the groin. The effect of drugs or exercise on this pressure may indicate if there is significant arterial disease proximal to the recording site. When stenoses are present this method detects a greater than expected fall of pressure in response to exercise or vasodilation.

Angiography is the mainstay of investigation of the patient with occlusive arterial disease. Two routes of introduction of contrast are available, translumbar or retrogradely via a catheter introduced into the common femoral artery. In the translumbar method, indicated when aorto-iliac atheroma is present, the patient is under general anaesthesia, prone, and a needle is introduced via the left loin into the aorta at or above the renal arteries. In retrograde aorta-arteriography, the catheter is introduced by the Seldinger technique under sedation and local anaesthesia. In either method, a radio-opaque, iodine-containing compound (e.g. Hypaque) is injected and a series of radiographs is taken, delayed so as to visualize the various arteries down to the calf vessels. Since the various compounds contain iodine, the patient must be questioned for prior iodine sensitivity. From the resultant radiographs the presence and the extent of stenoses or occlusions can be defined. These occlusions tend to fall into patterns clinically described as 'high', e.g. aorta or iliac where the arterial disease is proximal to the inguinal ligament, or 'low' where the superficial femoral, profunda femoris, or popliteal arteries are involved. The patterns of disease present determine the suitability of the patient for reconstructive surgery.

Other available methods of investigation are directed toward assessment of the functional incapacity of the patient. These methods include exercise tests on a treadmill or on a bicycle or pedal ergometer where some measure of objective asessment is available for what is otherwise a subjective symptom. Blood flow can be measured plethysmographically or by isotope washout. These methods are of some value in assessment of response to various drug regimens but have little place in the management of a particular patient.

Treatment

General advice to the patient includes advice about weight reduction if the patient is clinically overweight and advice to reduce smoking, which if taken, will improve claudication distance.

Surgical treatment of a direct nature is directed to reboring a stenosed or occluded artery — endarterectomy — which is now reserved only for young patients with local aorto-iliac disease or to bypassing the blocked artery using autogenous tissue — reversed long saphenous vein — or synthetic Dacron prostheses.

Surgical treatment of an indirect nature is surgical sympathectomy (q.v.).

Vasospastic conditions

Whereas in occlusive arterial disease there is an organic mechanical stenosis or occlusion, in the vasospastic conditions the pathological process is vasospasm which is initially reversible.

Raynaud's phenomenon

Raynaud's phenomenon describes the initial pallor then cyanosis of fingers or toes with exposure to cold; pain presents within minutes of the onset of the colour changes. A number of associated factors have been identified, including cryoglobulins, scleroderma and vibrating tools. In more than 50% of patients with these symptoms, however, no associated disease condition is encountered and the patients are given advice about keeping hands and feet warm in the winter and avoiding immersion in cold water. Reducing exposure to cold often significantly reduces the inconvenience of the phenomenon. Electrically heated gloves help considerably.

Acrocyanosis and erythrocyanosis

In these conditions the vasospasm is sustained and is not episodic as in Raynaud's phenomenon. The skin of the digits is purplish blue or red but this can be differentiated from the discolouration of an ischaemic limb since there is a brisk capillary return in response to pressure on the skin. These conditions look serious for viability of the tissues, though they are associated with a good prognosis. They respond well to sympathectomy.

Raynaud's disease

This extension of Raynaud's phenomenon is differentiated by the progress of the disease to produce tissue loss. More marked in the fingers than in the toes, the disease produces painful ulcers, atrophy of the skin and subcutaneous tissues of the pulp, paronychia, and in some cases, gangrene of digits. Although originally attributed to overactivity of the sympathetic innervation, there is now evidence that patients with Raynaud's disease have abnormal blood viscosity, digital vessels which are abnormal in their response to cold, and disturbances of basal metabolic rate and temperature control.

Sympathectomy may produce a temporary remission of symptoms in some patients and is usually undertaken for disabling symptoms or pregangrene. The response is, however, often only short-lived.

Sympathectomy

Sympathetic denervation has been used in peripheral arterial disease, in frostbite and related phenomena, in Raynaud's phenomenon and disease and related vasospastic disorders, and in hyperhidrosis.

Sympathectomy interrupts both the cholinergic and the adrenergic efferent fibres. The result of a successful sympathectomy is initially hyperaemia, raised skin temperature and a dry skin. Vascular tone is, however, soon regained, usually within 14 days, and the skin temperature approaches the control non-sympathectomized temperature (Fig. 10.4). The skin does not respond to central temperature changes though there is still present

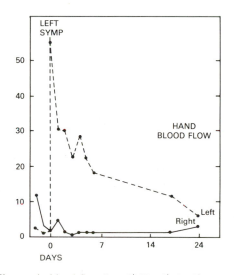

Fig. 10.4 Changes in blood flow (in ml/100 ml/min) in the sympathectomised left hand compared with the normal right hand. After sympathectomy, the temporary increase in blood flow is very large, but the permanent increase is small. (Walker, A. J., Lynn, R. B. & Barcroft, H. (1950). *St. Thomas's Hosp. Rep.* **6**, 18.)

the local response to change in temperature. Sweating remains permanently abolished.

Tests to detect completeness of sympathectomy are based either on this lack of response to central temperature changes, or on the lack of sweating. Such tests either employ a thermocouple to measure temperature or utilize a hygroscopic dyestuff or a measurement of skin electrical resistance to detect the absence of sweating.

Upper limb sympathectomy may be achieved via a number of routes (anterior, posterior or transthoracic) and consists in surgical excision of the lower tip of the stellate ganglion and the upper three or four thoracic sympathetic ganglia. Lower limb sympathectomy is achieved usually by a retroperitoneal route and involves removal of the 3 or 4 lumbar sympathetic ganglia. For both upper and lower limbs, sympathectomy may also be achieved by injection of phenol or alcohol into the tissues surrounding the appropriate sympathetic chain.

When applied in peripheral arterial disease, sympathectomy may be of benefit to patients with skin ischaemia, rest pain or pregangrene though it should be appreciated that, by virtue of a shunting effect, some patients may be adversely affected. Sympathectomy has no place in the management of intermittent claudication.

In frostbite and in immersion foot, sympathectomy may be of value in the later hyperaemic phase of recovery when there may be an element of vasospasm present.

In incapacitating Raynaud's phenomenon and in Raynaud's disease, sympathectomy may give relief to some patients though the signs of sympathetic denervation often remit within one year.

In hyperhidrosis, sympathectomy produces a complete remission of the symptom although, particularly for lower limb hydrosis, the sweating symptom may be replaced by a symptom comprising painful swelling of the dependent foot due to the increased tissue pressure consequent on vasodilatation.

Aneurysms

Aneurysms are local dilatations of major arteries. The underlying process producing the local dilatation is usually weakness of the vessel wall.

In the thoracic aorta, aneurysms were in the past usually due to syphilitic aortitis with disruption of the elastin in the wall. The weakened wall gradually stretched due to the intra-aortic pressure.

In the abdominal aorta, aneurysms are usually produced by arteriosclerotic weakening of the wall. The commonest site, in the infrarenal aorta, may also be related to reflection of the pulse pressure wave from the aortic bifurcation. The additive effect of an incident and a reflected pressure wave may cause locally-high wall pressure and this is considered to contribute to the formation of abdominal aortic aneurysms.

In the peripheral arteries, the popliteal artery is a relatively common site and there may be an association between abdominal aortic and popliteal artery aneurysms. Popliteal artery aneurysms are usually arteriosclerotic.

Embolization of infected vegetations in bacterial endocarditis may cause focal arteritis and mycotic aneurysm formation.

In some disease states associated with a defect in the structure of collagen, e.g. Marfan's syndrome, Ehlers-Danlos syndrome and Behçet's syndrome, there may be aneurysm formation because of relative weakness of the artery wall. In some patients, congenital defects in the formation of the media of the cranial arteries may cause local aneurysm formation, again because of focal weakness of the artery wall.

In trauma, or in relation to abnormal structures, e.g. cervical rib, damage to the media of the artery may predispose to aneurysm formation.

The physiological effect of an aneurysm is a damping of the pulse pressure wave but this is rarely important. Thrombus may form within the sac of the aneurysm and this may occlude the lumen or embolize distally. Progressive weakening of the wall of the sac, aggravated by systemic hypertension and promoted, in physical terms, by the Law of Laplace, may eventually lead to rupture of the wall and catastrophic haemorrhage.

Aneurysms may be detected clinically by palpation, or radiologically by angiography. Ultrasonic scanning of the abdomen is a simple non-invasive method of detecting aneurysms and has the virtue that the true dimensions of the aneurysm can be defined. Angiography has the disadvantage that it only defines the calibre of the lumen of the aneurysms and this may be much less than the size of the aneurysm if there is clot adherent to the wall. The surgical importance of this is the relationship of the size of an aneurysm to the likelihood of rupture. It has now been shown that abdominal aortic aneurysms of greater than about 6 cm diameter have an unacceptably high risk of rupture and therefore surgical resection if usually advised if an aneurysm greater than 6 cm is detected.

Varicose veins

Venous return to the heart is aided by the presence of bicuspid valves in the superficial and deep venous systems of the limbs. Movement of blood from superficial to deep systems is directed by valves in the communicating 'perforating' veins. Since the vascular system is closed and not open to the atmosphere at any point, any hydrostatic disadvantage in the venous system, due to dependency of a limb below the level of the heart, is offset by the hydrostatic gain in energy of blood in the arterial system. There would, however, be a gain in pressure due to the hydrostatic effect and this could expose the capillary beds to pressures which would affect their normal function. The presence of valves in the venous system of the limbs, in particular from the common femoral vein peripherally in the lower limb, reduces the hydrostatic pressure of blood and allows the capillaries to function with normal pressures.

Congenital defects of the main valve at the junction of the long saphenous vein with the femoral vein may account for early development of varicosity of the long saphenous vein. Increase in the pressure in the long saphenous vein causes it to be distended and tortuous, and distension of the vein at the site of a competent valve eventually causes incompetence of the valve. Symptoms are experienced when the high venous pressure affects the tissue tension.

A patient with symptoms of varicose veins must be assessed to determine if the problem is valve disruption of the superficial or the deep venous system. If the defect is in the superficial system, localization of the valves affected will determine if the whole long saphenous vein must be stripped out or if local ligation or injections of sclerosant agents may be appropriate. Incompetence of valves in the deep venous system is not amenable to surgical treatment.

Localization of incompetent valves on perforating veins may be made clinically by palpation and compression of the veins proximal to the presumed site of a perforator.

Other methods include use of thermography or fluorescein which is injected into the deep venous system via veins on the dorsum of the foot and then is detected with ultraviolet light if it re-enters the superficial system. Doppler ultrasonic flow detectors have also been used to detect sites of reversed flow due to passage of blood from deep to superficial systems. Finally, venography will detect perforator incompetence though identification of the surface markings of the perforator from a single plane X-ray film may be difficult.

Venous thromboembolism

Venous thrombosis is a common pathophysiological disorder of considerable surgical importance. With improved diagnostic techniques it is now appreciated that there is an incidence in excess of 30% postoperatively, in some categories of general surgical patients. For the most part there are no sequelae of these thrombi when confined to the calf veins. Where valves suffer damage due to the thrombi, a state of deep venous insufficiency may result. When the thrombus embolizes to the pulmonary circulation, a spectrum of sequelae occurs from fatality in massive embolism to pulmonary infarction when a small pulmonary artery branch is occluded.

The postulates of Virchow still apply to the aetiological factors:

1. Changes in the blood
2. Changes in the characteristics of flow of the blood
3. Changes in the vessel wall

The changes in the blood comprise the quantitative and qualitative changes in platelets which occur in malignancy and postoperatively: there is also a change in the coagulation mechanism and the fibrinolytic mechanism which results in a tendency to thrombus formation.

Changes in the characteristics of flow of blood peroperatively refers to the marked stasis which has been shown to occur in the calf circulation in anaesthetized, relaxed patients.

Changes in the vein wall are predominantly mechanical, related to the trauma to calf veins by compression in bed or on the operating table. There may be an additional electrostatic change in the vein wall, in response to trauma.

While these factors apply in varying degrees in many categories of patients, those patients with for example myocardial infarction or trauma and limb injury, have already been exposed to the factors predisposing them to venous thrombosis before admission to hospital. There are, however, a large group of patients undergoing elective procedures in whom the time of onset of their thrombosis is related to the arranged time of the procedure. In these patients, prophylactic measures can be instituted preoperatively. Such prophylactic measures have recently been intensively investigated with the advent of improved diagnostic methods.

Venous thrombosis may be diagnosed radiologically, ultrasonically, plethysmographically, or by radio-isotope localization.

Venography remains as the mainstay of the diagnostic methods for thrombosis of the deep venous system. Radio-opaque contrast is injected into veins on the dorsum of the foot and directed into the deep venous system with an ankle tourniquet. Progress up the limb is followed by screening and appropriately delayed radiographs. In some instances, pelvic veins are not well demonstrated and so contrast may be injected intraosseously into the greater trochanter of the femur; this method requires general anaesthesia. Venography remains the definite method of diagnosis though is clearly invasive, requires deployment of trained staff and expensive equipment and cannot be used in large trials or repeatedly in the same patient.

Ultrasonic detection of deep venous thrombosis may be performed non-invasively and repeatedly if required. The rationale of the method is that thrombus in a vein will obstruct or change the pattern of flow in the vein. In practice, the probe of a Doppler velocity detector is placed over the femoral vein in the groin. To detect thrombus peripheral to the probe, the calf is manually compressed and an augmented flow noise should be 'heard' over the femoral vein. If thrombus is present there is no increase in flow and no change in noise. To detect thrombus proximal to the probe, the fluctuation in iliac vein flow due to respiration is listened for and exaggerated by asking the patient to perform a Valsalva manoeuvre. If thrombus is present, the normal fluctuations in flow are not present and there will be no change in flow due to the Valsalva manoeuvre. The advantage of this method is its ease of application. The disadvantage is that non-occlusive thrombi are not detected nor are thrombi in calf veins.

Plethysmographic methods using in particular changes in electrical impedence in the limb due to the presence of thrombi, have been evaluated but remain predominantly of research interest.

Radio-isotope localization is the method of diagnosis which has increased the awareness of surgeons to the incidence of venous thrombosis and has permitted evaluation of a number of prophylactic methods. Fibrinogen labelled with a radio-isotope of iodine is injected intravenously into an arm vein. If thrombi form after this labelled fibrinogen has equilibrated with the pool of circulating fibrinogen, then the thrombus will comprise some labelled fibrin. Isotope localization meters can detect this and give a measure of the deposition of labelled fibrinogen relative to other parts of the same limb and relative to the comparable site on the contralateral limb. Such localization has been compared with venographic evidence of thrombosis and has been shown to have a high degree of correlation. The method is essentially non-invasive and can be used for up to 7 days in individual patients before decay of the radioactivity of the isotope. The method has been employed in large clinical trials and has enabled evaluation of a variety of methods of prophylaxis.

The various methods of prophylaxis can be discussed in relation to each of Virchow's postulates. Those designed to prevent or offset the changes in the blood are principally heparin and Dextran 70.

Heparin has been shown to be effective in 'low-dose' given subcutaneously. Therapeutic anticoagulation is not achieved, but in the dosages employed, e.g. 5000 u s.c. every 8 or 12 hours, it has an effect on enzymes contributing to the 'cascade' of the coagulation process. Of all the methods of prophylaxis, low dose subcutaneous heparin has been the most extensively investigated and has now been shown to be effective in reducing both deep vein thrombosis and fatal and non-fatal pulmonary embolism.

Dextran 70, a solution comprising a range of polysaccharides with an average mol.wt of 70 000, has been shown to be effective in the prophylaxis of deep vein thrombosis. In relation to postoperative changes in the blood, Dextran 70 exerts a disaggregating effect on red blood cells which minimizes the normal increased postoperative viscosity.

The methods aimed at preventing the reduction in blood flow are intermittent pneumatic compression or intermittent electrical stimulation of calf muscles. These methods increase venous flow and have been shown experimentally to reduce deep vein thrombosis. Other methods aimed at increasing blood flow are early mobilization, elevation of legs and application of elastic stockings, and these methods may offer some benefit. Dextran 70 also affects blood flow by its effect as a plasma expander. Circulating blood volume is increased and venous stasis minimized.

Methods aimed at minimizing vein wall trauma comprize careful application of leg rests, and use of cushions to elevate the heels and reduce pressure on the calf.

Although there are a number of effective methods, some do have possible disadvantages, e.g. heparin and Dextran 70 may increase operative bleeding and increase postoperative haematoma, and there has been a reluctance to use prophylactic methods widely. 'At risk' groups have been defined to attempt to minimize complications of treatment when there is only a small risk of venous thrombosis. Such 'at risk' factors are the presence of malignancy, obesity, presence of varicose veins, previous thromboembolism, the presence of infection and age over 40 years. These are some of the factors which can help to categorize patients into 'at risk' groups so that prophylactic treatment can be used.

Treatment of an established deep vein thrombosis may be with heparin, streptokinase or by thrombectomy which is the surgical removal of thrombus usually with a balloon Fogarty catheter. The method selected will depend on the size and extent of the thrombus, point in time relative to the operation, and the presence of pulmonary embolism. Venography is usually necessary to define the extent of the thrombus. If heparin is chosen as the method of anticoagulation, therapy may be switched to an oral anticoagulant, e.g. warfarin, and continued for several weeks or months.

When pulmonary embolism occurs the symptoms experienced vary with the size of the embolus. Large emboli obstruct the right ventricle outflow tract, producing acute right heart failure with marked elevation of central venous pressure and dyspnoea related to the severity of the ventilation perfusion defect. Smaller emboli may produce tachycardia, mild right heart failure and dyspnoea, or may lead to pulmonary infarction with pleuritic pain, pleural effusion and haemoptysis some days after the embolic incident. Clinical diagnosis requires awareness of the possibility of pulmonary embolism. Helpful investigations are chest X-ray and electrocardiography. Confirmatory tests are radioisotope lung scan and pulmonary angiogram. Treatment varies with the size of the thrombus and in particular the time of the incident relative to the initial operation. Heparin, streptokinase or pulmonary embolectomy may be used, the latter usually requiring cardiopulmonary bypass. Recurrent pulmonary embolism may lead to pulmonary hypertension as the pulmonary circulation is progressively obliterated. This can be prevented in appropriate cases by the insertion of an umbrella-shaped filter into the vena cava via the femoral or jugular veins.

FURTHER READING

Eastcott H H G 1973 Arterial surgery 2nd edn. Pitman Medical, London

Gillespie J A (ed) 1970 Modern trends in vascular surgery Butterworths, London

McDonald D A 1974 Blood flow in arteries 2nd edn. Edward Arnold, London

Nicolaides A N (ed) 1975 Thromboembolism. Medical & Technical Publishing, London

Roberts C (ed) 1972 Blood flow measurement. Sector Publishing Ltd, London

Strandness D E, Sumner D S 1975 Haemodynamics for surgeons. Grune & Stratton, New York

REFERENCES

Chambers R, Zweifach B W 1944 Topography and function of the mesenteric capillary circulation, American Journal of Anatomy 75:173

Whelan R F, De La Lande I S 1963 Action of adrenalin on limb blood vessels. British Medical Bulletin 19:125

Goldblatt H, Linch J, Hanzl R F and Summerville W W (1934) Studies in experimental hypertension. Journal of Experimental Medicine 59:347.

Blood

Blood has two compartments: a cellular compartment comprizing the formed elements, erythrocytes, granulocytes, monocytes, lymphocytes and platelets, and a non-cellular compartment, the plasma, in which these cellular elements are suspended. This chapter is concerned in the main with the role of the cellular components in normal physiology, and to some extent in disease. Some of the constituents of the plasma compartment require to be considered in the accounts of haemostasis and blood transfusion.

HAEMOPOIESIS

For many years there has been disagreement over the precise cellular source of the formed blood elements. It is now clear that all blood cells, including almost certainly monocytes and lymphocytes, are formed in bone marrow from single primitive haemopoietic stem cells, rather than from a progenitor stem cell for each cell line. The function of the stem cell is to divide, maintain its own numbers, and subsequently develop into one specific blood cell line. Stem cells represent a very small fraction of the total marrow cell population, and although at present they are morphologically unrecognizable, much evidence suggests their appearance is very similar to the small lymphocyte. Thus, primitive stem cells mature within the marrow to give the morphologically recognizable erythroid, myeloid and megakaryocyte precursor cells which further mature before release into the circulation as red cells, granulocytes, and platelets. However, there is also much evidence to suggest the presence of an intermediate cell population committed to develop down only one particular cell line but still maintaining many of the properties of a stem cell. Although lymphocytes and probably also monocytes arise in bone marrow from a similar or even identical stem cell, the bulk of lymphocyte production occurs in extramedullary tissue.

Although much information is now available about stem cells and haemopoiesis, the factors which control division and maturation of haemic cells are poorly established. Genetic and environmental factors are both involved, as are humoral factors which probably act at many stages of cell development, particularly the unipotential committed stem cell. There may well be distinct humoral control systems for each cell line. Erythropoiesis is dependent to a large extent on the hormone erythropoietin and several hormones affecting granulopoiesis have been described, but attempts to isolate and characterize thrombopoietic substances have been much less successful.

ERYTHROPOIESIS

Site of formation of erythrocytes

The site of red cell formation varies with age and according to red cell requirements. In the embryo, blood cells are first seen at the 2.5 mm stage in the blood islands of the yolk sac ('mesoblastic period'). By the 5–7 mm stage of embryonic development, haemopoiesis shifts to the liver and spleen where for the first time all the formed elements can be identified ('hepatic period'). The liver is the main haemopoietic site by 12–16th week, but by the 20th week of intra-uterine life the bone marrow has taken over as the main site of production, and by birth very little haemopoiesis occurs outside the marrow.

Throughout the period of active growth (Fig. 11.1), the red marrow occupies the whole of the medulla of all bones, but towards puberty this begins to be replaced by inactive

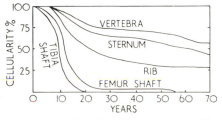

Fig. 11.1 Changes in the cellularity of bone marrow with age. (Whitby L E H, Britton C J C 1963 Disorders of the blood, 9th edn. Churchill, London).

fatty marrow. This change begins peripherally in the small bones of the hands and feet and spreads centrally. In the adult, red marrow is limited to the ribs, sternum, vertebrae, shoulder girdle, pelvic girdle and to proximal ends of the long bones, especially the femur and tibia.

When increased red cell production is required in response to anaemia, particularly chronic anaemia, the sequence is reversed and haemopoietic activity extends again distally into the shafts of the long bones. In certain diseases haemopoietic activity may also reappear in liver and spleen. This is seen in children where marrow output is grossly inadequate and in adults with primary marrow disease, e.g. aplastic anaemia or myelofibrosis, where the marrow's haemopoietic activity is severely impaired. In myelofibrosis particularly, splenic haemopoiesis may be of some importance and this must be considered carefully if splenectomy is proposed.

Haemopoietic marrow tissue has a high blood flow. The arterial supply is principally through osteal vessels via the nutrient artery. Blood passes to the marrow sinusoidal system and leaves by a central longitudinal vein. Blood cells develop extravascularly and in health only mature forms are released into the circulation. The mechanism and control of cellular release is poorly understood, but the vascular wall of the marrow sinuses would appear to serve as a major barrier controlling transcellular migration between the marrow and circulation. This control mechanism may break down in hyperproliferative marrow states and situations where there is an 'irritant' infiltration of the bone marrow with foreign tissue, when immature myeloid and erythroid cells pass into the circulation, often in large numbers. Such an anaemia with immature cellular precursors in the circulation is termed leucoerythroblastic anaemia. The common causes of a leucoerythroblastic anaemia include secondary carcinoma of bone, myelofibrosis, multiple myeloma and malignant lymphoma.

Maturation of erythrocytes

Although the committed erythroid stem cell is the earliest cell of the erythroid series, the pronormoblast is the earliest cell which is morphologically recognizable. Maturation proceeds through the successive stages of basophilic or early normoblast, polychromatic or intermediate normoblast, and orthochromatic or late normoblast until the cell becomes a reticulocyte and finally mature red cell or erythrocyte (Fig. 11.2). With conventional Romanowsky stains, the cytoplasmic colour of the erythocyte percursors changes from basophilic to polychromatic and then to orthochromatic due to the accumulation of haemoglobin. This progressive haemoglobination of the cytoplasm along with diminution in cell size and ripening of the nucleus as manifested by loss of nucleoli and condensation of chromatin is characteristic of the process of normoblastic maturation. The time for maturation from pronormoblast

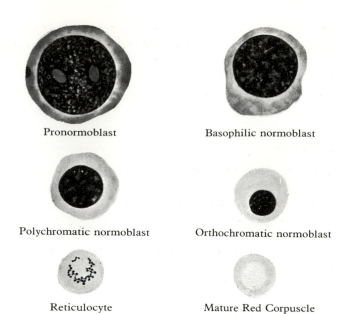

Pronormoblast   Basophilic normoblast

Polychromatic normoblast   Orthochromatic normoblast

Reticulocyte   Mature Red Corpuscle

Fig. 11.2 Maturation of red cells (After Garven H S D 1957 A students histology. Livingstone, Edinburgh).

to mature erythrocyte is approximately 6 days; during the first half of this period three to four mitotic divisions occur which result in 8–16 mature red cells per pronormoblast.

Pronormoblasts

These are round or oval cells 12–20 μm in diameter with scanty basophilic cytoplasm and a large nucleus with a finely reticular chromatin pattern and several nucleoli. Very few of these cells are seen in normal marrow.

Basophilic normoblasts

These are round cells 10–16 μm in diameter with plentiful deeply basophilic cytoplasm. The nucleus has no nucleoli and is still slightly reticular, though the nuclear chromatin is thicker and more deeply staining which gives it a coarser appearance. These cells form about 4% of nucleated red cells in the marrow.

Polychromatic normoblasts

These cells vary in diameter from 8–14 μm and have a smaller nucleus containing coarse clumps of deeply staining chromatin. The cytoplasm is beginning to be haemoglobinized and takes on an acidophilic tint which becomes more marked as the cell matures. These cells account for about 30% of the nucleated red cells in the marrow.

Orthochromatic normoblasts

These cells have a diameter from 8–10 μm and a dark

condensed nucleus which as the cell matures becomes a blue-black homogenous mass and occupies a slightly eccentric position in the cell. The cytoplasm is acidophilic as the cell has nearly its full haemoglobin complement, but a faint polychromatic tint persists. These cells account for about 65% of the nucleated red cells in the marrow.

Reticulocytes

These are flat, disc-shaped cells with no nucleus but containing traces of RNA which by supravital staining can be seen as a reticulum in the cell, or after fixation as a diffuse basophilia. Reticulocytes are slightly larger than mature red cells being 7–10 μm in diameter, and as they mature they decrease in size and lose the reticulum (or basophilia). The reticulocyte is the erythroid form which enters the circulation from the marrow, and requires about 2 days in the circulation to mature finally to an erythrocyte. Reticulocytes do not normally exceed 2% of the circulating red cells. A sustained reticulocytosis higher than 5% is evidence of increased erythropoiesis and is found in haemolytic anaemia, in the response to haemorrhage and in the response to appropriate haematinic therapy.

Erythrocyte

The mature erythrocyte is a non-nucleated, round biconcave disc with a diameter of 6.6–7.7 μm. The cell membrane is a tri-laminar structure the outer covering of which is mainly lipoprotein. This protein layer has several functions, one of the most important being to maintain the shape of the cell. The lipid coat also acts as a semipermeable membrane for the cell and is impermeable to large molecules and protein. Damage to the lipid coat may result in haemolysis because of escape of haemoglobin from the cell. Thereafter the empty stromal framework, or red cell ghost, may circulate for a short period before removal by the reticulo-endothelial system. Another important function of the membrane is its remarkable deformability which permits passage of red cells through the microcirculation.

Control of erythropoiesis

A wide variety of factors are necessary to establish and maintain normal erythropoiesis. Normal numbers of stem cells in a favourable marrow micro-environment as discussed are very important. However, hormonal factors are also involved and one of the most important is the regulatory hormone erythropoietin.

Erythropoietin

The fundamental stimulus to erythropoiesis is tissue hypoxia. Hypoxia itself cannot transmit a direct signal to the bone marrow to increase erythropoiesis, but acts through the humoral intermediary, erythropoietin. Although not yet fully characterized, erythropoietin is known to be a glycoprotein with an estimated molecular weight around 46 000. Although in vitro assay systems are available, activity is usually measured in an animal bioassay system, and in health hormonal activity is normally present in urine and plasma. The kidneys are the major source of the hormone, but bilateral nephrectomy does not completely eliminate erythropoietin activity, and other organs, particularly the liver, are probable sources. The juxtaglomerular apparatus within the kidney has been suggested as the major source of the hormone, but a diffuse tubular origin appears more probable, although a specialized zone of maximal excretion cannot be excluded. Indeed the kidney probably does not excrete active erythropoietin but a renal erythropoietic factor or erythrogen which reacts with a plasma substrate possibly of hepatic origin, to produce the active hormone.

Erythropoietin influences a wide range of biochemical processes in red cell precursors. It rapidly increases RNA synthesis in both committed erythroid stem cells and recognizable red cell precursors, and also increases the rate of DNA synthesis. The biochemical consequences that follow the increased RNA synthesis are a rapid increase in enzymes concerned with haem synthesis, particularly ALA synthetase, and increased iron uptake from transferrin. The principal kinetic effect of erythropoietin is to increase the proliferative activity and rate of conversion of erythroid committed stem cells to pronormoblasts. Cell cycle and maturation time of red cell precursors are also reduced and there is an accelerated release of reticulocytes from the bone marrow giving increased numbers of young basophilic erythrocytes which are known as 'shift erythrocytes' or skip cells.

In situations where erythropoietin production is increased haemoglobin synthesis will be accelerated and the time required for an individual cell to produce a normal complement of haemoglobin reduced. Accelerated haemoglobin production may be the explanation of the peripheral blood macrocytes which are seen with a stimulated marrow. When a critical haemoglobin concentration is achieved in an erythroid cell, it is probable that a feedback mechanism shuts off further nucleic acid synthesis and hastens maturation and marrow release. Thus, an accelerated rate of haemoglobin synthesis and a shortening of the time of differentiation, as is likely in a stimulated marrow, produces the critical cell haemoglobin concentration earlier, with the result that a terminal cell division is skipped and a larger cell, or macrocyte, is released.

In a different context, if there is a limiting factor for haemoglobin synthesis such as iron deficiency, the rate of cell maturation decreases and the interval to achieve the critical cell haemoglobin concentration is lengthened; additional cell division will occur and in the end a small cell, or microcyte, will be produced.

Elevated plasma erythropoietin levels are present in many congenital and acquired anaemias. Low levels are found in polycythaemia rubra vera but in other conditions with erythrocytosis very high levels are found often due to inappropriate production. As yet erythropoietin is not available for clinical use, but obviously would be great value in the treatment of certain anaemias such as occur with chronic renal failure.

Endocrine factors

Oestrogens are known to suppress erythropoiesis while androgens have a stimulatory effect. Both hormones are known to affect erythropoietin but androgens may also have a direct effect on erythroid bone marrow precursors. This hormonal effect in part accounts for the sex differences in haemoglobin and red cell count between males and females.

Other control factors

Many disorders of red cell production cannot be readily explained by hormonal factors alone, and there is now much evidence to suggest that cell to cell interactions are of major importance in regulating erythropoiesis. Phagocytic cells such as monocytes and lymphoid cells, particularly T-cells, are important in modulating normal erythropoiesis. This action may be effected by direct cell to cell contact or by secretory products.

Nutritional requirements for erythropoiesis

Many of the substances required for red cell production are obtained from the body's general metabolic pool, and are required in such small quantities that deficiencies rarely occur. Certain deficiencies however may lead to defects of erythroid proliferation or maturation and result in anaemia.

Amino acids

An adequate supply of first-class protein is required to provide the essential amino acids for synthesis of haemoglobin. Only in severe malnutrition, such as occurs with kwashiorkor in children, is this a factor.

Minerals

Iron is the major nutritional requirement for normal erythropoiesis and, if deficient, rapidly leads to anaemia. The role of several other minerals is uncertain although cobalt is known to stimulate erythropoiesis probably by increasing erythropoietin production.

Vitamin B₁₂ and folic acid

Both are required for normal nuclear development and deficiency results in megaloblastic erythropoiesis and megaloblastic anaemia.

Vitamin C

Ascorbic acid is required for normal erythropoiesis and for normal folic acid metabolism.

The B vitamins

Deficiencies of riboflavin, nicotinic acid, and pantothenic acid do not appear to cause anaemia in man. Pyridoxine (vitamin B_6) appears to be necessary for normal iron metabolism and if given in large doses, may correct the abnormality in certain sideroblastic anaemias. These rare anaemias are characterized by abnormal iron accumulation in the mitochondria of the erythroblasts which gives a positive Perl's reaction for iron in a ring distribution round the nucleus; this is called a ring sideroblast.

Erythrocyte metabolism

The red cell loses many of its metabolic and synthetic capabilities during its development from stem cell to mature erythrocyte. However, although appearing inert, the red cell remains metabolically very active. The biochemical capacity of the red cell serves several different functions which require a constant supply of energy. Energy comes principally from intracellular anaerobic glycolysis, the mature red cell lacking the normal cellular mitochondrial organelles required for oxidative phosphorylation. Although anaerobic glycolysis is less efficient, a non-oxidative metabolism is really necessary. The primary role of the erythrocyte is to transport oxygen. Any oxidative metabolism, such as Kreb's Cycle, might therefore utilize some of the transport oxygen.

Glucose metabolism thus provides the energy for several important activities. Energy is required to maintain red cell shape and membrane integrity, and for defence against exogenous influences. Especially important is energy for maintaining oxidation-reduction homeostasis within the cell to preserve haemoglobin and other proteins in their reduced functional state. The erythrocyte lacks large intracellular energy stores and thus is very dependent on freely available glucose. This renders it metabolically unstable and vulnerable in a hypoglycaemic environment.

Metabolic activity within the red cell gradually declines with age, with a fall in activity of most glycolytic enzymes.

For normal survival, the red cell must constantly regulate its volume, surface area, and, accordingly, its general shape by actively controlling its electrolyte and water content which also decreases with age. Within the cell there is a high concentration of macro-anion molecules particularly haemoglobin, producing osmotic forces which if unopposed would create an inwards gradient for water and consequently cellular swelling and lysis. Although water can freely permeate the red cell membrane and the transmembrane movement for physiological anions is almost as rapid, the selective character of the cell membrane limits the movement of the principal cations sodium and potassium, despite large differences in concentration of these cations between cells and plasma. The movement of sodium is so restricted that the red cell, utilizing energy from intracellular anaerobic glycolysis can 'pump' out sodium into the plasma against a concentration gradient. Similarly, the intracellular potassium concentration is regulated by active transport into the cell. Calcium cations pass into erythrocytes very slowly under normal conditions and more rapidly when glycolysis ceases.

The energy for the various metabolic processes including the sodium pump comes mainly from the high energy compound adenosine triphosphate (ATP) which is synthesized by the anaerobic Embden-Meyerhof pathway of glycolysis within the cell. Glucose is metabolized through a number of intermediate compounds to lactate, each step being catalysed by an enzyme. The conversion of glucose to two-three diphosphoglycerate (2,3 DPG), the phosphate which is present in greatest concentration in erythrocytes, actually utilizes two molecules of ATP. However, the second stage is the conversion of 2,3 DPG to lactate which yields four molecules of ATP. Thus each molecule of glucose metabolized gives a net gain of two molecules of ATP. High energy phosphate for red cell metabolism is thus supplied by ATP which then returns to the glycolytic cycle as adenosine diphosphate (ADP) for rephosphorylation. Glucose is also metabolized by the oxidation hexose monophosphate pathway (HMP). Usually only up to 10% of glucose is metabolized by this pathway, although under certain conditions this proportion can be increased. The primary function of this pathway is the production of reduced nicotinamide-adenine dinucleotide phosphate (NADPH).

The vital oxidation-reduction homeostasis within the red cell depends on the active formation of reduced pyridine nucleotides. Reduced NADH from the Embden-Myerhof pathway is essential for maintaining haem iron in the reduced functional form. NADPH from the HMP pathway is important to maintain the tripeptide glutathione in the reduced state. Reduced glutathione (GSH) maintains the integrity of red cells by reducing sulphydryl groups of haemoglobin, membrane proteins, and enzymes which have been oxidized. This protection is necessary to prevent auto-oxidation and precipitation of haemoglobin which would result ultimately in premature cell death. Any enzyme defect or chemical poison which interferes with the metabolic pathways of glucose or glutathione also threaten the red cell's integrity. The commonest enzyme defect is a genetic deficiency of glucose 6-phosphate dehydrogenase. Deficiency of this enzyme leads to impaired glutathione metabolism and leaves the cell very liable to damage from any oxidant stress, particularly drugs.

Red cell function

The red cells are the chief agents in the transport of oxygen and they play an important part in the transport of carbon dioxide. Of the large amounts of these gases carried by the blood, only a very small fraction is carried in chemical combination. Most of the oxygen is carried within the cells as oxyhaemoglobin; most of the carbon dioxide is carried in the plasma as bicarbonate, but a small amount is carried in the red cell as bicarbonate and as carbaminohaemoglobin.

Oxygen transport

Fully oxygenated arterial blood can carry up to 20 ml of oxygen per 100 ml blood, with nearly all the oxygen in combination with haemoglobin and only 0.3 ml in solution in plasma. Haemoglobin has the ability to take up and release oxygen rapidly according to the physiological situation. Thus it takes up oxygen almost to saturation point within the lungs and readily yields oxygen within the capillaries of the body tissues. The way whereby oxygen is taken up and released by blood is shown by the oxygen dissociation curve (Fig. 11.3) which is not linear but S-shaped, this S shape being much accentuated by normal flunctuations in carbon dioxide content. The curve illustrates the excellent adaptation of the red cell for oxygen transport. Within the lungs, where oxygen tension is 100 mmHg, uptake is about 96% of saturation, and is only slightly reduced by a fall in oxygen tension. In the tissues however, where oxygen tension may be 40 mmHg or less, saturation falls to 70% and small decreases in oxygen tension cause haemoglobin to yield large quantities of oxygen.

The shape and position of the oxygen dissociation curve are affected by several factors. If the curve is shifted to the left, then less oxygen is released at a given oxygen tension, and if shifted to the right more oxygen is released at equivalent oxygen tension. A small reduction in pH leads to more oxygen being given up at a more rapid rate. Thus in the tissues, the fall in pH associated with carbon dioxide production leads to a greater yield of oxygen from haemoglobin. This effect of pH in shifting the dissociation curve

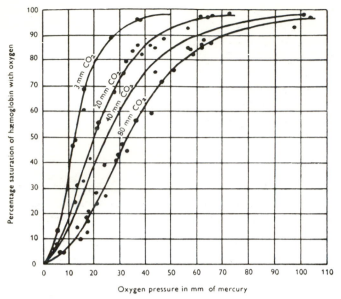

Fig. 11.3 Oxygen dissociation curve of haemoglobin at various pressures of oxygen and of carbon dioxide (Bell G H, Davidson J M, Scarborough H 1961 Textbook of physiology and biochemistry, 5th edn. Livingstone, Edinburgh).

is termed the Bohr effect. A rise in temperature has a similar result. Thus during exercise or with pyrexia, the fall in pH and rise in tissue CO_2 and temperature all decrease oxygen affinity and increase oxygen release.

The shape of the dissociation curve is also greatly influenced by the glycolytic intermediate 2,3 DPG. The addition of 2,3 DPG to haemoglobin decreases its oxygen affinity by binding to a specific site only available on deoxyhaemoglobin, shifting the curve to the right. Thus by lowering oxygen affinity, 2,3 DPG tends to make oxygen available to tissues more readily. The level of 2,3 DPG is important in a number of situations. In adapting to alterations in attitude, the higher 2,3 DPG levels which develop following hypoxia and respiratory alkalosis, are important in lowering the oxygen affinity of red cells. 2,3 DPG also has an important developmental role as it does not bind to fetal haemoglobin thus shifting its dissociation curve to the left of that of adult haemoglobin. In clinical practice, stored blood has low 2,3 DPG levels, and so where large amounts of blood are given, as in cardiac surgery, the raised oxygen affinity might theoretically exacerbate tissue hypoxia.

Fully saturated haemoglobin can carry 1.34 ml of oxygen per gram, or just over 20 ml per 100 ml of blood, although in life saturation is never complete. In venous blood the oxygen content is about 15 ml/dl so about 5 ml of oxygen is released to the tissues by each 100 ml of blood. With exercise the oxygen release may double, partly meeting the increased oxygen demand. However, although the increased yield of oxygen is in the order of two-fold, the increased demand may be five- or ten-fold. The additional oxygen is obtained not so much by increasing

the efficiency of extraction as by increasing the rate of blood flow. Clinically, oxygen affinity is assessed by measuring the tension of oxygen required to half saturate the haemoglobin (PO_{50}) rather than constructing a dissociation curve. The PO_{50} is normally 26–28 mmHg.

The inhalation of oxygen increases both the oxygen saturation of haemoglobin and the amount of oxygen carried in solution in the plasma. With normal respiratory function, the amount of oxygen dissolved in the plasma is about 0.25 ml/dl when breathing air; 1 ml when oxygen is given in an oxygen tent; 2 ml when oxygen is given by face mask; and about 4 ml when oxygen is given at a pressure of 2 atmospheres.

These concentrations of oxygen in the plasma reflect the various methods of administration, and are in fact proportional to the partial pressure of oxygen obtained in the lung alveoli. The actual gain in the amount of oxygen transported may appear small, but is to be compared with the normal extraction rate of oxygen which at rest is only about 5 ml per 100 ml of arterial blood.

Carbon dioxide transport

Less than 3 ml of carbon dioxide per 100 ml of blood is carried in simple solution, and about 20 times this amount is carried in chemical combination. Of this large amount, about two-thirds is carried in the plasma (as sodium bicarbonate) and about one-third in the red cells (partly as potassium bicarbonate and partly as a carbamino compound of haemoglobin).

The formation of bicarbonate requires the combination of carbon dioxide with water, producing carbonic acid. The enzyme carbonic anhydrase greatly accelerates this slow reaction. The hydrogen ion then released by this weak acid is mopped up by haemoglobin itself. The bicarbonate formed diffuses freely across the red cell membrane and a portion is exchanged with plasma chloride, a phenomenon called the 'chloride shift'.

The carbamino compound of haemoglobin results from the combination of carbon dioxide with a free amino group of globin and has the form NHCOOH. This compound is labile, and moreover, is readily formed by reduced haemoglobin but not by oxyhaemoglobin. It follows that the carbamino-haemoglobin formed in the tissues breaks down in the lungs. Although the total amount of carbamino-haemoglobin is small, it can alone transport most of the carbon dioxide formed by tissues at rest.

Just as oxygen transport is facilitated by changes in the concentration of carbon dioxide so carbon dioxide transport is facilitated by changes in oxygenation. Oxyhaemoglobin is a stronger acid than reduced haemoglobin, and tends to displace the weak carbonic acid; as a consequence of this, there is a tendency of increased elimination of carbon dioxide in the lungs, and of increased acceptance in the tissues.

The erythron

The total erythroid tissue, or the erythron, consists of the erythroid marrow cells and the circulating red cells. In the normal individual the erythron is maintained fairly constant by the production of mature red cells in the marrow in sufficient numbers to replace the aged red cells as they are removed by the reticulo-endothelial system.

It is estimated that about 1% of the circulating red cell mass is regenerated by the marrow each day and this is represented in the blood by a reticulocyte count of 1–2%. The reticulocyte count records the red cells which have been recently released from the marrow and gives an indication of the proportion of these cells compared with the fully mature red cells in circulation. Such a red cell production is sufficient to maintain a normal haemoglobin level and optimal tissue oxygenation. When optimal tissue oxygenation is not achieved, the marrow is stimulated to increase the red cell mass which in turn increases the blood's oxygen carrying capacity in an attempt to correct the defective tissue oxygenation. This response is mediated by an increased output of erythropoietin. If there is a defect in any part of the erythron, anaemia may develop. Within a few days of moderate anaemia developing, red cell production may increase to five times normal, and in cases of severe haemolytic anaemia increases of up to 10 times normal have been recorded. Such increased marrow production may be sufficient to maintain a normal haemoglobin i.e. the 'anaemia' has been compensated.

Abnormalities of the erythron can be of three broad types, according to the developmental level of the defect. They can occur: (i) during proliferation, (ii) during maturation in the marrow and (iii) during the life of the mature red cell in the circulation. Using this concept, anaemia may be classified on a functional basis.

Functional classification of anaemia

1. Defects of erythroid proliferation
   Erythropoietin deficiency
   Erythroid marrow failure
   Iron deficiency
2. Defects of erythroid maturation
   Nuclear abnormalities
   Cytoplasmic abnormalities
3. Defects affecting the erythrocyte
   Haemolysis
   Haemorrhage

Disorders of erythroid proliferation

These are conditions where the normal increase of erythroid precursors is less than expected for the degree of anaemia. This occurs:

1. With inadequate erythropoietin output as in renal disease and probably with endocrinopathies, protein malnutrition and infection
2. In marrow hypoproliferation as in hypoplastic anaemia
3. In iron deficiency where an inadequate supply of iron limits the increase in erythroid activity, despite high erythropoietin levels.

Disorders of erythroid maturation

There are disorders of red cell development which lead to abnormal maturation and consequently excessive destruction before release into the circulation. This occurs:

1. In the defective nuclear development of megaloblastic erythropoiesis where nuclear development lags behind cytoplasmic development
2. In the cytoplasmic abnormality of chronic iron deficiency where there is reduced haemoglobinization of the cells
3. In the sideroblastic anaemias

Defects affecting the erythrocyte

These are disorders in which the red cell is:

1. Prematurely destroyed, as in haemolytic disease or
2. Lost from the circulation, as in haemorrhage

ANAEMIA

Anaemia in physiological terms exists when the oxygen carrying capacity of the blood is below that required to maintain adequate tissue oxygenation. In haematological terms it exists when the haemoglobin level of the blood is below the lower limit of normal for sex and age (Table 11.1).

Table 11.1 Normal haemoglobin values

	g/dl
Adult males	13.5–18.5
Adult females	11.5–16.5
Children 10–12 years	11.5–15.0
Children 1 year	11.0–13.0
Infant 3 months	10.0–11.0
Cord blood	up to 20

Anaemia has already been classified on a functional basis according to the type of disorder causing the anaemia. It is also classified on a morphological basis according to the average volume and the average haemoglobin concentration of the red cells.

Morphological classification of anaemia

1. *Normocytic anaemia*: The red cell volume is in the normal range of 76–96 fl. Most normocytic anaemias are normochromic, i.e. the individual cells contain a normal concentration of haemoglobin.

2. *Microcytic anaemia*: The average red cell volume is below the normal range.

3. *Macrocytic anaemia*: The average red cell volume is greater than the normal range. Most macrocytic anaemias are normochromic.

4. *Normochromic anaemia*: The red cell haemoglobin concentration is normal.

5. *Hypochromic anaemia*: The red cell haemoglobin concentration is below normal. Most hypochromic anaemias are microcytic.

Such a morphological classification of anaemia can be made after simple haematological investigations and the examination of a stained peripheral blood film. Once defined in those terms it is often possible to suggest a pathogenetic mechanism for the anaemia.

Anaemia can therefore be classified in three ways as set out below, according to the pathogenetic mechanism, according to the morphological pattern of the red cells, or according to the functional abnormality of the erythron.

Comparative classification of anaemia

Pathogenetic mechanism	Morphological classification	Functional classification
Acute blood loss	Normocytic, normochromic	Red cell defect
Haemolysis	Normocytic, normochromic	Red cell defect
Chronic blood loss	Microcytic, hypochromic	Defect of erythroid proliferation and maturation
Iron deficiency state	Microcytic, hypochromic	Defect of erythroid proliferation and maturation
Marrow aplasia	Normocytic, normochromic	Defect of erythroid proliferation
Vitamin B$_{12}$ or folic acid deficiency	Macrocytic, normochromic	Defect of erythroid maturation
Infection	Normocytic, normochromic	Defect of erythroid proliferation
Liver disease	Normocytic, or macrocytic normochromic	Defect of erythroid proliferation
Renal failure	Normocytic, normochromic	Defect of erythroid proliferation

Posthaemorrhagic anaemia

After a single large haemorrhage the erythrocytes are reduced in number but are morphologically normal. If there is no nutritional or haematinic deficiency nor any complication which will suppress erythropoiesis, the marrow responds very rapidly to the blood's fall in 'oxygen carrying capacity' and quickly replaces the lost red cells.

Thus the normochromic anaemia is associated with a reticulocytosis and, as evidence of stimulation of the other haemopoietic cell lines, a modest polymorph leucocytosis and thrombocytosis.

Anaemia of chronic blood loss

If the blood loss is chronic the iron stores will become depleted, and what was initially a normochromic normocytic anaemia will become a microcytic hypochromic anaemia when iron deficiency develops. Such an anaemia may be the first evidence of occult bleeding from a 'silent' gastrointestinal neoplasm. Iron deficiency requires detailed consideration.

Iron deficiency anaemia

Iron metabolism

The total iron content of the body is usually estimated at 4–5 g, and approximately two-thirds of this is present as haemoglobin. The remainder is mainly storage iron which is contained in the reticuloendothelial tissues and the parenchymal cells of the liver. The rest of the body iron, about 5%, is present in muscle as myoglobin, and about 1% is in the plasma as transport iron. Very small amounts of iron are present in cellular enzymes, cytochromes, and peroxidases.

Dietary iron

A normal mixed diet supplies 10–15 mg of iron, of which only 1–2 mg is actually absorbed. Absorption is slightly greater in women than in men. Chief dietary sources are meats, eggs, green vegetables and fruit. The availability of iron present in different foodstuffs varies, being poorly absorbed in the presence of phosphates and phytates. Iron is only absorbed in the ferrous form and thus absorption is enhanced by reducing agents including gastric acid. Absorption of iron from meat is unaffected by these factors.

Iron absorption

Iron is absorbed principally in the upper 40 cm of the small intestine. Haem iron and inorganic iron are absorbed by different mechanisms; haem iron enters the gut epithelium and the iron is split from the haem within the cell while inorganic iron absorption is regulated by the epithelial cells lining the intestine. Immediately following uptake the iron is bound to an intracellular protein resembling transferrin. Some iron may be required by the cell itself, but the remaining iron is either absorbed through to the portal blood or held within the cell by apoferritin. When the body requires iron and the ferritin content of the epithelial cell is low, all the iron entering the cell is absorbed. However, if the body has sufficient iron stores, ferritin is produced and the incoming iron is trapped within the epithelial cell. Thus at the end of its life span of 3–4 days, the epithelial cell is shed into the gut lumen with its entrapped iron. This theory of iron absorption has been called the 'mucosal block'.

While iron absorption is closely related to body iron stores, the rate of erythropoiesis is also an important factor. When erythropoiesis is active, iron absorption is increased while the opposite occurs when erythropoiesis is depressed. Other less important factors which influence iron absorption are diet, pancreatic and gastric secretions.

Storage iron

Healthy males have about one-quarter of the body iron in stores, but many healthy women have little demonstrable iron stores. Iron is stored either as haemosiderin or ferritin. Haemosiderin is insoluble and is visible by ordinary light microscope as golden yellow intracellular granules, which stain an intense Prussian blue with the potassium ferrocyanide of Perl's stain. The demonstration of haemosiderin in bone marrow particles is a useful guide to iron stores.

Ferritin consists of a variable amount of ferric iron within a spherical protein shell, apoferritin. Each ferritin molecule is made up of 24 subunits and may contain up to 5000 iron atoms. Six channels communicate with the exterior and iron can pass readily in and out of the shell, the most recently entered iron being the first to leave. Plasma ferritin measured by an immunoradiometric assay gives a useful clinical guide to body iron stores, but its significance in several disease states, especially of a neoplastic nature remains unclear.

Plasma iron transport

Between 3 and 4 mg of iron are present in the plasma carried on a specific protein, a beta globulin known as transferrin. The function of transferrin is to transport iron between alimentary tract, marrow, and storage sites. Transferrin is synthesized in the liver, and each molecule is capable of carrying two atoms of ferric iron. Normally transferrin in the plasma is about one-third saturated. The total iron binding capacity of transferrin is usually in the range 45–77 μmol/l. The normal plasma iron level is approximately 18–45 μmol/l in males and 14–32 μmol/l in females, and has a diurnal variation.

Characteristic changes occur in the iron biochemistry in various pathological states. Serum iron rises in pernicious anaemia, haemolytic anaemia, aplastic anaemia, haemochromatosis and haemosiderosis, but as the total iron binding capacity of the serum is not elevated, the percentage saturation will also increase. The serum iron level is also elevated in infective hepatitis, and the rise appears to be correlated with the degree of parenchymal necrosis. In patients with iron deficiency anaemia, the characteristic finding is a subnormal plasma iron with an increase in total iron binding capacity. With infection, the plasma iron and total iron binding capacity may be lower than normal. The transferrin level may be reduced in some patients with disturbed protein metabolism, such as the nephrotic syndrome and chronic parenchymal liver disease.

Daily iron loss

There is no excretory pathway for iron and the body iron content is controlled only by regulating absorption from the gastrointestinal tract. In men and postmenopausal women a very small amount is lost daily (about 0.6 mg) from the skin by desquamation, from urine and in the stools from bile. In considering iron losses in premenopausal women, the amount lost in menstrual blood varies between 0.1 mg and 1.4 mg daily and the average amount of iron required to provide for red cell expansion during pregnancy, fetal growth and the placenta is approximately 800 mg. If the normal obligatory iron losses during the period of gestation are considered, a mean daily iron balance of 3.8 mg must therefore be achieved in order to stay in balance. Since, however, most of the iron required for increase of the red cell mass in the mother is returned at the end of pregnancy, the over-all iron balance can be maintained if the mean absorption is 2.7 mg daily.

This figure will naturally vary with such factors as the amount of bleeding during parturition and the size of the fetus. In calculating iron in relation to blood loss it is useful to remember that 1 ml of blood represents approximately 0.5 mg of iron.

The iron loss in the stools represents unabsorbed iron, the iron in occult blood and desquamated mucosal cells, and the iron excreted in bile. Losses from the urinary tract are fixed and of little significance in normal subjects; large amounts of iron can be excreted in the urine in clinical syndromes associated with intravascular haemolysis and in such instances haemosiderin is found in the urine. There is controversy about how much iron can be lost via the skin.

In brief, iron balance is generally satisfactory in men and postmenopausal women, but precarious in premenopausal women. The conservation of iron is generally advantageous but physiological mechanisms can only rid the body of a small amount each day; when intake is excessive, for example as a result of repeated blood transfusion, parenteral injection of iron or abnormal absorption from the intestine, the accumulation of iron which develops may have serious consequences.

Iron deficiency states

Iron deficiency anaemia is widespread in the United Kingdom and throughout the world and is by far the most common anaemia in clinical practice. In tropical and subtropical areas it is an even greater problem because of the additional blood loss due to hookworm infestation. Approximately 10% of women in Western countries have iron deficiency anaemia and about 20% have a latent iron deficiency.

In the development of iron deficiency, there are various stages of negative iron balance. In the first stage there may be complete utilization of stores without any fall in serum iron or change in the total iron binding capacity. In the next stage evidence of tissue depletion of iron appears with mild anaemia and a fall in the serum iron and a rise in the total iron binding capacity, though the red cells may still be normochromic and the haemoglobin still above 12 g/dl. In the last stage of actual deficiency and, of course, this occurs in varying degrees, there is the fully developed picture of hypochromic microcytic anaemia with tissue signs. The symptoms of iron deficiency anaemia include the general symptoms of anaemia — tiredness, lassitude, lack of energy and dyspnoea. The tissue signs are atrophic glossitis with loss of the normal tongue papillae, cheilosis at the angles of the lips and flaking and longitudinal ridging of the nails. In a very severe example, koilonychia or spoon-shaping of the nails may occur. Other changes include dysphagia with a web at the pharyngo-oesophageal junction and achlorhydria.

The diagnosis is made on the basis of anaemia and a hypochromic microcytic blood film. It is important to remember that the majority of normal blood films show some failure of haemoglobin staining in the centre of the cell but the hypochromia of iron deficiency is much more marked with only a residuum of haemoglobin round the edges of the red cell envelope.

The serum iron will be reduced and the total iron binding capacity elevated giving a low percentage saturation of transferrin, usually below 15%. It is seldom necessary to proceed to bone marrow examination but if this is done then stainable iron will be absent from the marrow.

The importance of iron deficiency anaemia is not only the chronic disability which it causes but the lead which it may give to underlying disease associated with chronic blood loss such as occult gastrointestinal neoplasm, hiatus hernia, salicylate ingestion, diverticulitis and haemorrhoids. In any unexplained iron deficiency anaemia the alimentary tract requires study by appropriate radiology and endoscopy and occasionally by an isotopic estimation of blood loss. In considering the aetiology of blood loss, enquiry should be made as to blood donation for trans-fusion purposes. There may well be malabsorption of iron for a number of reasons. Partial gastrectomy, and, to a lesser extent, gastroenterostomy lead to malabsorption of iron as do the more classical malabsorption syndromes including adult coeliac disease. Histamine-fast achlorhydria, probably because of the lack of acid, may well lead to impaired iron absorption.

In certain physiological situations increased iron requirement is a feature. In infancy, especially if prematurity has occurred, or twinning, then there is an increased iron requirement. Iron deficiency in infants may be aggravated by late onset of mixed feeding as milk is a poor source of iron; in adolescence, with active growth, iron deficiency may become obvious. Pregnancy causes iron deficiency, especially in the second and third trimesters.

Although this is a textbook of surgical physiology, there are aspects of management of these patients which are important in relation to the physiology of iron. Because of the aetiological factors, recurrence is very common and in hospital practice in this country about one-third of the patients reappear with recrudescence of the problem. Therefore the cause, where possible, must be removed and the iron deficit replaced; a good response would be represented by a haemoglobin rise of 0.1–0.2 g/dl daily. Ferrous sulphate is the cheapest preparation but the tablets have a bad reputation for side-effects. This is probably dose-related because the standard tablets contain large amounts of iron, but at the same time it is also probably partly psychological. Nausea, vomiting, abdominal pains and constipation are features of a patient who is apparently intolerant of iron therapy and various oral preparations should be tried before changing to parenteral therapy.

Full dosage should be continued for 6 months after the haemoglobin has been restored to normal in order to replenish iron stores and should be continued indefinitely if the cause cannot be removed. If iron therapy fails to be effective then it may be because the tablets are not taken, because of malabsorption or because of infection.

The surgeon also has to have some knowledge of the implication of parenteral iron therapy, whether this be intramuscular or intravenous. The indications for intramuscular iron therapy are failure or intolerance of oral iron therapy.

For parenteral therapy the intramuscular route is preferable. Two preparations are available: (i) iron sorbital citrate (Jectofer), a small molecule which diffuses rapidly from the injection site and which has a 30% urinary and saliva loss, and (ii) iron dextran (Imferon) which is a larger molecule with slower diffusion from the injection site and no urinary loss. These give the same rate of haemoglobin response as oral iron. Skin staining occurs with both preparations but is more common with iron dextran; allergic reactions are commoner with the dextran preparation. Both preparations, where inappropriately applied, either in excessive dosage or where no iron deficiency exists, can lead to excessive tissue iron or haemosiderosis.

Parenteral iron can also be given intravenously by a total dose infusion of iron dextran in saline. Major side-effects are rare but the use is probably only justified in selected cases; for example, in states of severe recurrent or continuous blood loss which cannot be controlled by conventional therapy. It may also be used where parenteral therapy is indicated but only small muscle mass is available for the intramuscular injection.

Iron overload

In contrast to iron deficiency, this is of course, rare, and is a direct reflection of the amount of iron available from the diet and the mucosal control of iron absorption. Iron overload may result either from long-term excessive absorption, excessive administration of parenteral iron, or from repeated blood transfusions. These conditions may result in the accumulation of over 25 g total body iron, compared to the normal of 3–5 g.

Menstruating women are partly protected from the effects of iron overload and it presents more frequently in males. The pathological effect of excessive iron in the body depends on the tissue localization of the iron, parenchymal iron being particularly liable to cause tissue damage, whereas reticuloendothelial iron is less harmful.

Parenchymal iron overload occurs particularly in idiopathic haemochromatosis where excess quantities of iron are absorbed from a normal diet, as a result of an inborn error of metabolism. The clinical effects of iron accumulation are usually first seen in males between 45 and 60 years of age. Parenchymal iron accumulation leads to hepatic cirrhosis with portal hypertension, hepatic failure and hepatoma may occur. Skin pigmentation due to excess melanin and iron is common. Diabetes mellitus, cardiac failure, testicular atrophy and other endocrine defects are also seen.

Plasma iron level is almost invariably raised as is transferrin saturation. Liver biopsy is the best diagnostic procedure allowing an assessment of iron deposition and extent of fibrotic change. Serum ferritin is also useful in assessing storage iron. Treatment requires removal of excess iron by venesection. Venesections of 500 ml at weekly intervals are continued until serum iron and saturation are normal. As only approximately 200 mg of iron are removed with each venesection, treatment requires to be continued for up to 2 years. Other complications such as diabetes mellitus or cardiac failure may also require treatment.

Other causes of excessive iron accumulation lead to haemosiderosis. Significant iron overload can occur if the diet contains a marked excess of iron, as in the Bantu population in South Africa who drink homebrewed beers which are heavily contaminated with iron. Multiple blood transfusions which are often required for beta-thalassaemia major, or refractory anaemias, also lead to excessive iron accumulation and haemosiderosis. Cardiac failure and other tissue effects may occur especially in younger children. Venesection is impracticable but continuous infusions of the chelating agent desferrioxamine might be worthwhile in young children with thalassaemia major. Very ill-advised and injudicious parenteral iron therapy will also produce similar results.

Megaloblastic anaemias

Vitamin B_{12} and folic acid deficiency

Our understanding of the physiology of vitamin B_{12} and folic acid has largely been acquired from study of the megaloblastic anaemias and it is impossible to give an account of the physiology of these two substances without a consideration of the megaloblastic anaemias. Megaloblastic anaemias are the morphological expression of any biochemical defect leading to slowing of deoxyribonucleic acid (DNA) synthesis, and occur particularly when vitamin B_{12} or folic acid, or both, are deficient or their action has been interfered with by competitive inhibition.

These anaemias are characterized by an abnormal type of red cell production and the erythropoiesis is megaloblastic as opposed to normoblastic; this is a descriptive term revealing characteristic cytological features in the developing nucleated red cells. An essential feature is nuclear-cytoplasmic disproportion. In the normoblastic series as the cell matures and becomes haemoglobinated, the nucleus is then relatively small in size and the chromatin material very dense. In the megaloblastic series the nucleus lags behind the cytoplasmic development so that a large nucleus with open chromatin is seen in a cell which contains much haemoglobin. This erythropoiesis arises when vitamin B_{12} or folic acid, or both, are deficient or their action has been interfered with by competitive inhibition.

Although the clinical syndromes of vitamin B_{12} or folic acid deficiency are dominated by anaemia other cellular components of the body are also affected. Leucopoiesis is affected so that leucopaenia results and the neutrophils are morphologically abnormal. Thrombocytopaenia is also a feature; furthermore, the morphological changes can be seen widely throughout other tissues, for example in the tongue and buccal mucosa. Vitamin B_{12} deficiency may cause the neurological syndrome of subacute combined degeneration of the cord.

In man, an abnormality of vitamin B_{12} or folic acid may result from defective intake, defective absorption, defective utilization or excessive requirement. Vitamin B_{12} and its analogues are found mostly in foods of animal origin such as meat, liver, eggs and milk. Vitamin B_{12} forms a complex with intrinsic factor which is secreted by the gastric parietal cells, and absorption of the complex occurs in the lower ileum. The normal daily need is about 2 μg, which is a very small amount. Folic acid and its analogues are found in animal liver but also in other animal products; it is also present in green vegetables and plants. Absorption occurs in the upper small intestine, and no intrinsic factor type of mechanism is involved. The physiological daily requirement is much greater than that of vitamin B_{12}, being in the order of 50 μg. Vitamin B_{12} and folic acid, once absorbed, are altered within the body to active forms, co-enzyme vitamin B_{12} and 5-methyltetrahydrofolic acid (5-methyl THF). Vitamin B_{12} is essential to convert 5-methyl THF to tetrahydrofolic acid (THF) which is essential for thymidilate synthesis for DNA. It is postulated the pathogenesis of megaloblastic anaemia in vitamin B_{12} deficiency is due to trapping of folate as 5-methyl THF thus producing secondary folate deprivation. This 'methyl-folate trap' hypothesis offers a reasonable explanation for the clinical and biochemical similarities of vitamin B_{12} and folate deficiency in man.

As already indicated, most of our knowledge about vitamin B_{12} and folic acid has been acquired from the study of a variety of clinical syndromes, all of which have megaloblastic erythropoiesis as a common factor. When trying to establish a diagnosis within this group it is essential that the clinical and laboratory data be combined and that the investigational procedures be selected as relevant to the particular clinical situation. Patients with this sort of anaemia usually have the general symptoms of anaemia, but may complain more specifically of other symptoms, such as those resulting from the neuropathy of vitamin B_{12} deficiency; this can cause painful paraesthesiae and symptoms resulting from posterior column damage and pyramidal tract damage. Points of importance in the clinical consideration are the age of the patient, any family history of anaemia, the dietary status, drug ingestion, intestinal symptoms and gastrointestinal surgery. On physical examination, particular attention is paid to the tongue, the abdomen and the central nervous system. In any severe megaloblastic anaemia, fundal haemorrhages may be seen.

Pernicious anaemia (Addisonian anaemia)

This is the commonest of all the megaloblastic anaemias and is a consequence of vitamin B_{12} malabsorption, due to gastric atrophy with lack of secretion of the intrinsic factor. The disease is uncommon under 40 years of age but is by no means rare. It is more common over 60 years of age and a family history of this anaemia is often present.

The onset is often slow and insidious and the patient may have glossitis with a complaint of sore tongue and lemon-yellow skin. He may have anorexia and weight loss and there is clinical difficulty in differentiation from carcinoma of the stomach. There may be evidence of peripheral neuritis or subacute combined degeneration of the cord. Patients may present with predominantly neuro-logical features and only minimal anaemia. Examination of the peripheral blood film shows that there is very great variation in the size of the cells, some being very much larger than normal and a few being very small. It is the contrast between the very large macrocytic cells and the small cells which alerts the haematologist to the possibility of a megaloblastic anaemia. Examination of the marrow shows the characteristics of megaloblastic erythropoiesis and parallel changes in the myeloid cell series. In a severe megaloblastic anaemia the cytological differentiation of the features provides no difficulty. With minor degrees of megaloblastic change, however, great skill and experience may be needed in interpretation of the marrow. This is especially true where there is accompanying iron deficiency, when the features of megaloblastic erythropoiesis may be less apparent. When there is no great urgency in these situations, replacement of the iron deficiency and repetition of the marrow examination thereafter may well show characteristic megaloblastic change. Serum B_{12} when estimated by microbiological technique is low, and histamine-fast achlorhydria can be demonstrated. Antibodies to parietal cells and to intrinsic factor will commonly be found in the serum. Absorption of radioactive B_{12} will be subnormal, but normal if intrinsic factor is given with it. The assay of intrinsic factor in the gastric juice will give a low result.

Vitamin B_{12} deficiency may be the cause of infertility and it is not uncommon to find a young married patient with pernicious anaemia who is treated and then has her first pregnancy subsequent to correction of the vitamin B_{12} deficiency.

Malabsorption

Vitamin B_{12} deficiency may occur with malabsorption syndromes such as tropical sprue, Crohn's disease, tuberculosis, or lymphoma of the ileum, and rarely with gluten enteropathy. More often megaloblastosis in these diseases is due to folate deficiency, but both serum vitamin B_{12} and folate may be below normal depending on which part of the bowel is most affected. Other features of malabsorption such as steatorrhoea, iron deficiency, and skeletal abnormalities are frequently present. Absorption of radioactive vitamin B_{12} if abnormal is not corrected by the addition of intrinsic factor.

Megaloblastic anaemia of pregnancy

The introduction of prophylactic folic acid administration as an accompaniment to the administration of oral iron to pregnant women has reduced the occurrence of this condition, which previously was not uncommon. It is best regarded as folic acid deficiency mainly due to excessive requirement aggravated by deficient intake. Malabsorption may occasionally be a factor in a small number of patients.

The condition is usually found clinically in the last trimester of pregnancy but may not be apparent until the puerperium. It is more common in multiple pregnancies and there is usually a poor dietary intake. It is often found in subsequent pregnancies. Serum folate when estimated is low.

Postgastrectomy megaloblastic anaemia

This is invariable after total gastrectomy and these patients should be given prophylactic vitamin B_{12}. Megaloblastic anaemia occurs, of course, after partial gastrectomy and the condition is best regarded as 'surgical pernicious anaemia'. The main fault is lack of intrinsic factor leading to B_{12} deficiency but folate deficiency may also occur due to inadequate diet and to some measure of steatorrhoea.

Dietary megaloblastic anaemia

Because of the very small amounts of vitamin B_{12} required at a physiological level, dietary deficiency of vitamin B_{12} is excessively rare, but has been recognized to occur in a group of ultravegetarians called vegans; they do not eat any animal produce and develop vitamin B_{12} deficiency. Folate deficiency can develop in elderly subjects much more readily when on poverty diets. If a healthy volunteer is starved of folate then megaloblastic change begins to appear in 3–6 months.

'Loop' megaloblastic anaemia

This is very rare but of interest because of the aetiological mechanism. The anaemia is associated with a stagnant loop, cul-de-sac, stricture or diverticulum formation of the small bowel; organisms proliferate in the stagnant area and ingest the vitamin B_{12} in the bowel lumen depriving the host of the vitamin and causing B_{12} deficiency. A feature of such an anaemia is that absorption of radioactive vitamin B_{12} is subnormal but normal after sterilization of the gut by antibiotics.

Drug-induced megaloblastic anaemia

Several drugs may induce a megaloblastic anaemia by interference with the metabolism of vitamin B_{12} or folate. The best known in this respect are anticonvulsants, particularly phenytoin, and antimetabolites such as methotrexate. Megaloblastic anaemia related to folate deficiency is occasionally noted in patients taking oral contraceptives, and is commonly found in association with chronic alcohol ingestion. The use of nitrous oxide as an anaesthetic agent has also been linked with the acute onset of vitamin B_{12} deficient megaloblastic anaemia, while sudden onset of folate deficiency may be seen in severely ill patients who require parenteral nutrition.

Investigational procedures

Having established that a patient has a megaloblastic anaemia it is then necessary to establish the disturbance of physiology responsible for the anaemia. It is usually inappropriate to apply all the possible techniques to any one specific patient and the selection of tests to be employed is a matter of clinical judgement.

Serum B_{12} is estimated by microbiological or radioisotopic assay. Some antibiotics when administered concurrently invalidate microbiological assay; for example, sulphonamides and broad spectrum antibiotics because they interfere with the growth of the organism used in the assay. The normal range is 180–1000 ng per litre of serum and a level of less than 100 ng/l indicates vitamin B_{12} deficiency. The estimate of serum folate is also a microbiological or radioisotopic technique and more difficult than the estimation of vitamin B_{12}. Normal ranges vary widely from laboratory to laboratory but a value of less than 2 μg per litre of serum usually indicates deficiency. An assay of the folate content of red cells gives a better assessment of the individual's overall folate status as the serum folate level fluctuates according to daily variation in folate intake. The assay of red cell folate is carried out using similar techniques. The normal range is 165–600 μg per litre of blood. The radioactive vitamin B_{12} absorption tests are of major diagnostic importance and relatively simple to perform.

The oral Schilling test is the most widely used test of vitamin B_{12} absorption. In this test an oral dose of radiolabelled vitamin B_{12} is given followed 2 hours later by a 1000 μg of non-labelled vitamin B_{12} parenterally. This parenteral dose of vitamin B_{12} 'flushes' out part of the labelled vitamin B_{12} which has been absorbed and this can be measured in a 24 hour urine collection.

The extent of absorption can be assessed by comparing the amount of radioactivity excreted in the urine with the radioactivity of the oral dose. The test can be repeated giving oral intrinsic factor with the oral dose of labelled vitamin B_{12} to show if any malabsorption is corrected by the 'intrinsic' factor. Such a correction by intrinsic factor indicates intrinsic factor deficiency or pernicious anaemia. The two main shortcomings of the Schilling test are impaired renal function, and an incomplete urine collection. Absorption of vitamin B_{12} using radioactive techniques can also be carried out using a whole body monitor or by counting the non-absorbed vitamin B_{12} in the stools, or by measuring hepatic uptake by isotope counting over the liver.

Radioactive folate is available as a tritiated preparation and can be used in a similar fashion to study folate absorption, but the counting techniques are much more demanding than with vitamin B_{12} and are really only available as an experimental technique for the present.

Intrinsic factor in gastric juice can be assayed in vitro

by measuring its ability to bind vitamin B_{12}, but is rarely performed in everyday practice.

A specific biochemical abnormality found in vitamin B_{12} deficiency is an excess of methylmalonic acid in the urine but the estimation requires gas chromatography and at this point in time cannot be viewed as a routine biochemical procedure.

Treatment

In vitamin B_{12} deficiency states, such as pernicious anaemia, treatment with vitamin B_{12} only is required. Indeed the administration of folic acid alone to a patient with vitamin B_{12} deficiency can be very dangerous as it can precipitate the onset of, or aggravate pre-existing, neurological damage. For obvious reasons parenteral administration is necessary, and to replenish body stores five daily injections of 1000 μg of vitamin B_{12} will suffice. Vitamin B_{12} as hydroxycobalamin is better retained and can be used in preference to cyanocobalamin. Patients require a maintenance treatment for life of 1000 μg of vitamin B_{12} or hydroxycobalamin each month. Oral treatment of vitamin B_{12} deficiency is quite unsatisfactory. In folic acid deficiency a daily dose of 20 mg is adequate. Even in absorptive defects this dose ensures enough absorption to meet the body's needs. Duration of treatment depends on the cause; this may be for life in adult coeliac disease or until 2 weeks after delivery in pregnancy megaloblastic anaemia.

Because of the metabolic interrelationships of vitamin B_{12} and folic acid, a vitamin B_{12}-deficient patient may respond to a large dose of folic acid, and a folic acid deficient patient may respond to a large dose of vitamin B_{12}. This does not occur if physiological doses are used. In the case of vitamin B_{12} this physiological dose is 1 μg intramuscularly daily and in the case of folic acid 0.2 mg intramuscularly daily.

Further response to such doses occurs only when the need is being met; it is of diagnostic as well as therapeutic value. In academic studies of this type of anaemia, it is this order of dosage which should therefore be used to establish the characteristics of the deficiency.

At the clinical level in a desperately-ill patient after megaloblastosis has been established by blood film and marrow examination, treatment should not be delayed; after a blood sample has been obtained for vitamin B_{12} and folic acid assay the patient should be given vitamin and folic acid simultaneously. Many of the severely megaloblastic patients are also potassium deficient and it is important to give, in addition, potassium supplements. Various diagnostic tests can be performed retrospectively and taken with the pretreatment assay values, should lead to accurate diagnosis. Blood transfusion may be required but carries a risk of precipitating left heart failure. If used, a unit of concentrated red cells given over 12 hours is likely to tide the patient over until a reticulocyte response

occurs at about the fourth or fifth day after starting treatment. If blood is given, a diuretic should be given immediately prior to the transfusion. In severe cases exchange transfusion may be necessary. In the following lists the causes of folic acid deficiency and vitamin B_{12} deficiency are enumerated.

FOLIC ACID DEFICIENCY

Deficient intake
   Tropical nutritional anaemia
   Pregnancy
   Hepatic cirrhosis
   Postgastrectomy
   Alcoholism
Deficient absorption
   Sprue
   Coeliac disease
Deficient utilization
   Anticonvulsant therapy
   Folic acid antagonists
   Hepatic cirrhosis
   Scurvy
Excessive need
   Pregnancy
   Neoplasm
   Haemolytic anaemia
   Leukaemia

Vitamin B_{12} deficiency

Deficient intake
   Tropical nutritional anaemia
   Vegans
Deficient absorption
   Deficiency of intrinsic factor:
      Pernicious anaemia
      Postgastrectomy
   Organismal competition:
      Loop syndrome
   Lesions of intestine:
      Resection or bypass of ileum
      Sprue
      Coeliac disease
      Ileal disease
Defective utilization
   Anticonvulsant anaemia
Excessive need
   Pregnancy

Symptomatic anaemias

Symptomatic anaemia, or the anaemia of chronic disorders is a well recognized entity seen in a wide range of patients suffering from infections, inflammatory diseases, malignancy, and chronic renal failure. Typically the anaemia appears normochromic and normocytic, but when long-standing the red cells can become hypochromic and microcytic. Although the anaemia is associated with a decreased serum iron concentration, normal or increased amounts of iron are found in the reticuloendothelial stores. The serum iron binding capacity and transferrin saturation may also be decreased, but serum ferritin concentration is usually normal.

The pathogenesis of the anaemia of chronic disorders is complex, and a number of different factors may contribute. Red cell life span is typically reduced and is inadequately compensated by erythroid activity. The suppressed erythroid function may be a result of iron being 'blocked' within the reticulo-endothelial system and thus unavailable for erythropoiesis. Inadequate erythropoietic stimulation may also contribute, serum levels being very low in symptomatic anaemias.

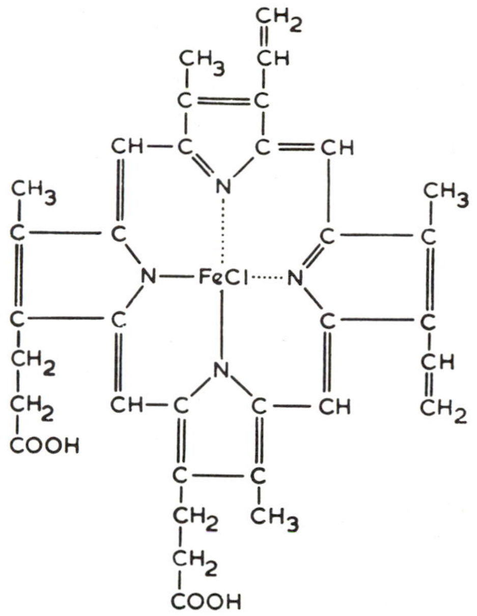

HAEMOGLOBIN

Haemoglobin is a conjugated protein with a molecular weight of approximately 65 000. It consists of a respiratory pigment (haem, an iron-porphyrin) conjugated to a specific globulin (globin). Haemoglobin synthesis is achieved by the synchronous production of globin chains and haem and the combination of these to form the final molecule. The globin part of the molecule is made up of four polypeptide chains, two alpha and two beta chains. Four haem groups are situated on the surface of the molecule in such a way that each is associated with a different polypeptide chain of the globin.

This molecule of haemoglobin can be regarded as an 'enzyme' with oxygen as one of its substrates and during oxygenation the beta chains of the globin move closer together. If there is an alteration in the amino acid composition of the globin's peptide chains, this chain movement which controls oxygen transport can be affected and the oxygen carrying capacity altered. This is seen in certain of the abnormal haemoglobins.

Haem

Haem, which constitutes about 4% of the weight of a haemoglobin molecule is an iron porphyrin. It has a porphyrin nucleus which is made from four pyrrol groups linked through carbon atoms, the whole forming a cyclic structure. Such porphyrin structures have the property of forming metal complexes and in haem each porphyrin nucleus is combined with one atom of ferrous iron. In this form haemoglobin is capable of transporting one atom of oxygen. Haem is the prosthetic group in haemoglobin, various cytochromes, catalases, peroxidase and other haem proteins (Fig. 11.4).

HAEM

Fig. 11.4 The chemical formula of haem. The iron atom is united to the nitrogen atoms of the four pyrrol rings which themselves form a large ring.

Haem synthesis

Glycine and succinyl CoA condense in the presence of the enzyme delta-amino laevulinic acid synthetase to form delta-amino laevulinic acid (ALA) This reaction has an important rate limiting role in the synthetic chain. Two molecules of ALA then unite to form a small ring-shaped molecule, a monopyrole porphobilinogen. Four porphobilinogen molecules then condense to form the colourless tetrapyrrolic compound uroporphyrinogen III which is then modified by the removal of four acetic acid side-chains to form corproporphyrinogen III. This colourless compound is rapidly auto-oxidized to the red protoporphyrin III. These reactions are carried out in mitochondria where the relevant enzymes are sited. Mature red cells which lack mitrochondria cannot continue haem synthesis.

Iron reaches the erythroblast bound to transferrin, is released at the cell membrane and transported to the mitochondria where under the influence of haem synthetase it is incorporated into protoporphyrin III to form haem. There is a close link between haem and globin synthesis to maintain the formation of haemoglobin in the cell 'in step'. Excess free haem in the cell, which can arise from delay in globin synthesis, depresses amino laevulinic acid synthetase activity and thus retards further haem formation. At the same time free haem in the cell serves to stimulate globin synthesis.

Globin synthesis

Normal globin is composed of two pairs of amino acid

chains called alpha and beta chains, the first comprising 141 amino acids and the second 146. The molecular weight of normal adult haemoglobin is 64 450. Different globins, and thus different haemoglobins, are evolved if the amino acid sequence of these peptide chains is altered. In normal adult haemoglobin, haemoglobin A (made of two alpha and two beta chains) comprises 98% of the total haemoglobin, and haemoglobin A_2 (made of two alpha and two delta chains) comprises 2%. In the fetus the globin of haemoglobin differs from the adult type and at birth 80% is HbF (made of two alpha and two gamma chains) and 20% HbA.

By the age of 4 months the HbF has fallen to 10% and by the end of infancy only traces persist. Over the last few years many different haemoglobins have been described, each new type having yet another variation in the amino acid sequence of a peptide chain in the globin.

Evidence suggests that beta-chain synthesis is directed by only one locus on the chromosome, but it appears likely that there are two loci for the alpha chain. The genetic information required for haemoglobin synthesis is carried by DNA, and transferred to messenger RNA. The different globin peptide chains are synthesized on the polyribosomes of the erythroblasts and are assembled in orderly fashion in pairs to give in normals the configuration of two alpha and two beta chain units. These then become associated with the haem units and haemoglobin is formed. All other protein synthesis is suppressed in the erythroblast to the extent that haemoglobin accounts for more than 95% of the erythroblast's protein production.

Haemoglobin degradation

The haemoglobin molecule's breakdown begins as an oxidative opening of the protoporphyrin ring to form verdo haemoglobin. The rate-limiting enzyme in this process is haemoxygenase. Then by cleavage of the iron and globin from the molecule, biliverdin is formed and is rapidly reduced to bilirubin. Bilirubin, which is insoluble in water, is transported in the plasma bound to albumin and is transferred to the hepatic cell where it is conjugated and excreted as a water soluble glucuronide.

On storage in the gall bladder, bilirubin slowly becomes oxidized to biliverdin which has a characteristic green colour. Oxidation does not normally proceed further, but when biliverdin is incorporated in gall stones it may very slowly oxidize to bilicyanin, a much darker pigment.

Bilirubin and also biliverdin when exposed to bacterial action are reduced to urobilinogen (stercobilinogen). Most of this is excreted in the faeces in the oxidized form of stercobilin and is responsible for the normal brown colour of the stools. A small proportion of the urobilinogen, however, is reabsorbed from the intestine, carried to the liver and re-excreted in the bile. A mere trace of the reabsorbed urobilinogen is normally excreted in the urine.

The nature of the bile pigment derivatives in the urine is of clinical importance. As the bilirubin normally present in the bloodstream is the prehepatic, water-insoluble form it cannot pass the glomerular membrane and appear in the urine; bilirubin is, however, excreted in the urine in obstructive jaundice because posthepatic water soluble bilirubin glucuronate accumulates proximal to the biliary obstruction and is absorbed from the bile into the blood.

Bilirubin in this posthepatic form passes the glomerular membrane and is found in the urine. Urobilinogen is normally present in the urine only in the trace amounts, and increased urobilinogen in urine suggests increased haemoglobin catabolism and haemolytic disease. In obstructive jaundice, bile pigments no longer reach the intestine, urobilinogen is no longer formed by intestinal putrefaction and urobilinogen consequently disappears from the urine. Occasionally in obstructive jaundice, urobilinogen may appear in the urine; this is indicative of cholangitis for the only site where bile pigment can be subjected to bacterial reduction is now proximal to the biliary obstruction.

THE HAEMOLYTIC ANAEMIAS

The fate of the red cell

The red cell's survival in the circulation depends on its ability to maintain its unique physical properties despite wide variations in the chemical composition of its environment and despite the continuous trauma which it experiences in the circulation. As the red cell's enzyme systems, which are essential to maintain the integrity of its membrane, age and become less effective, there comes a stage when the intact membrane can be no longer maintained and is destroyed. Furthermore, such a highly specialized, non-nucleated cell as the red cell is incapable of repair. Though a small number of red cells are destroyed in the bloodstream, the majority are removed by the spleen and the reticulo-endothelial system.

The aged red cell, which is becoming metabolically more unstable, when subjected to a short period of sequestration in the hypoglycaemic splenic sinusoids, is destroyed from failure of its enzyme systems to maintain its sodium pump. The normal red cell survives from 100–120 days in the circulation.

In disease, other factors may affect this orderly process of clearing the circulation of old red cells. The cell itself can be basically abnormal and more susceptible to lysis, or the plasma may contain abnormalities which damage the cell membrane from without and hasten its destruction. Thus, haemolytic disorders can be classified into intrinsic red cell (corpuscular) disorders, or extrinsic red cell (extracorpuscular) disorders.

Classification of haemolytic disease

Intrinsic red cell defects
    Hereditary spherocytosis (acholuric jaundice)
    Hereditary haemoglobinopathies and thalassaemia
    Hereditary non-spherocytic haemolytic anaemias
Extrinsic red cell defects
    Autoimmune idiopathic
    Autoimmune secondary to virus pneumonia
    Autoimmune secondary to lymphoid tumours
    Autoimmune secondary to systemic lupus erythematosus
    Autoimmune secondary to drugs (methyldopa)
    Haemolytic disease of the newborn
    Haemolytic anaemia due to drugs or chemicals
    Haemolytic anaemia of severe burns
    Microangiopathic haemolytic anaemia
    Hypersplenism

When increased red cell breakdown occurs, marrow output is increased and this may be able to compensate and prevent a fall in haemoglobin. Many mild cases of congenital spherocytosis are detected incidentally in later life and at no time have been anaemic. Increased red cell destruction leads usually to a raised serum bilirubin and clinical jaundice. In some cases, however, the liver can clear the increased bilirubin load and no bilirubinaemia occurs. The bilirubin is of the unconjugated or indirect reacting type and gives a positive indirect Van den Bergh reaction. Unconjugated bilirubin does not appear in the urine as its renal threshold is high and the haemolytic anaemias can be described as acholuric, i.e. without bile in the urine. Because of the increased bile cleared by the liver in haemolytic states, the faecal urobilinogen content is increased, and this is reflected in an increased urinary urobilinogen excretion.

Increased red cell destruction is followed by compensatory erythroid hyperplasia in the marrow. A healthy marrow can produce up to six times the normal output of cells, but marrow function can be depressed by infection, tumour infiltration or folic acid deficiency. Compensatory erythroid hyperplasia is reflected in the peripheral blood by a reticulocytosis and an elevated reticulocyte count which can be as high as 50%. In certain cases of long-standing haemolytic disease the marrow hyperplasia is sometimes sufficiently marked to cause bony changes. These are seen particularly in the skull and are a fairly constant feature in a chronic haemolytic state like thalassaemia major. Chronic haemolytic disorders may also commonly be complicated by biliary pigment calculi and episodes of biliary obstruction which might obscure the primary haemolytic state.

Also in the peripheral blood there are usually 'pre-haemolytic' red cell changes which suggest haemolysis — spherocytosis and red cell fragmentation. Both these changes suggest damage to the red cell. The spherocyte is a small globular cell as opposed to the biconcave disc of the normal erythrocyte. Red cell fragments take many shapes and can be triangular cells, helmet cells, crescentic cells or just distorted cell fragments or schistocytes. The red cell's integrity can be tested by exposing it to a range of concentrations of saline. Such a red cell osmotic fragility test is abnormal in most haemolytic states. The spherocyte is already swollen and when exposed to hypotonic saline has a greater tendency to lyse than the normal erythrocyte (Figs. 11.5 and 11.6).

The shortened red cell life span in haemolytic disease can be demonstrated by radioisotope studies. Red cells from the patient are labelled by the radioactive isotope of chromium (^{51}Cr) and their survival followed in the circulation by scintillation counting of serial blood specimens. If there is doubt about the presence of haemolysis on the basis of simple haematological tests, this very sensitive method of detecting shortened red cell survival can be very helpful. As an extension to this investigation, scintillation counting can be used to seek evidence of red cell sequestration in the spleen. If such red cell sequestration is demonstrated it suggests that the spleen has adopted a pathological role and should probably be removed (Fig. 11.7).

Haemolytic anaemias

Hereditary spherocytosis is inherited as a Mendelian dominant and is an intrinsic cell defect, probably of the glycolytic mechanism. It may be a relatively severe

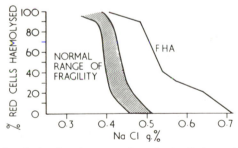

Fig. 11.5 Graph showing the proportion of red cells haemolysed in various concentrations of saline. The cross hatched area represents the range of normal. In a case of familial haemolytic anaemia (FHA) some of the red cells are very weak indeed, but a few are almost as tough as normal cells (After Whitby L E H, Hynes M 1935 The quantitative estimation of the fragility of the red corpuscles. Journal of Pathology and Bacteriology 40:219).

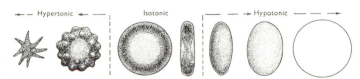

Fig. 11.6 The shape of red cells immersed in saline which is hypertonic, isotonic and hypotonic (Garven, 1957).

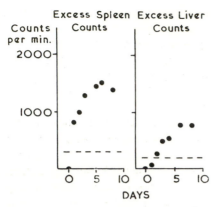

Fig. 11.7 Auto-immune haemolytic anaemia showing the results of surface counting over spleen and liver after tagging the patients own erythrocytes with Cr⁵¹. The broken lines indicate the upper limit of the normal range. The excess counts indicate active destruction of erythrocytes in both spleen and liver (Dacie J B 1963 The haemolytic anaemias Part II 2nd edn. Churchill, London).

disorder and present in early childhood, or it can be very mild and only be detected by chance investigation in late life. The blood film shows frequent, small, spherical erythrocytes or microspherocytes and a reticulocytosis. The spleen is usually slightly enlarged and should be removed.

Splenectomy does not correct the red cell abnormality but it does largely correct the shortened red cell survival and anaemia; clinical cure results from splenectomy. Of all the various indications for splenectomy this is the one in which splenectomy can be confidently recommended.

Certain hereditary haemolytic anaemias are characterized by the production of abnormal adult haemoglobin — the haemoglobinopathies. These constitute a large medical problem on a world scale and are broadly of two types. In the first, the normal adult haemoglobin, haemoglobin A, is replaced by a different haemoglobin according to an amino acid substitution in a peptide chain of the globin. Thus, there are haemoglobins S, E and C etc. Haemoglobin S is the most important one clinically, giving sickle cell disease in homozygous patients. Sickling of cells occurs with deoxygenation and eventually leads to irreversible damage and premature destruction. Sickle cell disease is a chronic haemolytic anaemia complicated by 'crises' affecting many organs. Treatment is mainly symptomatic, including adequate oxygenation, which is clearly essential during anaesthesia.

The second group of haemoglobinopathies are characterized by genetically-determined defects of globin chain synthesis. The result is imbalanced globin chain synthesis with normal haemoglobin A formation suppressed, as in the thalassaemia syndromes. The thalassaemia genes are transmitted as autosomal Mendelian dominants. Homozygous patients have severe chronic haemolysis while heterozygotes tend to be asymptomatic.

A small number of haemolytic anaemias have an auto-immune pathogenesis, i.e. an auto-antibody is present. In addition to the haematological findings already described such patients have in the serum an auto-antibody which reacts with a red cell antigen, generally a Rhesus antigen. The red cells are therefore coated with antibody or human immunoglobulin and give a positive reaction in the direct antiglobulin test or direct Coombs' test, i.e. such immunoglobulin-coated red cells when incubated with an anti-human globulin serum, agglutinate.

This antibody globulin coating of the red cell may be eluted and studied serologically to determine its antigenic specificity. Not all of the antibody may be bound to the red cell and often free antibody can be demonstrated in the serum by the indirect antiglobulin test or indirect Coombs' test. In this test a mixture of red cells, carrying among them most red cell antigens is incubated with the test serum and if antibody is present which has red cell specificity the cells carrying the appropriate antigen will be coated with immunoglobulin. This coating can be detected by adding anti-human globulin which brings about agglutination of these coated cells.

Such cases of autoimmune haemolytic anaemia may respond to steroid therapy; others, which have not responded to steroid therapy, may require splenectomy. In this instance, unlike congenital spherocytosis, splenectomy is likely to give a remission in only about half of the patients.

The majority of examples of autoimmune haemolytic anaemia are idiopathic; a certain percentage are, however, secondary to lymphoproliferative tumours.

Haemolytic disease of the newborn will be discussed in the section on blood transfusion.

A wide range of drugs are known to cause haemolysis. A few, such as methyldopa, do so by immunological mechanisms. More commonly, drugs which are oxidants, such as phenacetin or dapsone, produce Heinz bodies within the red cells and subsequent haemolysis. This occurs particularly in patients deficient in the enzyme glucose 6-phosphate dehydrogenase.

If blood passes through a fibrin mesh in vitro, red cells are caught and damaged by the fibrin strands and the blood which emerges shows red cell fragmentation. A similar morphological pattern with an associated haemolytic anaemia is found in conditions where there is disease and fibrin deposition in the small vessels — microangiopathic haemolytic anaemia (MHA). This was first described in the haemolytic uraemic syndrome of infants, and more recently has been found in a variety of renal diseases, in carcinoma of stomach and other malignancies, and in conditions with disseminated intravascular coagulation.

A similar pattern of red cell fragmentation may be met in patients with cardiac plastic valve prostheses. If a high pressure jet of blood is created by a leak in a faulty suture line around the plastic valve prosthesis, or if the cloth covering of the valve is damaged, damage to the red cells occurs and fragmentation and chronic haemolytic anaemia develop. Recent improvements in the design of cardiac plastic valve prostheses have greatly reduced the incidence of this complication.

LEUCOPOIESIS

Leucocytes are formed in the bone marrow from, it is believed, the same primitive stem cells as the erythrocytes. When mature, they are released into the circulation where they provide a defensive system which in health recognizes, localizes and eliminates 'foreign' material. The leucocytes can be subdivided functionally and morphologically into three cell series — the granulocytes or myeloid series, the lymphocytes or lymphoid series and the monocytes or monocyte series.

Granulocytes

Granulocytes are formed from myeloblasts in the bone marrow passing through stages of maturation and proliferation comparable to erythroid development. The stages of development after myeloblast are premyelocyte, myelocyte, metamyelocyte (or stab cell) and segmented polymorph (or mature granulocyte). As these cells mature in the marrow they develop cytoplasmic granules which stain characteristically in one of three ways and provide a further subclassification of the series into neutrophil, eosinophil and basophil granulocyte. The physiological function of these three types varies and as can be seen from the table of white cell values, the neutrophil granulocyte predominates numerically in the peripheral blood.

The neutrophil granulocyte's contribution to the overall immunological defence mechanism is phagocytosis. While other mechanisms to be described are largely responsible for recognising and attacking foreign material, the granulocyte, in particular the neutrophil polymorph, is attracted to the area, engulfs the foreign material, digests it and eliminates the breakdown products.

Neutrophils are attracted to an inflammatory response by various chemotactic principles including bacterial filtrates, antigen-antibody complexes, immunoglobulins and heat-labile complement components. Following adhesion to the vascular endothelium, the neutrophil emigrates between endothelial cells and into the tissues. Foreign particles are engulfed by pseudopodia from the granulocyte which fuse to surround it completely. Thus the foreign particle comes to occupy a vacuole in the cell which is lined by invaginated cell membrane. In effect this phagocytic vacuole still occupies an extracellular space, but the granules of the neutrophil then fuse with the membrane of the phagocytic vacuole resulting in discharge of the liposomal contents with consequent destruction and lysis of the ingested particle. All neutrophil killing functions are oxygen-dependent, while phagocytosis itself relies heavily on anaerobic glycolysis to produce sufficient energy. Neutrophil degranulation results in cell death with extracellular release of liposomal material producing tissue inflammation.

Numerous methods have been suggested to assess neutrophil function. In vivo, the inflammatory response is best assessed by using the skin-window response. In vitro chemotaxis can be evaluated using millipore filters by the Boyden technique, and a variety of tests of phagocytosis have been devised although none is ideal. Deficient enzyme activity, as occurs in chronic granulomatous disease can be detected by the nitro blue tetrazolium test (NBT test).

The eosinophil granulocyte's prime function is poorly understood. Like the neutrophil granulocyte, it passes quickly out from the blood into the tissues, where it has a similar amoeboid motion and the ability to phagocytose, but its general activity in these respects is more sluggish than its neutrophil counterpart. Eosinophils characteristically increase in allergic conditions and parasite infections, and it has been shown that antigen-antibody complexes provide a chemotactic stimulus for eosinophils and are then phagocytosed by them. In lymph nodes, eosinophils will be found at the site of antibody production arriving there at the earliest appearance of antibody. The phagocytic process is similar to the neutrophil, but is likely to be associated with the escape to the outside of eosinophil peroxidase and basic protein. The eosinophil peroxidase is a potent histamine release agent and in eosinophilia therefore, it is to be expected that histamine will be liberated from the mast cells.

Even less is known of the basophil granulocyte. Like the other granulocytes it passes rapidly out into the tissues, where it appears to be related functionally to the mast cells. Unlike the neutrophil polymorph the basophil, under certain stimuli, appears to discharge its granule content into the tissue spaces. Various agents are known to achieve this degranulation and the most important physiologically are eosinophil peroxidase and antigen-antibody reactions involving complement. Indeed, the main function of the basophil appears to be the discharge of its granules into the extracellular space, while the neutrophil is mainly concerned with phagocytosing particulate matter, and the eosinophil with the discharge of substances into the extracellular space.

Normal white cell values

Adults	$4.0–11.0 \times 10^9/l$
Children 8–12 years	$4.5–13.0 \times 10^9/l$
Children 4–7 years	$6.0–15.0 \times 10^9/l$
Infants at birth	$10.0–25.0 \times 10^9/l$

Normal adult white cell differential count

Neutrophils	40–75%	$2500–7500 \times 10^6/l$
Lymphocytes	20–45%	$1500–3500 \times 10^6/l$
Monocytes	2–10%	$200–800 \times 10^6/l$
Eosinophils	1–6%	$40–440 \times 10^6/l$
Basophils	0–1%	$0–100 \times 10^6/l$

Granulocytes can be regarded as occupying three phases in the marrow. The first is the phase of mitosis, where there is a rapid reproduction of cells up to the myelocyte stage. Then there is a phase of maturation and finally there is a phase of marrow storage. There is considerable overlap between these three phases. This marrow granulocyte store is made up of segmented polymorphs and metamyelocytes and it contains a considerably greater number of cells than the total granulocytes in the peripheral circulation. On demand, numbers of segmented polymorphs are released into the peripheral circulation and it is possible that this is mediated through a factor called leucocyte release factor. This factor has been demonstrated in animals, but not as yet in man. Once in the peripheral circulation the granulocytes can go to one of two pools, the marginal or the circulating pool. The marginal pool is a pool of granulocytes distributed throughout the vascular tree and adherent to the blood vessels. The largest part of this marginal pool is in the pulmonary vasculature. This pool is not static and cells move from the marginal pool into the circulating pool continuously, for it appears that the circulating pool is being constantly maintained from the marginal pool. This shift from the marginal pool can be greatly increased by exercise and by adrenaline.

It is the concentration of granulocytes in the circulating pool which is measured in a white cell count and there is no good means of estimating the marginal pool. These granulocytes in the circulation have a half-life of about 7 hours which, by comparison, is much shorter than the red cell. Indeed it could be said that granulocytes are not primarily blood cells, for they are merely in the blood for a short period, passing through en route to the tissues. Once in the tissues they rarely re-enter the circulation.

An increase in the number of granulocytes in circulation may be physiological, as is found in children and in pregnancy, or it may be the response to a pathological process.

Alterations in circulating polymorphs

Causes of polymorph leucocytosis

1. *Infection.* Infections with pyogenic cocci are the commonest causes of a high granulocyte count. Leucocytosis occurs, however, with many other and many non-pyogenic organisms.

2. *Haemorrhage and trauma.* When haemorrhage occurs, particularly into serous cavities, a neutrophil leucocytosis is common. Trauma, particularly if associated with tissue damage, fractures or surgical operations, also gives a leucocytosis in a matter of hours after the incident.

3. *Malignant disease.* Leucocytosis is not uncommon in malignant disease particularly with rapidly growing necrotic tumours. If these are infected this will be another cause for leucocytosis. Similarly, in active Hodgkin's disease, a modest polymorph leucocytosis is often found

4. *Myeloproliferative states.* In chronic myeloid leukaemia the leucocyte count is often very high, often amounting to 200 or 300×10^9 per litre, and many of the cells are only at the myelocyte stage of development. Basophils are also characteristically present in increased numbers. Polycythaemia rubra vera and myelofibrosis are also often accompanied by a polymorph leucocytosis with a left shift.

Causes of neutropenia

1. *Infection.* Viral infections, typhoid fever, brucellosis and rickettsial infections are frequently associated with reduced polymorph numbers.

2. *Marrow infiltration.* Involvement of the bone marrow by leukaemia, lymphoid neoplasms, or secondary carcinomas is a common cause of neutropenia, often severe, and results in an increased liability to infection.

3. *Hypoplastic anaemia.* Severe neutropenia may occur in both primary hypoplastic anaemias or if secondary to drugs or chemicals.

An elevation of the eosinophil leucocyte count may be found in allergic disorders, parasitic infestations, certain skin diseases, certain types of malignant disease, and after certain drugs.

LYMPHOCYTES

Lymphocyte production is more complex than the formation of other cellular blood elements and has proved more difficult to study. Although a certain amount of information is available from human studies, much of our understanding of this cell system's physiology in the human is derived from experimental studies in other animals.

Lymphocyte morphology

Morphologically, lymphocytes are usually divided into two classes, small and large lymphocytes. Small lymphocytes generally comprise about 90% of the total and have a diameter of 6–10 μm. The nuclear chromatin is dense and clumped and there is only a thin rim of clear cytoplasm, which may contain a few azurophilic granules. The large lymphocyte measures 12–16 μm in diameter and has a more generous rim of cytoplasm and a more open nuclear structure. Primitive lymphoid forms, lymphoblasts are not seen in health in the peripheral blood, but may appear in acute leukaemia. Normal lymphoblasts however are more likely to have the appearance of a transformed lymphocyte. Under certain circumstances such as viral infections, immune reactions and particularly with infectious mononucleosis, larger lymphocytes, 20 μm in diameter, with more abundant basophilic vacuolated cytoplasm and immature nuclei appear in the circulation. These 'blast' cells have been given a number of terms including virocytes and irritated or activated lymphocytes, but none is particularly ideal. Similar cells may be seen in lymphocyte cultures in vitro when exposed to mitogens like phytohaemagglutinin.

Lymphopoiesis

Lymphocytes are formed both centrally in the bone marrow and thymus and peripherally in the spleen, lymph nodes and Peyer's patches of the gut. There is now much evidence to show that the principal primary site of lymphocyte production is the thymus. In the lymph nodes, spleen and Peyer's patches of the gut, lymphocytes are formed usually in response to antigenic stimuli, but minor degrees of primary lymphocyte production could still occur in germinal centres.

In the thymus, small lymphocytes are actively formed, particularly in early life, but many of these disintegrate within the organ and never reach the general circulation. As a result of this selection the small thymic lymphocyte which emerges is immunologically competent and can recognize 'self'.

In the bone marrow the cellular sequence is not understood but it appears that marrow lymphocytes originate from the same fundamental stem cell as the other formed elements of the blood. Indeed, it has been postulated by some authors that a small marrow lymphocyte is indeed the primordial haemopoietic stem cell. No intermediate cells have been identified in marrow lymphopoiesis and the cell which leaves the marrow and enters the circulation is a small lymphocyte. The factors controlling marrow lymphopoiesis are obscure, but it is known that marrow lymphocyte production is not activated by antigenic stimulation, unlike lymphopoiesis in other areas.

Thymic (T) and bursal (B) lymphocytes

Lymphocytes are not only heterogeneous in their morphology, but also in functional activity which they can perform following appropriate antigenic stimulation. There would appear to be at least two distinct broad lineages of lymphocytes. One of these is derived from the thymus, comprises the T-lymphocyte and is concerned with cellular immunity. The other lymphocyte population is concerned with humoral immunity and are designated bursal or B-lymphocytes because of analogues with lymphocytes from the bursa of Fabricius in birds. No mammalian analogue

of the bursa of Fabricius has been demonstrated, but fetal liver or bone marrow are suggested sites. T- and B-lymphocytes are not distinguishable by light microscopy, but can be identified on the basis of differing surface markers. T-cells are identified by their ability to bind sheep erythrocytes and form rosettes (E rosettes), a property lacked by B-cells. Identification of B-cells depends on demonstrating a high density of surface immunoglobulin or a receptor for a fragment (Fc piece) of antibody molecules. A subpopulation of B lymphocytes also carries receptors for the third component of complement (C_3). Some recently described mononuclear cells have been shown to lack both T- and B-cell markers, and are known as killer or K-cells as they may be involved with various cytotoxic reactions in tumours and foreign grafts.

A recent major advance in the elucidation of lymphoid cells has been the development of monoclonal antibodies. These reagents are produced from clones of mouse lymphoid cells formed by the fusion of an antigen stimulated B lymphocyte and a continuously growing myeloma cell line. These reagents have already allowed identification and quantification of T-lymphocyte subsets and will doubtless provide much further information about other cell lines.

Lymphocyte circulation and life span

The majority of small lymphocytes probably survive for many years and are capable of extensive recirculation. It is difficult to give finite life span to lymphocytes as antigenic stimulation can occur at any time producing transformation, and thus ending life of that cell.

In lymph nodes recirculating small lymphocytes pass through post capillary venules into the paracortical area of the cortex, and leave the node via medullary sinuses which join the main lymphatic ducts. In the spleen the situation is less clear. Small lymphocytes migrate through gaps in the marginal sinus and enter periarterial lymphocyte sheaths, and probably exit via the marginal zone. Thymus and bone marrow are probably not sites of recirculation. The value of this large population of recirculating lymphocytes appears to be recruitment of immunologically competent cells into sites regionally stimulated by antigen.

Alterations in circulating lymphocytes

Lymphocytosis. An increase in the peripheral lymphocyte count is common with acute infections such as infectious mononucleosis, rubella, measles, mumps and other viral illness. A lymphocytosis may also occur with chronic infections such as tuberculosis, syphilis, or brucellosis and in malignant conditions such as chronic lymphatic leukaemia and non-Hodgkin's lymphomas.

Lymphopenia. A reduction in the peripheral blood lymphocyte count to below 1.0×10^9 may occur with leukaemia, aplastic anaemia, systemic lupus erythematosis and following chemotherapy or radiotherapy.

Plasma cells. Plasma cells are readily identifiable by their oval shape, characteristic basophilic cytoplasm and eccentric nucleus. Although not normally found in peripheral blood they are present in bone marrow and lymph nodes. Plasma cells are derived from B-lymphocytes and represent the final stage of development of this cell line. The function of plasma cells is to produce immunoglobulin.

Pathological proliferation of plasma cells results in multiple myelomatosis or a related disorder. These diseases are characterized by the production of an abnormal protein (paraprotein) of monoclonal origin. Infiltration of the bone marrow by the malignant plasma cells leads to anaemia, leucopenia and thrombocytopenia with a great propensity to pathological fractures of bone. The paraprotein itself may lead to hyperviscosity, renal failure or amyloidosis. Treatment with chemotherapy is now moderately successful in relieving symptoms and prolonging survival, while radiotherapy is a useful adjunct for local tumour masses.

Monocytes. Monocytes are closely related to the granulocyte series, sharing a common stem cell, which differentiates to promonocyte and on to mature monocyte. Monocytes are probably only produced within the bone marrow. They circulate for approximately the same time as polymorphs before passing into the tissues. In the tissue monocytes, or macrophages are phagocytic, but they also have a role in control of the immune system. A peripheral blood monocytosis may be observed in some chronic infections (tuberculosis, subacute bacterial endocarditis, brucellosis etc.), in Hodgkin's disease and in monocytic leukaemia.

LEUKAEMIA

The leukaemias are a group of disorders characterized by progressive uncontrolled proliferation of leucocytes with accumulation of immature cells in the bone marrow and blood. Although any leucocyte may be involved, most commonly it is either the lymphocyte or granulocyte, and both may present in acute or chronic forms.

Acute leukaemia

Acute lymphoblastic (ALL) and acute myeloblastic leukaemia (AML) are broadly similar conditions. ALL is more common in infancy while AML occurs more frequently in adults. Aetiology is unknown but radiation and certain chemical carcinogens have been implicated. Clinical features are usually a result of bone marrow failure or local tumour masses. Anaemia is almost invariable. Leucopenia leads to a marked propensity to infections which are often acute and fulminating, while purpura and bleeding due to thrombocytopenia is also frequently present. Enlarged lymph nodes, spleen and liver are frequently present on examination, while leukaemic infiltration can affect most organs of the body, particularly bone, skin or nervous system. Diagnosis is usually easily established by blood and bone marrow examination, often using special cytochemical stains to differentiate the different types of leukaemia. The recent application of monoclonal antibodies has resulted in greatly improved diagnostic accuracy and revealed marked heterogeneity within each major group.

The main principles of treatment are the use of combination chemotherapy to eradicate the leukaemic clone of cells combined with supportive measures to combat anaemia, infection, bleeding and metabolic disturbances such as hyperuricaemia. Combining two or more cytotoxic drugs has proven to be eminently successful, particularly in ALL in children. Over 80% of such cases now achieve remission using a combination of vincristine and prednisolone, while the addition of a third drug such as daunorubicin can increase remission rates to well over 90%. Unfortunately AML is not as sensitive to cytotoxic drugs, but remission should now be achieved in nearly two-thirds of cases. Following remission some maintenance chemotherapy is required for up to 2 years, while prophylactic craniospinal irradiation is essential in ALL to prevent CNS involvement. While a very large proportion of children with ALL remain in remission up to the end of treatment and for many years afterwards, the prognosis in AML is much poorer. Other approaches to therapy once relapse has occurred, such as bone marrow transplantation, may then be worthwhile.

Chronic leukaemia

Unlike the acute forms, the white cells in the chronic leukaemias have a significant capacity for differentiation. As before chronic myeloid leukaemia (CML) and chronic lymphatic leukaemia (CLL) are the most common forms, but are widely different in their clinical presentation and course.

Chronic myeloid leukaemia

Chronic myeloid leukaemia occurs mainly in middle age and tends to run a subacute course with a rapid terminal phase. Although the aetiology is unknown, cytogenetic studies have demonstrated a consistent chromosomal abnormality in the erythroid, myeloid and megakaryocytic cell lines in the bone marrow, the Philadelphia (Ph') chromosome. Initially, CML tends to follow a relatively benign course, the main problems being related to anaemia, hypermetabolism or the mechanical effects of an enlarged spleen. The blood picture shows an increase, often gross, in neutrophils and granulocyte precursors. Therapy with a single agent such as busulphan is usually highly effective but eventually the leukaemia becomes refractory or metamorphoses to a terminal acute phase. Overall survival times are very variable and may be 10 years or more, but a mean of around 3 years is much more common.

Chronic lymphatic leukaemia

Chronic lymphatic leukaemia (CLL) is a disease of the middle-aged and elderly characterized by widespread lymph node enlargement, hepatosplenomegaly, and the accumulation of mature small lymphocytes in the peripheral blood and bone marrow. Blood film examination also characteristically shows numerous smudge or smear cells. Patients with CLL have a great susceptibility to infection. However, the majority of patients survive many years as CLL generally runs a benign course. Treatment with cytotoxic drugs is only recommended for specific complications such as massive lymph node or splenic enlargement, impaired bone marrow function or auto-immune haemolytic anaemia. A few patients tend to run a more aggressive course, but unlike CML, there is rarely an acute terminal phase.

LYMPHOMAS

Primary malignant neoplasms of lymph nodes are lymphomas. These tumours embrace a wide pathological and clinical spectrum and have proved to be particularly difficult to classify. In general, two main groups are recognized: Hodgkin's disease, and all others known as the non-Hodgkin's lymphomas.

Hodgkin's disease

Hodgkin's disease is diagnosed on a pathological basis. The essential feature is the presence of Reed-Sternberg cells. Four different pathological forms of Hodgkin's disease are recognized and pathological type is an important feature in determining prognosis. Hodgkin's disease occurs more commonly in males and has a characteristic bi-modal age peak for presentation, at 25 years and 70 years. Commonest presenting feature is painless lymphadenopathy, and while this is most often in the neck, it can present with any group of nodes. Many other organs in the body may also be infiltrated with Hodgkin's tissue and systemic symptoms are also common (weight loss, fever, pruritus). It is essential to establish the precise clinical extent of the disease. While this may be possible by relatively non-invasive techniques, laparotomy and splenectomy are usually essential to establish abdominal node and organ involvement. Treatment of local disease with radiotherapy is very effective and many patients who present early with little tumour mass are almost certainly cured. More advanced disease is best treated by chemotherapy and excellent results are obtained using one of several schedules of four drugs in combination.

The non-Hodgkin's lymphomas

This term encompasses a wide variety of lymphomas which have proven difficult to classify on a pathological basis. They vary from relatively benign tumours such as some well-differentiated, lymphocytic lymphomas to aggressive, poorly-differentiated tumours. Lymph node enlargement is the commonest presenting finding and exact pathological diagnosis of an excised node is essential. The role of 'staging' these tumours like Hodgkin's disease is controversial. Treatment depends to a large extent on nature of the lymphoma. Many well differentiated tumours can be adequately managed with radiotherapy or single agent chemotherapy while the more aggressive tumours require combination chemotherapy regimes.

HAEMOSTASIS

Haemostasis embraces several physiological mechanisms required to arrest bleeding from injured vessels. When a vessel is severed, eventual haemostasis is secured by vascular factors, platelets, blood coagulation, and fibrinolysis, and depends in part on the size of the vessel involved.

In capillaries the bleeding may stop by adhesion of the collapsed walls. In arteries the arrest of bleeding may be aided by active and passive contraction of the vessel wall due to its content of elastic fibres and smooth muscle cells. As regards the components within the vascular compartment, the initiating influence is the reaction of platelets to the severed vessels. Platelets are attracted to the exposed collagen and by adenosine diphosphate (ADP) at the site of rupture of the vascular intima. When some platelets have become adherent, further platelets are encouraged to aggregate and adhere to the initial platelet aggregate by the release of intrinsic ADP from those platelets initially deposited. In this way, a platelet plug is built up which eventually completely blocks the severed vessel.

Neither the vascular factors, nor the platelet plug, however, is able to produce permanent haemostasis. Only when the coagulation mechanism provides fibrin for reinforcement of the platelet haemostatic plug does haemostasis become secure. Eventually haemostasis is finally secured by the processes of healing when fibrous tissue grows in to replace the haemostatic plug, and fibrin is removed by the fibrinolytic enzyme system. Any process which interferes with fibrin formation also interferes with wound healing. This is often seen in haemophilic wounds where the scar is disproportionate to the wound. Proper deposition of fibrin is important, not only in superficial wounds but in fractures and deeply incised wounds where it provides a suitable matrix for the ingrowth of fibrous tissue. In superficial wounds fibrin provides a protective scab.

It is also important to realize that thrombosis is misappropriately applied haemostasis and the mechanisms involved in the prevention of thrombosis work in balance with the haemostatic system. The structure of a thrombus has striking similarity to that of a haemostatic plug. The haemostatic plug consists of the platelet aggregation blocking the mouth of the severed vessel, reinforced behind with fibrin, the strands of which spread deep into the haemostatic plug of platelets. After a time interval fibrin can be seen in between individual platelets. A thrombus also consists of a head of platelets and a fibrin tail. The appreciation that these two mechanisms of haemostasis and thrombosis are so similar may well lead to advances in the prevention and management of thrombosis.

The vascular component

Active constriction is an important factor in securing haemostasis with blood loss from large muscular arteries. Capillaries have also been shown to contract when severed due to contractile filaments within the endothelial cells. The exposure of underlying collagen is important to initiate adhesion and aggregation of platelets, which also appear to have a role in maintaining integrity of vascular endothelium. Platelets contribute to the vascular component by releasing serotonin, a vasoconstricting substance which thus augments vascular contraction.

The blood coagulation component

The modern concept of blood coagulation is an expansion of the old theory that fibrinogen is converted to fibrin under the influence of thrombin derived from an inactive precursor prothrombin. The coagulation cascade (Fig. 11.8) now envisages a series of step-wise reactions. In each reaction an inactive precursor protein is converted to an active enzyme which in turn converts a further precursor to an active enzyme until fibrinogen is converted to fibrin. There are basically two pathways to activate the coagulation cascade, both of which are available to bring about the conversion of fibrinogen to fibrin. In the 'extrinsic' system the activating mechanism is tissue juice or thromboplastin which rapidly, in about 10 seconds, leads to blood clotting. The 'intrinsic' system requires contact with a foreign substance to trigger the coagulation sequence, such as collagen. Clotting by the intrinsic pathway occurs much more slowly, taking about 10 minutes. Both these systems require to be functioning normally for physiological haemostasis.

The whole object of the overall coagulation system is to generate biochemical activity in a controlled and localized fashion to bring about the conversion of the soluble plasma protein fibrinogen to the insoluble plasma protein fibrin, i.e. to form a blood clot. The extrinsic and intrinsic systems are both designed to generate prothrombin converting principle (also known as a thromboplastin) which acts on the plasma protein prothrombin to convert it to the proteolytic enzyme thrombin; this in turn acts on fibrinogen to form fibrin.

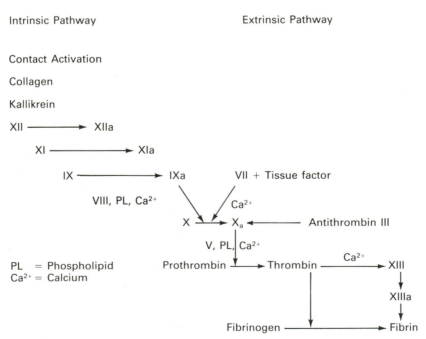

Fig. 11.8 The coagulation 'cascade'.

Fibrinogen-fibrin reaction

Thrombin is a proteolytic enzyme which is formed from prothrombin. It splits peptide units, the fibrinopeptides A and B, from fibrinogen leaving fibrin monomer. These fibrin monomers gel to form soluble fibrin and the fibrin gel polymerizes under the influence of factor XIII and forms fibrin strands large enough to be seen with a light microscope. These polymers can be seen as bands on fibrin strands under the electron microscope.

Although platelets form a major and important part of the haemostatic plug as described above, some will be caught in the interstices of the fibrin network, and fibrin strands radiating from clumped platelets may be seen. Within platelets there is a contractile protein thrombasthenin. When platelets are activated this protein is activated and retracts, drawing on the fibrin strands. This is the mechanism which brings about retraction of the clot.

The fibrinolytic component

As outlined in the introductory part of this section, once fibrin has formed it is eventually removed by the fibrinolytic enzyme system. The enzyme which dissolves fibrin is plasmin, and this arises from an inactive precursor in the plasma, called plasminogen. Whenever fibrinogen is laid down it carries associated with it sufficient plasminogen to ensure its subsequent lysis. The conversion of plasminogen to plasmin is brought about by plasminogen activators. There are two main types of plasminogen activator. One is plasma plasminogen activator which is formed in the endothelium of the small veins and released into the circulation; the other is tissue plasminogen activator which is present in tissues and is fixed in the tissues.

The activation of fibrinolysis is limited in the free circulation by a range of inhibitors. These have difficulty in gaining access to a clot and so the activators can act on the plasminogen within a clot without any major inhibition from inhibitors. The system can be outlined in the following diagram:

```
              PLASMINOGEN
                   |
ACTIVATORS  ———————+——— INHIBITORS
                   |
               PLASMIN
                   |
     FIBRIN  ——————————  FIBRINOGEN
                          DEGENERATION
                          PRODUCTS
```

Activation and inhibition of fibrinolysis can be induced therapeutically. Streptokinase and urokinase can be used as activators and epsilon amino-caproic acid, tranexamic acid and Trasylol as inhibitors.

Table 11.2 International nomenclature of coagulation factors

Factor	Synonyms
I	Fibrinogen
II	Prothrombin
III	Tissue factor, thromboplastin
IV	Ionized calcium
V	Proaccelerin
VII	Proconvertin
VIII	Antihaemophilic factor (AHF)
IX	Christmas factor
X	Stuart-Prower factor
XI	Plasma thromboplastin antecedent (PTA)
XII	Hageman factor
XIII	Fibrin stabilising factor

A number of these clotting factors require brief consideration (Table 11.2).

Factor I (fibrinogen)

Fibrinogen is a glycoprotein and is present in the blood at the highest concentration of any of the clotting factors, normally 1.5–4.0 g/l. Congenital absence of fibrinogen (afibrinogenaemia) or congenital fibrinogen variants (dysfibrinogenaemia) are very rare, but several different types have been described. Acute fibrinogen depletion may arise as an obstetrical emergency, e.g. in abruptio placentae, or following certain surgical procedures such as heart-lung bypass, or in operations involving stripping of tissue, e.g. dissection for removal of the rectum or dissection of malignant glands of neck. It is likely that most acute and many chronic defibrinations are due to disseminated intravascular coagulation (DIC) as a result of activation of the haemostatic system within the circulation. In same situations, however, excessive activation of the fibrinolytic enzyme system is the mechanism responsible for the defibrination, e.g. during the administration of streptokinase.

Many of the clinical problems of acute defibrination are short-lived 'storms', where the appropriate therapy is to ride out the storm with the transfusion of fresh blood and fibrinogen. In chronic defibrination, the commonest example of which is found in metastatic carcinoma, the fibrinogen depletion can be corrected by giving heparin which reduces the DIC and the fibrinogen consumption. Where there is a clearcut case of haemostatic failure from activation of the fibrinolytic enzyme system, e.g. during streptokinase therapy, then the fibrinolytic inhibitors mentioned above can be given, in particular epsilon aminocaproic acid. In so doing the clinician must appreciate that any fibrin subsequently laid down will be unlysable because it will have the fibrinolytic inhibitor incorporated in it.

Factor II (Prothrombin), Factors VII, IX, and X

These four factors are termed the vitamin K-dependent

coagulation factors. Synthesized in the liver as inactive precursor proteins, they require vitamin K to carboxylate the amino acid, glutamic acid. This is required for proper lipid and calcium binding which is essential for normal proteolytic action. These four factors become deficient following the administration of coumarin or indanedione oral anticoagulant drugs or when a patient has become vitamin K-deficient from malabsorption, obstructive jaundice or haemorrhagic disease of the newborn. These abnormalities can be corrected in a matter of 6–8 hours by the administration of vitamin K_1.

This particular preparation of vitamin K will reverse the deficiency of these coagulation factors, whether it is a true vitamin deficiency or one which has arisen as a consequence of administration of oral anticoagulant drugs. It is therefore the drug of choice in the management of these conditions. If the clinical situation does not permit a delay of 6–8 hours then the defect can be immediately corrected by giving a calculated dose of fresh frozen plasma or a factor IX concentrate (see blood products section).

Factor III (tissue extract)

This is present in all tissues and is usually prepared for laboratory study from brain or lung. It is important to appreciate that the tissues of a haemophiliac who dies of his disease are equally powerful in the coagulation of normal or haemophilic blood, as is tissue prepared from a normal subject. This stresses the importance in physiological haemostasis of the intrinsic blood thromboplastin system.

Factor IV (ionized calcium)

This is required at several stages in the coagulation mechanism. The commonest method to anticoagulate blood for laboratory investigation is to remove the ionised calcium by agents such as citrate.

Factor V

Factor V is a labile factor which does not survive well in stored blood and is consumed during the coagulation reaction. It has little clinical relevance.

Factor VIII (antihaemophilic factor)

This factor is deficient in haemophilia. It disappears rapidly on storage of blood and its concentration in normal blood can be quite markedly increased by exercise or by the injection of adrenaline. Factor VIII concentration is markedly reduced in haemophilia; it is zero in severe classical haemophilia with haemarthrosis, but is present in small concentration in the milder grades of haemophilia.

Factor IX (Christmas factor)

Like Factor VIII it is required for the formation of intrinsic thromboplastin but is more stable, and when it occurs as an isolated deficiency causes Christmas disease. Factor IX deficiency is more commonly met as part of the defect in coumarin drug therapy or vitamin K deficiency, as already indicated.

Factor X (Stuart-Prower factor)

The importance of this factor again is not because of genetic deficiency, but because it forms part of the II, VII, IX and X deficiency as already described.

Factors XI and XII

These factors are both concerned with the earliest stages of blood coagulation and it is remarkable that when blood is transferred from contact with vascular endothelium to contact with a glass surface it changes from a solution to a gel. The triggering of the reactions which result in this starts as activation of Factor XII or Hageman factor. Surprisingly, deficiency of Hageman factor is not associated with a haemorrhagic state.

Factor XIII

Factor XIII, which is a transglutaminase activated by thrombin, is essential to stabilize fibrin by forming covalent bonds between adjacent monomers. Without factor XIII, fibrin formed has different solubility characteristics and lacks tensile strength. Factor XIII deficiency is very rare and so of little clinical relevance.

Extrinsic and intrinsic coagulation systems

As indicated above, both of these systems are necessary for physiological haemostasis. An intact extrinsic system is not sufficient to provide haemostasis. Equally, a patient with, say, isolated factor VII deficiency as a genetic defect has a haemorrhagic state, demonstrating that a normal intrinsic mechanism is not adequate and that a normal extrinsic system also has to be present for physiological haemostasis.

In the laboratory the extrinsic system can be tested by the one-stage prothrombin time (OSPT), as described by Quick in 1935. In this test, plasma from the patient is clotted under the influence of a tissue extract and calcium, and the time taken compared with results from a normal. Such plasma will clot in 10–15 seconds. Prolongation indicates a deficiency of factor V, factor VII or factor X, or a combination of two or more of these; severe Factor II deficiency will also cause a prolongation of this result (Table 11.3).

Table 11.3 Scheme of simple investigations to screen for a coagulation disorder

Intrinsic coagulation system
  Kaolin cephalin clotting time (KCCT)
  Activated partial thromboplastin time (APTT)
Extrinsic coagulation system
  One stage prothrombin time (OSPT)
Fibrinogen-fibrin conversion
  Thrombin clotting time (TCT)

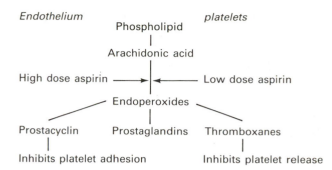

Fig. 11.9 Effects of high and low dose aspirin on platelet function.

The intrinsic system as a whole can be tested by taking plasma and clotting it under standard conditions of contact activation provided by kaolin and the addition of a standard amount of phospholipid which would normally be supplied to the blood from platelets. For this purpose an extract of brain cephalin is used. This test is called the kaolin-cephalin clotting time (KCCT) or activated partial thromboplastin time and provides a screening procedure for the intrinsic coagulation system. The range of results varies from laboratory to laboratory according to the different conditions used.

If the screening tests are abnormal then the defect has to be precisely localized in the coagulation system by carrying out specific coagulation factor assays. Thus in haemophilia, the KCCT would be abnormal and the OSPT normal. This points to a defect of the intrinsic coagulation system and should be followed up by specific assays of factor VIII and factor IX.

The platelet component

In one sense, platelets form the keystone of the haemostatic system and in a samilar way are thought now to have a vital role in the process of thrombosis. Platelets are derived from the megakaryocytes of the bone marrow and have an average survival time of 8–10 days in the peripheral circulation. When platelet numbers are seriously depleted spontaneous capillary bleeding will occur. A significant haemostatic abnormality may also occur if platelets are not functioning normally.

Normal platelet haemostatic function depends on several mechanisms. Immediately following trauma to a vessel, wall platelets become sticky and adhesion occurs to subendothelial fibres. Adhesion is then followed by platelet aggregation, induced by ADP and thrombin. This results in transformation of the normally-shaped discoid platelet into a small, reactive sphere allowing interaction with other platelets to form a tightly packed mass. Aggregation is then followed by the platelet release reaction where secretory granules release ADP, serotonin and other substances which can perpetuate the reaction and enlarge the haemostatic platelet plug. Recently prostaglandins have been shown to play a major role in platelet function. When platelets undergo the release reaction, arachidonic acid from the membrane phospholipid is converted to labile cyclic endoperoxides such as Thromboxane A_2 which is a powerful aggregating agent. This sequence is irreversibly inhibited by aspirin which has been employed as an antithrombotic agent. However, the endothelium of the vessel wall produces prostacyclin which inhibits platelet adhesion, and so aspirin at certain dosages may paradoxically inhibit an important physiological antithrombotic process.

Congenital defects of platelet function are rare, but defects of adhesion, aggregation and release have all been described. Acquired defects in platelet function have been found in several disorders such as uraemia, acute leukaemia, myeloproliferative disorders, and following extracorporeal circulation for cardiac surgery. The precise importance of such defects to the overall bleeding problems encountered is difficult to establish. Many drugs including aspirin (Fig. 11.9), indomethacin, alcohol, dextran and some antibiotics are also known to interfere with normal platelet function.

Role of local pressure

Appropriate measures of local pressure may provide the only available therapy for haemorrhage. For example, epistaxis in hereditary telangiectasia can usually be controlled by nasal packing. With any local measures in conditions of haemostatic failure the physician must always be aware of the relative advantages and disadvantages of the procedures adopted. In nasal packing in a generalized defect it is important not to produce new areas of trauma due to the packing. It is important that the packing should not be so tight as to produce areas of necrosis which later give larger bleeding surfaces; absorbable packing or gauze covered with petroleum jelly (e.g. Vaseline) may produce the least possible damage in that context. Local pressure may be even more dangerous in other haemorrhagic states, such as haemophilia, when external blood loss may be controlled but the bleeding continues and the blood travels backwards into the tissues with consequent pressure on vital structures.

Haemophilia (factor VIII deficiency)

Haemophilia A due to deficiency of factor VIII is the commonest congenital coagulation disorder. Recently it has been generally accepted that haemophiliacs have a qualitative rather than a strict quantitative defect. Assays show absence or severe reduction in the level of factor VIII coagulant activity, the level of which correlates well with the severity of the bleeding problem. However, immuno-logical tests show the presence of normal amounts of material antigenically similar to factor VIII but without normal coagulation function. Thus haemophiliacs produce an abnormal or incomplete factor VIII molecule.

Haemophilia is inherited as a sex-linked recessive disorder with an incidence of about 1 in 4000 male births. In about one-third of cases there is no family history with the disease probably arising by gene mutation. Female carriers with low factor VIII coagulant activity may occasionally be clinically affected.

The level of factor VIII is the most important factor in determining disease severity, and classical haemophilia occurs principally with a plasma factor VIII of less than 5% of normal. Spontaneous bleeding may occur when no factor VIII activity is present and haemorthrosis and muscle haemorrhage are the commonest clinical problems. Other common problems include haematuria, epistaxis, gastrointestinal tract bleeding, and intracranial haemorrhage which has a high mortality.

The basis of treatment is to raise and then maintain the plasma factor VIII to a level suitable for secure haemostasis. As the half-life of infused human factor VIII is of the order of 8–9 hours, daily or even twice-daily replacement therapy is required. Treatment will be required for several days or even weeks to ensure sound healing. Whole blood is of no value as a source of factor VIII, but transfusion is essential to maintain an adequate red cell mass. Unlike normal patients, a haemophiliac may develop massive 'latent' haemorrhage into tissue without any great external blood loss. Thus the blood transfusion requirement can be easily underestimated. It is not uncommon to see a haemophilic patient who has bled some four-fifths of his total blood volume into a large ileopsoas retroperitoneal haematoma without any blood being lost externally.

While fresh frozen plasma (FFP) can be used as a source of factor VIII, there are now several therapeutic concentrates available which have revolutionized management. Initially cryoprecipitate was the mainstay of therapy. Prepared from 'snap frozen' fresh plasma that is thawed slowly at 4°C, this insoluble protein precipitate dissolves on warming and is a rich source of factor VIII. Although simple and cheap to prepare it has to a large extent been superseded by lyophilized high purity concentrates which allow a large dose to be administered in a small volume. These products are exceedingly useful in surgical cases, young children, patients at risk from circulatory overload and in home treatment. Although very expensive to prepare, and also expensive in terms of the plasma required because of the low yield of factor VIII, their use is becoming very widespread.

The main risks of replacement treatment are circulatory overload, allergic reactions and hepatitis. While Hepatitis B remains the important clinical problem, other forms of hepatitis are becoming increasingly common following infusion of blood products.

Also over the last few years it has become apparent that blood and blood products can transmit the human T-lymphocyte retrovirus (HTLV III) which is thought to be the causative agent of the acquired immune deficiency syndrome (AIDS). While many haemophiliacs have already been exposed to the virus screening of blood donors and heat treatment of coagulation concentrates will hopefully prove effective in limiting the prevalence of this devastating disease.

An increasing problem in the management of haemophilia is the development of circulating inhibitors to factor VIII and this may, on occasion, render the patient virtually untreatable by replacement therapy. In such patients, it is likely that the factor VIII is viewed as a foreign protein and an antibody is developed. It may on occasion be possible to overwhelm the inhibitor, but in our experience this unhappily has frequently not been the result. Other approaches such as immunosuppressive therapy perhaps combined with plasma exchange or the use of 'activated' prothrombin complexes which bypass factor VIII in the coagulation cascade are often required for control of bleeding in patients with inhibitors.

Christmas disease (factor IX deficiency)

The management principles in this disorder are the same as in haemophilia. An adequate level of the missing factor must be obtained and sustained by daily intravenous infusion. The in vivo and in vitro survival of factor IX is greater than that of factor VIII and this makes therapy easier. Today factor IX concentrates are available in reasonable amounts and provide efficient replacement therapy. The DE FIX preparation is the most commonly used. This contains Factors II, IX and X. An alternative is the PPSB type of preparation. This contains Factor II, VII, IX and X but it is prepared from EDTA plasma and is available only in short supply. Fresh plasma can also be used for factor IX replacement therapy but this is limited by the large volumes required.

Von Willebrand's disease

This disorder is inherited as an autosomal dominant and so affects both males and females. It is characterized by a deficiency of factor VIII, a prolonged bleeding time, and a defect of platelet adhesion. Clinically the bleeding tendency is less severe than in haemophilia and characteristically haemorrhage occurs from mucous membranes, especially the nose.

The administration of cryoprecipitate, rich in factor VIII, results in an immediate rise of factor VIII and this is sustained and increased for 24–48 hours after infusion, suggesting that cryoprecipitate provides such patients with material which enables them to generate more procoagulant. Recent work has shown that factor VIII is made up of a high molecular weight component and a low molecular weight component. In Von Willebrand's disease the patient is unable to synthesize normal amounts of the high molecular weight component, while in haemophilia A, the low molecular weight component is deficient.

Acquired haemorrhagic disorders

Defibrination syndrome

A haemorrhagic state may arise because of a sudden or slow fall in fibrinogen concentration. This probably occurs most frequently as a consequence of intravascular coagulation but occasionally may occur because of excessive activation of the fibrinolytic enzyme system as happens, for example, during the infusion of streptokinase. The distinction between these two conditions is usually difficult and the laboratory investigations to discover the primary phenomenon take so long that it is likely to be of little therapeutic relevance.

It is probably wise to accept that the vast majority of the defibrination syndromes are due to intravascular coagulation, rather than excessive fibrinolysis.

Massive blood transfusion and cardiopulmonary bypass

In surgical practice, two clinical situations are recognized to be associated occasionally with abnormal bleeding. Haemostatic failure may arise following massive blood transfusion and after cardiopulmonary bypass. The pathogenesis of these defects is complex. Provided, however, that any surgical cause for bleeding has been corrected then the systemic abnormality, whatever its nature, is likely to be self-limiting. Fresh whole blood to keep up with the loss is the best available therapy. In both of these situations platelet deficiency is one of the features, and this can be modified by giving platelet concentrates. Calcium gluconate proportional to the transfused blood should be administered in both of these situations.

Naturally occurring anticoagulants

Haemophilia-like diseases can arise as acquired disorders due to the presence of a circulating anticoagulant. The commonest of these is a specific inhibitor of factor VIII

and effectively, therefore, these patients have haemophilia. A small addition of blood from one of these patients to normal blood prolongs the clotting time of the normal blood. These anticoagulants may arise unassociated with any underlying disease and no specific therapy is effective. However, as the inhibitor may spontaneously disappear there is a strong case for treating these patients as required by blood replacement. Such anticoagulants, for example, may arise in the puerperium and in systemic lupus erythematosis. The problem of specific inhibitors of factor VIII or factor IX arising in haemophilia and Christmas disease has already been discussed.

Deficiency of Vitamin K-dependent factors

In the therapy of these coagulation defects, the clinician should become competent in the use of vitamin K_1. The intravenous administration of 10 mg of vitamin K_1 will correct the coagulation defect in an adult with this deficiency in 5–6 hours — the time it takes for the liver to synthesize sufficient of the missing coagulation factors. In haemorrhagic disease of the newborn, 1–2 mg vitamin K_1 intramuscularly is the appropriate management. When the bleeding has arisen because of coumarin or indanedione therapy then the clinician has to take a decision whether he intends to continue therapy. If he gives a dose of 20 mg vitamin K_1 this will render the patient resistant to further therapy for 2 weeks. If a correction in the defect is required urgently as in a patient who is actively bleeding, then a dose of PPSB will correct the defect immediately.

If the patient is not bleeding but has an excessive anticoagulant effect, as judged by laboratory test, then the dose of vitamin K_1 should be 5 mg

Heparin

In bleeding from heparin, the appropriate dose of protamine sulphate is required. This may be determined by titration procedures but in routine clinical practice 1–2 mg protamine sulphate should be given for each 1 ml (100 units) of heparin administered. There are a number of variables which may require to be considered in the dose decision, including the time intervals since the intravenous administration of the heparin, and whether or not the heparin has been given intramuscularly.

Liver disease

The treatment of haemostatic failure in cirrhosis of the liver is very unsatisfactory. Fresh whole blood and fibrinogen supplements should be used. Despite the markedly increased fibrinolytic activity in cirrhosis of the liver, there is no convincing evidence that fibrinolytic inhibitors have a therapeutic role. PPSB containing factors II, VII, IX and

X can be used but should be used with great caution because of the risk of inducing DIC. Some PPSB preparations appear to contain certain amounts of activated coagulation factors which may trigger DIC.

Purpuras

The term purpura refers to a haemorrhagic skin rash which may develop in a range of conditions affecting either the platelets or the vascular endothelium. As a result purpura is described as (i) non-thrombocytopenic or vascular purpura and (ii) thrombocytopenic purpura

Vascular purpura

In vascular purpura the platelet count and platelet function are normal and the primary cause is pathology of the small skin vessels. Thus it may be associated with a vasculitis, as in Henoch-Schonlein purpura and systemic lupus erythematosis or be caused by a vessel wall defect, as in scurvy, or small vessel involvement, as in fat embolism or hyperglobulinaemia.

Thrombocytopenic purpura

Thrombocytopenic purpura is caused by a deficiency of platelets. This may arise from failure of production in the marrow, or from excessive destruction, utilization or sequestration which exceeds the marrow's capacity to produce platelets.

Decreased platelet production arises from disease affecting the marrow such as aplastic anaemia or secondary tumour infiltration. It also occurs in severe vitamin B_{12} and folate deficiency. The treatment is that of the primary disorder plus, on occasions, replacement therapy with platelet concentrates. Platelet replacement therapy has only a limited role to play in the long-term management as eventually the patient will become sensitized and develop platelet antibodies which will render further transfusions relatively ineffective. Generally speaking, unless the patient is actually bleeding from thrombocytopenia, platelet concentrates are not given if the platelet count is greater than 20×10^9 per litre.

One of the important causes of thrombocytopenia in adults is idiopathic thrombocytopenic purpura (ITP). This is presumed to be of an autoimmune aetiology but platelet auto-antibodies have only been detected in a certain percentage of cases. The definition of this condition remains imprecise because there is no specific test for this syndrome. The diagnosis is one usually reached by the exclusion of other causes of thrombocytopenia. Thrombocytopenia generally develops abruptly and the morphology of the megakaryocytes in the marrow may be abnormal and give a pointer to the diagnosis.

Platelet production may be poor in the marrow despite megakaryocytic hyperplasia. The choice of treatment in ITP lies between corticosteroids, splenectomy and immunosuppressive therapy. Corticosteroids should be tried first and may induce a remission which is maintained when the therapy is withdrawn. If the condition relapses when corticosteroids are withdrawn then splenectomy is indicated or if the condition fails to respond to corticosteroids then earlier splenectomy is indicated. Generally speaking, splenectomy should be carried out early, i.e. within 3 months of presentation. The majority of patients respond well to splenectomy though the results tend to be poorer in the older age groups. If splenectomy does not produce a satisfactory remission then immunosuppressive therapy should be tried (Fig. 11.10). Supportive therapy will be required for splenectomy in ITP cases. Firstly, corticosteroids will have to be re-introduced in preparation for surgery and these should be discontinued as rapidly as is physiologically possible after surgery. Secondly, platelet concentrates may be required postoperatively. These should be given after the splenic pedicle is tied. If given prior to this stage the platelets are likely to be lost in the spleen. At the time of surgery it is important to search for and remove any accessory splenic tissue. Failure to remove an accessory spleen is a possible cause of a delayed relapse after splenectomy.

After splenectomy the platelet count generally rises rapidly and by 24 hours is often higher than normal. This is a good prognostic sign for a permanent remission. In the first week after the operation the count generally falls back into the normal range. In other cases the platelet response may be much slower and in such cases replacement therapy with platelet concentrates may be required to control haemorrhage. In a very small number of cases

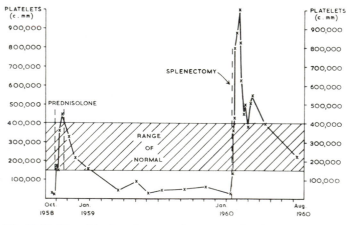

Fig. 11.10 Idiopathic thrombocytopenic purpura, showing the response of the platelet count to prednisolone and splenectomy. Remission of symptoms (menorrhagia, epistaxis and crops of petechiae) lasted for 5 months after the months course of prednisolone. Remission continued 4 years after splenectomy and there was no abnormal bleeding during pregnancy and confinement.

there is no response to splenectomy and platelet concentrates are required in quantity to control the bleeding problem.

Thrombocytopenia may also be caused by an immunological mechanism following the administration of certain drugs. The most important of these drugs in current use are quinidine, quinine, digitoxin, chlorothiazide, sulphonamides and rifampicin. The disorder is self-limiting when the drug is withdrawn.

Thrombocytopenia also arises from excessive consumption of platelets in DIC situations. Here the intravascular coagulation 'consumes' the platelets and leads to thrombocytopenia. A similar situation exists in the somewhat rare condition of thrombotic thrombocytopenic purpura. In such conditions heparinization is likely to control the intravascular coagulation and bring about a rise in platelet count.

Hypersplenism is another cause of thrombocytopenia. Here the platelets tend to be trapped in the spleen leaving a platelet deficiency in the peripheral circulation. Any condition leading to splenomegaly may lead to this and splenectomy will correct the platelet deficiency but not necessarily the basic disease process.

Thrombocythaemia

A modest increase in platelet count or thrombocythaemia is frequently met in situations of severe haemorrhage. Here the marrow has over-reacted slightly and produced excess platelets. In this situation there is no platelet functional defect. Increased platelet production is however a feature of the myeloproliferative syndrome and in this situation platelet function is often abnormal. The thrombocythaemia may be the only abnormality in which case it is known as essential thrombocythaemia or it may be part of the syndrome of polycythaemia rubra vera or chronic myeloid leukaemia.

Where there is pathological platelet proliferation this should be controlled by radioactive phosphorus therapy. Aspirin has been reported of value in control of some symptoms in thrombocythaemia. It is worth mentioning the effect of aspirin on platelets as the therapeutic prospect of 'anti-platelet' therapy with aspirin in occlusive arterial disease is the subject of a number of large clinical trials at present. After oral administration of aspirin most, but not all, recipients have a change in platelet reactivity to adenosine diphosphate (ADP). This change is imprinted on the platelet for its lifespan and may explain why, in some patients aspirin-induced gastric bleeding continues for some days. It is theoretically possible that such gastro-intestinal bleeding might be treated by fresh platelet-containing blood or platelet concentrates, when all the salicylate has been excreted.

The platelet count in peripheral blood after major operation or severe trauma follows a fairly typical pattern; there is a gradual rise to a point in time 10–14 days after the operation or trauma with the count usually returning to normal by the end of the third week.

At its peak during the second week the platelet count may be two or three times its pre-operative level. The extent of the rise tends to be proportional to the extent of the trauma. After splenectomy the rise may be unusually high and the count may remain permanently above the pre-operative level, although it tends to fall back towards the pre-operative level in a person with a platelet count which was previously normal.

Defences against intravascular thrombosis

Within the intravascular compartment the safety devices against intravascular thrombosis include the contact activation of factors XI and XII, inactivation of thrombin, and the fibrinolytic enzyme system.

Contact activation

It is remarkable that vascular endothelium is able to maintain blood fluidity and blood drawn carefully into non-wettable containers has very little tendency to coagulate. Coagulation is activated normally by contact with a wettable surface or with tissue. Contact activation depends on factors XII and XI; if factor XII is lacking, blood drawn into glass tends to behave like blood drawn into a siliconized tube.

The absence of contact, therefore, in the presence of healthy vascular endothelium tends to restrict the occurrence of thrombosis. It should be noted, however, that venous thrombosis has been reported in factor XII-deficient patients and coronary thrombosis occurs in haemophiliacs.

Antithrombin

Several different antithrombin mechanisms have been described, but the most important is antithrombin III (or heparin co-factor). Antithrombin III (AT III) is a single chain polypeptide synthesized in the liver, and has a molecular weight around 65 000. It rapidly complexes thrombin and inhibits the proteolytic activity, a function which is rapidly enhanced in the presence of heparin. The concentration of AT III in blood is relatively high. A hereditary deficiency of AT III has been described and is associated with a hypercoaguable state characterized by recurrent spontaneous venous thrombosis. Low levels are also encountered in hepatic failure, disseminated intravascular coagulation, and women receiving oral oestrogen containing contraceptive pills.

Conclusions

The haemostatic mechanism is a complicated chain reaction in which constituents of the vessel wall, platelets and plasma factors participate. After injury for a few seconds a cut vessel is provided with loose platelet aggregates through which the outflowing blood penetrates at irregular intervals. The time interval between the injury of the vessel and the haemostatic plug becoming impermeable to the blood flow amounts to a few minutes and is equal to the primary bleeding time. The transformation of the temporary haemostasis into permanent haemostasis takes hours to days. If this fails, there is recurrence of bleeding.

BLOOD TRANSFUSION

The history of blood transfusion falls into three phases:

1. The early developmental phase, 1900 to the late 1930s: the recognition of the ABO blood group antigen system followed by the Lewis, MN and P antigen systems.

2. The main developmental phase, 1940 to the early 1960s: the recognition of the Rhesus antigen system, the Kell, Duffy and other antigen systems.

3. The blood component phase, early 1960s to present time: the development of the technology of blood products and the development of their therapeutic applications.

After the initial development, there was a rapid expansion in blood transfusion during and immediately after the Second World War. As surgery advanced, more and more blood was required and this increasing demand continues today. It is important now that as many donations as possible are fully utilized to prepare blood products. For the past few years many varied components from whole blood have been prepared and it must now be the aim in transfusion practice to separate as many units of blood as possible into therapeutically useful components. Each donation will thus benefit several recipients. Blood transfusion practice at present is largely concerned with providing red blood cells which are compatible with, and acceptable to, the patient. Red cells can be provided in the form of whole blood or, preferably from the point of view of providing plasma components, as red cell concentrates. By preparing a red cell concentrate, the plasma is removed from the blood after settling or centrifugation of the whole blood and used for the preparation of other blood components. The red cell concentrate which is left in the residual plasma has a packed cell volume (PCV) of approximately 70%.

Another function of blood transfusion practice is to provide material for plasma volume replacement. In the past whole blood and then reconstituted dried plasma were largely used for this purpose. However, albuminoid fractions of plasma such as plasma protein fraction (PPF) are now more widely available and have several advantages

Table 11.4 Blood products for plasma volume expansion

Plasma protein in fraction (PPF)
Lyophilized plasma
Lyophilized fresh plasma

Table 11.5 Albumin preparations

Plasma protein fraction
Salt poor albumin

over other volume expanders (Table 11.4). PPF solution contains calculated quantities of protein and electrolytes, is pasteurised during manufacture rendering it free from serum hepatitis, is easily stored, has a long shelf-life, and is quick and easy to use. PPF does not, however, contain any coagulation factors or immunoglobulin which may require to be replaced in some situations such as in extensive burn injuries. Albumin can also be prepared in a salt-poor concentrated form (Table 11.5). This can be useful in the treatment of hypoalbuminaemia associated with the nephrotic syndrome, liver disease or starvation.

With the rapid advances which have occurred in recent years in protein purification a second generation of products has become available for the treatment of haemostatic disorders and has enabled much more selective low volume therapy to be provided. If plasma is separated without delay after blood donation, snap frozen and stored frozen, then its coagulation factors remain relatively stable for several months. This fresh frozen plasma (FFP) can be used for non-selective replacement therapy in coagulation factor deficiencies, or as the basic material for the preparation of purified coagulation factors. The main disadvantage of FFP is that it can only produce minor improvements in a coagulation factor deficiency without producing circulatory overload.

More purified and more concentrated low volume products are therefore necessary. Cryoprecipitate was an early low volume concentrate prepared by thawing FFP to 4°C and collecting the precipitated cryoglobulins. This product contains approximately 50% of the factor VIII of the original donation concentrated into a volume of about 10 ml and is also rich in fibrinogen. Further purification and concentration of factor VIII from fresh plasma can be made by techniques of fractionation with ether, alcohol or polyethyleneglycol precipitation to produce a low volume lyophylized concentrate of factor VIII, which stores well. Each of these products can be used effectively to correct the Factor VIII deficiency in haemophilia during a haemostatic challenge.

Although cryoprecipitate has been the mainstay of factor VIII replacement therapy for many years, it has several disadvantages. The factor VIII content of cryoprecipitate can be very variable and it is somewhat time consuming to reconstitute. Over the last few years concentrated freeze

Table 11.6 Blood products for haemostatic disorders

Product	Main Indication
Fresh frozen plasma (FFP)	Mixed coagulation deficiencies
Cryoprecipitate	Factor VIII deficiency
	Fibrinogen deficiency
Factor VIII intermediate concentrate	Factor VIII deficiency
Commercial factor VIII concentrates	Factor VIII deficiency
Animal factor VIII	Factor VIII inhibitors
DE FIX	Factor IX deficiency
Commercial factor IX concentrates	Factor IX deficiency
Lyophilized fibrinogen	Fibrinogen deficiency
Platelet concentrate	Thrombocytopenia

dried preparations of factor VIII (Table 11.6) have become much more widely available and are now used extensively in place of cryoprecipitate. Lyophilized preparations are easily stored and reconstituted, are of known and standardized potency and can be administered in small volumes. They are thus particularly useful during surgical operations on haemophiliac patients and with home therapy which is becoming an increasingly widespread practice. In the authors' experience, the factor VIII intermediate concentrate prepared by the Scottish National Blood Transfusion Service Protein Fraction Centre and the commercial factor VIII concentrates shown in Table 11.6 are very efficient in correcting a factor VIII deficiency and should be used where large amounts of factor VIII have to be administered.

The factor IX deficiency in Christmas disease can be corrected by the administration of FFP, lyophylized fresh plasma or factor IX concentrate. As in factor VIII deficiency, it is desirable to use a concentrate rather than FFP to correct a deficiency and as can be seen from the table several factor IX concentrates are available. The DE FIX concentrate prepared by the Scottish National Blood Transfusion Service Protein Fraction Centres is, in the authors' experience over several years, very satisfactory in the management of factor IX deficiency. This is prepared largely from the plasma supernatant of cryoprecipitate production, illustrating a further step in the utilization of whole fresh plasma. PPSB, the other factor IX concentrate shown in Table 11.6, contains factor VII in addition to factors II, IX and X which are the factors in DE FIX. It is therefore suitable for replacement therapy where there is a deficiency of the vitamin K-dependent factors as in liver disease and as in coumarin overdosage. It should be used with caution, however, in severe liver disease because in this situation PPSB has been suspected in some instances to be associated with DIC. It is possible that certain PPSB preparations contain activated coagulation factors which precipitate DIC.

A lyophilized concentrate of fibrinogen can be prepared from pooled plasma and this can be used in haemostatic problems with hypofibrinogenaemia. Cryoprecipitate is also rich in fibrinogen and is probably the preparation of choice where fibrinogen replacement is required. Hypofibrinogenaemia occurs most commonly in obstetrical situations particularly accident retroplacental haemorrhage. In this situation there may be a fairly sudden depletion of fibrinogen by intravascular coagulation. This should be treated by fresh blood transfusion and fibrinogen.

In addition to concentrated red cells, concentrated platelets and concentrated leucocytes can be prepared. By centrifugation, platelet concentrates can be prepared as a by-product of the preparation of plasma for other blood components. These platelets can be pooled and used for the haemostatic problem in thrombocytopenia. The role of such platelet replacement therapy is limited because, despite ensuring their ABO compatibility with the patient, platelet antibodies will eventually develop and seriously limit their usefulness. Broadly speaking, they should be reserved for short-lived thrombocytopenic haemostatic emergencies, and particularly for the intensive care of patients undergoing cytotoxic therapy for acute leukaemia or malignancy.

Leucocyte concentrates are now being prepared in a number of centres. Availability of white cell concentrates has been greatly facilitated by the development of continuous flow cell separators. Using such machines heparinized whole donor blood is centrifuged at high speeds. The blood is separated into red cell, plasma and buffy layer components. The buffy coat which principally contains leucocytes is removed and the remainder of the blood returned to the donor. As with platelet concentrates, leucocyte concentrates have at present limited application and should be reserved for replacement therapy in short-lived agranulocytic situations, such as the intensive cytotoxic therapy of leukaemia and other malignancies (Table 11.7).

Table 11.7 Blood products — cellular components

Red cell concentrates
Leucocyte free red cell concentrates
Washed red cell concentrates
Frozen red cell concentrates
Leucocyte concentrates
Platelet concentrates

Pooled immunoglobulin is prepared by alcohol and ether fractionation and contains mainly IgG. This can be used prophylactically to protect against certain virus infections. It is given to children under 1 year to protect against measles, to women exposed to rubella in the first 4 months of pregnancy and to children unimmunized and exposed to poliomyelitis. It has also been recommended for protection in exposure to infective hepatitis. In cases of hypogammaglobulinaemia it is given regularly as replacement therapy (Table 11.8).

Table 11.8 Blood products — immunoglobulin preparations

Normal human immunoglobulin
Immunoglobulin anti-Rh (D)
Immunoglobulin anti-vaccinia
Immunoglobulin anti-tetanus
Immunoglobulin anti-hepatitis B
Immunoglobulin anti-zoster
Immunoglobulin anti-rabies

As can be seen from Table 11.8, a variety of special immunoglobulins can be prepared. These are prepared from the plasma of hyperimmune donors and are used to give passive immunity. Those shown on the table are currently available from the National Blood Transfusion Service but some can be obtained commercially.

Perhaps the biggest advance in this field has been in Rhesus prophylaxis. Today by giving anti-Rh(D) immunoglobulin to unimmunized Rh(D) negative mothers at the time of delivery of a Rh(D) positive child, Rhesus haemolytic disease of the newborn is largely prevented. Other specialized immunoglobulins have been prepared for prophylaxis against vaccinia, tetanus, serum hepatitis, zoster and rabies.

The recent expansion of blood component therapy has only been made possible by several technical improvements including the introduction of plastic bags giving a closed sterile system. Another advance has been the development of more suitable anticoagulant preservative solutions. In the past the anticoagulant most suitable for red cell donations was acid citrate dextrose (ACD), but it has been replaced to a large extent by citrate phosphate dextrose (CPD) anticoagulant. CPD allows a full 28 day storage life at 4°C compared to 21 days for ACD. It also conserves better the 2.3 DPG levels within the red cells thus maintaining good gas transport efficiency. CPD also reduces the risk of metabolic acidosis that can develop following massive transfusion. The addition of adenine nucleotides and purine derivatives such as guanosine or inosine is also thought to improve the storage properties of blood, but toxicity problems have limited their usefulness.

Another recent development is the use of frozen red cells, employing glycerol as a cryopreservative and storing at temperatures of around minus 160°C. Such techniques have been shown to prolong the storage life of blood to several years and have many other advantages such as preventing transmission of viral hepatitis, aiding component therapy, collection of rare blood groups and aiding supply of blood in times of shortage. However, there are also several drawbacks (cost, time, short shelf life of reconstituted cells) which have limited the development and usefulness of this technique.

The expansion of blood component therapy has reduced the supply of whole blood. At the present time, the indications for the use of whole blood are becoming fewer.

Whole blood has a definite place in the management of surgical and traumatic haemorrhage. For small losses in the operating theatre, red cell concentrates, supplemented if necessary with a plasma volume expander, are to be preferred. Likewise, both pre-operatively and postoperatively, red cell concentrates should be used if blood transfusion is required. At all times it is preferable that 'anaemia' should be treated wherever possible by the appropriate haematinic. The practice of 'topping up' with blood is to be discouraged; as mentioned above it exposes the patient unnecessarily to the hazard of serum hepatitis.

Even in cases of chronic anaemia such as aplastic anaemia, blood transfusion should be minimized. Many such patients can achieve a reasonable activity with a haemoglobin level of between 9 and 10 g/dl. Patients on regular dialysis therapy adjust to a haemoglobin level of between 6 and 7 g/dl and require only very occasional transfusion. By accepting these low haemoglobin levels, such patients are not unnecessarily exposed to the risk of serum hepatitis.

BLOOD GROUPS

Antigens

Human red cells carry on their surface an array of antigens. The development of these antigens is genetically controlled and they remain throughout life. Many well-defined blood group systems have been described including the ABO, Rhesus, MNSs, P, Lutheran, Kell, Lewis, Duffy and Kidd systems. The two of major clinical importance, the ABO and the Rhesus systems, will be discussed here. These antigens are of large molecular size and are basically polysaccharide-amino acid complexes. Similar substances are to be found in certain plants and simple animals.

Antibodies

Antibodies are immunoglobulins which appear in the plasma as the result of stimulation by the antigen, and react specifically with that antigen in some observable way. In blood transfusion serology they are IgM or IgG, or occasionally IgA immunoglobulins. They can be of two types, naturally occurring or immune. Naturally occurring or spontaneous antibodies occur without any obvious antigenic stimulus and the iso agglutinins of the ABO system belong to this group. These probably develop from exposure to antigen in the first few months of life, for at birth they are not detectable.

Immune antibodies result from stimulation by a blood group antigen which is not present in the patient's cells or body fluids. This can arise from blood transfusion, from injections of blood or from transplacental haemorrhage.

Antibodies can also be classified according to their

serological characteristics. They may be complete (saline agglutinating antibodies) and, as such, can agglutinate red cells bearing the appropriate antigen in a saline medium. They can be incomplete (albumin antibodies) and, as such, only coat the red cells bearing the appropriate antigen in a saline medium.

To produce agglutination as the end point of the reaction, a high molecular weight protein like albumin has to be added, or the red cells have to be rendered more antigenically reactive by treatment with a proteolytic enzyme such as papain or ficin. Such cells coated with antibody can also be detected in the antiglobulin test by the use of anti-human globulin, which, added to the globulin-coated cells, will bring about agglutination and achieve a visible end point.

The ABO system

The ABO system was the first system to be described and remains clinically by far the most important. It consists of four main blood groups, A, B, AB and O, which are determined by the presence or absence on the red cell of the antigens A and B. Thus, group A possesses only the A antigen, group B only the B antigen, group AB both antigens, and group O neither antigen. The serum contains naturally occurring antibodies directed against the antigens of this system lacking on the red cells. Thus, a group A individual lacks the B antigen on the red cells, and his serum will contain anti-B agglutinins. Similarly group B has anti-A agglutinins in the serum, group O both anti-A and anti-B agglutinins in the serum and group AB no agglutinins in the serum. These agglutinins are saline agglutinating and are IgM immunoglobulins.

These ABO groups can be further subdivided but for practical purposes only the subgroups of A are important. In Europeans, four-fifths of group A individuals belong to the subgroup A_1, and one-fifth to the subgroup A_2; similarly, four-fifths of AB individuals belong to the subgroup A_1B and one-fifth to the subgroup A_2B.

For most purposes the A_2 antigen can be regarded as a weak form of the A_1 antigen but in 1% of group A_2 and 25% of A_2B, an anti-A_1 will be present, which is active at 37°C and will destroy transfused A_1 red cells.

Universal donors and universal recipients

Group O donors have in the past been regarded as 'universal' donors because they lack both the A and B antigens. This concept is, however, dangerous because group O donor blood contains anti-A and anti-B in the plasma which, if in high titre, can react with A or B antigens on the patient's own cells. There may also be reactions involving other blood group systems if group O blood is used universally. Similarly, the concept of group AB as a universal recipient is unsatisfactory, for such patients, if

transfused with blood of high anti-A or anti-B titre, may also have transfusion reactions.

Association between disease and ABO group

In several diseases, notably gastric carcinoma and duodenal ulcer, the frequencies of the various ABO groups differ from the frequencies found in the general population. Among the patients with gastric carcinoma there is an excess of individuals of group A, and in duodenal ulcer there is an excess of individuals of group O.

The rhesus system

This is the red cell antigen system, second in importance to the ABO system.

It is now recognized that it is made up of at least three sets of alternative antigens: D or d, C or c, E or e. The D antigen is by far the strongest and is the most important in clinical practice. Patients are classified broadly into two groups, rhesus (D) positive and rhesus (D) negative, according to their D status.

Approximately 83% of the British population are Rh(D) positive, and 17% Rh(D) negative. Practically all Rhesus antibodies result from immunization. This can arise from the transfusion of Rh(D) positive blood to an Rh(D) negative person, or by the passage of Rh(D) positive cells from a fetus across the placenta into an Rh(D) negative mother. When a Rhesus negative person has been so immunized, transfusion of Rhesus positive blood can result in a haemolytic transfusion reaction which may be fatal. It is worth mentioning that unlike the ABO system there are no naturally-occurring antibodies against the C, D, E, c, d, e antigens of the Rhesus system. If a Rhesus antibody is found it will have been acquired. These antibodies are of the complete or incomplete variety, and are largely IgG immunoglobulins. The other antigens of the Rhesus system are much less antigenic than D and are of little clinical importance.

However, occasionally anti-E, anti-C, anti-c and, very occasionally, anti-e may occur as a result of a transfusion or pregnancy. Sensitive techniques are required for their detection. These other Rhesus antibodies may develop in Rh(D) positive patients, according to the phenotype.

At all times, it is desirable that a Rhesus negative patient is given Rhesus negative blood, but because of shortages of Rhesus negative blood, this is not always possible and Rhesus positive blood may have to be given. This will produce no problem at the time of the first transfusion because there are no naturally occurring Rhesus antibodies but it is likely to lead to the production of Rhesus antibodies which will complicate further blood transfusion. While such practice in males and in postmenopausal females is acceptable, it is quite unacceptable in females of, and below, the reproductive age. Such a change of blood group may bring about Rh(D) immunization and is likely to prejudice any further pregnancies and could render the female unable to have any live children.

Haemolytic disease of the newborn

When an Rh(D) negative woman has an Rh(D) positive baby, during the pregnancy, and particularly at the time of placental separation, a small transplacental haemorrhage of the baby's Rhesus positive cells may occur.

This is likely to sensitize the patient and at a second pregnancy, if a transplacental haemorrhage of Rh(D) positive cells occurs, detectable Rhesus antibodies may develop. These antibodies are IgG immunoglobulins directed against the Rhesus D antigen and are small enough molecules to cross the placental barrier from the mother's circulation in subsequent pregnancies. The larger IgM immunoglobulins such as the naturally occurring isoagglutinins cannot cross the placenta. If the next baby is Rh(D) positive, the antibody will coat the baby's D positive cells and may lead to haemolytic disease of the newborn. If severely affected, this will lead to intra-uterine death; if moderately affected, this will lead to haemolytic disease of the newborn (Fig. 11.11).

The management of severely affected fetuses and babies remains a difficult problem. Intra-uterine transfusion into the fetal peritoneal cavity has greatly reduced the incidence of intra-uterine deaths while exchange transfusion remains the basis for managing affected neonates. Recently, intensive plasmapheresis has been introduced in the management of severely affected fetuses but the precise value of this adjunct to standard treatment remains to be established.

As has been previously mentioned, it is most important that anti-D is not produced unnecessarily in females of or below reproductive age by the transfusion of Rhesus positive blood for surgical procedures or in the management of anaemia.

Anti-D immunoglobulin

As has been described, sensitization of a Rhesus negative

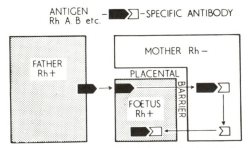

Fig. 11.11 Diagram showing how Rh isoimmunisation in the mother leads to an antigen-antibody reaction in the foetus. (Redrawn from Bell G H, Davidson J N, Scarborough H 1961 Textbook of physiology and biochemistry, 5th edn. Livingstone, Edinburgh.)

mother is usually brought about by the transplacental haemorrhage of Rh(D) positive cells at birth. These can be rendered antigenically inactive by the intramuscular injection of anti-D IgG in the first 72 hours after delivery.

Recent extensive clinical trials of this blood product have established its efficiency in protecting Rhesus negative mothers against sensitization. Sensitization can also occur from fetal maternal haemorrhage at the time of abortion or termination of pregnancy. Anti-D immunoglobulin prophylaxis should therefore also be given to all Rh(D) negative mothers at the time of abortion or termination of pregnancy.

Anti-D immunoglobulin is presently obtained mainly from female donors by plasmapheresis who were sensitized to the D antigen during pregnancy before the advent of anti-D prophylaxis. The success of the prophylaxis is such that very few females will be available in the future. Rh(D) negative male volunteers are therefore being immunized to maintain the supplies of this most valuable blood product.

Choice of donor blood for transfusion

It is first necessary to determine the ABO and Rhesus group of the recipient. This is carried out on the patient's red cells using a range or specific antisera. The ABO group is always confirmed by testing the patients serum for iso-agglutinins in a system incubating serum against red cells of known ABO groups.

It is also important to investigate the patient's serum for irregular antibodies, for if no irregular antibodies are present it is unlikely that there will be any difficulty with a subsequent blood compatibility test. In the screening test for antibodies, the patient's serum is tested by a variety of techniques designed to cover most types of clinically important antibodies, against a mixture of red cells carrying all the clinically important red cell antigens (other than ABO). Thus, if an anti-D, an anti-E or an anti-Kell is present, this antibody screening test will be positive and further investigation can be carried out to identify the antibody. If an antibody is present, knowledge of its specificity assists in the provision of compatible blood. When the ABO and Rhesus group have been determined, blood of an identical group should be drawn from the blood bank for the patient. It is not essential that it be ABO and Rhesus identical, but it is highly preferable. The donor blood is grouped at the Regional Blood Transfusion Centre before issue. The final test required before issue to the patient is a compatibility test in which donor cells are tested against patient's serum by a range of sensitive techniques to detect any antibody reaction with donor cells. It has been said that, provided a sensitive antibody screening test is negative, homologous ABO and Rhesus blood may be given without the final compatibility test.

This is a recommendation which few haematologists are prepared to follow, because in the compatibility test matching donor cells against recipients serum serves as a last, final, direct test of compatibility before release to the patient.

Blood can be supplied at four levels of safety and compatibility according to the urgency of the clinical situation. The four levels are:

1. Unmatched ABO and Rhesus homologous blood
2. Unmatched ABO and Rhesus homologous blood in a patient with a negative antibody screening test
3. ABO and Rhesus homologous blood with an emergency compatibility test
4. ABO and Rhesus homologous blood with a full-time compatibility test

Blood at levels 1 and 2 can be supplied in 5–10 minutes; at level 3 in 45 minutes and at level 4 in $1\frac{1}{2}$ hours. Where at all possible, blood should always be supplied at the level of a full-time compatibility test and for practical purposes should be ordered from the transfusion laboratory a full 24 hours in advance of requirement. Only if the urgency of the clinical situation warrants it, should blood of a lesser compatibility level than a full-time compatibility test be used.

Adverse reactions to blood transfusion

The majority of blood transfusions are given without any untoward effects. In the small percentage where complications do occur, the majority are of a trivial nature. However, in careless hands blood can be one of the most dangerous drugs to be prescribed.

One of the main hazards of blood transfusion is the risk of transmitting serum hepatitis. The risk of transmitting serum hepatitis by blood donation has recently been reduced significantly by the development of the techniques for the detection of hepatitis B antigen (HbAg). All blood donations are now screened for HbAg and any positives are discarded. The majority of cases of post-transfusion hepatitis are now due to other causes, probably other viruses. In the past any donor with a history of jaundice was rejected. Recent practice suggests that any donor with a history of jaundice can be accepted providing the clinical illness occurred more than 12 months previously and the serum can be shown by a sensitive method not to contain HbAg. A past history of malaria or syphilis is, however, still a cause for rejection as a donor.

Table 11.9 Adverse reactions to blood transfusion

Early	Delayed
Febrile reactions	Transmission of:
Haemolytic reactions	Viral hepatitis
Allergic reactions	Syphilis
Reactions to platelet antigens	Cytomegalovirus
Reactions to leucocyte antigens	Malaria
Bacteraemia	Brucellosis
Citrate toxicity	Haemosiderosis
Air embolism	Haemolytic disease of
Circulatory overload	the newborn

As can be seen from the table (Table 11.9) of adverse reactions to blood transfusion, the possible range of reactions is wide but fortunately the incidence of these reactions is very small. Blood transfusion reactions arise most commonly because of faulty patient identification. It is essential that accurate comprehensive patient identification is given on the blood transfusion request and on the blood specimen for the compatibility test. If the identification is unsatisfactory then it is in the patients' best interest for the haematologist to refuse the request.

FURTHER READING
General Haematology

Hardisty R M, Weatherall D J 1982 Blood and its disorders, 2nd edn. Blackwell Scientific, Oxford
Thomson R B 1977 Disorders of the blood. Churchill Livingstone Edinburgh
Clinics in Haematology Volume 1–14 Saunders, London
Hoffbrand A V, Lewis S M 1981 Postgraduate haematology, 2nd edn. Heinemann, London

Haemostasis

Biggs R 1977 Human blood coagulation, haemostasis and thrombosis, 3rd edn. Blackwell Scientific, Oxford
Pollez L 1977 Recent advances in blood coagulation. Churchill Livingstone, Edinburgh

Blood Transfusion

Mollison P L 1983 Blood transfusion in clinical medicine. 7th edn. Blackwell Scientific, Oxford.
Wallace J 1977 Blood transfusion for clinicians. Churchill Livingstone, Edinburgh

Spleen

Studying spleen function is complex because the organ shares cellular components and functions with other organs, especially the bone marrow, the liver and the lymph nodes. The precise contribution of the spleen to the total function of these cellular systems is difficult to know with certainty. At a clinical level, the spleen seldom attracts attention except when palpably enlarged from a diversity of pathological conditions and as a cause of deficiency of cellular conponents in the peripheral blood. It is important, however, for research to continue towards improving understanding of splenic function in relation to

blood diseases, disorders of the immune state, the therapeutic suppression of immune responsiveness and, therefore, to the whole field of organ transplantation.

The normal spleen in the adult varies considerably in size between individuals and at various times in the same individual, the organ becoming smaller with age. The structure of the spleen can be regarded as consisting of a framework of connective tissue vascular channels, lymphatic channels, lymphatic tissue, phagocytes and autonomic nerves (Fig. 12.1).

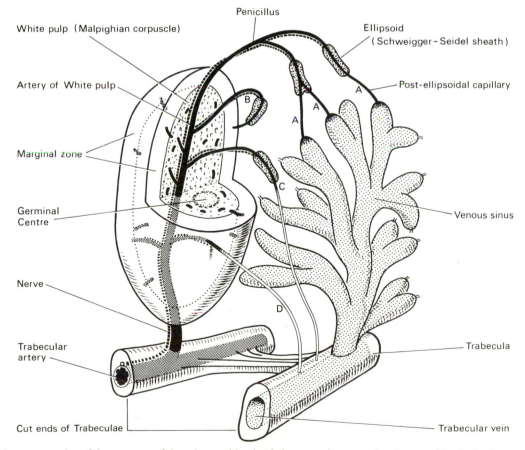

Fig. 12.1 Schematic representation of the structure of the spleen and its circulation: note, however, that the route blood takes between the penicilli and the splenic veins is still uncertain. (Garven H S D 1957 A Student's Histology. Livingstone, Edinburgh)

STRUCTURE OF THE SPLEEN

The spleen is encased in a dense connective tissue capsule. Extending from this into the splenic pulp and carrying blood vessels are an interconnecting lacework of trabeculae. The collagen of the capsule and trabeculae is continuous with the dense network of reticular fibres which provide the supporting system of the splenic pulp.

Structurally and functionally the spleen consists of three regions, the red pulp, the white pulp and interposed between, a marginal zone. The vascular supply is unique in that blood of the systemic circulation is brought into close relationship with lymphatic tissue. The splenic artery divides into trabecular branches which further subdivide within the spleen until they form very small vessels which are embedded in a lymphatic tissue sheath. This is made up of a periarterial collection of lymphocytes but also includes plasma cells, reticulum cells, macrophages, and granulocytes. This lymphocyte accumulation lacks the typical organization of most lymphatic tissue, but eventually comes to merge with characteristic lymphoid tissue with typical germinal centres. Lymphocytes of the periarterial sheath are principally T-lymphocytes, while those of the germinal centre are usually B-lymphocytes. This lymphoid tissue is the white pulp of the spleen.

The marginal zone between the red and white pulp contains lymphatic vessels which represent the efferent side of the lymphatic circulation through the spleen. The precise anatomy of the arterioles which pass through the white pulp has provided one of the principal dilemmas of the circulation through the spleen. Some may terminate within splenic venous sinuses, but free terminations within the splenic pulp appear to be more frequent and probably provide the principal source of flow.

The main area of splenic pulp, the red pulp, forms the space external to the venous sinuses. The red pulp consists essentially of spaces within the reticulum meshwork, with thin cellular linings composed of reticular cells and fixed macrophages. Under normal conditions less than 5% of the blood passing through the spleen traverses these cords in the red pulp, the remainder being shunted through to the sinuses. During passage through the splenic cords any damaged or effete red cells are removed (culling function) while any intracellular particles within intact red cells are removed without destroying the cell (pitting function).

There are quite marked variations in the extent and configuration of the lymphatic component of the spleen which are partly, though inconstantly, dependent on the age and probably on the immune experience of the individual. The principal variations are in the cellular composition of the germinal centres which may show very few reticulum cells and occasionally are composed entirely of small lymphocytes. The distinction between the zone of small lymphocytes and the perifollicular layer may also be difficult to make in some cases. In addition to the fixed structural components of the spleen, such as endothelial cells of the arterioles and sinuses, and those which like the lymphocytes and lymphoid nodules are potentially mobile but in organized formation, there is a significant population of free cells mainly derived from the blood.

FUNCTIONS OF THE NORMAL SPLEEN

The normal spleen has a multiplicity of functions, although removal from a normal adult is generally well tolerated, adequate compensation being effected by other organs.

Extramedullary haemopoiesis:

Although the spleen is an active site of haemopoiesis in the foetus, this has almost ceased by birth. However, the spleen retains the capacity to support haemopoiesis in abnormal circumstances. Compensatory extramedullary haemopoiesis is seen principally with chronic haemolysis, especially in infants and young children, and in adults with myelofibrosis.

Blood storage in the spleen

Many mammals show significant red cell storage in the spleen, but there is no evidence for this in man. The normal content of red cells in the spleen is 20–40 ml. However, isotope studies suggest the presence of a splenic platelet pool, comprising 20–40% of the platelets available to the circulation. The relationship of the spleen to the circulating granulocyte is not totally clear, but normal subjects do not appear to have an intrasplenic granulocyte pool.

Phagocyte function

Phagocytosis of particulate material is a major function of the spleen. This function is aided by the unique vascular structure of the red pulp. The spleen removes red cell inclusions from intact red cells (pitting function), such as Howell-Jolly bodies, Heinz bodies and siderotic granules before returning the undamaged red cell back to the general circulation. The spleen is also very sensitive to any increase in red cell rigidity and so spherocytes, antibody-coated cells, and cells with damaged membranes are all effectively removed (culling function).

Senescent red cells and platelets are also destroyed within the spleen. However, splenectomy does not alter red cell life span, and so the spleen can be neither unique nor indispensible in this role. Almost certainly removal of senescent red cells is a function carried out throughout the reticulo-endothelial system.

Lymphopoiesis

The abundant mitoses found in the germinal centres of the spleen provide some ground for belief that the spleen is an active site of lymphopoiesis. It has become clear that the lymphocyte population is heterogeneous with respect to life span. The spleen appears to contain principally the long lived lymphocytes, for which the required rate of replacement must be very low. The bulk of evidence suggests that the majority of lymphocytes appearing in the organ are there by migration from sites of production elsewhere. Some lymphocytes are almost certainly formed in the spleen, although numerically these must provide only a minor contribution to the total lymphocyte economy.

IMMUNE RESPONSES

Antibody production to intravenously administered antigen is found to be greatest in the spleen and bone marrow. However, intramuscular and intradermal administration of antibody invoke little response in the spleen. The common observation of acute enlargement of the spleen in septicaemic states clearly reflects the hyperplasia evoked by the presence of blood-borne antigens.

SPLENOMEGALY

Disease involvement of the spleen almost invariably results in its enlargement. The spleen is usually clinically palpable when twice its normal size. Splenomegaly is found in a wide range of haematological disorders, including haemolytic anaemias, haemoglobinopathies, leukaemias, lymphomas and myeloproliferative disorders. Other causes of splenomegaly include infective, inflammatory and granulomatous conditions, lipid storage diseases, neoplastic diseases, cysts and amyloid. Portal hypertension and congestive heart failure frequently lead to congestive splenomegaly.

Anaemia in splenomegaly

Splenomegaly may lead to anaemia by a variety of mechanisms. Firstly, splenomegaly may be associated with significant red cell pooling. Secondly, there is often increased destruction of red cells with reduced red cell survival and thirdly, an expansion of plasma volume is commonly found in patients with splenomegaly. Peripheral blood indices may thus not accurately reflect the total red cell volume, and isotope studies of blood volume may be required to gauge this better.

Hypersplenism

Hypersplenism is a syndrome comprising of splenomegaly, reduction in one or more peripheral blood elements and a normal or hypercellular bone marrow. Splenectomy should result in return of the peripheral blood elements to normal values, although this does not occur with all cases. Hypersplenism may occur in a wide range of conditions (Table 12.1).

Table 12.1 Principal diseases frequently associated with hypersplenism

Primary hypersplenism
Congestive splenomegaly
Myelosclerosis
Felty's syndrome
Leukaemias and lymphomas
Lipid storage diseases
Sarcoidosis
Thalassaemia major
Chronic infections, e.g. malaria, brucellosis

INDICATIONS FOR SPLENECTOMY

The majority of surgical splenectomies have been done to facilitate other major surgery, usually of the upper gastrointestinal tract, occasionally of the colon or kidney. Gastric surgical procedures necessitating splenectomy are now performed less frequently. A considerable number also are removed because of traumatic rupture; spontaneous rupture is very rare in temperate climates. The spleen may be removed in portal hypertension, but is usually only done in these circumstances as part of a shunt procedure, usually a splenorenal shunt.

Splenectomy is often of value in a very wide range of haematological disorders. It may be performed for the treatment or correction of hypersplenism, persistent local discomfort, recurrent splenic infarction, portal hypertension, or local splenic disease. Splenectomy may also be performed for diagnostic purposes for staging of Hodgkin's disease and other lymphomas.

Probably the clearest indication for splenectomy is the condition of hereditary spherocytosis where clinical cure of the condition can be guaranteed, although the red cell abnormality persists. Patients with other hereditary haemolytic anaemias may also require splenectomy, but the overall indications are not so clear as with hereditary spherocytosis, and in some is of no value. In autoimmune haemolytic anaemias the case for splenectomy is also less definite, but frequently is of value in cases resistant to corticosteroid therapy. Similarly, splenectomy may also be of benefit in chronic autoimmune thrombocytopenic purpura unresponsive to conservative measures. The operation is only rarely needed in acute cases.

Effects of splenectomy

Splenectomy in a healthy adult is not followed by significant sequelae, and this has tended to reduce the appreciation of the hazards of this procedure in other circumstances. However, the overall mortality rate of splenectomy in haematological diseases is about 8%, although it is significantly less than 1% in uncomplicated cases such as hereditary spherocytosis or staging of Hodgkin's disease. Splenectomy in haematological diseases should be carried out when the patient is relatively fit and not physically impaired by extensive disease.

Venous thrombosis

Venous thrombosis occurs more frequently after splenectomy than after other upper abdominal operations. One important factor is the marked thrombocytosis which occurs after splenectomy. The two commonest sites are the peripheral veins and the tributaries of the portal vein. Prophylactic measures to counter postoperative thrombo-embolic complications are therefore important.

Infection

Many reports have suggested a predisposition to infection following splenectomy. This is a rare event in otherwise healthy adults, but there is a significant risk in childhood. The frequency of severe bacterial infections is highest following splenectomy in infancy, but after 1 year the incidence lessens although the mortality is still great. Overall, the risk appears to be greatest for the first 2 years after the operation. Pneumococcal infections, often fulminating and fatal, are most common but there is also an increased incidence of streptococcal infections. Prophylactic antibiotics are of value in children for up to 2 years after splenectomy.

Malaria may also be reactivated in previously infected patients. The explanation of these findings is unclear, but altered immune function, including immunoglobulins, has been noted.

Other complications

A wide range of postoperative problems is seen after splenectomy including haemorrhage, pulmonary complications, ileus and pancreatic trauma. In myeloproliferative disorders the postsplenectomy thrombocytosis may lead to a haemorrhagic disorder often with gastrointestinal bleeding, while in thalassaemia major, splenectomy may result in greater iron deposition within the liver and thus hepatic parenchymal damage.

Peripheral blood changes

Following splenectomy characteristic changes are noted in the peripheral blood. Howell-Jolly bodies are invariably present within the red cell, and there are increased numbers of target cells and schistocytes. A leucocytosis occurs within hours following splenectomy and is maximal within a week. This gradually falls over several weeks, but in a significant proportion it may persist for much longer. The platelet count also rises to a peak between the 4th and 14th days, and gradually subsides over the ensuing 3 months. A proportion of patients, usually those with persisting anaemia or a myeloproliferative disorder, may show a continuing thrombocytosis. Such cases have an increased frequency of thrombotic complications.

Central nervous system

INTRODUCTION

Although neurological surgery is a specialist subject, many aspects of disordered neural function impinge on other disciplines. The outcome of a patient who has been resuscitated from shock or who has undergone successful surgery using cardiopulmonary bypass may be dominated by the disabling sequelae of brain hypoxia. Compression of the brain or spinal cord may complicate head injury, metastatic tumours or systemic infection and command attention in general surgical wards. The mechanisms by which these conditions produce death or disability are, in general, poorly understood. The rapidity with which they may progress is often not appreciated and misdiagnosis and delay in treatment can have tragic results. Another problem with which general surgeons are frequently confronted is severe and intractable pain as a complication of malignant disease. An understanding of the principles involved in localization and control of pain is invaluable in the management of these unfortunate patients.

The apparent complexities of neuroanatomy and neurophysiology deter many who seek tc understand the often dramatic signs of brain and spinal cord compression but, in fact, many of the processes involved are primarily mechanical or haemodynamic rather than neurophysiological in character.

The topics which form the substance of this chapter have been selected not only for their clinical importance, but also because they illustrate the principles governing the maintenance of the stable physicochemical milieu which is essential to the function of the central nervous system. Knowledge of some simple neuroanatomical principles along with an appreciation of the mechanisms involved in energy supply to the brain, control of the cerebral circulation of both blood and cerebral spinal fluid (CSF), and of intracranial pressure, facilitates effective care of patients with brain and spinal cord lesions.

ENERGY SUPPLY TO THE BRAIN

The brain's energy requirements are considerable. Virtually all of the energy supply must be derived from the oxidative metabolism of glucose and, since there is no reserve supply of oxygen in the brain and only a small glucose reserve, the availability of these substrates in cerebral blood must be plentiful and constant. The brain uses about 60 mg of glucose and 45 ml of oxygen per minute; these rates account for a quarter and a fifth respectively of whole body glucose and oxygen utilization.

Carriage of glucose and oxygen to the brain is determined by tissue perfusion (cerebral blood flow) and by those factors which govern the content of oxygen in the blood, including arterial oxygen tension (Po_2), pH, body temperature, and haemoglobin concentration. The energy derived from oxidative glucose metabolism is supplied as adenosine triphosphate (ATP), 38 molecules of this high energy phosphate for each mole of glucose. In the absence of oxygen, glucose may be converted anaerobically to lactate resulting in a much lower energy yield, 2 moles of ATP for each mole of glucose.

Energy is required by the brain for establishment of the ionic gradients across membranes necessary for neuronal transmission, for the synthesis, release, uptake and destruction of neurotransmitter substances necessary for synaptic transmission, and for preservation of cellular structures in the central nervous system including the complex processes of lipid metabolism involved in myelinization of neurones. Energy is also required for protein synthesis involved in information storage, for CSF formation and for the metabolic processes of the astroglia. These processes together represent what we accept as normal brain function.

The consequences of interruption of energy supply to the brain are immediate and dramatic. Consciousness is lost within 15 seconds of onset of total brain ischaemia. In severe hypoglycaemia the process is only a little slower. These dramatic clinical events are accompanied by electroencephalographic (EEG) changes, presumably reflecting disturbed neurophysiological function but appear to be at variance with reports which show that brain mitochondrial function can be preserved even when brain tissue P_{O_2} is as low as 0.3 kPa (2 mmHg), and that ATP production may be fully restored after prolonged brain ischaemia. A possible explanation for the discrepancy is that the neurotransmitter substances in the brain are very sensitive to even relatively mild hypoxia. For example, tyrosine hydroxylase, which is a rate-limiting enzyme in the synthesis of noradrenaline and dopamine, becomes reduced as soon as arterial P_{O_2} falls below 9.3 kPa (70 mmHg). Dopamine, acetylcholine and noradrenaline levels in the brain are all reduced in hypoxia. Only when oxygen lack is more prolonged and severe do changes associated with structural damage occur: a decrease in brain lipids involved in membrane structure, such as phosphatidylinositol, and an efflux of potassium from neurones and influx of calcium, both reflecting and causing breakdown in the membrane transport systems or of the membranes themselves (Tables 13.1, 13.2 and 13.3).

Interruption of the energy supply to the brain may therefore produce effects ranging from purely functional

Table 13.3 Cerebral effects of hypoglycaemia

Blood sugar level	Changes
2.2 mmol/l (40 mg/dl)	Consciousness preserved EEG normal, but behaviour may change
1.9 mmol/l (35 mg/dl)	Confusion, drowsiness EEG slowing appears
1.4 mmol/l (25 mg/dl)	Convulsions, EEG grossly abnormal Cerebral ATP normal
0.8 mmol/l (15 mg/dl)	Coma, EEG pattern flat ATP level falls. Death imminent Pathological damage in boundary zones

changes, manifest as alteration in personality, judgment, memory, or impaired tolerance of drugs or alcohol, to profound coma. The latter may be accompanied by evidence of damage to the ultrastructure of nerve cells in the form of oedema due to membrane breakdown, abnormal cells containing vacuoles representing the swollen remnants of the mitochondria, and total cell necrosis. There are regional variations in the severity of hypoxic brain damage. Cell damage is most pronounced in the Purkinje cells of the cerebellum, in the cells of the third, fifth and sixth layers of the cerebral cortex particularly in the occipital region, and in the cells of the Sommer

Table 13.1 Effects of hypoxic cerebral hypoxia

Arterial P_{O_2}	Biochemical change in brain	Physiological change
6.7 kPa (50 mmHg)	Glycolysis starts with production of lactate Phosphocreatine and ATP still normal Serotonin, noradrenaline, dopamine and acetylcholine levels fall	Cerebral blood flow increases Minor changes in the EEG Memory impairment on testing
4.7 kPa (35 mmHg)	Glycolysis pronounced Phosphocreatine levels fall but ATP still normal	EEG clearly abnormal Judgement and behaviour impaired
2.7 kPa (20 mmHg)	ATP levels fall Brain lipid metabolism impaired	EEG slowing (1–2 Hz) or absence of activity Coma (response only to pain)
0.7 kPa (< 5 mmHg)	Mitochondria cease function, cell damage (cerebellum, cerebral cortex and hippocampus)	Death from cardiovascular failure

Table 13.2 Effects of total brain ischaemia

Duration	Biochemical changes in brain	Physiological changes
0–20 sec	Ratio of NADH/NAD increases	EEG slows into 0–4 Hz range Consciousness lost after 15 seconds
1–12 min	Decrease in oxygen and glucose consumption Decrease in serotonin and noradrenaline Reduction in protein synthesis Increase in brain lactate, free fatty acids and in cyclic AMP and GABA (inhibitory transmitter)	EEG activity ceases completely Brain stem reflexes absent Pupils dilated and fixed

20–60 min	Energy metabolism ceases
	RNA activity and protein synthesis stop
	Visible evidence of damage to mitochondria and other
	   organelles
	Cell damage in boundary zones or cerebral cortex,
	   cerebellum and hippocampus
		Brain death — widespread irreversible neuronal damage

sector of Ammons horn in the hippocampus. When the hypoxic insult is due to ischaemia produced by systemic hypotension, brain damage is most pronounced in the boundary zones between the territories of distribution of the anterior and middle cerebral arteries, of the middle and posterior cerebral arteries and of the superior cerebellar and posterior inferior cerebellar arteries.

In any given area of the brain the energy status is most accurately expressed in terms of the relative proportions of ATP, adenosine diphosphate (ADP) and adenosine monophosphate (AMP) present at that time or in terms of the ratio between nucleotide adenophosphate (NAD) and nucleotide adenophosphodehydrogenase (NADH). Since these measurements involve exposure or sampling of brain tissue, clinicians have access only to less direct indices of brain oxygenation.

Information can be obtained by sampling jugular venous blood (assuming that this represents cerebral venous drainage) and making measurements of cerebral venous P_{O_2}, oxygen saturation and content. If arterial blood is sampled simultaneously, measurements can be made of the cerebral arteriovenous differences for oxygen and carbon dioxide content and for glucose, lactate and pyruvate (Table 13.4). However, such measurements have great limitations. Uptake or production of a substance by the brain is the product of the arteriovenous difference and the blood flow through the brain (Fick Principle). While it is possible to measure cerebral blood flow, either through the entire brain or in specified regions, the real problem is uncertainty about the degree to which jugular venous blood relates to cerebral venous drainage in different regions of the brain.

Table 13.4 Typical cerebrovascular values

Measurement	Value
Jugular venous P_{O_2}	5.3 kPa (40 mmHg)
Jugular venous O_2 saturation	65%
Cerebral A–V O_2 content difference	6 ml/dl
Cerebral V–A CO_2 content difference	6 ml/dl
Cerebral A–V glucose difference	0.6 mmol/l (10 mg/dl)
Cerebral V–A lactate difference	0.2 mmol/l (1.5 mg/dl)
Mean cerebral blood flow	50 ml.min^{-1}.100 g^{-1}
Cerebrovascular resistance	1.8 mmHg.ml.min^{-1} 100 g^{-1}
Cerebral oxygen uptake	3 ml.min^{-1}.100 g^{-1}

When the brain is evenly perfused with blood and a uniform hypoxia or ischaemia occurs (e.g. reduced cardiac output) jugular venous P_{O_2} values correspond fairly well with brain oxygenation. In such circumstances, intellectual impairment and minor EEG abnormalities develop as venous P_{O_2} falls below 4.0 kPa (30 mmHg). Consciousness is lost and EEG frequencies slow into the delta range (1–4 Hz) as jugular P_{O_2} falls to 2.0 kPa (15 mmHg). As venous P_{O_2} nears 1.3 kPa (10 mmHg) death is imminent.

This simplified schema is of limited clinical value however, because most brain disorders are focal and cerebral blood flow is not homogeneous but shows wide regional variations. Severe focal brain ischaemia may fail to be reflected in low jugular venous P_{O_2} levels. For example, sudden occlusion of one internal carotid artery can produce severe ischaemia in the ipsilateral cerebral hemisphere in one patient in five, sufficient to produce contralateral hemiplegia. Yet jugular venous P_{O_2} values during carotid occlusion in such patients often give no indication of the tissue hypoxia. Once an area of the brain has ceased to function, any blood flowing through that area will have no oxygen extracted from it and the venous effluent from the area will consist of bright red, well-oxygenated blood. This phenomenon of 'red veins' is known to occur around cerebral infarcts and brain tumours, although in the latter case it may be due to development of abnormal arterio-venous shunts.

Measurements of brain oxygenation based on sampling of jugular venous blood are therefore useful only in limited circumstances where the brain is subject to global hypoxia or ischaemia.

With the advent of computerized X-ray tomography, photon emission tomography and now positron emission tomography, it is possible to measure glucose and oxygen consumption through the intact skull in any region of the human brain. This technique requires short-lived, cyclotron-produced isotopes and is consequently available in only a few centres.

CEREBRAL BLOOD FLOW

The brain has a rich, well-regulated blood supply. Four main arteries (carotid and vertebrals) feed into the circle of Willis, which is anatomically incomplete in 50% of cases. The basic pattern of blood supply to the brain (and spinal cord) is of ventral perforating branches to midline structures and dorsal encircling vessels which in turn give off penetrating vessels from the surface. In the 20% of patients in whom occlusion of one carotid artery results in contralateral hemiplegia the anastomotic circulation at the circle of Willis is functionally inadequate; in the remainder the collateral circulation is evidently sufficient. Although there are no large anastomotic vessels distal to the circle of Willis some cortical arterial anastomoses exist at the edge of the territories of distribution of the anterior, middle and posterior cerebral arteries. These are not functionally adequate because the cerebral circulation is particularly vulnerable to ischaemic hypoxia at the 'watershed' areas between the territories of the main distributing arteries.

The capillary network is of the continuous reticular type with a density which varies according to the tissue supplied. Grey matter, both cortical and deep, has a capillary density three to four times that of white matter.

Cerebral venous drainage is via two systems — a deep, periventricular system draining into the great vein of Galen, the straight sinus and torcular, and a superficial system draining via cortical veins into the sagittal and lateral sinuses. In addition, there are copious anastomoses between cerebral and cephalic venous systems at the base of the skull via the petrosal and cavernous sinuses and on the surface via the emissary veins of the skull. The principal intracranial-extracranial arterial anastomosis is between the ophthalmic branch of the internal carotid and the facial branches of the external carotid.

It is possible to measure cerebral blood flow (CBF) in the human subject by an ingenious modification of the Fick Principle. For the latter the quantity of a tracer taken up by or cleared from the brain and its concentration in arterial and cerebral venous blood require to be known. By using a metabolically inert, freely diffusible substance with a known partition coefficient between blood and brain it is possible to estimate the brain concentration of tracer from the cerebral venous level, provided that full tissue saturation has been achieved. Blood flow may then be expressed as flow per unit weight of brain, calculated solely from arterial and venous values of tracer. In the arterio-venous method total CBF is measured, so far as jugular venous blood is representative of cerebral venous blood. Suitable tracers for this technique are nitrous oxide, argon or hydrogen in low concentrations.

Using these techniques a normal CBF value of 50 ml $min^{-1}.100 \ g^{-1}$ is obtained, equivalent to about 750 ml min^{-1} in a normal adult brain. This is 3 times resting myocardial blood flow but only 60% of resting renal blood now. As blood flow falls progressively, a series of thresholds of dysfunction and disorder is crossed: the first is the threshold for neuroelectrical dysfunction at 20 $ml.min^{-1}.100 \ g^{-1}$; at 15 $ml.min^{-1}.100 \ g^{-1}$ potassium begins to leave the cell and at 10 $ml.min^{-1}.100 \ g^{-1}$ brain oedema begins to form as the cell membrane pump mechanisms fail and calcium ions enter the neuronal cell body, triggering off a series of processes that produce free oxygen radicals that are destructive to the cell membrane.

If the normal cerebral arterio-venous oxygen content difference is 6 ml/100 ml cerebral metabolic rate or uptake of oxygen ($CMRO_2$) can be derived from the product of blood flow and arterio-venous difference, thus:

$$CMRO_2 = CBF \times AVD = \frac{50 \times 6}{100}$$

$$= 3 \text{ ml } O_2.min^{-1}.100 \ g^{-1}$$

This value is one and one-half times resting myocardial oxygen consumption and three times renal oxygen consumption. When the value of $CMRO_2$ throughout the brain is reduced below 1 ml min^{-1} 100 g^{-1} in the whole brain, coma occurs and if not drug-induced, death will follow cessation of spontaneous respiration. Cerebral metabolic rates for glucose, amino acids, ketone bodies, lactate and pyruvate and many other substances can be calculated by the same technique. Since all derive from measurements from jugular venous blood, however, considerable caution has to be exercised in interpretation in patients who may have focal derangements of cerebral blood flow and metabolism.

By using gamma-emitting radioisotopes of inert gas tracers which can be monitored in the brain by multiple external radiation detectors, cerebral tissue concentrations of tracer can be measured and cerebral venous values calculated. If the cerebral washout of isotope is measured following an intracarotid bolus injection, arterial concentration of isotope during washout will be zero provided the chosen tracer is rapidly eliminated by the lungs and tracer recirculation is minimal. $^{133}Xenon$ gas dissolved in saline is an inert, freely diffusible tracer which has these properties. Since concentration of tracer in the brain, arterial and cerebral venous blood can be measured, assumed and calculated respectively, all factors for the Fick Equation are known, permitting a solution in terms of volume of blood flowing through a unit weight of brain per minute. By placing multiple shielded external radiation detectors around the head, a multiregional 'map' of cerebral blood measurements can be obtained.

If cerebral washout curves and the expired air curve of radioisotope concentration are monitored during and after a period of inhalation of $^{133}Xenon$ gas, the head curves can be corrected for recirculated isotope and regional cerebral blood flow calculated using a small computer. This atraumatic method of measuring regional cerebral blood flow is the most widely used today.

If cerebral blood flow is measured by externally detected isotope clearance methods, when the clearance curve of radioactive tracer from the brain is plotted graphically it can be seen that in normal individuals the washout curve is that of a two compartment system in which one component has a fast flow of 75–100 $ml.min^{-1}.100 \ g^{-1}$ and the other a much slower flow of 20–25 $ml.min^{-1}.100 \ g^{-1}$. These flow rates correspond to the relative degrees of vascularity of grey and white matter, and it is generally agreed that they represent flow in these two tissues. When the brain is damaged, however, or when overall slowing of the cerebral circulation has occurred it may be no longer possible to distinguish these two flow components clearly and most workers prefer to express cerebral blood flow as an average value regardless of the estimated proportions of grey or white matter flow.

Control of cerebral blood flow

Although the exact mechanism by which blood flow is adapted to the needs of different areas of the brain is not known, there is now good evidence that such local adap-

Table 13.5 Factors affecting cerebral blood flow

Decrease	Increase
Hypocapnia	Hypercapnia
Hyperoxia	Hypoxia
Hypothermia	Hyperthermia
Hypothyroidism	Hyperthyroidism
Barbiturates	REM sleep
Neuroleptanalgesics	Volatile anaesthetic agents

tation occurs and the general responses of the cerebral circulation to many physiological and pharmacological stimuli are now well established (Table 13.5).

Interregional variation and local control of blood flow

By using multichannel radioisotope detector systems in man, or multiple implanted blood flow probes in animals, selective increases in blood flow can be recorded in areas of the brain which are physiologically stimulated, e.g. the lateral geniculate nucleus or occipital cortex during photic stimulation, or the motor cortex during contralateral arm exercise. Anaesthesia appears to abolish or attenuate such interregional flow changes. It appears, therefore, that cerebral blood flow is highly adapted to fulfil local neuronal metabolic requirements.

Arterial blood pressure

In the range of mean arterial pressure 60–140 mmHg the brain has a well-developed capacity for maintenance of cerebral blood flow within a narrow normal range. When arterial pressure falls, cerebral arteries and arterioles dilate, vascular resistance is reduced and flow returns rapidly (within seconds) to normal. During moderate increases in arterial pressure, vasoconstriction occurs in the resistance vessels and blood flow remains constant. The exact mechanism of this regulatory process is not known but probably resides in the cerebral arteriolar muscular coat. On this basis it is generally referred to as 'autoregulation' since the mechanism is intrinsic to the brain. This is only partly true, however, for there is now evidence that this myogenic mechanism is 'set' by both neurogenic and metabolic factors at different levels of the cerebrovascular tree, with neurogenic factors active proximally on extra-parenchymal vessels and metabolic effects acting on the small vessels within the brain.

When arterial pressure falls below 60 mmHg further vasodilation is not possible and CBF falls and produces cerebral ischaemia. When arterial pressure is severely raised it appears that cerebral resistance vessels can no longer contain the pressure and CBF increases abruptly, a process termed 'breakthrough of autoregulation'. Autoregulation within the normal pressure range is impaired or abolished by a variety of insults including brain trauma,

ischaemia and hypoxia and also by hypercapnia when there is a more powerful vasodilator stimulus. The clinical implications are considerable, e.g. a patient with a head injury (and impaired autoregulation) will be less able to withstand arterial hypotension due to other injuries.

With information on cerebral blood flow, arterial and cerebral venous pressure, it is possible to derive values for cerebral vascular resistance (CVR) because the difference between arterial and cerebral venous pressure is the cerebral perfusion (CPP). Thus:

$$CVR = \frac{CPP}{CBF}$$

$$= \frac{\text{Arterial} - \text{cerebral venous pressure}}{CBF}$$

The value of cerebral venous pressure that is required is, however, not jugular venous pressure, but that in the veins within the cranial cavity. This is difficult to measure directly but fortunately is closely approximated by the intracranial pressure (ICP). When ICP increases, cerebral venous rises in a parallel manner, remaining 1–4 mmHg higher than ICP. Therefore:

$$CVR = \frac{\text{Arterial} - \text{intracranial pressure}}{CBF}$$

$$= \frac{100 - 10}{50} = 1.8 \text{ mmHg} \cdot 100 \text{ g}^{-1} \cdot \text{ml}^{-1} \cdot \text{min}^{-1}$$

Carbon dioxide

This is probably the most potent physiological stimulus to the cerebral circulation. CBF doubles as arterial P_{CO_2} rises from 5.3–10.6 kPa (40–80 mmHg), and halves when arterial P_{CO_2} falls from 5.3–2.7 kPa (40–20 mmHg). If hyperventilation is taken to lower levels of P_{CO_2} there is little further reduction in CBF, but CSF lactate values increase and there is cerebral dysfunction, manifest by drowsiness and EEG slowing, that can be reversed by administration of oxygen. It has been proposed, therefore, that profound hyperventilation causes cerebral tissue hypoxia and that hypoxic cerebral vasodilatation (q.v.) is counteracting the vasoconstrictor effects of hypocapnia. Evidence that such hypoxia can proceed to structural damage is lacking and the dangers of hyperventilation have probably been overstressed. The cerebral circulation is at its most sensitive to variations in arterial P_{CO_2} around the normal range. The effect of CO_2 is probably mediated by changes in extracellular pH round the cerebral resistance vessels in the parenchyma. If this fluid is made acid using a micropipette technique local arterial vasodilatation occurs and if the extracellular fluid is made alkaline the appropriate vessels constrict.

Responsiveness of cerebral vessels to changes in arterial P_{CO_2} is attenuated and eventually lost when the brain is damaged by trauma or ischaemia or when competing vasodilator stimuli are present, e.g. severe hypoxia or arterial hypotension.

Oxygen

Changes in arterial oxygen tension within the range 6.7 to 66.5 kPa (50–500 mmHg) have little effect on cerebral vessels. When P_{O_2} in arterial blood falls below 6.7 kPa there is a pronounced cerebral vasodilatation. This corresponds to the point in the oxygen dissociation curve where saturation levels fall steeply with decreasing oxygen tension and it can be presumed that the vasodilatory mechanism is aimed at the preservation of an adequate oxygen delivery to the brain.

The high partial pressures of oxygen which can be achieved by administration of 100% O_2 under hyperbaric conditions have more complex effects on the cerebral circulation; when arterial P_{O_2} rises from 106.4 to 159.6 kPa (800–1200 mmHg) there is a mild cerebral vasoconstriction, even when arterial P_{CO_2} and blood pressure are constant, and CBF falls by 20–25%. With higher levels of arterial P_{O_2} (more than 159.6 kPa) CBF is unchanged. It has been proposed that such high levels of oxygen result in metabolic damage of brain cells possibly causing a rise in P_{CO_2} in brain tissue and in the extracellular fluid of the brain and thus counteracting the vasoconstrictor effects of oxygen. Administration of carbon dioxide will certainly reverse the vasoconstrictor properties of oxygen. As with blood pressure and carbon dioxide effects on the cerebral circulation, the responses to oxygen excess and lack are abolished by brain trauma, brain oedema and other forms of damage.

Anaesthesia

Anaesthetic agents may affect cerebral blood flow either by direct action on the cerebral vessels or, secondarily, either by depressing brain metabolism or by altering blood pressure or intracranial pressure. Barbiturate agents such as sodium thiopentone or pentobarbitone reduce CBF. Volatile agents such as halothane or trichloroethylene cause cerebral vasodilatation.

In addition, agents which depress respiration, such as morphine or pethidine, may produce secondary effects on the cerebral blood vessels through elevation of arterial P_{CO_2}.

Autonomic influences

Stimulation of the sympathetic chain in the neck causes a small decrease in resting CBF and sympathectomy may produce a small increase in flow by changing the calibre of larger cerebral vessels. These effects are slight, however, when compared with the effect of carbon dioxide on the intraparenchymal vessels. It has been suggested that the role of the parasympathetic and sympathetic innervation of cerebral vessels, which undoubtedly exists, is to modify the response to changes in arterial blood pressure, P_{CO_2} and P_{O_2} than with haemorrhagic hypotension. The threshold above which arterial hypertension produces 'breakthrough' is increased during sympathetic stimulation. Patients with chronic hypertension show the same elevation of both the lower and upper autoregulation thresholds.

While it is agreed generally that the effects of the peripheral autonomic nervous system on cerebral blood flow are relatively slight (as compared with effects of CO_2 for example) much current interest revolves around a central autonomic pathway from brain stem into the cerebral hemispheres. The central noradrenergic pathway which emerges from the locus caeruleus seems to be involved not only with the cerebrovascular response to CO_2 but possibly regulation of water transport across cerebral capillaries as well.

Intracranial pressure

The interactions of CBF and intracranial pressure are complex because an increase in CBF with cerebral vasodilatation may produce an increase in ICP, and in other circumstances a rise in ICP can produce a fall in CBF. This is considered in more detail in the section on intracranial pressure (q.v.).

CEREBROSPINAL FLUID AND BRAIN WATER

Cerebrospinal fluid (CSF) is produced largely by the choroid plexuses within the brain and circulates through the ventricular system from the lateral ventricles via the foramina of Monro, third ventricle and aqueduct of Sylvius (iter) to the fourth ventricle, through the foramina of Luschka into the cerebellopontine cisterns and to a lesser extent via the midline foramen of Majendie into the cisterna magna. Subarachnoid CSF may then circulate round the spinal cord towards the lower end of the dural sac or upwards to the ambient cisterns at the level of the mid-brain and tentorial notch. After passing this isthmus fluid passes up over the cerebral hemispheres to be absorbed into the cerebral venous system via arachnoid granulations in or close to the superior sagittal sinus (Fig. 13.1.).

The production of CSF is a complex process, requiring energy, so that production rates are reduced in hypothermia, old age and after administration of several drugs, notably acetazoleamide, frusemide and probably digoxin. CSF production is not apparently affected by CSF pressure

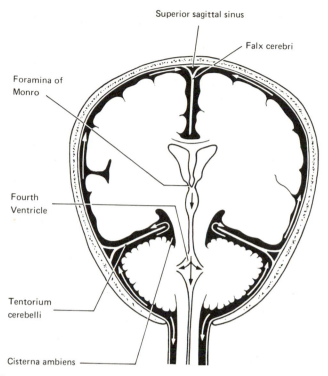

Superior sagittal sinus

Falx cerebri

Foramina of Monro

Fourth Ventricle

Tentorium cerebelli

Cisterna ambiens

Fig. 13.1 Normal CSF circulation. CSF passes through the foramina of Monro into the third ventricle aqueduct and fourth ventricle from whence it reaches the subarachnoid space. The fluid in the cranial cavity circulates upwards through the cisterna ambiens between the tentorium cerebelli and the mid-brain, over the surface of the hemisphere to the superior sagittal sinus.

anisms. Disturbances of the CSF content of protein, sugar, electrolytes and cells are of considerable diagnostic value. Elevation of CSF protein is seen below a spinal CSF block, and in the presence of certain tumours and in most inflammatory processes. In bacterial or viral infections, the cell content of CSF rises also. Polymorphs predominate in acute bacterial infection, mononuclear cells in viral and chronic bacterial infections. In tuberculous meningitis and severe carcinomatous meningitis, the sugar content of CSF is reduced, sometimes to undetectable levels. When the blood sugar level is increased, CSF sugar rises also. The acid-base balance of CSF is also finely regulated bearing in mind that there is little buffering capacity in this fluid. Evidence continues to accumulate that CSF pH, normally in the range of 7.30–7.35, i.e. more acid than arterial blood and not quite as acid as cerebral venous blood, is at least partially responsible for regulating respiration and the calibre of small intraparenchymal cerebral resistance vessels (Fig. 13.2.).

The brain has a high water content, 80% in grey matter and just under 70% in the white matter where the fat content is higher. Water is contained not only in the cells but also in the extracellular or brain interstitial space. This latter volume is now thought to be as much as 10% of total intracranial volume; previous lower estimates were artefactual due to swelling of astrocytes in the processes of fixation. Brain extracellular fluid content is thought to be in equilibrium with CSF so that some investigators regard the CSF pool as an extension of the brain extracellular fluid space with a role equivalent to that of the lymphatic system in other organs. A well-developed barrier system (mainly located at the tight junction between adjacent cerebral capillary endothelial cells) limits the passage of substances (and water) from the cerebral blood pool into the extracellular fluid space, so that regulation of the content of the extracellular fluid exists. Even within the CSF space, however, marked differences exist both in the content of

and in a normal adult remains constant at 0.3–0.5 ml/min until ICP becomes so high that the brain becomes ischaemic, at which point CSF production is reduced. Absorption of CSF is, however, strongly related to CSF pressure, in particular to the pressure difference between CSF and venous blood at the absorption site and it has been proposed that CSF and its contained protein and cellular elements pass into the bloodstream by bulk flow via pressure-sensitive, valvular tubules.

The volume of CSF, which is about 150 ml in normal man, is determined by the balance struck between production and absorption and, as will be seen, this is one of the several factors which determine intracranial pressure. The CSF volume is decreased by space-occupying processes within the cranium. It may be increased (hydrocephalus) either by an increase in production rate (exceptionally rare) or by blockage of the CSF circulatory processes which lead to CSF absorption, within the narrower portions of the ventricular system (e.g. foramina of Monro, aqueduct), in the subarachnoid space at the base of the brain or mid-brain, or at the level of the tubules leading to the venous system.

The content of CSF is tightly controlled by barrier mechanisms which prevent large molecules escaping from the choroid plexus vessels and by active, transport mech-

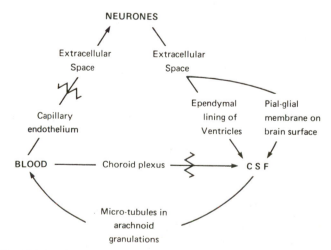

NEURONES

Extracellular Space

Extracellular Space

Capillary endothelium

Ependymal lining of Ventricles

Pial-glial membrane on brain surface

BLOOD —— Choroid plexus ⇒ C S F

Micro-tubules in arachnoid granulations

Fig. 13.2 Barriers in the CNS.

solutes and in acid-base status between ventricular, cisternal and lumbar subarachnoid CSF.

Clearly the CSF system is complex with multiple functions ranging from the mechanical buffering of the CNS from trauma and the equilibration of pressure differentials in the craniospinal axis to the finely tuned metabolic regulation of specific areas in the brain. It is a system which above most others must be thought of in terms of dynamic equilibria with respect to content, volume and pressure.

INTRACRANIAL PRESSURE

The contents of the craniospinal axis, invested by the relatively rigid dural membrane, are largely fluid. Brain and spinal cord tissue (approximately 75% water) accounts for 70% of total volume; intravascular blood volume, CSF and extracellular fluid each account for about 10%. In the adult, the cranial dura being applied to the rigid skull cannot expand; distension is possible in the child with unfused cranial sutures. The spinal dura can expand into the spinal epidural space displacing blood from the epidural venous plexus.

Since cranial contents are fluid they are also incompressible. Additions to cranial volume must therefore be compensated by expulsion of an equivalent volume of blood or CSF from the cranium or the intracranial pressure (ICP) will rise. This proposition is generally known as the Monro-Kellie Doctrine.

The ICP can conveniently be recorded from the CSF space (lateral ventricle, cisterna magna, lumbar subarachnoid space), but recordings are also possible from transducers introduced directly into the cerebral extradural or subdural spaces. Under normal conditions the pressure ranges from 0 to 10 mmHg (0–136 mmH$_2$O) relative to the right atrium in the recumbent position and the pressure waveform exhibits arterial and respiratory pulsations (the latter related to changes in intrathoracic and central venous pressure) (Fig. 13.3). Under pathological conditions, however, ICP may rise over 100 mmHg until it becomes equal to arterial pressure.

The causes of raised intracranial pressure can be related to increases in the volume of one or other of the normal intracranial constituents or an addition to them such as tumour, haematoma or abscess. Increases in blood volume may be caused by arterial vasodilatation (hypoxia, hypercapnia) or to venous obstruction. Increases in CSF volume (hydrocephalus) are produced by ventricular or subarachnoid blockage. Increases in brain water content (brain oedema) may be produced by vascular damage (ischaemia, trauma, around tumours and abscesses) or by swelling of cells or myelin sheaths (severe hypoxia, tissue poisons) (Fig. 13.4.).

Multiple causes for raised intracranial pressure are frequently present, for example in oedema surrounding tumours, and the net effect of such increases in volume on intracranial pressure is a function of the total increase in volume and the degree of volumetric compensation which can be produced by expulsion of CSF and blood from the cranial cavity. It has been estimated that 65% of the volume compensation available for an expanding intracranial mass is provided by expulsion of CSF into the spinal canal and dural distension into the spinal epidural space. The remaining 35% comes from compression of cerebral blood and fluid volume. These compensatory processes are of limited capacity however, and the intracranial pressure-volume relationship can be represented by a curve which is flat at first then inflected towards the pressure axis more and more steeply as the compensatory mechanisms are exhausted (Fig. 13.5). When a patient reaches the steep part of the pressure-volume curve an addition of only 1 ml to the intracranial contents may increase ICP by as much as 15 mmHg. Thus, the pressure-volume relationship determines the extent of increase in ICP which will result from any given change in volume.

The clinical effects of increased intracranial pressure are difficult to dissociate from other effects produced by the process which causes the increase in pressure. Swelling of the optic nerve head (papilloedema) is a direct effect of raised intracranial pressure, and if unchecked may progress to optic atrophy and blindness. Headaches and vomiting may be related more to brain shift (q.v.) or dural distension than to raised ICP per se. Bradycardia and elevation of the arterial pressure are almost certainly related to brain shift and are late events.

When ICP is increased, subarachnoid cerebral venous pressure rises to maintain venous pressure just above ICP (otherwise, the thin-walled veins would collapse). In this way, effective cerebral perfusion pressure falls during intracranial hypertension. When ICP reaches the level of arterial pressure, cerebral perfusion pressure falls to zero and cerebral blood flow ceases, producing brain death. This is the mode of death in many patients with severe head injury and subarachnoid haemorrhage.

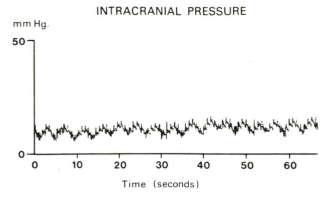

INTRACRANIAL PRESSURE

mm Hg.

Time (seconds)

Fig. 13.3 Recording of intracranial pressure from a catheter placed in the lateral ventricle, showing both arterial and respiratory fluctuations in pressure.

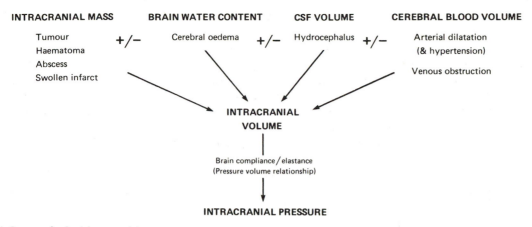

Fig. 13.4 Causes of raised intracranial pressure.

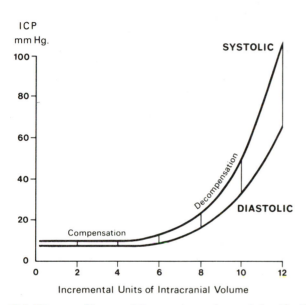

Fig. 13.5 Diagram of intracranial pressure — volume relationship. The curve is flat at first, with no rise in ICP despite addition of volume to the intracranial cavity because of compensatory shifts of CSF and blood. As compensation becomes exhausted and the process continues, both mean ICP and the pulse pressure of ICP begin to rise steeply and to resemble an arterial pressure record.

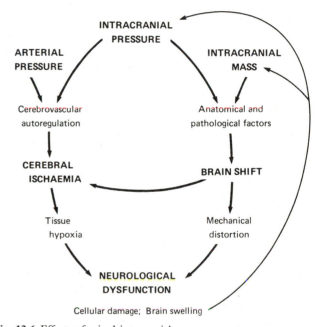

Fig. 13.6 Effects of raised intracranial pressure.

Smaller increases in ICP are tolerated without reductions in flow, however, by the same autoregulatory mechanism which protects the brain against falling blood pressure. A critical point is reached, however, when ICP is within 40 mmHg of arterial pressure; beyond this point CBF is reduced (Fig. 13.6). If autoregulation is already impaired CBF may be decreased to critical levels by lesser degrees of intracranial hypertension.

The relationship between ICP and CBF therefore is a double one. Primary increases in CBF are associated with a passive increase in ICP, the extent of which is a function of the volume of blood added to the cranium and of the steepness of the pressure-volume curve at that point. Primary increases in ICP are associated with a reduction in CBF when ICP is within 40 mmHg of arterial pressure, or at an earlier stage when autoregulation is disturbed.

BRAIN COMPRESSION, BRAIN SHIFT AND PRESSURE CONES

Many sources of increased intracranial pressure, e.g. tumour, abscess, haematoma, brain contusion or infarct, are focal, generating a disturbance in one area of the brain.

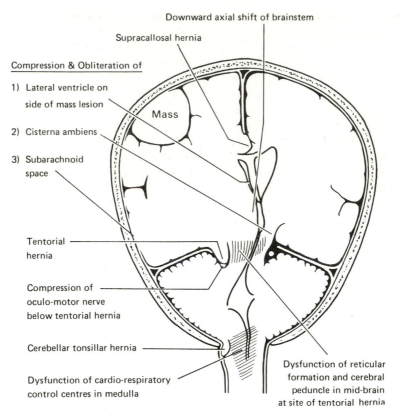

Fig. 13.7 Effect of brain compression by a supratentorial mass lesion.

Since the brain is essentially incompressible, this introduces another variable into the set of factors which determine overall brain function in disease states. As a localized lesion expands, the surrounding brain becomes deformed and shifts away from the mass towards the exit foramen of the skull, the foramen magnum. Brain shifts occur in a fairly predictable way and produce certain recognisable clinical signs, many of which have in the past been erroneously attributed solely to increased intracranial pressure (Fig. 13.7).

When a unilateral mass expands in the supratentorial compartment, brain shifts occur in two directions. Brain in the affected hemisphere will herniate under the falx, and in doing so may entrap the anterior cerebral artery(ies) producing contralateral or bilateral leg weakness. This, then, is one of the causes of 'cerebral paraplegia' which may lead the physician to seek in vain for a spinal lesion to explain the patient's problem. The second type of brain herniation is of more immediate clinical importance. As a unilateral mass expands and compensatory volume is used up by compression of the subarachnoid space and the lateral ventricle, the medial portion of the ipsilateral temporal lobe starts to herniate through the tentorial hiatus with dramatic effects on brain function. With a lateral type of herniation the mid-brain is compressed producing loss of consciousness due to distortion of the central reticular

formation and contralateral hemiplegia and decerebrate rigidity due to pressure on the cerebral peduncle. As the compression proceeds, decerebrate rigidity becomes bilateral. With this lateral type of herniation, which occurs with temporoparietal masses, the advancing temporal lobe impinges on the oculomotor (third cranial) nerve producing an ipsilateral pupillary dilatation with loss of light reflex, ptosis and lateral deviation of the eye (due to unopposed action of the sixth cranial nerve). When the compressing lesion is bilateral or frontal or occipital the tentorial herniation is posteriorly placed, resulting also in depression of consciousness but accompanied by bilateral ptosis and failure of upward gaze due to compression of the tectal (quadrigeminal) plate, particularly the superior colliculi. This most valuable clinical sign is also present in severe hydrocephalus. These processes may be variously termed tentorial herniation, temporal lobe herniation or tentorial coning.

As the process of brain compression progresses the cerebellum is pushed down by pressure on the tentorium from above, and the brain stem is also forced caudally towards the foramen magnum. The cerebellar tonsils impact in the foramen magnum (tonsillar herniation), compressing the medulla oblongata and the vascular supply of the entire brain stem is imperilled since the deep ventral perforating branches from the basilar artery are stretched. This combination produces the well-known bradycardia and arterial hypertension of the 'Cushing vasopressor response' and also produces respiratory irregularity and ultimately apnoea. Death in unrelieved brain compression is almost invariably due to respiratory arrest. Brain compression must be relieved within minutes if spontaneous ventilation is to return. Institution of artificial ventilation without relief of the brain compression may result in continued cardiac function for many hours but death is inevitable. For this reason patients who suffer severe inoperable brain compression, e.g. due to overwhelming subarachnoid haemorrhage, are often considered as organ donors. What then constitutes total irreversible loss of brain function ('brain death') must be clearly defined and will be discussed in the next section.

When the origin of brain compression is in the posterior cranial fossa there may be little warning before total apnoea occurs since none of the warning signs of pupillary dilatation or gradual depression of consciousness, or hemiparesis and decerebration will be present prior to tonsillar herniation (also known as cerebellar coning).

Appreciation of the dynamics of brain compression is of importance if the urgency of diagnosis and treatment is to be understood. To await bradycardia, arterial hypertension and irregular respiration is to permit the preterminal stage of brain compression to be reached in which minutes, rather than hours, count. The finding of a fixed, dilated pupil means that the brain has already herniated through the tentorial notch. The cardinal observation is that of depression of the conscious level, and this entails sequential, objective neurological assessment.

As an intracranial mass first expands, ICP is initially elevated equally throughout the craniospinal axis, but as tentorial or cerebellar tonsillar herniation occurs, the free transmission of ICP in the CSF spaces is lost. Pressure differentials develop in which supratentorial pressure becomes progressively higher than that recorded in the lumbar subarachnoid space, which may actually return to normal. This differential or gradient will actually serve to accelerate the process of brain herniation. Lumbar puncture in such circumstances is not only misleading because of an erroneous recording of low ICP but also dangerous since continued leakage of CSF through the small hole in the lumbar arachnoid will further reduce pressure below the tentorial or foramen magnum block and encourage further herniation. Thus fatal 'coning' may occur immediately or more often several hours after lumbar puncture in patients with intracranial mass lesions.

In patients with mass lesions who are close to decompensation and at the steep portion of the intracranial pressure volume curve the addition of any factor which increases volume of the intracranial constituents such as hypoxia, hypercapnia, intracranial haemorrhage or brain swelling may suffice to tip the balance towards massive supratentorial intracranial hypertension and brain hernia-

tion. Neurological deterioration in such cases is often so sudden that the clinician frequently, but usually erroneously, invokes haemorrhage into the cerebral lesion to explain the dramatic clinical change. These patients require the closest of observation, the best of intensive care and urgent decompression.

Relief of raised intracranial pressure and brain shift

Knowledge of the processes responsible for intracranial hypertension can be turned to therapeutic profit in devising methods for reducing increased ICP and alleviating brain shift. Surgical decompression can be achieved by removing mass lesions or by removing the overlying skull and allowing the brain to bulge into the bone defect. This will reduce ICP and correct brain shift, although bony decompression is now frowned upon as it tends to encourage further swelling of the involved brain. If surgical decompression is not feasible, reduction of ICP can be achieved by withdrawing CSF from the lateral ventricles or by inducing cerebral vasoconstriction by hypocapnia (hyperventilation). Brain water content can be reduced either by intravenous hypertonic agents (urea, mannitol, glycerol) or by powerful glucocorticoids (betamethasone, dexamethasone). The non-surgical forms of decompression have less effect on brain shift, particularly hyperventilation and hypertonic solutions, which exert most effect on normal brain. In these critically ill patients, however, the withdrawal of only a few millilitres of fluid from the cranium may produce dramatic lowering of ICP and improvement in neurological function.

CONSCIOUSNESS AND COMA

Consciousness may be thought of as including the phenomena of arousal and awareness, the latter implying the capacity to recognize changes in the external environment and to respond appropriately. Its anatomical substrate is the ascending reticular formation of the brain stem and the complex interconnections between this system and the thalamus, hypothalamus and cerebral cortex. Sleep is a special state, incompletely understood, in which increased activity of part of the reticular activating system produces the eye closure and synchronisation of the EEG typical of sleep. During sleep, however, episodes occur during which the EEG is desynchronized, cerebral vasodilatation occurs and there are rapid spontaneous eye movements. Intracranial pressure tends to increase at such times, and if the patient already has intracranial hypertension the further rise in ICP may be severe. In patients undergoing prolonged monitoring of ICP, this is twice as likely to increase at night as by day. For this reason, continuous monitoring of ICP must always include at least one overnight recording.

Table 13.6 The Glasgow Coma Scale

Testing	Function	Response
Arousal	Eye opening	Spontaneous To command To pain None*
Awareness	Motor response (best obtained from arms)	Obeys commands Localises pain* Flexor withdrawal* Abnormal flexion* Extension* None*
Awareness	Verbal response	Fully orientated Disorientated Words only Sounds only* None*

* = within the definition of coma

Loss of consciousness (coma) can be produced by general depression of all cerebral neurones due to ischaemia/hypoxia or toxins, by direct damage to the reticular formation, by brain stem haemorrhage for example, or by deafferention of the brain stem by widespread subcortical damage as occurs in high speed acceleration/deceleration head injury.

Clinical evaluation of the state of consciousness should include assessments of arousal, awareness and brain stem function. Arousal is indicated by eye opening, awareness by the best motor response to command or pain of which the patient is capable and by the verbal response. These have been assembled into the widely-used Glasgow Coma Scale (Table 13.6). On this scale, coma is defined as a state in which there is no eye opening to any stimulus, inability to obey commands or to utter recognizable words. Brainstem function is tested by the pupillary light responses and the eye movement reflexes in response to passive head rotation (oculocephalic reflex) and irrigation of cold water in the ears (oculovestibular reflex).

THE CONCEPT AND DEFINITION OF BRAIN DEATH

Two recent developments have led to a demand for definitive criteria of the state of severe, irreversible loss of brain function in which life would be extinct but for the use of life support systems, in particular artificial ventilation. These are the advent of the modern, intensive care unit and the success of organ transplantation, particularly of kidneys. It is now possible to support the cardiovascular system for many hours after all other brain function has ceased, eventually to a stage of liquefaction necrosis of the brain, hypothermia, arterial hypotension and renal failure before cardiac arrest finally occurs. Fruitless prolongation of intensive supportive care when all hope of recovery has passed is undesirable because it is distressing to the family of the patient, wasteful of the limited resources of the intensive care unit and renders body organs unfit for use in transplantation. A decision should be made, therefore, to terminate mechanical ventilation at a stage when the cardiovascular system is still capable of producing adequate organ perfusion.

The following should be regarded as the essential criteria necessary to make this decision. The cause of brain damage must be established, e.g. trauma or intracranial haemorrhage, and the condition considered beyond treatment. The possibility of hypothermia or drug ingestion must be excluded. Spontaneous respiration must be demonstrably and persistently absent. This is best demonstrated by allowing the arterial P_{CO_2} to rise by over 5.3 kPa (40 mmHg) during temporary cessation of mechanical ventilation. Severe hypoxaemia is prevented by airway insufflation with 100% oxygen which provides adequate oxygenation by diffusion during the apnoeic period. Clinical examination demonstrates the absence of supratentorial and brain stem function. There should be total absence of response to visual or auditory stimuli and no response from facial muscles or arms to painful stimuli applied to supraorbital ridges, sternum, arms and nail bed of fingers. There must be no response on testing brain stem reflexes — no pupillary light reaction, no corneal reflex, no oculocephalic response (eye movement in response to head turning), no oculovestibular response (eye movement in response to irrigation of both ears with ice-cold saline), and no gag or cough reflex (to manipulation of the endotracheal tube). When all these responses are absent there may still be some lower limb movement in response to painful stimulation. This does not imply cerebral activity but rather release from it with activity in spinal reflex arcs. On the same basis tendon reflexes in the limbs may persist after all supratentorial and upper brain stem function has ceased.

These clinical criteria, when verified twice by two physicians, are sufficient for the diagnosis of brain death and a decision to terminate mechanical respiration. Corroborative evidence is not essential but may be sought in various ways. Most commonly employed are the demonstration of complete absence of cerebral activity on an EEG recorded at maximum gain, and absence of evoked responses (visual, auditory, somatosensory). If radio-opaque dye is injected into the carotid arteries it may fail to enter the cerebral circulation or may pass through extremely slowly — a transit time of more than 15 seconds is said to be critical. Arrest or slowing of the cerebral circulation is usually ascribed to severe intracranial hypertension though other factors such as capillary obstruction by red cells sludging or astrocytic swelling may also play a part. If a radioisotope tracer is injected into the internal carotid artery it may either fail to reach the brain or fail to clear from it. In the rare cases where brain death has been determined clinically but where cerebral blood flow appears to persist at normal levels, measurements of jugular venous blood show high levels of oxygen tension, saturation and content with correspondingly low values of arterio-venous oxygen difference and cerebral oxygen uptake. Reduction of $CMRO_2$ from 3 to 1 ml min^{-1} 100 g^{-1} has been cited as critical.

Finally it must be emphasized that when deep coma is due to hypothermia or barbiturate or other drug overdosage *none* of these clinical or laboratory criteria of brain death are valid. With intensive supportive care and detailed monitoring of body systems clinical recovery is possible even from the deepest of drug comas and vigorous therapy must *always* be based on this premise.

SPINAL CORD

The contents of the spinal canal — cord, cauda equina and nerve roots — are vulnerable to compression within the bony confines of the canal in the same way that the brain may be compressed within the skull. The spinal cord may also be damaged by direct trauma, by vascular lesions — haemorrhagic and ischaemic — and by various disease processes. Because of the relatively simpler organization of the fibre tracts and cell groups in the spinal cord, areas of damage may be fairly accurately localized by neurological examination. In general, a lesion of the spinal cord can cause two sets of signs; those due to long tract interruption consisting of an upper motor neurone lesion and sensory loss below the level of the lesion, and less frequently, a lower motor neurone lesion and girdle pain due to root and anterior horn involvement at the level of the lesion. Voluntary movement is lost below a complete cord lesion, but muscle tone and tendon reflexes are increased, although in acute cord lesions there may be a temporary period of several days during which all muscle activity is absent. Below a root lesion, voluntary power, tone and tendon reflexes are all lost. Fasciculation and wasting of involved muscles develops later.

In partial lesions of the spinal cord, knowledge of the disposition of the main fibre tracts is essential for localization (Fig. 13.8). Motor fibres from the left cerebral hemisphere decussate at the level of the pyramids and pass down the lateral white columns on the right side of the spinal cord, the lower motor neurones connected with these fibres pass out in the anterior roots of the right side of the cord. In parallel, the proprioceptive fibres from the right leg enter the right posterior roots, ascend in the right posterior white columns and cross at the sensory decussation in the medulla. Thus sensory and motor pathways concerned with movement of trunk and limbs follow the same pattern in their route in the cord. By contrast, sensory fibre pathways for pain, temperature and light touch entering the right posterior root cross the midline

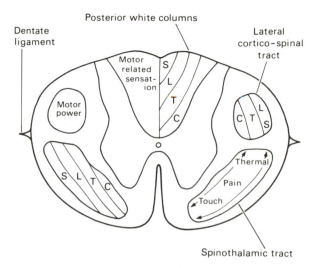

Fig. 13.8 Section of cervical cord. Distribution of main motor and sensory tracts.

in the anterior white decussation immediately, or within three segments, to reach the left anterior lateral quadrant of the cord and ascend on the left side of the cord in the spino-thalamic tract. This pathway is considered in more detail in the section on pain.

Laterally placed lesions of, or compressing, the cord produce the Brown-Séquard syndrome in which motor power and proprioception are lost on the side of the lesion and pain, thermal sensation and light touch are lost on the opposite side. Often the neurological picture is incomplete, but the basic pattern of most motor loss on one side and most sensory loss on the other is very common. Anterior cord lesions affect pain, thermal and touch sensation predominantly, while posterior lesions mainly alter proprioception distal to the lesion. Small central cord lesions selectively impair pain and temperature since these fibres are closest to the centre of the cord at the anterior white decussation. Larger central cord lesions which involve touch fibres may still produce sparing of sacral sensation since these fibres lie most laterally in the spinothalamic tracts.

In the adult the bony spinal canal is much longer than the spinal cord. This means that there is an increasing discrepancy between bony and neurological levels of spinal lesions. Upper cervical cord segments are covered by the appropriate spinous processes. Cord segment T_2 is covered by the spine of C_6 vertebra, cord segment L_2 is covered by the spine of T_{10} and cord segment S_2 by the spine of T_{12}. The tip of the conus medullaris lies between L_1 and L_2 vertebral levels. This is why lumbar puncture is normally performed at $L_{3/4}$ or $L_{4/5}$ levels.

When the spinal lesion is at the level of the lower end of the spinal cord the neurological picture is more complex. This is because at this level the cord is surrounded by nerve roots which must run within the spinal canal for several segments before exiting at the root foramina. Down to a cord level of L_5 there may be a mixed picture of upper motor and lower motor neurone signs, or at lower levels a combination of impairment of bladder, bowel and sexual function with lower motor neurone signs. Lesions which cause compression of the nerve roots in the centre of the cauda equina, such as a central disc protrusion, produce a characteristic neurological picture which is all too often misdiagnosed. This consists of numbness confined to the 'saddle' area ($S_{2,3,4}$) and retention of urine; depending on how far lateral the compressing lesion extends there may or may not be signs in the legs. If surgical decompression is not carried out within hours of onset, bladder dysfunction is permanent even when motor power and sensation return to the limbs. Lateral lesions of the lower spinal canal produce the characteristic picture of sciatic pain with motor, sensory and reflex loss related to the involved root or roots. In 95% of cases of lumbar disc protrusion the involved levels are either $L_{4/5}$, compressing the L_5 root and causing sensory disturbance on the outer aspect of the lower leg and dorsum of foot and weakness of dorsiflexion of the foot and toes, or L_5/S_1, compressing the S_1 root and causing numbness of the outer border of the foot and depression of the ankle jerk.

The vascular supply of the spinal cord comes mainly from penetrating branches of the anterior spinal artery which supply the anterior two-thirds of the cross-sectional area of the cord (Fig. 13.9). The remaining posterior third is supplied by short branches from the encircling arteries which arise from the two posterior spinal arteries. Ischaemia may be limited to one or other territory resulting in loss of power, pain and temperature sensation but preservation of proprioception in anterior spinal artery occlusion, and the reverse picture when ischaemia affects the posterior vessels.

As the anterior and posterior spinal arteries pass down they receive blood from radicular arteries which are especially prominent at the mid-cervical, mid-thoracic and lower lumbar levels. The spinal cord is particularly susceptible to ischaemia at the watershed between these territories of vascular supply — in the upper thoracic and upper lumbar levels. Some of the syndromes of spinal cord damage which have been ascribed to cord compression in cervical spondylosis and spinal trauma may be related to spinal cord ischaemia. In the central cord syndrome, there is severe motor and sensory involvement of the arms with relative sparing of the lower limbs. Reference to figure 13.8 makes it clear why this should be the case. Figure 13.9 shows how anterior spinal artery ischaemia could explain this syndrome, a not uncommon sequel of hyperextension injuries of the neck. Spinal cord infarcts can result from damage to radicular arteries and may be a complication of aortography, dissecting aortic aneurysm or thoracotomy.

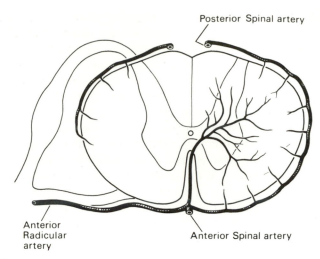

Fig. 13.9 Section of cervical cord. Arterial blood supply.

At the microvascular level the spinal cord circulation behaves in the same way as the cerebral circulation. The mean value for blood flow is lower because of the greater proportion of white matter to grey but the vessels dilate with hypercapnia and hypoxia as do cerebral vessels, and constant flow is preserved by an autoregulatory mechanism during moderate changes in arterial pressure. Elevations of spinal venous pressure act in the same way as elevations of intracranial pressure with preservation of blood flow by arterial dilatation as the effective perfusion pressure falls, again within physiological limits and provided that spinal cord damage has not impaired the autoregulatory mechanism.

PAIN

Pain, normally a protective mechanism, becomes a neurosurgical problem when it has ceased to act as a warning and becomes a clamant symptom which has begun to disable the patient; when simple analgesics fail to bring adequate or prolonged relief; and when medication controls pain only by depressing the level of consciousness to the point where the patient can no longer function normally. While surgery is sometimes employed to relieve pain arising within the nervous system (e.g. trigeminal neuralgia) it is most commonly used with the aim of producing analgesia in a part of the body afflicted by some intractable, often malignant pathology.

The surgical control of pain is an exercise in applied neuroanatomy and neurophysiology with the constraint that knowledge of the location and extent of pain pathways and the pain mechanisms in the CNS is incomplete. Nevertheless, understanding is growing and this is in no small part due to the experience gained from pain surgery.

Pain has been described as a modality in search of an

end organ. Although pain sensations can be shown to come from arborized endings in the skin these are not exclusive in transmitting pain. Excessive stimulation of any sensory receptor will ultimately be interpreted as pain and when pain has been present for a considerable time removal of the affected extremity may not remove the pain, which now appears to be 'imprinted' in some way in the pain pathway. Damage to peripheral nerves may also produce sensations of pain in the area served by the nerve. An extreme form of this is causalgia, often dramatically relieved by sympathectomy. Pain from viscera transmitted by sympathetic pathways initially may be referred to the somatic area served by the same segmental level — referred pain. Examples of referred pain include pain in the left arm or throat produced by cardiac ischaemia and diaphragmatic pain referred to the top of the shoulder (C3, 4). Damage within the brain itself may also result in pain in the limbs, 'thalamic pain' sometimes seen after cerebrovascular lesions is an example.

It was realised early in the history of pain surgery that the basic neuroanatomical model of sensory pathways was inadequate. Thus although the majority of 'pain fibres' ran in a certain tract or direction, a few exceptions to the rule could vitiate the results of surgery.

Somatic pain pathways are differentiated into those arising from the trunk and limbs reaching the brain via the spinal cord and those arising from the head which reach the brain via the cranial nerves, mainly the trigeminal, glossopharyngeal and vagus nerves. Visceral pain pathways are mainly sympathetic but parasympathetic nerves also carry many afferent fibres and may therefore transmit sensations although the capacity for such sensation to attain consciousness as pain may be limited.

Pain arising from the trunk and limbs is thought to reach the CNS by smaller poorly myelinated C and A delta fibres. The older concept of unmyelinated fibres is now outmoded — even the smallest fibres carry some investment of myelin, provided by Schwann cells in the periphery and by the oligodendroglia in the CNS. The sensory fibres have their cell body in the dorsal root ganglion and enter the spinal cord in the lateral bundle of the dorsal root and pass into Lissauer's zone. However, some fibres which transmit pain enter in the medial bundle and some may even enter the cord in the anterior motor root, a substantial proportion of which has recently been shown to consist of afferent fibres. Most fibres cross the substantia gelatinosa and enter the nucleus proprius of the posterior grey horn of the spinal cord and synapse with the second order neurones and processes which cross to the opposite side of the cord in the anterior white commissure. For the most part this crossover is achieved within three segments of the level of entry at the dorsal root. Some first order fibres may however ascend for a longer distance in Lissauer's tract on the side of entry prior to entering the posterior horn proper.

The bulk of the second order fibres after decussation ascend in the lateral spinothalamic tract in the anterior quadrant of the spinal cord. This tract is generally pictured as lying medial to the anterior spinocerebellar tract and to exhibit lamination with sacral fibres most posterolateral and cervical fibres anteromedial. There is also considered to be functional localisation with thermal sensory fibres lying most posterior, up to the level of the dentate ligament, pain fibres in the middle and light touch anteriorly, blending with the anterior spinothalamic tract. As the lateral spinothalamic tract ascends it moves dorsally to lie superficially on the posterolateral aspect of the medulla dorsal to the olive. At the level of the midbrain the tract lies just ventrolateral to the colliculi.

The lateral spinothalamic tract terminates in the thalamus. Most sensory fibres synapse in the ventral posterolateral nucleus of the thalamus, but pain fibres are thought to terminate in the centrum medianum. From the thalamus third order neurones communicate with the cortex.

The central pain pathway is much more diffuse than the above description implies. The entire anterior quadrant of the spinal cord is transversed by pain fibres, and the lateral spinothalamic tract gives off collaterals as it ascends to the tectum, tegmentum and reticular formation, some of which cross over the midline again.

Pain from the face travels with the fibres of the three divisions of the trigeminal nerve to the trigeminal ganglion. The sensory root from the trigeminal ganglion enters the lateral aspect of the pons. Pain and temperature fibres travel caudally into the ipsilateral trigeminospinal tract, lying superficially on the dorsolateral aspect of the medulla in line with Lissauer's tract. The fibres synapse in the spinal trigeminal nucleus, which lies in direct continuity with the substantia gelatinosa and extends down to C3 level where the first division (ophthalmic) fibres are lowest while the mandibular area extends up to the pons. From this long spinal nucleus the second order neuronal processes *decussate*, the lowest in the anterior white commisure and the upper fibres in the median raphe ventral to the fourth ventricle. From here they pass up to the ventral posteromedial nucleus of the thalamus. At this stage pain fibres from cranial nerves 7, 9 and 10 have joined.

Management of pain

This term implies the interaction between the patient, his pain and his treatment. Thus, the personality of the patient not only influences the way he responds to his pain but also the frequency with which he requests medication, its effectiveness and the way in which the demands of the patient are met by medical and nursing staff. It must also be appreciated that the longer the duration of pain the lower the threshold which can be borne equally. In such circumstances, the substitution of pain by some disagreeable sensation, such as numbness or paraesthesia, may be almost as unpleasant for the patient.

If surgical treatment is to be successful the aim must be to produce analgesia well beyond the anatomical limits of the source of pain, because the area of analgesia produced by surgery is generally smaller than expected and recedes with time.

Peripheral nerve section is a poor procedure: motor and all sensory function is lost and division of the nerve may itself give rise to pain.

Dorsal nerve roots may be cut just prior to entry into the spinal cord. This requires laminectomy and at least three levels above and below the site of the pain must be included. All sensation is lost, so that it is most suitable for painful lesions of the trunk.

In view of the number of afferent fibres in the anterior root, removal of the dorsal root ganglion may be a more logical way to remove all sensory input. Although either form of surgery preserves motor fibres, this may be less useful than expected because of the loss of proprioceptive information.

An intrathecal injection of phenol 5–10% is often successful in abolishing pain without impairment of motor power or other forms of sensation. This differential effect is evidently related to the size and degree of myelination of the fibres. If stronger solutions are used total paralysis and sensory loss occurs. Hypertonic saline has been used in a similar manner. Local injections of alcohol or localized radio-frequency lesions also destroy neural function and can be placed in suitable specific sites such as the trigeminal sensory root.

Lateral spinothalamic tractotomy constitutes the procedure of cordotomy in which incision of the cord is made just anterior to the dentate ligament to a depth sufficient to reach the anterior grey horn (4–5 mm deep). For lower limb pain the cordotomy can be made at the upper thoracic level on the opposite side of the spinal cord. This is to ensure that all delayed crossings of fibres have occurred and because the level of analgesia drops with time. Cordotomy is now usually performed by a percutaneous technique again using the dentate ligament at C1–2 (identified by radiological means) as a landmark. Analgesia may be taken up to C1, but the level again tends to fall with time. Bilateral high cervical cordotomy interferes with respiratory function by abolishing proprioceptive input so that patients may become apnoeic when they fall asleep. Medullary and mesencephalic tractotomy have largely been abandoned, partly because of the hazards of surgery in this area and mainly because of their limited effectiveness, which may be related to the branching which occurs as the lateral spinothalamic tract ascends through the lower brain stem. Efforts have been made to place lesions in the centrum medianum of the thalamus to control pain. These

need to be bilateral and carry a risk of severe sensory deficit if placed too far lateral. Finally, destructive lesions have been made in the subcortical white matter, all of which tend to alter the patient's response to pain rather than alter sensation of the pain itself. This approach has lost favour because of the alteration of personality and affect produced.

Similar principles underlie the treatment of facial pain. Operative procedures can start with the blocking or sectioning of peripheral nerves in the face (supraorbital, infraorbital, inferior dental), section of all or part of the sensory root of the trigeminal nerve or division of the tract at medullary level. Percutaneous radio-frequency lesions can be sited in the trigeminal ganglion to produce analgesia in the specific areas of the face according to the site of the pain. While a number of patients are relieved only after repeated lesions, this is usually the most appropriate initial surgical procedure when trigeminal neuralgia cannot be controlled by carbamezapine.

In recent years a different approach has been used for pain relief based on the observation that stimulation of large calibre fibres entering the spinal cord inhibits the sensations transmitted by the smaller fibres. To this end various forms and sources of stimulus of large nerve fibres have been used ranging from transcutaneous vibrators and electrical stimulators, to stimulators placed over the dorsal columns of the spinal cord or even centrally in the thalamus or periaqueductal grey matter. The value of these devices for the long term control of pain has not yet been established.

One of the most exciting recent developments in the neurosciences has emerged from the need to explain the presence of stereospecific morphine receptors in the mammalian brain. This led to the discovery of naturally-occurring, morphine-like substances — α and β endorphins and enkephalin — in the brains of animals. A longer chain parent polypeptide — β-lipoprotein — is produced by the pituitary gland. The morphine-like action of these agents on smooth muscle is antagonized by naloxone. The pain relief produced by deep grey matter stimulation and acupuncture but not hypnosis, are also antagonized by naloxone. It appears, therefore, that the brain possesses its own mechanisms for manufacturing and releasing morphine-like substances. Furthermore, in CNS sites where the putative specific pain neurotransmitter, substance P, is emitted, there are also opiate receptors. So for every pain transmitter mechanism in the CNS, there may also be a pain inhibitor. This system is now being successfully exploited for the long-term relief of intractable pain.

CONCLUSION

The surgeon has a great opportunity to make valuable

observations at the bedside and in the operating theatre. The uniqueness of the human brain and spinal cord makes the neurological surgeon privileged indeed. Opportunities favour the prepared mind — understanding of current physiological concepts is the stepping stone to fresh knowledge.

FURTHER READING

Bond M R, 1979 Pain — its nature, analysis and treatment. Churchill Livingstone, Edinburgh

Bain W H, Taylor K M 1983 Handbook of intensive care. Wright, Bristol

Crockard A, Hayward R, Hoff J T 1985 Neurosurgery: The scientific basis of clinical practice. Blackwell, Oxford

Haymaker W 1969 Bing's local diagnosis in neurological diseases. C V Mosby, St Louis

Jennett B, Teasdale G 1981 The management of head injuries. Davies, Philadelphia

King R B 1979 Principles of pain management. Journal of Neurosurgery 50: 554–559

Langfitt T W 1969 Increased intracranial pressure. Clinical Neurosurgery 22: 76–105

Melzack R 1973 The puzzle of pain. Penguin, London

Miller J D 1975 Volume and pressure in the craniospinal axis. Clinical Neurosurgery 22: 76–105

Miller J D 1982 Physiology of trauma. Clinical Neurosurgery 29: 103–130

Plum F, Posner J H 1980 The diagnosis of stupor and coma, 3rd edn. Davis, Philadelphia

Scientific American 1979 The Brain. 241: 44–232

Peripheral nerves

The surgeon's interest in peripheral nerves is focused on the effects of injury. He has a general interest in the phenomena of degeneration and regeneration and a particular interest in the effects of nerve injury on skin and muscle, in the electrodiagnostic techniques used in their investigation, in the quality of the recovery that may be expected after various types of nerve injury, and finally in causalgia. The literature in relation to the subject is now encyclopaedic and for further reading the monographs by Sunderland (1978) and Seddon (1975) should be consulted.

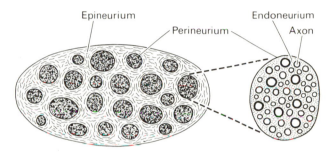

Fig. 14.1 Diagrammatic cross section of a typical peripheral nerve trunk to show the distribution of supporting tissues.

THE STRUCTURE OF NERVE TRUNKS

The essential unit in a peripheral nerve trunk is the axon, or nerve fibre, which may be myelinated or non-myelinated, and is closely related in development to a continuous sheath of Schwann cells. The endoneurium is the connective tissue binding together groups of axons and their associated Schwann cells into fasciculi or bundles (Fig. 14.1). It includes the collagenous sheaths of the nerve fibres as well as the associated fibroblasts, mast cells and blood vessels. Individual fascicles are bounded by a lamellated perineurium of flattened mesothelial cells and collagen. There is some evidence that this functions as an endothelium forming a physiological barrier to diffusion in a similar manner to the blood/brain barrier. Groups of fasciculi are enclosed in a loose, connective tissue epineurium to form the nerve trunk.

An axon is an enormously elongated process derived from a cell lying in the central nervous system or in a paravertebral ganglion. It consists of semifluid protoplasm showing evidence of longitudinal striation. Moreover, the constituent protein molecules are believed to be longitudinally orientated, and disturbance of this orientation, after minor violence, may account for transient arrest of nerve conduction. After violence sufficient to sever the axon, the arrest of conduction is prolonged, for the distal portion of the axon degenerates. It is doubtful if the axon possesses a true limiting membrane, but the surface layer

of its protoplasm acts like a semipermeable membrane with remarkable properties. Like other cell membranes it is permeable to Na^+ and K^+, but is able to 'pump out' the Na^+ actively using energy from enzymatic splitting of ATP. The result is that within the fibre there is a relative deficiency of Na^+ and a relative excess of K^+. In other cells the internal excess of K^+ counterbalances the external excess of Na^+, and there is no electrical potential across the membrane. In nerve fibres, and also in muscle fibres, the amount of Na^+ extruded is very slightly increased to the extent of one sodium ion in about 10 million. The slight ionic imbalance that results from this is sufficient to make the interior of the resting fibre about 90 mV negative as compared with its surface. Also, during the transit of an 'action potential', the surface layer momentarily leaks, admitting Na^+ and allowing K^+ to emerge.

A myelin sheath is present around all axons of a diameter greater than 1–2 μm, which includes all the somatic efferent and some somatic afferent fibres. The smaller, but numerically greater, non-myelinated fibres include the majority of the somatic afferents and all the autonomic efferents. Myelin consists of alternate layers of protein and lecithin and its 'insulating' effect is thought to favour the more rapid propagation of nerve impulses. The myelin does not form a continuous tube, but is broken into segments at the nodes of Ranvier with a Schwann cell lying at the centre of each internode. The intimate relationships between the Schwann cells and the axons have been clarified by recent electron microscope studies (Eames & Gamble, 1970). Both types of axon during development become invaginated into the cytoplasm of a Schwann cell carrying with them a double layer of surface membrane to form a mesaxon. In myelination a single Schwann cell secretes a double myelin layer at its surface membrane in the mesaxon, which becomes wrapped spirally around a single axon. In contrast, multiple non-myelinated axons are related to a single Schwann cell, either lying in furrows in its surface membrane or in contact with cytoplasmic outgrowths from its surface.

The various supporting tissues in a nerve trunk are of great surgical importance. The endoneurium or neurilemma sheath persists indefinitely even though its axon has degenerated and it forms a tube down which a regenerating axon can be led to the periphery. The perineurium, which binds the nerve fibres into fasciculi, is important because it may proliferate (especially after traction injuries) and form a mechanical barrier to regeneration. The epineurium, which forms a stout sheath to the nerve trunk, is technically important in the repair of divided nerves.

The standard method of repairing a divided nerve consists in accurately suturing the epineurium, so that the proximal and distal stumps are neatly apposed without being rotated. In a freshly divided nerve the epineurium is freely mobile, and can easily be drawn down from the position to which it has retracted. In old injuries the epineurium becomes adherent in its retracted position, and before it can be sutured the protruding portion of the nerve trunk must be discarded.

Attempts have been made to improve the quality of nerve repair by more accurate realignment of the individual nerve bundles. This technique of 'fascicular repair' depends on suturing the perineural sheaths as a preliminary to the standard repair of the epineurium and demands special instrumentation as well as high power microscopy of the operative field.

The blood vessels of the nerve trunks form a longitudinal anastomosis reinforced at intervals from neighbouring arteries. This well developed anastomosis protects the peripheral nerve from ischaemia particularly in surgical mobilisation of long segments. However, Nicholson and Seddon (1957) have cautioned against excessive mobilisation of the distal segment of divided nerves since the descending vessels are much larger than the ascending. This vascular arrangement makes nerves particularly susceptible to pressure and stretching which may result in permanent functional deterioration.

THE STRUCTURE OF CUTANEOUS SENSE ORGANS

The cutaneous sense organs include free, beaded networks of fine non-myelinated fibres, networks around the bases of hair follicles and specialized end-organs or 'corpuscles'. The three basic types of cutaneous sensation subserved by this wide variety of receptors are touch or pressure, temperature and pain. Several types of corpuscle can be distinguished but they conform to the same general plan, having an outer connective tissue sheath and a protoplasmic core, from which the branches of at least two nerve fibres ramify. It is agreed that the free beaded networks subserve pain, and that the networks around hair follicles contribute to touch, but it is doubtful if there are specific types of corpuscle for the sensations of touch, cold and warmth (Weddell & Miller, 1962).

The punctate nature of cutaneous sensibility is well known, but it is important to recognize that the various end-organs are dispersed in depths as well as in area. The networks subserving pain, formed by interlocking arborizations of fibres, lie not only between and beneath the basal cells of the epidermis but also more deeply in the dermis itself. Again, groups of corpuscles (forming, for example, a single 'cold spot') are distributed in small clusters at varying depths in the dermis. Such a dispersal in depth has two advantages over dispersal in a single plane. A greater number of end-organs underlies any given area of skin. Secondly, as a stimulus applied to the skin surface becomes more intense, it can activate end-organs lying more and more deeply. Dispersal of the end-organs in depth is therefore favourable both for the accurate localization of a stimulus and for appreciation of its intensity. A stimulus applied to even a small area of the skin must excite a large number of end-organs, and (bearing in mind the double innervation of corpuscles) an even larger number of nerve fibres. Until this concept of multiple innervation was developed it was difficult to suggest a morphological basis for the zone of hypo-aesthesia which is one of the consequences of nerve injury. It is now clear that the zone of hypo-aesthesia is accounted for by destruction of a proportion of the many nerve fibres serving that area of skin. This diminished sensation may also result from the inappropriate connections which may occur in the regeneration following nerve section as compared with nerve crushing, where the sensory neurones reform peripheral connections to the same skin receptors (Jabaley et al, 1976).

RATE OF CONDUCTION IN NERVE

The factors which govern the rate of conduction in nerve are beginning to be important clinically now that methods have been developed for measuring conduction rates in man. In health, the factors of chief importance are fibre size, temperature, age and the individual nerve concerned. Pathological slowing of conduction occurs chiefly when nerves are compressed and in diseases which lead to demyelination. The normal conduction rate in motor fibres ranges from 40–70 m/sec.

Fibre size

Peripheral nerves contain fibres of different diameters, varying from as much as 20–0.2 μm or even less, and in general the rate of conduction is directly proportional to diameter and the presence of a myelin sheath. On the basis of rate of conduction, the fibres are classified as 'A' (fast), 'B' (intermediate) and 'C' (slow). The 'C' fibres include all the non-myelinated dorsal root afferent and autonomic efferent axons.

Among efferent fibres, the 'A' fibres include the very fast α fibres which are motor to skeletal muscle, and the moderately fast γ fibres which are motor to the intrafusal muscle fibres of the muscle spindles. The 'B' fibres are myelinated, preganglionic, sympathetic fibres.

Among afferent fibres a further subclassification is based directly on size: Group I (20–12 μm diameter), Group II (12–4 μm), and Group III (less than 4 μm). The largest and fastest fibres carry impulses concerned with postural tone, the Group IA fibres carrying impulses from the annulospiral rings in muscle spindles, and the Group IB fibres carrying impulses from the Golgi endings in tendon. Slower fibres of Groups II and III carry impulses concerned with other modalities of sensation from muscles, joints and skin. There is no doubt that at least one component of pain sensation, described as dull or 'aching' is carried by slow and small fibres of type 'C' termed Group IV. It is probable that the other components of pain, particularly the 'sharp', well-localized sensation is carried by the fast fibres of Group III conducting at 5–30 m/sec.

Temperature

Cooling retards conduction. Lambert (1962) quotes retarding by about 2.4 m/sec for each reduction of 1°C for the ulnar nerve. The temperature gradient along the course of a nerve in man is difficult to measure exactly, but it leads to conduction being slower towards the extremity of a limb unless the limb is artificially heated.

Age

In newly-born infants, conduction rates are about half those quoted as normal in adults, but the normal rates are gained at 3–5 years of age. Conduction rates fall progressively after middle age and are reduced by 10% in both motor and sensory fibres after the age of 70.

Rates in different nerves

Conduction rates are generally faster in the upper limb

Table 14.1 Conduction rates (motor)

	Mean rate (m/sec)
Median to abductor pollicis brevis	57.2
Ulnar to abductor digiti quinti	56.2
Ulnar to first dorsal interosseous	55.0
Lateral popliteal to extensor digitorum brevis	49.7
Medial popliteal to abductor hallucis	43.2

than the lower, but apart from this there are minor differences from one nerve to another, as in Table 14.1 (Thomas et al, 1959).

Conduction rates in disease

Measurable slowing of motor conduction and presumptive evidence of slowing of sensory conduction were first found in nerve subjected to compression.

Slowing of motor conduction was first demonstrated by Simpson (1956) in the median nerve at the wrist in the 'carpal tunnel syndrome'. He found that the time interval between stimulating the median nerve above the wrist and the onset of the action potential in opponens pollicis was increased from the normal 3–5 msec to 6–14 msec. Similarly, in late ulnar palsy from cubitus valgus, Simpson found delayed motor conduction; the delay occurred only in the segment of nerve which was subject to compression at the elbow. Later, the knee-ankle conduction time was shown to be prolonged in the lateral popliteal nerve in patients recovering from drop foot of acute onset (Gilliatt et al, 1961).

Presumptive evidence of delayed sensory conduction can be obtained by the technique of evoked nerve action potentials (Dawson, 1956). Normally after applying a single brief stimulus to an electrode encircling the base of a finger or toe an action potential can be recorded from an electrode either overlying or inserted near the appropriate nerve trunk. However, no action potential in the nerve trunk can be detected in 50% of patients where the median nerve is compressed at the wrist, or where the lateral popliteal nerve is compressed at the neck of the fibula. In another 35% of the patients there is a prolongation of the latency of the evoked sensory nerve action potential, making the technique slightly more sensitive than motor nerve conduction (Thomas et al, 1967). It should be noted that these sensory potentials are of a thousand times smaller magnitude than muscle action potentials and may easily be missed.

The mechanism of the slowed conduction rates in compression neuropathy is not entirely certain, though it seems to be a combination of local demyelination of the larger fibres and ischaemia from microvascular damage (Denny-Brown & Brenner, 1944). This is reflected in the clinical findings of some immediate improvement in nerve function after surgical release of the external constriction, followed by a slower recovery of the remaining function as remyelination occurs. Delayed motor and sensory conduction has been demonstrated in many other forms of peripheral neuritis with demyelination of the nerve fibres as the common factor.

The conduction rates in motor nerves, which have regenerated following division and suture, never return to normal. Even under the most ideal conditions, where the nerve is crushed but not divided, this is still 25% below normal at 12–16 months (Cragg & Thomas, 1964). This probably reflects a failure of regeneration in the larger, myelinated fibres.

Sensory conduction rates may be used in the investigation of traction lesions of the branchial plexus, since this function is normal where the postganglionic fibres are intact (Bonney, 1959). In practice it is easier to use the technique of histamine-induced axon reflexes to determine whether the site of damage is proximal or distal to the posterior root ganglia.

It is well known that local anaesthetics abolish the sensation of pain before touch. In contrast, after minor trauma such as a 'crutch palsy', pain is usually retained despite muscular paralysis. It can be concluded that the small 'C' fibres subserving pain are particularly sensitive to local anaesthetics, but relatively resistant to trauma.

Finally, the effects of experimental ischaemia induced with a tourniquet have been examined by Nathan (1958). He finds that in the arm there is an early phase of tingling paraesthesiae lasting from about the third to the sixth minute of arterial occlusion; in the leg, this phase is slight or lacking. Normal sensation is then recovered till the onset of anaesthesia and paralysis, usually at about 25 minutes in the arm and about 30 minutes in the leg. On release of the tourniquet there is an immediate but brief recovery of normal sensation, followed by several minutes of severe pain and paraesthesiae. During the early phase of painless paraesthesiae (in the arm) the sensation of touch is retained but the sensation of pain is greatly dimmed or lost. In the stage of continuous pain and severe paraesthesiae following removal of the tourniquet, all forms of peripheral sensitivity are lost. It is of interest that during these phases of paraesthesiae, electrical stimulation at the periphery still gives rise to action potentials proximal to the site of application of the tourniquet, even though these stimuli do not enter consciousness. It appears therefore that when the nerve fibres are firing spontaneously any additional impulses they transmit from the periphery are incapable of being interpreted.

ELECTROMYOGRAPHY

The recording of action potentials from muscle is becoming increasingly important as a diagnostic procedure in many diseases of muscle and nerve. The techniques and applications of electromyography have become increasingly complex and have largely superseded the simple strength duration curves for this purpose (Desmedt, 1973).

For some purposes it is sufficient to record muscle action potentials from a pair of electrodes applied to the skin, the small test electrode being applied over the muscle and the larger 'indifferent' electrode elsewhere. More detailed information, particularly in denervation, requires the insertion of a pair of needle electrodes directly into the muscle. In a routine test, records are made both with the muscle relaxed and during sustained voluntary contraction; sometimes further records are made following electrical stimulation of the motor nerve. Action potentials are normally triphasic with two small positive deflections separated by a larger negative one.

At rest, normal muscle is quiescent after a preliminary burst of activity in response to the injury of inserting the needle electrodes. In denervated muscle, fibrillation gives rise to unremitting but irregular action potentials with a low amplitude of the order of 100 μV compared with the normal average of 2 mV (Fig. 14.2). It is sometimes possible to diagnose partial division of the motor nerve by demonstrating that some parts of a muscle are fibrillating whereas other parts show normal quiescence. These fibrillation potentials do not appear until some 2–3 weeks after the onset of denervation.

During voluntary contraction of a normal muscle, action potentials are well sustained. The amplitude of the potentials is held to be proportional to the size of the 'motor units', that is to say the average number of muscle fibres innervated by each nerve fibre. In peripheral muscles the average motor unit is of the order of 100 muscle fibres. Motor units tend to be smaller in muscles concerned with finely coordinated repetitive movements, such as the external ocular muscles and the small muscles of the hand, where the motor units are less than ten muscle fibres. By contrast there may be 300–350 fibres in the motor units of muscles such as gluteus maximus, which are characterized by slow sustained contractions of high tension. The skilled observer requires to know what amplitude of action potential is normal for the muscle he is testing. The amplitude is reduced if the muscle is partially denervated, or if there is primary disease of muscle (see Fig. 14.2). Giant action potentials are present in muscles supplied by a motor nerve which is recovering from division and suture; these giant potentials are believed to result from the regenerated nerves now supplying many more muscle fibres than their normal quota. In myasthenia gravis, the action potentials on sustained voluntary contraction are initially about normal, but soon fade; their amplitude rapidly increases if an anti-cholinesterase is given.

A single short electrical stimulus applied to a normal motor nerve is followed by a burst of muscle action potentials which is brief and compact. In nerves subjected to

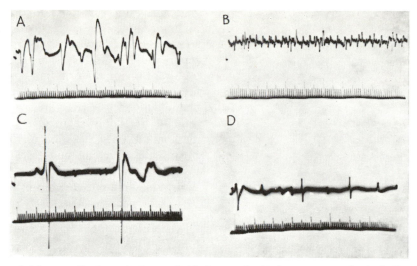

Fig. 14.2 Action potentials recorded from needle electrodes in muscle (during sustained voluntary contraction in A, B and C). Time marked in msecs. A, *normal muscle*. B and C, *myopathy*: in type B the reduced amplitude indicates that the motor units contain fewer muscle fibres than normal, whereas in type C the reduced frequency indicates loss of whole motor units. D, *denervated muscle*, showing unremitting fibrillation. (Courtesy of Dr P. Bauwens, London.)

pressure, and in peripheral neuritis. the nerve fibres are conducting at widely-dispersed rates, and the burst of muscle action potentials is correspondingly prolonged. Again, the rate of motor conduction in nerve can be calculated by successively stimulating the nerve at points a known distance apart and comparing the time intervals that elapse before the onset of the muscle action potentials.

NEUROMUSCULAR TRANSMISSION

Although the mechanism of neuromuscular transmission and the use of muscle relaxants concern primarily the anaesthetist, the surgeon should have some notion of his colleague's problem.

Resting potentials and action potentials

When a micro-electrode is inserted into a resting nerve fibre or resting muscle fibre, the interior of the fibre is found to be about 90 mV negative with reference to its exterior, and the surface membrane can therefore be said to be polarized. If a subthreshold stimulus is applied, this resting potential can be reduced by about 30 mV without leading to any propagated electrical disturbance. If, however, the resting potential is reduced by more than about 30 mV, polarization suddenly breaks down, giving rise to an action potential. As this action potential successively depolarizes the nearby membrane, it is self-propagating. The action potential is attributed to a sudden and brief inrush of Na^+ and sometimes Ca^{2+} ions from the surface, followed by a slower counterbalancing egress of K^+ and followed finally by restoration of the original state.

Both in nerve and in muscle an action potential can lead to a brief reversal of electrical sign, the exterior of the fibre becoming 20–30 mV negative instead of the interior being about 90 mV negative as at rest. Over the motor end-plates however the sign never becomes reversed, and a maximal end-plate potential results merely in the resting potential being abolished.

Motor end-plates

The end-plates comprise a neural element (the terminal fibrils of the motor axon) and a non-neural element which may be of glial origin (the nucleated protoplasm of the 'sole-plate'). An end-plate is a small discoid structure encircling about one-third of the circumference of a muscle fibre, but occupying only a tiny fraction of its length. When the motor nerve reaches its muscle fibre its outer-most sheath, the sheath of Henle, fuses with the outer layer of the sarcolemma. The myelin sheath ends abruptly. The axon divides into expanded fibrils which fan out into the substance of the sole-plate (Fig. 14.3). Within the protoplasm of the sole-plate, electron microscopy reveals many tiny vesicles, each thought to consist of a 'packet' of about 1000 molecules of acetylcholine. The sole-plate is separated from the underlying sarcoplasm by a very delicate membrane which is thrown into such deep folds that it resembles a palisade. It is probably this palisade membrane which is depolarized during neuromuscular transmission.

When an action potential in the motor nerve reaches the end-plate it is held to release one or more of the 'packets' of acetylcholine. This acetylcholine briefly depolarizes the membrane of the end-plate before being rapidly destroyed

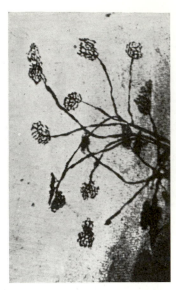

Fig. 14.3 Normal sole-plates in striated muscle. (Untouched photograph of a beautiful preparation of structures not easily displayed.) (Courtesy of Mr F. W. Gairns, Department of Physiology, University of Glasgow.)

by cholinesterase. The brief depolarization of the end-plates sets off an ionic disturbance involving shifts of Na^+ and K^+ in the nearby muscle membrane, and this disturbance is propagated along the muscle as an action potential. Before another action potential can be propagated, both the end-plate and the muscle fibre must regain their resting potential.

Muscle relaxants

The 'competitive' relaxants block neuromuscular transmission by competing with acetylcholine for its receptor sites at the end-plate and thus prevent depolarization. Typical examples are tubocurarine and quaternary ammonium compounds such as gallamine tri-ethiodate. Their action is uniform in all muscles and can be reversed by increasing the local concentration of acetylcholine by the use of anti-cholinesterase substances such as neostigmine.

The 'depolarizers' are a group of relaxants which block neuromuscular transmission by preventing the end-plates from regaining their resting potential. Most are quaternary ammonium compounds, such as suxamethonium and decamethonium, which resemble acetylcholine but are resistant to hydrolysis by cholinesterase. The paralysis they produce is preceded by the stimulant effects of depolarization with spontaneous fasciculations and uncoordinated muscle contraction. Their blocking action is not easily antagonized and is increased by the administration of anti-cholinesterases, such as neostigmine. In some animals, but probably not in man, they may have a 'dual' action when their initial depolarizing action may be succeeded by a competitive block (Churchill-Davidson, 1963).

In practice, the competitive relaxants tubocurarine and

gallamine are generally used for the production of prolonged relaxation, particularly for abdominal operations. Suxamethonium is the most used of the depolarizers because of its very short action, which is particularly useful for giving the brief but complete relaxation required for intubating the trachea or manipulating a fracture. If the manipulation of a fracture proves to be unexpectedly difficult, it is unwise to give several injections of suxamethonium: each injection of the depolarizer is followed by muscle twitching and fasciculation before the block becomes complete, and repeated injections can be followed by troublesome muscle pain in early convalescence.

DEGENERATION OF NERVE (WALLERIAN DEGENERATION)

If a nerve is divided, the whole of the distal portion degenerates, and in addition, there may be some degeneration of the proximal stump and chromatolysis of the parent nerve cells. Functionally, the nerve ceases to transmit impulses a few hours after injury, though some irregular compound action potentials may persist in the distal stump up to 3 days.

Degeneration of the distal portion of the nerve begins within a few hours of injury, and is marked by the end of 7–10 days. The axons first break up into short segments, and the myelin into droplets. These are later removed by macrophages which become stuffed with fatty debris, and therefore appear as 'foam cells' in sections treated with fat solvents. The Schwann cells multiply and become fusiform from the accumulation of protoplasm. The outgrowth of Schwann cells and fibrous tissue from the proximal end of the distal stump gives rise to a 'false neuroma' (in contradistinction to the 'true neuroma' of the proximal stump). Finally, it should be noted that the endoneurial tubes persist indefinitely as 'ghosts' but their diameter gradually shrinks, and because of this shrinkage the fully degenerated nerve trunk is reduced to about one-third of its normal diameter.

Retrograde degeneration of the proximal stump is a variable feature and is greater in non-myelinated than in myelinated fibres. It is usually slight after simple crushing, but may extend for as much as 3 cm if the nerve has been violently torn across. The changes are the same as in the distal stump.

Chromatolysis of the parent nerve cells may occur, especially if the axons are divided close to the cells. The Nissl granules disappear and the nucleus becomes swollen and eccentric. Normal appearances are regained within 3–4 weeks.

REGENERATION OF NERVE

The course of regeneration is greatly influenced by the

nature of the original injury. After injury by simple crushing, termed 'axonotmesis' (where the fluid axons are disrupted, but the membranous endoneurial sheaths remain intact), the regenerating axons are led directly to the end-organs they previously innervated, and the final result is therefore usually excellent. After division of a nerve trunk, termed 'neurotmesis', the gap must be bridged before the growing axons start their progress towards the periphery. In the process of bridging, some axons make contact with endoneurial tubes which lead them to appropriate end-organs, but some are led to end-organs where they cannot function and others go astray in the scar between the nerve stumps. In consequence, the end-result, even after accurate suture of a divided nerve, is always imperfect. This is particularly true in 'mixed' nerves as compared with those containing mainly motor fibres such as the radial. After traction injuries, there is usually a combination of complete rupture of some fibres with mere axonal rupture in others. Fibres which have been completely torn across do not usually regenerate because the ends are widely retracted, but any axons lying in intact endoneurial tubes regenerate well. The end-result therefore depends on the violence of the original traction.

Regeneration after crushing

Regeneration may begin within a few days of injury. In the early stages it appears that the protoplasm of the axon — which is a viscous fluid — slowly flows onward into the endoneurial tube which is ready to receive it. In the later stages, when fresh protoplasm must be built up, it is uncertain whether this is synthesized locally at the growing tip, or centrally at the parent cell which may force it distally down the endoneurial tube like water down a hosepipe. The rate of advance of the growing tip, as determined by direct measurement in experimental animals, is of the order of 4 mm per day, slowing down somewhat in the more peripheral part of a limb. It must be remembered, however, that the axons, when they first reach their end-organs, are very slender and poorly myelinated. They must thicken and acquire myelin before they can function usefully by carrying action potentials at correct speeds. This process of maturation begins centrally and gradually extends towards the periphery. When regeneration is judged by functional recovery, the rate of regeneration is usually rather less than 2 mm per day.

Regeneration after nerve division

The initial bridging of the gap between the nerve ends is carried out by proliferation of Schwann cells and fibroblasts growing from both stumps, but especially from the distal stump. The rate of advance is so rapid that a narrow gap is bridged in a few days. There is no evidence that the proliferating cells are directed at the opposite stump, and

it seems that they merely grow along the line of least resistance. These bands of Schwann cells are therefore liable to go astray in the granulation tissue unless the stumps have been apposed accurately by careful suture of the epineurium. After a good repair, the bridge is narrow, crossed by longitudinally-orientated Schwann bands, and contains a minimum of fibrous tissue. The next stage is the crossing of the bridge by axons growing from the proximal stump. This may begin within a few days, or may be delayed for 3–4 weeks, depending on the extent of retrograde degeneration. Each axon divides into a large number of branches — as many as 50 or 100 — and these appear as strands, spirals and rings which sprout in all directions. Many of these outgrowths are abortive and are later absorbed, but some persist as the neuroma of the proximal stump.

In favourable cases, many of the sprouting axons grow along these bands of Schwann cells to the peripheral stump, where they enter endoneurial tubes. In the early stages there may be as many as 30 branches of various axons within a single endoneurial tube, but as growth proceeds all but one are suppressed. The surviving axon may find itself within a tube which leads to a suitable end-organ, but many axons are led to unsuitable end-organs or occupy tubes which are too narrow to allow of maturation. For these reasons, only a proportion of fibres which have successfully negotiated the bridge between the nerve ends can eventually function, and the end-result, even after careful surgical repair of a divided nerve, can never be perfect. Short of perfection, however, good results can often be obtained. Functional recovery is due in the main to the prolific branching of the axons growing from the proximal stump, which increases the chance that a high proportion may find their way to suitable end-organs despite the unavoidable random criss-crossing at the bridge.

Regeneration after traction injuries

In the usual type of traction injury, the nerve trunk is not completely severed, but within the trunk some fibres are completely torn across while others suffer division of their axons within intact endoneurial tubes. Regeneration takes place only in fibres lying in intact tubes, because the ends of divided fibres retract widely. It is important to note that the levels at which different fibres are torn are distributed over a distance of several centimetres of the nerve trunk. Excision of the whole of the damaged segment would, therefore, leave a gap too wide to allow the stumps to be sutured, and a direct attempt at surgical repair is seldom feasible.

Similarly, in the comparatively few cases when violent traction leads to complete severance of a nerve trunk, operative repair usually fails because of extensive intraneural damage.

NERVE GRAFTS

A nerve graft can occasionally be used to bridge a gap in a nerve trunk when loss of tissue prevents direct end-to-end suture. In selected cases, particularly in patients under the age of 15 years, the reported results have been almost as good as repair by suture (Seddon, 1963). However, there are serious practical limitations on its use arising from three main causes: (i) the graft must be obtained from the patient himself; (ii) the distal stump of the nerve to be repaired must not have suffered ischaemic fibrosis; and (iii) the graft must either be sufficiently slender to obtain nutriment by diffusion from its new bed or must carry its own blood supply.

Nerve autografts survive well. Nerve homografts excite the usual immunity response and few have succeeded in man though occasional survival of the graft has been claimed in animals. The need to work exclusively with autografts is a serious limitation, for there are only a few cutaneous nerves, such as the medial cutaneous of the forearm and the saphenous, which can be spared. These nerves must be taken proximal to their area of distribution to avoid the problem of diameter discrepancy. The slenderness of the grafts obtained from these nerves, of average diameter 2–3 mm, makes them especially suitable for repairing slender nerves. The principal applications of nerve grafting are in repairing the digital nerves of the fingers, the nerves of the arm and forearm, and the facial nerve in its course through the facial canal where it may be accidently divided during an operation to drain the mastoid air sinuses. 'Cable grafts', consisting of many strands of cutaneous nerve, have occasionally been used to repair a defect in a large nerve trunk, but seldom with much success.

The state of the distal stump of the nerve to be repaired is of critical importance for the success of the graft. If the stump has been subjected to prolonged ischaemia it becomes converted to dense collagenous tissue which is quite impervious to the passage of regenerating nerve fibres, and so the graft must fail. For this reason a biopsy of the distal stump should be carried out at an early stage of the operation, and grafting proceeded with only if the distal stump is found to be healthy. It must be remembered that the nerve trunks commonly run in company with the principal vessels, and that the kind of soft tissue injury which carries away a segment of nerve is particularly apt to destroy vessels and lead to ischaemia.

The nutrition of a newly-inserted graft is not critical in the case of a slender nerve graft, which can obtain nutriment by diffusion from the vascular tissue of its bed, but is a limiting factor in the use of large grafts. Lengths of up to and over 15 cm have been used successfully but the diameter is more critical: that of the radial nerve is satisfactory but the common peroneal is too large for survival.

The survival of a transplanted graft can be improved if it is predegenerate, presumably because the metabolic requirements following Wallerian degeneration are less. Occasionally large nerve trunks become available from a limb that requires amputation, and might be used in another limb whose main nerves are damaged. Unfortunately, the free grafting of a large nerve trunk from one limb to another fails through ischaemic necrosis of the graft. There is, however, an ingenious method of obtaining a pedicled nerve graft for repairing the median nerve when both the median and the ulnar have been divided with loss of tissue. At the first operation the proximal stump of the median is sutured to the proximal stump of the ulnar, and in order to allow the median fibres to cross the suture line the ulnar nerve is crushed at a higher level. Four to five weeks later, when a vascular anastomosis has developed across the suture line, the ulnar nerve is cut across and its distal portion swung down to bridge the gap in the median.

RESULTS OF SECTION OF CUTANEOUS NERVES

Several workers have described the results of deliberate section of cutaneous nerves in themselves. An outstanding account was given by Trotter and Davies in 1909. They extended the earlier work of Head and others and showed that the hypothesis of 'protopathic' and 'epicritic' sensibility was based on the results of faulty observation. It is indeed remarkable that this hypothesis was to remain current for many years after it had been shown to be untenable.

The cutaneous nerves contain not only afferent sensory fibres, but also efferent fibres destined for blood vessels, sweat glands and hair follicles. After section of a cutaneous nerve, there is a central zone of skin in which the loss of sensory and motor function is complete, surrounded by a zone in which the loss is partial. The central zone corresponds with the autonomous distribution of the nerve, and the surrounding intermediate zone with the area of overlap with adjacent intact nerves. It is important to recognize that there is no abrupt transition from normal sensation to hypoaesthesia, or from hypo-aesthesia to anaesthesia, but merely a gradually deepening loss of function as the autonomous zone is approached. This progressively deepening loss of function is found with all modes of sensation — touch, warmth and cold, and pain — and with all modes of motor activity — vasomotor, pilomotor and sudomotor.

Touch

Two boundaries of impaired tactile sensation can be recognized. The outer boundary is best found by the patient stroking the skin with his own finger; when the boundary is crossed, the sensation evoked, though difficult to describe, is recognized as abnormal — it is said to be 'smoother' and less liable to tickle. The inner boundary marks the limit within which stroking with a fine brush or a wisp of cottonwool can no longer be appreciated. This is the boundary commonly determined clinically, because of the ease with which it can be mapped out. Detailed examination with graduated von Frey hairs shows that in passing from the outer to the inner of these boundaries there is a deepening hypo-aesthesia, for successively heavier hairs must be used for effective stimulation. As might be expected, the heaviest hairs can be appreciated for a short distance within the boundary marked by brush strokes.

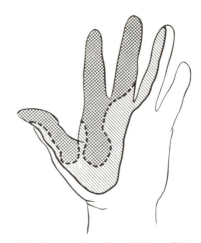

Fig. 14.4 Impaired pain sensation after division of the median nerve: the cross-hatched area indicates anaesthesia, and the lined area indicates hypo-aesthesia. (After Trotter & Davies 1909 Journal of Physiology **38**: 134)

Heat and cold

Normal skin is capable of a range of discrimination covering the sensations hot, warm, indifferent, cool and cold. Temperatures within 5 or 6°C of the skin temperature (i.e. a total range of 10 or 12°) are indifferent. Warmth and coolness are believed to be pure thermal sensations, whereas hot and cold are regarded as admixtures of thermal sensation and pure pain. After division of a cutaneous nerve, there is a central area of thermal anaesthesia, surrounded by a zone of hypo-aesthesia. In the zone of thermal hypo-aesthesia, the impairment is both quantitative and qualitative. Thus the range of temperature regarded as indifferent may be increased from the normal 10°C to about 20°C and temperatures which on normal skin appear hot or cold now appear warm or cool. Detailed examination shows that the areas of impaired sensation of heat and of cold do not exactly coincide, the area of impaired cold sensation being somewhat the smaller.

Pain

There is again a central zone of analgesia surrounded by an intermediate zone of hypo-aesthesia (Fig. 14.4). The zone of hypo-aesthesia cannot be demonstrated in routine clinical testing by freehand use of a needle (which gives only maximal stimulation) but it can be demonstrated easily if the needle is attached to von Frey hairs so that the intensity of stimulation can be graded. The demonstration of hypo-aesthesia is somewhat complicated by the occurrence of hyperaesthesia at various times. Hyperaesthesia may be present during the first 24–48 hours after nerve section, again during the third and fourth weeks, and yet again during the process of re-innervation.

Vasomotor disturbance

Vasoconstrictor fibres derived from the sympathetic system are distributed with the main somatic nerves and their branches, but their distribution is by no means uniform over the body surface. The main distribution of vasoconstrictor fibres is peripheral, and there is a pronounced vascular disturbance after division of the median, ulnar or sciatic nerves. After division of cutaneous nerves in the upper arm or in the thigh, the vascular disturbance is slight.

For some 3 weeks after section of a nerve distributed to the periphery of a limb, the skin is hot, flushed and dry, and this full vascular dilatation is maintained even on exposure to cold. Thereafter, the skin temperature becomes dependent on the environment, and in cool or temperate climates the skin is cold. In the absence of re-innervation this cold state is permanent. Whether the limb is in the initial 'hot phase' or the later 'cold phase', it takes no part in the regulation of the body temperature, and there is no local increase in skin temperature on immersing indifferent limbs in hot water (see Fig. 14.5). Nevertheless, full vasodilatation can be induced by metabolites liberated locally. Reactive hyperaemia is still to be found on releasing an arterial tourniquet, and full dilatation occurs in response to local sepsis. The well-known tendency of denervated skin to develop intractable ulcers cannot indeed be attributed to any failure of the hyperaemic component of the inflammatory response. Intractable ulceration is probably due in part to oedema of a limb which is often allowed to hang dependent and idle, and in part to the fact that in skin which is insensitive, the initial damage may be unduly severe and later damage may be suffered inadvertently.

The temperature changes which have been described are usually more obvious in the hands than in the feet, because the hands are uncovered but the feet protected. Again, there is considerable overlap in the vascular territory

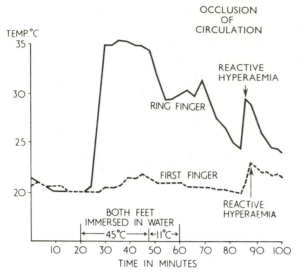

Fig. 14.5 Temperature responses in denervated skin (first finger) and normally innervated skin (ring finger). The denervated finger lacks the normal rise and fall of temperature in response to immersing the feet in hot and cold water, but retains the normal response to the release of a tourniquet. (After Richards R L 1946 The Peripheral Circulation in Health and Disease. Livingstone, Edinburgh)

controlled by adjacent nerves. Thus, in isolated lesions of the median nerve the vascularity of the thumb and ring fingers usually remains normal, and in isolated ulnar lesions the ring finger is again normal.

The vascular changes which follow division of a peripheral nerve have a general resemblance to the effects of sympathectomy. The initial phase of full dilatation is common to both, and lasts about 3 weeks. The skin temperature then falls, in the case of division of a somatic nerve to about the environmental temperature, and in the case of sympathectomy to a stable level, commonly 23–25°C. The difference in final outcome is due to several factors, of which the chief is probably disuse of a limb handicapped by division of a somatic nerve: in this connection, it must be remembered that disuse alone, as in hemiplegia, leads to coldness, cyanosis and oedema. Again, on exposure to cold the total blood flow to a limb can still be reduced after division of a peripheral nerve for the innervation of many of the limb vessels is still intact. Finally, the loss of axon reflexes after degeneration of cutaneous nerves may play a part.

Pilomotor paralysis

The area of skin showing pilomotor paralysis corresponds approximately with the area of anaesthesia to brush strokes. The skin is abnormally smooth because of absence of tone in the muscles surrounding the hair follicles. The hairs, instead of lying for the most part in the same direction, lack orientation and, when displaced, tend to remain in the new position. Surrounding the zone of complete

paralysis there is an area in which the hairs respond weakly to reflex stimulation.

Sudomotor paralysis

Absence of sweating is complete over an area corresponding approximately with the area of analgesia to pinprick. It is best demonstrated by immersing the indifferent limbs (e.g. the feet, in a patient with a nerve lesion of the arm) in water at 45°C. Within 10–20 minutes, glistening beads of sweat can be seen easily on normal skin, but are absent from skin which has been denervated. Clinically, considerable use has been made of this absence of sweating during recent years. The method used is to dust the limb with a powder, such as quinizarin, which changes colour on becoming moist (Fig. 14.6). Unexpected areas of anhydrosis are sometimes found, and further testing of these areas usually shows derangements of sensation which have been previously overlooked.

The foregoing consideration shows that, following division of a cutaneous nerve, derangements of sensation and derangements of motor function follow the same general pattern. There is a central area in which the loss of function is complete, surrounded by an area where the loss is partial. The areas over which the various functions are lost correspond in a general way, but for no pair of functions does the area of loss coincide exactly.

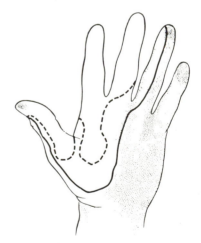

Fig. 14.6 Loss of sweating in denervated skin demonstrated with a special dusting powder. The powder remains pale over dry skin in the territory of the intact ulnar nerve. The broken and continuous lines indicate areas of sensory loss as in Figure 14.4 (After Trotter & Davies, *loc. cit.*)

Sensory changes during recovery after section

The recovery of sensation in a denervated area depends chiefly on regeneration of the injured nerve. In addition, in the early phase, there is some concentric shrinking of the area of abnormal sensation attributable to the ingrowth of fibres from neighbouring cutaneous nerves.

The area of altered sensation is maximal immediately after the nerve injury, and begins to shrink within a few days. Concentric shrinking of the area of sensory loss is rapid during the first few days, but after 2 or 3 weeks becomes very slow. The total shrinkage may amount to 1–2 cm or even more. Shrinkage is best seen after crude injuries such as gunshot wounds and is least evident after clean surgical section of a nerve trunk. Accordingly, shrinkage is believed to be due in part to the resumption of function in fibres of neighbouring nerves which have suffered damage short of division. In part, however, the shrinkage is due to the actual ingrowth of new fibres. Weddell and others (1941) established that fibres from adjacent nerves could be shown to pass in the direction of the central area of anaesthesia. These fibres were fine, usually beaded and resembled the undifferentiated normal endings subserving pain sensation. Histologically, the advancing front of these fibres corresponded very closely with the limit of pain sensation previously marked by tattooing the skin. This ingrowth of fibres subserving pain may account in part for the well-known observation that the area of analgesia is always smaller than the area of tactile anaesthesia. However, the overlap between neighbouring nerve territories is always greater in respect of pain than for other forms of sensation, as can be shown by temporarily blocking one nerve with novocain.

The onset of recovery by regeneration of the injured nerve is always delayed for many weeks. Thus, Trotter and Davies (1909) found that after simple section of a cutaneous nerve the first evidence of regeneration appeared between 10 and 14 weeks, and the delay may be greater if a long length of nerve trunk requires to be re-formed. Recovery begins at the proximal part of the denervated area and extends distally; this is a rule applicable to all nerves supplying the distal portions of the limbs, but in the proximal portions of the limbs there are a few exceptions of which the concentric recovery after lesions of the axillary circumflex is a notable example.

The recovery of appreciation of pain, touch and cold all begin at about the same time and extend slowly distally at about the same rate. Recovery of the sensation of heat is rather slower. The clinical impression that recovery of pain precedes the recovery of touch and cold is not borne out by critical examination. It must be remembered that routine clinical testing for pain is carried out by freehand pricking with a needle — a maximal stimulus — whereas touch is tested with a wisp of cotton-wool or a brush, and cold with a test tube containing water at perhaps 15–20°C, both of which are sub-maximal stimuli. When these submaximal stimuli are replaced by maximal stimulation with heavy von Frey hairs and ice-cold water, it is found that recovery of pain, touch and cold advance more or less together.

The quality of sensation in the recovering area remains abnormal and often unpleasant for several months and, indeed, after recovery following suture, the quality of sensation may remain abnormal permanently.

Tinel's sign is often used as an indicator of the level of nerve regeneration. It is positive when percussion over a nerve results in a sensation of 'pins and needles' or a painful 'electric shock', both locally and in the peripheral distribution. Henderson (1948) evaluated its use in a large series of nerve injuries not treated by surgery. He found that it took at least 4 months for the sign to appear and that good recovery could only be expected where the distal response at the level of regeneration was as strongly positive as at the level of injury.

EFFECTS OF DENERVATION OF MUSCLE

The most obvious effects of denervation of muscle are flaccid paralysis dating from the moment of nerve injury, atrophy beginning within a few days and eventually fibrosis and contracture. Biopsy of the denervated muscle reveals a striking series of histological changes. The responses of the muscle to electrical stimulation are altered, and these alterations are important both in diagnosis and treatment.

Paralysis, atrophy and contracture

Flaccid paralysis of the denervated muscles can be demonstrated by simple clinical testing, and a consideration of the distribution of the affected muscles usually indicates the site of the nerve lesion. Sometimes the identification of the paralysed muscle is made difficult by the development of trick movements, while conversely paralysis may occasionally be simulated in hysteria. Paralysis continues throughout the period of denervation. During recovery after re-innervation, the power of voluntary contraction is regained progressively, beginning with a barely perceptible tautening of the muscle. It has been found useful to grade the power of the recovering muscles according to the following numerical convention, whose use is now general:

0 — Complete paralysis
1 — Flicker of contraction
2 — Movement, but not against gravity
3 — Movement against gravity
4 — Contraction against gravity and some resistance
5 — Contraction against powerful resistance

Atrophy in muscles which have been denervated begins about the third or fourth day, progresses rapidly during the first few weeks, and thereafter more slowly. The cause of the atrophy is generally held to be simple disuse, and the abolition of resting tone as well as voluntary contraction accounts for the atrophy being more profound than in a healthy muscle immobilized, for example, in a plaster splint. Another characteristic of denervated muscle is the presence of fine fibrillation. These spontaneous contractions of individual muscle fibres appear a few days after denervation and continue for some months, although they decrease with increasing atrophy of the muscle. They were thought by Tower (1939) to be responsible for atrophy as they are accompanied by increased oxygen consumption indicative of catabolic activity. However, the atrophy can be shown to precede fibrillation and continues when fibrillation is blocked by quinidine.

The eventual development of a fixed contracture in a denervated muscle is a phenomenon of variable occurrence. It is common in muscles which lie in a shortened state in the position of rest, and is particularly common in the long flexors of the wrist and fingers, and in the intrinsic muscles of the hand and foot. It does not occur in muscles which are stretched by the action of gravity and is unknown in the deltoid or in the dorsiflexors of the ankle. Contracture is seldom evident in less than 2–3 months from the time of nerve injury and is slowly progressive. It is of interest to note that the contracture is not relaxed by anaesthesia, local asphyxia, or even by death. If re-innervation should occur before the contracture is fully established, partial or even complete recovery is possible, but in established contracture the muscle comes to resemble tendon, and no recovery is possible.

Histological changes in denervated muscle

The histological changes following denervation were well reviewed by Bowden and Gutmann (1944) and only minor modifications have resulted from electron microscopy studies. In the muscle fibres, changes are evident at about 2 weeks, when the nuclei become round instead of elongated, and dispersed through the fibres instead of lying under the sarcolemma. By the end of a month the nuclei are swollen, vesicular and many are beginning to disintegrate. The apparent increase in the number of nuclei visible at this time is probably due to concomitant atrophy of the sarcoplasm, so that an abnormally large number of fibres is present in each microscopic field. At about 6 months the remaining nuclei of the muscle fibres resume their elongated shape, but they remain dispersed through the fibres. From about this time also the sarcoplasm, which is already atrophic, begins to lose its cross-striation though the longitudinal striation persists. In addition, the interstitial fibrous tissue increases in amount, and the muscle eventually becomes modified to a tissue intermediate between scar tissue and tendon.

Although motor end-plates can be shown to persist for at least a year after denervation there is a progressive fibrocytic infiltration from the termination of the endoneural tube. This may block re-innervation unless the level of axon division is close to the muscle allowing early reconnection between the new fibre and the end-plate. When fibrosis blocks the ingrowth of the regenerating motor nerve fibres these may run parallel with the muscle fibres

and form new end-plates at other sites. Other inappropriate sensory and autonomic fibres fail to establish connections with the fibres and merely intermingle with them sometimes resulting in muscle tenderness. For these reasons the re-innervation after nerve suture is never complete, though good function may follow axonotmesis in the distal part of a nerve. The return of muscle contractility always lags behind re-innervation and is preceded by the appearance of action potentials on electromyography.

Superimposed on the generalized and orderly progress of atrophy and fibrous replacement, there may from time to time be acute focal necrosis. Free mononuclear cells accumulate round groups of muscle fibres which become oedematous and disintegrate. Focal necrosis is quite irregular in occurrence, but may be a conspicuous feature of biopsy material obtained between 3 and 9 months after denervation. Its cause is unknown, but pressure sores and systemic infections are believed to be predisposing factors.

Electrical stimulation of denervated muscle

The response of denervated muscle to electrical stimulation is of diagnostic and therapeutic importance. During the first week the muscle can be stimulated directly or through its nerve, but early in the second week the nerve becomes too degenerate to convey impulses. During the second week also, the type of contraction and the excitability of the muscle become abnormal. A delayed, sustained contraction makes its appearance as the characteristic response of denervated muscle. Again, the muscle becomes increasingly sensitive to mechanical stimulation or to chemical stimulation (e.g. with acetylcholine). Electrical stimulation with galvanic current remains effective, but faradic (induced) current ceases to be an adequate stimulus when the nervous elements have degenerated. Numerous electrical tests have been used in diagnosis including the classical 'reaction of degeneration' and 'strength-duration curves'. However, more detailed information can be obtained from electromyography, which has largely superseded them.

The reaction of degeneration has two main features: a slow, sustained contraction in response to galvanic stimulation and an absence of response to faradism. The results of this technique can be fallacious and it is now rarely used.

The determination of strength-duration curves is a logical extension of the classical reaction of degeneration. In this technique a long-duration square wave electrical impulse is applied to the muscle and the amount of current required to elicit a minimal contraction (rheobase) is measured in milliamps or volts. The duration of the impulse is progressively shortened and the intensity of current required to produce a minimal contraction determined for each time and recorded on a curve. Typical strength-duration curves for normal and denervated muscle are

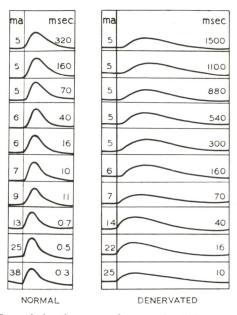

ma	msec.
5	320
5	160
5	70
6	40
6	16
7	10
9	11
13	0.7
25	0.5
38	0.3

NORMAL

ma	msec.
5	1500
5	1100
5	880
5	540
5	300
6	160
7	70
14	40
22	16
25	10

DENERVATED

Fig. 14.7 Strength-duration curves for normal and denervated muscle. Note the prolonged duration of stimulus required in the case of denervated muscle. (Doupe, 1943.)

shown in Figure 14.7, where it will be seen that for a given strength of current, the time required for effective stimulation is much longer in denervated than in normal muscle. It will be appreciated that the strength-duration curve and the classical reaction of degeneration have the same basis, but the newer test is the more delicate. Thus, the strength-duration curve begins to be abnormal within 3–4 days of denervation and on recovery begins to return to normal up to 3–9 weeks before the return of voluntary contraction.

In the past, electrical stimulation of denervated muscles has been used therapeutically in an attempt to limit atrophy pending re-innervation. The concept was based on observations in experimental animals reported by Guttmann and Guttmann (1944). However, Doupe et al (1943) investigating the use of galvanic stimulation in the treatment of radial nerve lesions concluded that it could not prevent atrophy when given several times a week. They also showed that electrical stimulation of healthy muscle was much less effective than a voluntary contraction in inducing increased muscle blood flow. The practical limitation of its use is the need to apply strong repetitive stimuli for a prolonged period on a daily basis to achieve any measurable benefit. Most patients would find such treatment too painful and inconvenient.

CAUSALGIA

The term causalgia was introduced by Weir Mitchell (1872) to describe the severe burning pain that may occur as a rare complication of injury of the peripheral nerves. Its original description related to experience in the Amer-

ican Civil War and its most common occurrence is in relation to gunshot injuries. Causalgia is commonest after an incomplete lesion of the median or sciatic nerve, especially when the lesion involves the plexus or the main nerve trunk at the root of the limb. In a review of the published literature, Richards (1967) found an incidence of 1.8–13.8% in all war nerve injuries. It usually begins within a few hours of the injury, lasts for many months, and tends gradually to become less severe. Its characteristics have been listed by Barnes (Medical Research Council Report, 1954) as follows:

1. It is severe, spontaneous and persistent
2. It usually has a burning quality
3. It may spread beyond the territory of the injured nerve or nerves
4. It is invariably aggravated by both physical and emotional stimuli

A fifth characteristic might profitably be added: it can be relieved by sympathetic nerve block.

From time to time, attention has been drawn to a number of physical changes in the causalgic digits, but none of these is constant. The skin may be shiny, cyanosed or dusky red, either dry or persistently sweating, the bloodflow may be increased and the bones may be rarefied. Causalgia may, however, be present without these changes and again posttraumatic disturbances of nutrition are common without causalgia.

The site of origin of the painful stimuli may be either peripheral or at the site of the nerve lesion. For example, in causalgia of the fingers consequent upon a partial lesion of the median nerve in the upper arm, it is found in some cases that the pain can be temporarily abolished by blocking the main nerves at the wrist with procaine (peripheral causalgia), whereas in other cases relief is obtained only by blocking the main nerves at the level of the lesion (proximal causalgia).

The painful impulses must enter the cord by the posterior roots (Doupe et al, 1944), for the pain can be abolished by a spinal anaesthetic, carefully given to block the posterior roots (as evidenced by cutaneous anaesthesia) without blocking the sympathetic outflow (as evidenced by absence of vasodilatation). Nevertheless, the pain can also be abolished temporarily by a paravertebral procaine block of the sympathetic chain and permanently by sympathectomy. The benefit obtained from sympathectomy is dramatic if the nerve lesion involves a main nerve trunk, but unfortunately, results are poor in high lesions of the brachial or lumbosacral plexus. In deciding whether individual cases would benefit from surgery a diagnostic trial using a systemic sympathetic paralysant such as trimetaphan may be of value.

Why sympathectomy relieves causalgia is uncertain. Relief was formerly attributed to the abolition of arterial spasm, or to improve nutrition of the skin. Recently, a rather more elaborate concept has been developed. It is now thought that causalgia results from the stimulation of somatic nerve fibres by activity in adjacent sympathetic fibres which may release acetylcholine, or by release of neurokinins in the periphery. The frequency with which causalgia is associated with incomplete nerve lesions, particularly related to high velocity missiles, may be significant as these may produce rupture of the basement membrane without interruption of the axon itself. According to this view the relief of causalgia by sympathectomy results from protection of the somatic fibres from unnatural stimulation at the site of injury.

REFERENCES

Barnes R 1954 Causalgia: A review of 48 cases. In: 'Peripheral nerve injuries'. Medical Research Council Special Report Serial No. 282, HMSO London

Bonney G 1959 Prognosis in traction lesions of the brachial plexus. Journal of Bone and Joint Surgery 41B: 4

Bowden R E M, Gutmann E 1944 Denervation and re-innervation of human voluntary muscle. Brain 67: 273

Churchill-Davidson H C 1963 Muscle relaxants. In: Hewer C L (ed) Recent Advances in Anaesthesia and Analgesia. Churchill Livingstone, London

Cragg B G, Thomas P K 1964 The conduction velocity of regenerated peripheral nerve fibres. Journal of Physiology 171: 164

Dawson G D 1956 The relative excitability and conduction velocity of sensory and motor nerve fibres in man. Journal of Physiology 131: 436

Denny-Brown D E, Brenner C 1944 Paralysis of nerve induced by direct pressure and by tourniquet. Archives of Neurology and Psychiatry 51:1

Desmedt J E 1973 New developments in electromyography and clinical neurophysiology. (In three volumes) S. Karger, Basel

Doupe J, Barnes R, Kerr A S 1943 Studies in denervation: effect of electrical stimulation on circulation and recovery of denervated muscle. Journal of Neurology and Psychiatry 6: 136

Doupe J, Cullen C H, Chance G Q 1944 Posttraumatic pain and causalgic syndrome. Journal of Neurology and Psychiatry 7: 33

Eames R A, Gamble H J 1970 Schwann cell relationships in normal human cutaneous nerves. Journal of Anatomy 106: 417

Gilliatt R W, Goodman H V, Willison R G 1961 The recording of lateral popliteal nerve action potentials in man. Journal of Neurology, Neurosurgery and Psychiatry 24: 305

Guttmann E, Guttmann L 1944 Effect of galvanic exercise on denervated and reinnervated muscles in rabbit. Journal of Neurology, Neurosurgery and Psychiatry 7: 7

Henderson W R 1948 Clinical assessment of peripheral nerve injuries. Tinel's test. Lancet ii:801

Jabaley M E, Burns J E, Orcutt B S 1976 Comparison of histologic and functional recovery after peripheral nerve repair. Journal of Hand Surgery, 1:119

Lambert E H 1962 Diagnostic value of electrical stimulation of motor nerves. Electroencephalography and Clinical Neurophysiology, Suppl. 22:9

Mitchell S W 1872 Injuries of Nerves. Philadelphia: Lippincott

Nathan P W 1958 Ischaemic and post-ischaemic numbness and paraesthesiae. Journal of Neurology, Neurosurgery and Psychiatry, 21:12

Nicholson O R, Seddon H J 1957 Nerve repair in civil practice: results of treatment of median and ulnar nerve lesions. British Medical Journal, 2:1065.

Richards R L 1967 Causalgia, a centennial review. Archives of Neurology, Chicago, 16:339.

Seddon H J 1963 Nerve grafting. Journal of Bone and Joint Surgery, 45B:447

Seddon H J 1975 Surgical Disorders of the Peripheral Nerves, 2nd edition. Edinburgh: Churchill Livingstone

Simpson J A 1956 Electrical signs in the diagnosis of carpal tunnel and related syndromes. Journal of Neurology, Neurosurgery and Psychiatry, 19:275

Sunderland S 1978 Nerves and Nerve Injuries 2nd edn. Edinburgh: Churchill Livingstone.

Thomas J E, Lambert, E G, Cseuz K A 1967 Electrodiagnostic aspects of the carpal tunnel syndrome. Archives of Neurology, Chicago, 16: 635

Thomas P K, Sears T A, Gilliatt R W 1959 The range of conduction velocity in normal motor nerve fibres to the small muscles of the hand and foot. Journal of Neurology, Neurosurgery and Psychiatry, 22:175

Tower S S 1939 The reaction of muscle to denervation. Physiological Reviews, 19:1

Trotter W, Davies H M 1909 Experimental studies in the innervation of skin. Journal of Physiology, 38:134

Weddell G, Guttmann L, Guttmann E 1941 The local extension of nerve fibres into denervated areas of skin. Journal of Neurology and Psychiatry, 4:206

Weddell G, Miller S 1962 Cutaneous sensibility. Review of Physiology, 24:199

Bone

The physiology of bone is of practical importance to the surgeon concerned with the management of injuries and disorders of the skeleton. In particular, a knowledge of the mechanisms of bone healing and its use as a graft material is fundamental to the treatment of fractures and local bone disease. As a calcified tissue it forms the major endogenous source of calcium in the body and is actively involved with its homeostasis. The physiological control of calcium metabolism depends on the interaction of the endocrine glands and exogenous vitamins. Disturbances of these mechanisms may have surgical implications, while disease of the intestinal or urinary tracts may upset the balance between mineral intake and output producing secondary effects on the skeleton.

Although this chapter is concerned with bone physiology, an understanding of the normal structure of the tissue and its development are fundamental to the subject.

THE STRUCTURE OF BONE

Bone is not a homogenous tissue but has a structure which varies with its site and function in the skeleton. It can be classified on its macroscopic appearance or microscopic organization.

Macroscopically, the compact bone forming the cortex of long bones can be distinguished from the more porous cancellous bone, with its characteristic trabecular structure, which is found in the axial skeleton and the metaphyseal region of long bones.

At a microscopic level the types of bone are distinguished by the arrangements of their collagen fibres, cells and vascular channels. The collagen, which forms 20% of the dry weight of bone and constitutes 90–95% of its organic matrix, is a fibrous protein showing a characteristic cross-banding on electron microscopy at intervals of 640 Å units. It provides the bone with its elasticity and strength and is arranged in irregular coarse fibre bundles in woven bone and in parallel or concentric sheets in mature lamellar bone. This reaches its highest level of organization in the Haversian systems or osteones of compact bone where it is formed in concentric layers around a central vascular channel.

Collagen is a unique protein since all the hydroxyproline in the body is contained in it. This amino acid is derived from the enzymatic hydroxylation of proline, a process which is dependent on a number of co-factors. These factors include oxygen, ferrous iron, alpha-ketoglutarate and ascorbic acid. This provides a tool for the investigation of collagen metabolism and therefore bone turnover, since radioactive-labelled proline can be used as a tracer to determine synthesis while the excretion of hydroxyproline in the urine reflects breakdown. After hydroxylation the collagen molecule undergoes maturation from a soluble to an insoluble form. This process begins in the cell when three polypeptide chains wind around each other in a triple helix to form a tropocollagen molecule. After extrusion from the cell these molecules aggregate by cross linkages into the mature collagen fibres and, as a result of their overlapping, produce the characteristic cross-banding. Five distinct collagen types have now been identified in the body; type I is predominant in bone and type II in cartilage (p. 4). Some collagen diseases and inherited disorders of bone, such as osteogenesis imperfecta, may result from a failure of normal formation of the collagen molecule, or the molecular cross linkages in the fibres (Prockop et al, 1979).

The remaining non-collagenous fraction of the bone matrix is made up of carbohydrate-protein complexes of two types termed glycosaminoglycans (mucopolysaccharides) and glycoproteins. The main glycosaminoglycan found in cortical bone is chondroitin sulphate which forms the amorphous ground substance in which the collagen fibrils lie. The predominant glycoprotein is a sialoprotein which has a strong affinity for heavy metals but no proven physiological function.

The inorganic material which comprises 65–70% of the bone by weight consists largely of crystalline hydroxyapatite with a smaller amount of amorphous calcium phosphate. The crystals of hydroxyapatite, with a chemical

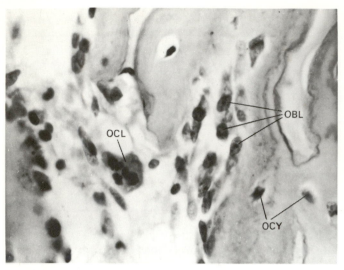

Fig. 15.1 Histology of embryonic human metaphyseal bone to show main cell types. ×440. OCL — Osteoclasts, OBL — Osteoblasts, OCY — Osteocytes. (Courtesy of Professor R. Scothorne, University Department of Anatomy, Glasgow.)

formula corresponding to $Ca_{10} (PO_4)_6 (OH)_2$, are found in mature bone deposited in a well-ordered spatial relationship within the collagen fibril. They may contain traces of other elements and because of their large surface area, allow a continuous dynamic interchange of ions between their surface and the intercellular fluid bathing them.

Three main types of cell are found in bone; the osteoblast, osteocyte and osteoclast, all of which are of mesenchymal origin (Fig. 15.1). The formation of new bone requires the presence of the osteoblast which is responsible for the production of the organic matrix or osteoid. When 'active' it is a plump cell, showing deeply-basophilic staining due to its high content of alkaline phosphatase. The cells are found closely applied to surfaces of new bone formation and occur in rows in the deep layers of the periosteum covering the bone and in the endosteum lining it. Pritchard (1972) compared their arrangement to an epithelial membrane, with the ability to secrete collagen on one side and maintain ion exchange with the intercellular fluid on the other. Osteoblasts are also found lining the Haversian canals and on the surface of the trabeculae of cancellous bone. When they become inactive, or 'resting', the cells become more flattened and pale staining and once entrapped in their own calcified matrix, form osteocytes.

The osteocyte is no longer capable of secreting organic matrix but plays an important part in its nutrition. These cells intercommunicate with each other and with the capillaries of the Haversian system by fine cellular processes lying in canaliculi in the bone. There is some evidence from the work of Belanger (1969) that osteocytes can be activated by parathyroid hormone to resorb bone matrix without the intervention of osteoclasts, the process

being termed osteocytic osteolysis. This removal of perilacunar bone is insufficient to produce structural change, but may play an important part in the metabolic control of calcium homeostasis (Rasmussen & Bordier, 1974).

Osteoclasts are the characteristic acidophilic, multinucleate giant cells found at the sites of active bone resorption. The cell type has been described in detail by Hancox (1972) who was able to relate their electron microscopic structure to their resorptive function. He demonstrated the 'brush' border of finger-like processes arising from the cell membrane adjacent to the resorbing bone surface. Between the cytoplasmic processes are channels adjacent to intracellular vacuoles which are thought to secrete the lysosomal enzymes produced in the cell and absorb bone salts and fragments of digested collagen fibres. These large cells are usually found in shallow depressions on the resorptive surface, termed Howship's lacunae, but may sometimes appear to be engulfing the ends of bony trabeculae undergoing resorption. The factors controlling the osteoclastic activity have not been fully elucidated but are thought to include parathyroid hormone and prostaglandin E.

All these cells and others found in bone, such as the flattened fibroblasts of the superficial layer of the periosteum and the chondrocytes of cartilage, were thought to arise from a common mesenchymal stem cell. Hall (1970) suggested that this basic osteoprogenitor cell differentiates in response to factors within its environment. Hyperoxia, mechanical pressure or tension, and hyperaemia stimulate the production of osteoblasts and osteocytes, cells capable of forming collagen. Conversely, hypoxia and ischaemia stimulate cell differentiation into the chondrocyte series, characterized by the synthesis of glycosaminoglycans. An alternative theory has emerged for the origin of osteoclasts, which are now thought to be a separate cell line derived from circulating macrophages. Evidence in support of this hypothesis was provided by Buring (1975) who studied the fate of these circulating cells after radioactive labelling by the use of crossed circulations in parabiotic rats.

DEVELOPMENT AND GROWTH OF BONE

The majority of the bones of the skeleton are formed initially during embryonic development as cartilaginous models which are later replaced by bone tissue. This type of bone production is described as endochondral ossification, in contrast to the formation of bone by the process of intramembranous ossification without passing through a cartilaginous stage.

The embryonic bones first appear as a condensation of mesoderm in which the cells differentiate to form cartilage cells or chondroblasts which secrete an organic matrix of glycosaminoglycans. The cartilaginous model is covered by a condensed mesenchymal membrane termed the perichondrium and is able to increase in length by interstitial growth and in width by appositional growth. At the centre of the cartilaginous model the chondroblasts become hypertrophic and the intercellular matrix thins and becomes calcified. Capillaries then invade the perichondrium converting it to periosteum as its deeper cells differentiate into osteoblasts and form a thin shell of bone on the surface of the shaft. The formation of a primary ossification centre results from a progressive replacement of the degenerate hypertrophied cells of the calcified cartilage by invasion of osteoblasts from the periosteum. This is accompanied by the ingrowth of capillaries which assist in the removal of the calcified organic matrix to form a marrow cavity. Bone is deposited on the surface of the remains of the calcified cartilage matrix in the region of hypertrophic cartilage cells proximal and distal to this cavity. As the medullary cavity expands towards the ends of the bone there is a simultaneous increase in thickness of the periosteal bony collar to form the bony shaft or diaphysis. The secondary centres of ossification then appear in the central portions of the cartilaginous ends of the bone. Here the cells again become hypertrophic with calcification of their matrix and a resultant invasion by capillaries and osteoblasts to deposit bone. The centrifugal enlargement of these secondary ossification centres in combination with the longitudinal enlargement of the medullary cavity results in the formation of a zone of uncalcified cartilage cells and matrix between them, termed the epiphyseal or growth plate (Fig. 15.2). The chondrocytes of the growth plate line up in vertical rows and differentiate to form zones with distinct histological appearances. Immediately adjacent to the bone end or epiphysis containing the secondary centre of ossification are the small chondrocytes of the resting zone. These multiply rapidly to form columns of flatter cells in the zone of proliferation before maturing and enlarging in the hypertrophic zone. As they degenerate the hypertrophic cells become surrounded by calcified matrix and are then removed by the osteoclasts and macrophages carried in by capillary invasion from the metaphysis.

There is a continual growth in length of bones until the age of puberty by interstitial division of the cartilage cells in the epiphyseal growth plate. The continued production of chondrocytes and their degeneration and replacement by bone on the diaphyseal side of the plate is the process of endochondral ossification. The physiological control of this process is not entirely understood but it is certain that growth hormone production by the pituitary and the secretion of sex hormones at puberty are interrelated in its maintenance. Growth hormone has been shown to act indirectly through somatomedin or sulphation factor produced in the liver. Thyroxine is also an important early stimulus for growth plate function and deficiency states in cretinism can result in severe stunting and dwarfism. Of the sex hormones, testosterone appears to stimulate carti-

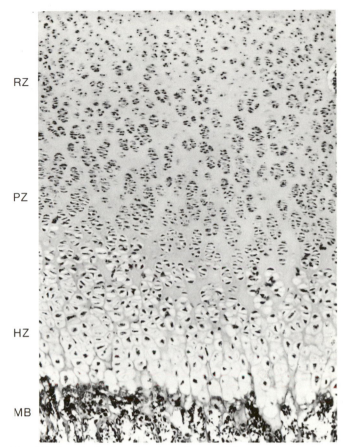

Fig. 15.2 Longitudinal section through part of the growth plate in an embryonic human long bone. ×80. RZ — resting zone, PZ — proliferative zone, HZ — hypertrophic zone, MB — metaphyseal bone. (Courtesy of Professor R. Scothorne, University of Glasgow.)

lage growth and matrix elaboration, whereas oestrogens increase matrix calcification which accompanies cessation of epiphyseal growth. The interrelationships are uncertain but offer an explanation for the earlier closure of epiphyseal plates in girls at the time of puberty. At puberty, when the growth in length of bone is complete, the proliferation of chondroblasts in the growth plate slows down and eventually ceases. When no cartilage remains separating the diaphysis from the bony portion of the epiphysis, the centre of ossification is said to be closed or fused. Occasionally, under conditions of hyperpituitarism the cartilage cells may persist and even re-activate resulting in continued growth in length and the condition of gigantism. Similarly, a deficiency of pituitary growth hormone may lead to premature closure of the growth plate with resultant dwarfism.

The shafts of long bones also grow in width by continued appositional bone formation as the osteoblastic cells in the deeper layers of the periosteum lay down bone directly on the outer surface of the cortex by a process of intramembranous ossification. There is a simultaneous resorption of bone from the inner or endosteal surface which enlarges the diameter of the marrow cavity.

Until puberty the epiphyses at the ends of long bones continue to enlarge by hemispherical growth at their surface. This occurs by a similar sequence of endochondral ossification to that seen in the epiphyseal growth plate. This process which occurs in the subchondral region of the articular cartilage may account for as much as 5% or more of the total growth in length of long bones. The absence of a medullary cavity in the epiphyses means that the diameter of long bones in their epiphyseal and metaphyseal ends is much greater than that in the diaphysis or shaft.

During normal growth, or even in conditions of postfetal osteogenesis as occur in fracture healing, the shape and contour of bones respond to local mechanical stresses. Prior to growth plate closure there is some anatomical restraint by the integrity of the periosteum. This can be demonstrated by experimental circumferential division of this membrane which will result in a temporary acceleration of longitudinal bone growth. A similar effect may be seen following a fracture of a long bone in childhood and may result in limb length discrepancy.

Any local increase in the stresses acting on an area of bone, either from muscle action or transmission of weight, results in an increase in bone formation. Similarly, a decrease in stress within a bone leads to bone resorption and a condition of disuse osteoporosis may result. The mechanism of this mechanical stimulus to bone formation is not fully understood though the theory has been advanced by Bassett (1968) that it is related to the piezo-electric effects of the bone mineral crystal. The crystals are thought to function as transducers converting mechanical forces into electrical and biological signals with resultant local changes in the hormonal control of bone turnover. This theory has formed the basis of new experimental treatments for delayed and non-union, using implanted electrodes to produce low-voltage currents or by external coils to induce electro-magnetic fields in the bone.

Hyperaemia is another local stimulus to increased bone formation, probably through a change in tissue oxygen tension or local pH. Stimulation of epiphyseal growth may occur in the prepubertal long bone from congenital arteriovenous fistulae or the hyperaemia associated with metaphyseal infections, resulting in limb length discrepancies. Hyperaemia has also been noted to stimulate fracture healing, though there has been some controversy as to the tissue gas tensions resulting from this circulatory change. Heppenstall et al (1975) suggested that new bone formation occurs under anaerobic conditions and demonstrated low oxygen tension with increased blood flow at the site of experimental fractures.

SKELETAL RENEWAL AND BONE TURNOVER

After the cessation of longitudinal bone growth at puberty the skeleton continues to renew itself by a process of balanced formation and resorption or bone 'turnover'. This process occurs at a microscopic level in both cancellous and cortical bone and allows the mineral to participate in the normal process of calcium homeostasis. The process is under complex physiological control from general metabolic factors affecting the whole skeleton, but can be modified by local stimuli such as fractures, infection or tumours.

As the tissue of bone is replaced its architecture is altered as well, reflecting the local stimuli acting at that site in the skeleton. In cortical bone the existing Haversian systems are remodelled by the ingrowth of new osteones. These are preceded by a 'cutting cone' of osteoclasts creating resorption cavities, which are then filled in by osteoblasts laying down collagen and osteoid which is subsequently mineralized. A similar process occurs in cancellous bone with the resorption of old trabeculae and the formation of new osteoid on their surfaces. At sites of active bone formation the calcified matrix is covered by an unmineralized osteoid 'seam' or layer averaging 6–10 μm thickness. These become thicker in conditions of impaired mineralization, such as rickets or osteomalacia, where the stimulus to matrix calcification is lacking.

The biochemical changes in osteoid preceding calcification are not fully understood but may be related to the maturation of collagen fibrils. Initially the bone mineral is deposited as amorphous calcium phosphate, which is either converted directly to apatite crystals or indirectly through the formation of another crystalline form, octocalcium phosphate. The extracellular fluid is normally fully saturated with respect to calcium and phosphate and once crystal deposition is initiated, a process termed nucleation, a process of crystal growth continues indefinitely. It is thought that this nucleation is inhibited by the presence of pyrophosphate which is itself broken down by the phosphatases released from the osteoblasts. Another inhibitory factor may be the excess of the glycosaminoglycan chondroitin sulphate, which disappears from the osteoid just prior to calcification. In new bone the process of primary calcification occurs rapidly and is 70% complete in a few hours. The remaining 30% of inorganic mineral is deposited by a slower process of accretion over several weeks or months and is less directly under osteoblast control. There is some experimental evidence that the primary bone mineral is less stable and more available for 'exchange' than the fully mature or secondary mineral.

The physiological process of skeletal renewal can be studied by various in vivo techniques which may be used to provide the surgeon with a knowledge of the process in the whole skeleton or at one particular bone site. The use of radioactive isotopes for tracer studies and skeletal scintimetry has been reviewed by Bauer (1968). Isotope tracers, such as calcium-45 and -47, can be used to study the kinetics of mineral turnover in the skeleton using balance studies and whole body counters. The collection

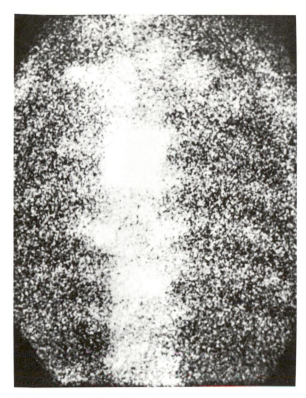

Fig. 15.3 Technetium-99m diphosphonate gamma camera scan of thorax and spine in patient with multiple metastases in ribs and vertebrae from bronchial carcinoma. (Courtesy of Dr P. Horton, Western Infirmary, Glasgow.)

and interpretation of data are difficult and time consuming since tracer retention is of two types; the 'exchangeable' calcium pool in the extracellular fluid and primary bone mineral and the 'non-exchangeable' calcium in fully mature bone. Of more practical value is the use of gamma-emitting isotopes such as strontium-85 and -87 m, fluorine-18 and the technetium-99m polyphosphates which can be detected using an external scanner or camera, containing a sodium iodide crystal. This bone scan will identify the sites of new bone formation in relation to infection or tumours which may not be visible by conventional radiography (Fig. 15.3).

Invasive techniques can be used to study the process of bone formation and resorption in a biopsy taken from a particular site in the skeleton. In addition to conventional histology the differences between areas of 'primary' and 'secondary' mineralization can be studied using micro-radiography. Additional evidence can be obtained if the patient is given intravital dyes, such as the tetracyclines, prior to biopsy. These have been shown by Harris et al (1962) to be preferentially localized in all bone-forming surfaces at the time of their administration and indicate those sites by fluorescence when undecalcified sections are examined under ultraviolet light. If two dissimilar tetracyclines are used at different periods a comparison of bone formation with time can be obtained. The areas of active

bone formation can be expressed as a percentage of the total bone area in the section and allow extrapolation to provide formation rates against time. However these can only provide rough data for activity in the skeleton as a whole because of the problem of heterogeneity in the sites of formation and resorption. What is known is that cancellous bone remodels at a much faster rate than cortical bone and probably accounts for 50% of the turnover in only one-fifth of the skeletal mass.

FRACTURE HEALING

An understanding of the normal mechanisms of fracture healing enables the surgeon to select the most appropriate treatment, either conservative or operative, for any type of bone injury.

Secondary bone healing

The majority of fractures are treated by conservative methods using external splintage and heal spontaneously by a process of secondary bone healing. This is characterized by the production of a callus of vascular granulation tissue which ensheaths the two broken fragments of bone. This is later replaced by cartilage and trabecular bone prior to final bony union and remodelling. The steps are shown diagrammatically in Figure 15.4.

The granulation tissue bond was originally thought to derive from cellular differentiation within the haematoma formed between the two broken ends but recent work summarized by Ham and Harris (1971) suggests it arises from the periosteum and endosteum. The cells in the deeper osteogenic layers of the periosteum proliferate, as do those from the endosteum of the Haversian canals and marrow cavity, to invade and replace the resolving blood clot at the fracture site. When the thickened periosteum has joined across the fracture line it forms the fusiform external callus. The osteogenic cells in the deeper layers differentiate to become osteoblasts forming trabecular bone while more superficially they resemble chondrocytes and deposit cartilage ground substance.

The local conditions at the fracture site, particularly the blood supply and the degree of movement between the bone ends, determine to what extent this granulation tissue weld differentiates into cartilage, woven bone or fibrous tissue. Excessive movement or loss of the blood supply to one or both fragments produces local ischaemia with a consequent low oxygen tension which predisposes to the formation of excessive amounts of cartilage or even a fibrous tissue 'non-union'. The new bone finally forms a bridge across the cortical fragments showing more coarse trabecular bone towards the outside and on the endosteal surface. In the final stages of fracture healing this external callus is remodelled by the conversion of the trabecular

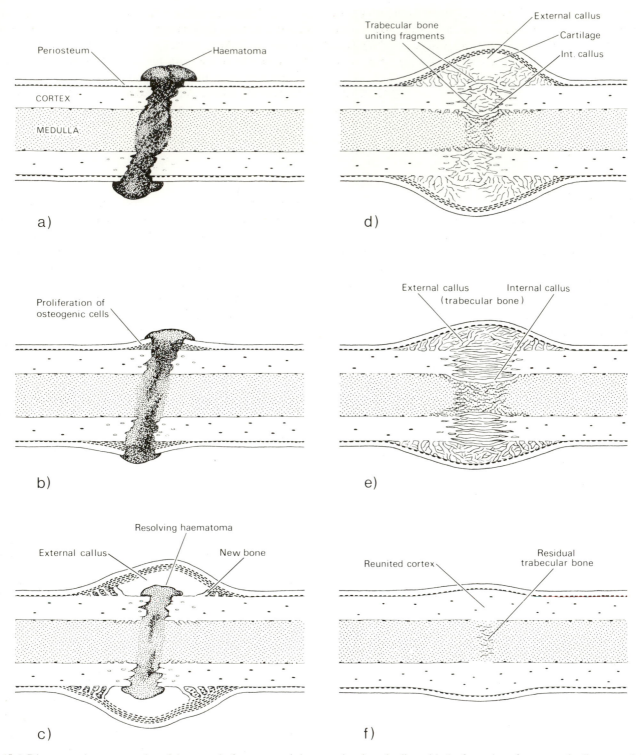

Fig. 15.4 Diagrammatic representation of the stages in fracture repair by secondary bone healing with the formation of an external callus around the bone ends.

bone to compact lamellar bone uniting the cortical fragments after the dead bone at their ends has been resorbed. This bony union takes several months to occur in cortical long bones, but may be a more rapid process in young children or in cancellous bone because of the richer blood supply and better osteogenic potential. Excessive external callus is slowly removed and the mechanical forces acting at the site of the healing fractures are mainly responsible for restoring the normal anatomy when overlapping or angulation has occurred. They produce resorption on the convex side and increase bone formation on the concave side with resultant re-alignment of the Haversian systems in the lines of stress.

In fractures of cancellous bone, medullary osteogenesis plays the major role in healing but in cortical long bones the periosteum is the most important structure and its soft tissue attachments must be preserved as much as possible in any surgical approach.

Primary bone healing

This is a less common event and only occurs when the two bone fragments are held in rigid contact by axial compression fixation techniques. Under these conditions, which have been investigated in experimental and clinical states by Perren et al (1969), no external callus is formed. Initially the minimal gap between the bone ends becomes filled with woven bone, deposited by cells growing in from the periosteal and endosteal surfaces (Fig.15.5). This is followed by a remodelling phase in which Haversian systems grow directly across the fracture line from one cortex to the other. These ostcones remove bone by an

osteoclastic 'cutting cone' action and then deposit new bone from the osteoblasts lining the Haversian canal. The time taken to heal a fracture by this method is probably no quicker than that achieved by secondary bone healing and the lack of callus may make radiological assessment of union difficult. The advantages of rigid internal fixation are to permit early mobility of the fractured bone thereby reducing the risk of joint stiffness and immobilization osteoporosis.

Delayed union

This may occur in fractures when one or both fragments are deprived of their blood supply, in excessive comminution with loss of bone contact, from interposition of soft tissue, or when infection supervenes in open injuries. These factors can be minimized by careful handling and reduction of the fragments to maintain bony contact and prevent further damage to the periosteum and soft tissues. This should be combined with adequate immobilization, particularly if one fragment has lost its blood supply, since revascularization must occur by creeping substitution across the fracture line.

General factors rarely result in impaired fracture healing though this could occur in gross vitamin C or vitamin D deficiency states and these should be excluded, particularly in elderly patients.

BONE GRAFTING

The use of bone grafts was first described by McEwan in 1880 and is now well established in the practice of orthopaedic surgery. They may be used to stimulate osteogenesis in the treatment of ununited fractures, to fill defects in bone due to tumours or chronic infections, and to produce an arthrodesis of a joint by bridging the gap between the bones of the articulation.

The two types of bone used for grafting are either chips of cancellous bone or slabs of compact cortical bone. Cancellous bone has the advantages of being easily available from the iliac crest and conforms readily to the space to be filled. Compact bone has the ability to provide some degree of mechanical stability and can be fixed in place with screws or wire, but is more difficult to obtain as an autogenous transplant. Both types of graft may be removed from the patient's own skeleton when they are termed autografts. They may be obtained from another human donor, allowing storage if required, and are then described as allografts or homografts. Bone grafts removed from species other than man are termed xenografts or heterografts and some attempts have been made to use them in clinical practice.

Bone grafting was well established as a practical surgical procedure before the immunological aspects of transplan-

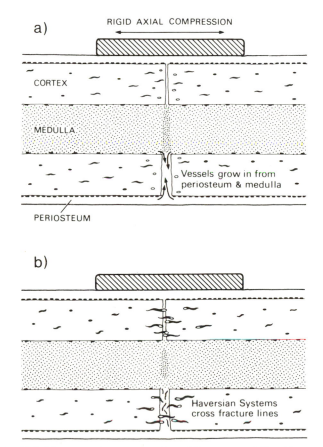

Fig. 15.5 Diagrammatic representation of fracture repair by primary bone healing where fixation by rigid compression has resulted in no gap or a minimal space between the bone ends.

tation became known. However, knowledge of these mechanisms is important in considering the choice of graft and has led to a clearer understanding of the earlier clinical observations on bone transplantation. The other problem on which research has been concentrated is the source of the osteogenic stimulus provided by the graft and whether the cells of the donor bone are able to survive transplantation.

The viability of compact bone is dependent on an intact blood supply and the few cells buried in its dense, calcified matrix cannot survive free transplantation. After a few days the osteocytes in an autologous graft of compact bone become pyknotic, many lacunae are empty and the graft is effectively dead. Nevertheless, it still provides an osteogenic stimulus to the bed in which it is placed, causing the osteogenic cells of the host tissue to proliferate. These first anchor the graft and then gradually invade it by revascularization of the old Haversian systems to remove dead bone by osteoclastic activity and replace it with new living bone formed by the osteoblastic cells.

In contrast, cancellous bone contains relatively more cells near its surface and in the case of adherent marrow these may be markedly pluripotent. In addition, the spaces between the trabeculae are larger and lend themselves more readily to the ingrowth of the new blood vessels. Although many of the cells fail to survive free transplantation, there is strong evidence that the more superficial cells remain viable by diffusion of nutrients from the tissue fluids. The histological studies of Gallie and Robertson (1920) using compact and cancellous grafts to the back muscles of dogs, first drew attention to these differences in behaviour. The ability of these superficial cells to undertake osteogenic activity has been confirmed by more recent work using the technique of labelling with tritiated

thymidine for cell division and by demonstrating tetracycline fluorescence in the newly formed bone. These surface cells have the ability to proliferate and differentiate into osteoblasts, which lay down new bone on the surface of the dead fragments within a few days of transplantation. By 3 weeks the cancellous graft is largely replaced by new bone, in contrast to compact bone which only achieves the same state after a period of about 3 months. Thus, autologous cancellous bone is preferable to compact bone where osteogenesis is required and mechanical stability can be added by the use of the metallic implants.

When allografts are used a new factor of the immune mechanism is introduced. Chalmers (1959) compared the behaviour of autologous and allogeneic cancellous bone grafts transplanted into the muscles of the rat. He showed that the initial behaviour at 6 days was identical in both grafts, with immature new bone laid down by the surviving osteoblastic cells on the surface of the dead implants. However, after 10 days the new bone in the allograft showed marked degenerative changes when compared with the autologous transplant (Figs 15.6a and b). The bone-forming cells became pyknotic and there was a heavy infiltration with mononuclear cells suggesting a cell-mediated allograft reaction. In the later stages of graft rejection there was an almost total resorption of the allogeneic bone after 3–4 weeks. Allografts of compact bone produce a less severe rejection reaction, presumably because they present a smaller cell population, provide less antigenic stimulus, and are less exposed to the host tissues.

Attempts have been made to lessen the antigenic properties of allogeneic bone grafts by cell destruction using triple freezing or freeze drying to leave the intercellular matrix intact. The sterilization of stored allografts is also a problem since boiling, autoclaving or deproteinization all

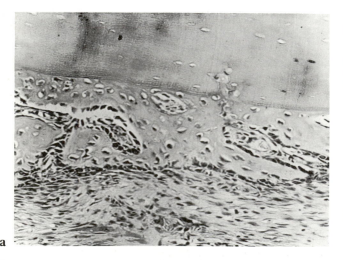
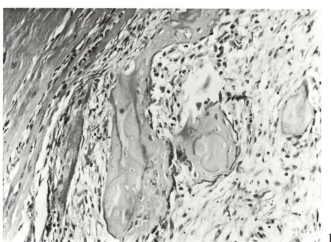

Fig. 15.6a Histology of autogenous bone graft after 10 days. ×175. The original graft is largely acellular but there is vigorous proliferaton of new bone from its surface; b Histology of homologous bone graft after 8 days. ×175. The surface layer of osteoblasts on the new bone are more flattened and basophilic while osteoclastic resorption is commencing. (Courtesy of Mr J. Chalmers, Edinburgh, and the Editor of the Journal of Bone and Joint Surgery.

reduce its inductive capacity. The types of allogeneic and xenogeneic graft available and the results of their use in experimental and clinical practice have been reviewed by Burwell (1969). Xenografts of calf bone have been prepared by methods designed to reduce their antigenicity, either by freeze drying (Boplant) or by deproteinization (Kiel). These enjoyed a brief popularity in clinical practice but have now been largely discarded because of the loss of osteogenic capacity produced by their preparation. The best bank bone available for clinical use is freeze dried allogeneic cancellous bone sterilized by irradiation.

Allografts of cartilage will, of course, survive transplantation since chondrocytes do not require a blood supply and the intercellular substance, which allows diffusion of nutrients, prevents antibodies or activated lymphocytes from reaching them.

CALCIUM HOMEOSTASIS

Of the calcium contained in the body, 99% is held in the mineral phase of the body skeleton as hydroxyapatite. The remaining 1% is found in the body fluids in both ionized and non-ionized form. The normal plasma calcium level is 2.2–2.6 mmol/l (8.8–10.4 mg/100 ml) of which approximately 1.1–1.2 mmol/l is in ionized form and the remainder is bound to the plasma protein, albumen. At normal albumen concentrations 50–60% of the total plasma calcium is in bound form. The ionized calcium concentration is dependent on the pH and the concentration of the anions with which it combines, especially phosphate. Any increase in phosphate concentration will decrease the ionic calcium level, as will a rise in plasma pH which increases the association of the two ions. This divalent cation is essential for many normal body functions including nerve conduction, muscle contraction, the structural integrity of cell membranes, and adhesion between cells. In addition it participates in many enzyme reactions, including the blood clotting mechanism, though the concentrations required for these is less crucial.

To preserve these normal functions the calcium concentration must be maintained within a close range and elaborate homeostatic mechanisms exist in the body to ensure this. As the dietary intake is intermittent the bone of the skeleton must provide calcium to maintain the plasma levels, which can also be regulated through excretion and re-absorption of the ion by the kidney. In the last decade there has been a major expansion of research in this field which has yielded a great deal of new information on the factors controlling calcium metabolism. The old concept of control by parathyroid hormone alone has been changed by the discovery of other calcium-regulating hormones, notably calcitonin and the active metabolites produced from vitamin D. A diagram of the current concept of calcium homeostasis and these hormonal interactions is shown in Figure 15.7.

In the normal diet three-quarters of the calcium is provided by milk and dairy products, with the exception of butter, together with bread which, in Britain, is made from flour artificially supplemented with calcium. The average daily intake required for adults is 600–800 mg, but in periods of active bone formation in growing children or pregnant women or during prolonged lactation, the demand may rise to 1.5–2 g daily. To this dietary calcium the bile and intestinal secretions add a further 500–700 mg so that in intestinal dysfunction rapid and heavy loss may occur. It is absorbed throughout the intestine and although this mechanism is most efficient in the duodenum the bulk is absorbed from the small intestine because of the longer exposure time. Despite the large daily intake the net absorption from the intestine is only about 150 mg.

Vitamin D has been known to be an essential factor for the normal intestinal absorption of calcium for many years, but its mode of action was less certain. The recognition that vitamin D_3 or cholecalciferol, derived from the diet or by ultraviolet irradiation of the skin, underwent metabolic changes in the body led to a knowledge of its hormonal function. The current views on calcium homeostasis have been described by De Luca (1975) who also observed the stimulation of calcium absorption by the active metabolite 1,25-dihydroxy vitamin D_3. Other factors may influence calcium absorption which is decreased by alkalinity because this stimulates the formation of insoluble calcium salts, such as phosphate and phytate. This may also be the mechanism in steatorrhea, though bulky stools and intestinal hurry also contribute to the loss. The phytic acid in some cereals may precipitate calcium with loss of absorption as will a high intake of dietary phosphate, the standard experimental technique for inducing a deficiency state in the rat.

The amount of calcium excreted in the urine varies with the degree of tubular re-absorption. It is estimated that 5000–8500 mg of calcium per day is filtered and over 90% of this is re-absorbed. Parathyroid hormone (PTH) is known to stimulate calcium and inhibit phosphate re-absorption. Normal calcium loss ranges from 100–300 mg but may fall to less than 100 mg if the dietary intake is reduced for a few days.

PHOSPHORUS METABOLISM

The dietary phosphorus content is normally high and deficiency states from inadequate intake are virtually unknown. The daily requirement of 1–1.5 g is easily met since all animal and vegetable cells are rich sources of the mineral. About two-thirds of the dietary intake is absorbed from the intestine by an active transport mechanism while the remainder is lost in the faeces as insoluble phosphate

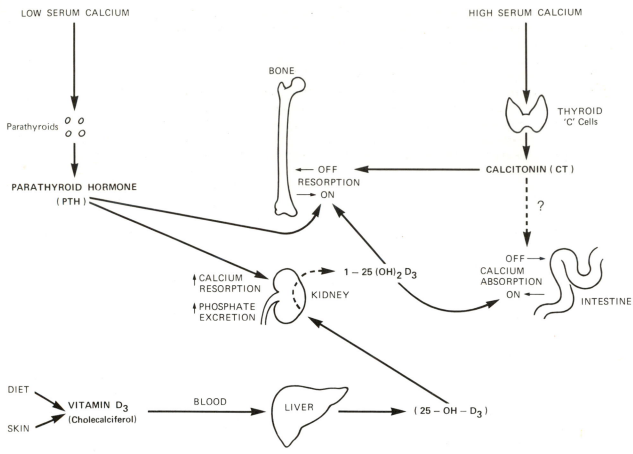

Fig. 15.7 The biological factors concerned with the maintenance of calcium homeostasis.

salts. The absorption of phosphorus, like calcium, is impaired in vitamin D deficiency and there is a resultant increase in faecal calcium phosphate. Excessive intake of aluminium hydroxide as an antacid may result in formation of insoluble aluminium phosphate in the gut with symptoms of clinical depletion such as muscle weakness.

The total plasma phosphate of 3.9 mmol/l is made up of two forms; an organic component averaging 2.8 mmol/l largely bound to lipids and a smaller inorganic fraction of 1.1 mmol/l. It is this inorganic phosphate which is normally estimated clinically and reported as the serum phosphate with a normal range of 0.8–1.5 mmol/l the (2.5–4.8 mg/100 ml). The normal values, as with calcium, vary from laboratory to laboratory as well as being higher in infancy and after meals or exercise. Hypophosphataemia may result from deficient gut absorption and has also been reported in surgical patients on prolonged intravenous hyperalimentation with phosphorus-free, high carbohydrate fluids.

The commonest cause of a clinical deficiency state is failure of renal tubular reabsorption of phosphate. Normally more than 80% of the phosphate in the glomerular filtrate is reabsorbed in the proximal tubule under the control of parathyroid hormone and calcitonin. An increased urinary phosphate excretion may occur in hyperparathyroidism as well as congenital or acquired tubular reabsorption defects. Advanced nephritis with glomerular failure will impair excretion and increase the plasma concentration of phosphate. Other causes of hyperphosphataemia are metastatic carcinoma of bone, blood transfusion, haemolysis, muscle damage and hypoparathyroidism.

PHOSPHATASES

The enzymes which hydrolyse phosphate esters in the tissues of the body are classified into acid and alkaline phosphatases from a knowledge of their optimum pH. The alkaline phosphatases act between pH 8 and 10 and are derived from bone, liver, kidney, gut and placenta. The acid phosphatases which are most active at pH 4.5–5 are present in the prostate, spleen, kidney, liver and red cells.

The activity of the enzymes in the serum can be estimated by techniques which utilize the liberation of phenol from artificial phosphate esters, such as sodium monophenyl phosphate, under standard conditions. The reaction is performed at pH 9.1 for alkaline phosphatase and pH 4.8 for acid phosphatase. The result is normally expressed in King-Armstrong (KA) units, where one unit is equivalent to the amount of enzyme which liberates 1 mg of phenol from the substrate under the standard conditions. Newer, automated techniques of phosphatase estimation use paranitrophenyl phosphate as the substrate and the results may be expressed in new international units with a normal range from 40–165 units per litre in the 18–65 age group. It should be noted that these new values do not bear a linear relationship with the old system of King-Armstrong units.

Alkaline phosphatase

The normal level of serum alkaline phosphatase in adults is 3–13 KA units/100 ml, though much higher levels are found in children. Thus, the results in suspected childhood diseases are more difficult to interpret because of the wide range of normal with an upper limit of at least 30 KA units. Elevated levels of the enzyme may result from diseases of the liver or occur in generalised bone disorders such as Paget's disease. Electrophoretic techniques can be used to separate the liver and bone enzymes in the serum, though a more simple method is heating to 50–60°C for 15 minutes which inactivates the bone enzyme.

The associated clinical disorders are usually indicative of the source of the elevated serum enzyme level and have been reviewed by Kaplan (1972). The bone enzyme, which is thought to function as a pyrophosphatase, can be identified by histochemical staining in relation to areas of potential or active bone formation. It is found extensively in developing bones at the site of the epiphyses, particularly in relation to the hypertrophic cartilage cells. In adult bones it is largely confined to the deep layers of the periosteum but whenever new bone formation occurs, such as in fracture healing, it can be identified within the osteoblasts and young osteocytes as well as the new matrix. It is not associated with mature osteocytes or osteoclasts. Its presence is thought to be associated with the local production of phosphate required for the normal process of calcification to deposit bone mineral in any new osseous matrix. The serum levels are elevated in fracture healing, rickets and osteomalacia, osteogenic sarcoma, some metastatic bone tumours and may reach very high levels of 100–200 units in generalized Paget's disease. Its concentration in skin is normally low but becomes markedly elevated in the granulation tissue of healing wounds where it can be demonstrated in relation to fibroblasts and newly formed fibrous tissue.

The serum alkaline phosphatase may also be elevated in liver disease and is important in the differential diagnosis of jaundice, where levels above 30 KA units are indicative of an obstructive rather than a hepatogenous aetiology. It is thought to be present in the intestinal mucosa for the normal absorption of calcium and phosphate and elevated levels over 50 KA units are common in steatorrhea and some other forms of malabsorption.

Acid phosphatases

When blood is withdrawn for estimation of the serum acid phosphatase care must be taken to avoid haemolysis which liberates this enzyme from the red cells. If this is avoided the serum acid phosphatase is largely derived from the prostate with a small contribution from the osteoclasts of bone. The level is normally 0–4 KA units/100 ml but may be elevated above 5 units in prostatic carcinoma, particularly when this is associated with extensive bone metastases. The concentration of the serum enzyme can be decreased by castration or oestrogens and is sometimes used to monitor treatment of the neoplasm by these techniques.

BIOLOGICAL FACTORS IN MINERAL HOMEOSTASIS

Vitamin D and its metabolites

The fat-soluble vitamin D influences calcium homeostasis through its active metabolites which function as steroid hormones with the intestine and bone as the two target organs. The natural vitamin D_3, cholecalciferol, occurs in the diet and is also formed in the skin when it is exposed to ultraviolet light. Foods which are particularly rich in the vitamin are milk, eggs and fatty fishes and their liver oils. Vitamin D_2, calciferol, is produced artificially by ultraviolet irradiation of sterols and has a similar potency to the natural vitamin. Both are defined in terms of an international unit which is equal to 0.025 μg of the pure crystalline substance. The daily requirement in adults is of the order of 100 international units, while children may require from 200–400 international units. As the vitamin is fat-soluble it is poorly absorbed in coeliac disease and sprue and from its affinity for mineral oils may be excessively excreted in over-purgation with liquid paraffin.

After absorption into the intestine the vitamin is transported to the liver, where it is hydroxylated in the endoplasmic reticulum by an enzyme reaction to form 25-hydroxy vitamin D_3 (25-OH D_3). This metabolite is the main circulating form of the vitamin in the blood with a normal level, probably maintained by a feed-back enzyme mechanism, at 25–50 ng/ml. It is carried bound to an alpha 2-globulin in the plasma and has only weak biological activity. In the kidney the mitochondria of the renal cells induce a further hydroxylation to produce the biologically active metabolite 1,25-dihydroxyvitamin D_3 (1,25-$(OH)_2D_3$). The enzyme reaction for its production is controlled through a negative feed-back mechanism by the serum calcium concentration, which stimulates increased secretion of parathyroid hormone.

The action of 1,25-$(OH)_2D_3$ on the intestine is to stimulate calcium and phosphate absorption, though the exact mechanism is uncertain. Using radioactive tagged metabolite it has been shown to enter the columnar epithelial cells of the villi probably in the nuclear fraction. It has been suggested that it interacts with the nuclear DNA to stimulate the formation of the RNA necessary for the synthesis of a specific calcium binding protein. However, no quantitative correlation can be demonstrated between the rate of calcium transport across the intestine and the quantity of binding protein present. Alternatively 1,25-$(OH)_2D_3$ may bind to a cytoplasmic receptor to form a larger receptor which in turn binds to nuclear material. Its presence is known to be necessary for the transfer of calcium ions across the brush border of the intestinal epithelial cell and it may activate a calcium dependent enzyme adenosine triphosphatase in the brush border itself.

Clinical or experimental low calcium diets will elevate the rate of intestinal calcium absorption, presumably by stimulating production of 1,25-$(OH)_2D_3$ through an increased secretion of parathyroid hormone. This effect persists after return to a normal diet until any bone demineralization has been fully corrected. The dietary phosphorus level is also important as deprivation of this has been shown to stimulate the synthesis of 1,25-$(OH)_2D_3$, though the mechanism is again unclear.

Experimental work in vivo and in vitro has shown the action of 1,25-$(OH)_2D_3$ on bone is to induce mobilization of calcium from previously formed mineral. The mechanism may again be through the stimulation of bone cells to produce a messenger RNA for the production of a transfer protein, as the effect can be blocked by previous administration of the antibiotic actinomycin D. In vivo experiments also suggest that parathyroid hormone is necessary for this process and if one or other of these two factors are absent the calcium mobilisation from bone will fall.

Commercial preparations of the metabolite 1,25-$(OH)_2D_3$ and a synthetic analogue 1,α-OHD_3 are now available and are being evaluated in the treatment of osteomalacia and vitamin D resistant renal rickets.

Parathyroid hormone

For many years it was known that surgical removal of the parathyroid glands was followed by a profound fall in blood calcium resulting in convulsions and tetany, which were in turn relieved by calcium infusions. Collip in 1925 first prepared an extract from bovine parathyroid tissue which could reverse these symptoms in parathyroidectomized dogs. McLean (1957) postulated that production of the hormone was controlled by a feed-back mechanism and that hypocalcaemia stimulated its production while hypercalcaemia suppressed it.

Work by Potts et al (1971) has fully evaluated the biosynthesis, secretion and metabolism of the parathyroid hormone which differs slightly in structure from species to species. The human hormone is made up of a sequence of 84 amino acids with a molecular weight of 9500. The first 34 sequences of amino acids from the amino terminal have been synthesized and show nearly as much biological activity as the natural hormone. It is thought that a precursor, proparathyroid hormone, with a molecular weight of 11 500 is converted in cells of the parathyroid gland prior to secretion into the circulation. The circulating hormone is thought to undergo cleavage, probably in the peripheral tissues, into two biological fragments which are immunologically separate and can be used to differentiate types of clinical hyperparathyroidism. The larger of the two, based on the carboxy terminal, has a molecular weight of 7000, while the smaller amino terminal fragment may be more biologically active.

The primary site of action of parathyroid hormone is thought to be on renal tubular reabsorption to maintain plasma calcium levels. Its other main action is to stimulate calcium mobilization from the bone by increased osteoclast and possibly osteocyte activity. The hormone also acts on the kidney to stimulate the enzymatic conversion of the vitamin D metabolite 25-OHD_3 to 1,25-$(OH)_2D_3$, resulting in an increase of intestinal absorption of calcium. Its action on the kidney and bone is mediated through an intermediary nucleotide, cyclic adenosine 3,5 monophosphate (AMP). This is produced when the polypeptide hormone binds to a specific cell membrane receptor with an increased secretion of an intracellular enzyme, adenyl cyclase.

Calcitonin

The discovery of a calcium-lowering hormone, calcitonin, by Copp (1961) rapidly advanced the knowledge of the mechanism for close control of plasma calcium levels. He based his claim on perfusion experiments in which the passage of high-calcium blood through the thyroid and parathyroid glands was shown to cause a prompt fall in plasma calcium. The hormone responsible is formed by the cells of the embryonic ultimo branchial body, which in later life form the parafollicular or 'C' cells of the thyroid gland. These cells can be recognized by their characteristic fluorescent histochemical staining and in man are also found in the thymus and parathyroid glands. It is possible that production of calcitonin, unlike parathyroid hormone, falls off in the elderly and may be one of the many factors in the production of senile osteoporosis. No clear clinical deficiency state has yet been demonstrated in man and it is possible that the hormone provides a mechanism to control the occasional high levels of calcium in the blood or may only be operative in lower animals.

The structure of this peptide hormone is now known,

consisting of a sequence of 32 amino acids with a molecular weight of 3400 (Potts et al, 1971). It has been synthesized and used in the treatment of conditions with excessive bone resorption, such as Paget's disease or the hypercalcaemia of metastatic bone carcinoma. It acts on the bone and kidney as its two target organs. In bone it inhibits osteoclastic bone resorption, both in vivo and in vitro, probably by blocking the action of parathyroid hormone. The less important renal effect is to increase the urinary excretion of calcium and sodium by a direct action on the tubular cells. This is accompanied by an increased phosphate excretion. It blocks the absorption of phosphate, but not calcium from the gut. Its mode of action at a cellular level remains uncertain although Talmage et al (1973) postulated that it is primarily a hormone for the control of phosphate metabolism. They suggest that it stimulates the transfer of phosphate into the cells and fluid of bone with a secondary inhibition of calcium outflow to the extracellular fluid. Like parathyroid hormone, calcitonin is thought to act through cyclic AMP as an intermediary.

Adreno-cortical hormones

The adrenoglucocorticoids, such as hydrocortisone, have actions on the skeleton, which may form part of the normal physiological control of growth or may sometimes induce pathological states when present in excess. Prolonged steroid medication in rheumatoid arthritis and other collagen disorders may produce bone changes indistinguishable from those seen in Cushing's syndrome. In this disease there is a state of endogenous hypersecretion induced by a tumour of the adrenal cortex or indirectly through an excessive production of corticotrophins by a tumour of the anterior pituitary. The changes are maximal in the axial skeleton with similar spinal changes to those of severe idiopathic osteoporosis with bulging intervertebral discs and vertebral body collapse and fracture. Jowsey et al (1965) showed with a microradiography study that the condition results from an imbalance between the increased bone resorption rate and a depressed bone formation rate. The serum levels of calcium and phosphate are normal though the alkaline phosphatase may sometimes be slightly elevated and there is a high urinary calcium excretion leading to a negative calcium balance. The mechanism of the steroids in reducing bone formation is uncertain though experimental evidence suggests that they inhibit protein synthesis, including RNA, by osteoblasts.

Sex hormones

Experimental work in vitro by Atkins et al (1972) suggests that the oestrogens oppose the action of parathyroid hormone on bone thereby reducing bone resorption. Whether this provides sufficient evidence to support the concept that the relative osteoporosis in post-menopausal women is due to oestrogen deficiency rather than a physiological ageing process remains uncertain. In a prospective study with a 2-year follow-up Horsman et al (1977) showed that oestrogen treatment would prevent the expected bone loss in normal post-menopausal women compared with non treated controls. The treatment group showed preservation of bone mass measured by photon densitometry and a diminished endosteal resorption in standardised metacarpal radiographs. Large doses of oestrogen have been shown to induce premature epiphyseal closure in experimental animals and these hormones may interact with growth hormone at puberty to terminate growth at the epiphyses in long bones.

The androgens have a less clear-cut action on bone but some related anabolic steroids have been used to induce a general increase in nitrogen retention and gain in body weight.

Growth hormone

The growth hormone produced by the anterior lobe of the pituitary controls body growth as a whole including that of the long bones through the epiphyseal growth plate. Clinical deficiency states in childhood may result in pituitary dwarfism, the biochemical recognition of which has been described by Kaplan et al (1968). With newer immuno-assay techniques for human growth hormone and its production for therapeutic use, the effects of deficiency should prove reversible if diagnosis is established early. Experimental and clinical studies by Daughadey et al (1959) showed that the hormone acts through circulating plasma sulphation factors, termed somatomedins, which are produced by the liver. These have been shown to have a direct effect on cartilage, stimulating the production of glycosaminoglycans, protein and nucleic acids. In addition these have non-specific, insulin-like effects on other non-skeletal tissues.

Thyroid hormones

A deficiency in thyroid hormone decreases structural remodelling in bone and also reduces its blood flow. Bone formation and resorption rates are both reduced to subnormal levels and though plasma calcium and phosphate levels remain normal, the urinary hydroxyproline concentration is reduced. These changes are seen in the hypothyroid condition of cretinism and are associated with retarded osseous development characterized by thickened abnormal epiphyses unlike the pituitary dwarf where these are normal in proportion.

In adult thyrotoxicosis the excess production of thyroid hormones stimulates both bone formation and resorption. Biochemically it is often associated with elevation of the serum calcium, increased urinary re-absorption of phosphate, hypercalciuria and a negative calcium balance.

There is a marked osteoporosis, sometimes complicated by pathological fractures, and morphologically, Adams et al (1967) have demonstrated an increased rate of bone resorption with the normal or increased bone formation. The mechanism of action of the thyroid hormones is not certain but may be to produce a general increase in metabolic activity of the mesenchymal cells.

Vitamin C (ascorbic acid)

Severe dietary deficiency of vitamin C results in the disease of scurvy which has been recognized for over 200 years. It was common in the age of exploration when long sea voyages were made without access to fresh vegetables or citrus fruits. The condition was characterized by excessive bruising, bleeding gums, delayed wound healing and even the breakdown of old previously healed scars. Haemorrhages occur in the skin and other soft tissues while in severe cases there may be delayed healing of fractures or arrest of bone growth. Experimental work on the mechanism of the vitamin deficiency was hampered by the lack of suitable experimental animals since most are able to synthesize the vitamin in their gut. The exceptions who lack this mechanism are man, the other primates and the guinea pig.

Follis (1943) has described the changes of experimental and clinical scurvy in growing bones. In the growth plate there is normal chondrocyte division with formation of a calcified matrix in the hypertrophic zone. However, this is not resorbed in the normal manner but becomes broadened and excessively fragile, a condition which often results in spontaneous epiphyseal separation. The sparse osteoblasts in the metaphyseal region lie in an oedematous connective tissue due to a failure of normal osteoid synthesis. Collagen fibres cannot be recognized in the ground substance and the few fibres present resemble reticulin on staining. Subperiosteal haemorrhages may occur with elevation of the periosteum in which new bone formation is also inhibited. In adult bones the cortex is thinned and osteoporotic, and fractures are slow to unite with persistent haematoma formation and slow organisation into non-specific fibrous tissue. The teeth themselves may be hypoplastic and are frequently loose in the spongy gums which bleed readily from any minor trauma.

The basic defect in vitamin C deficiency appears to be a failure by specialized cells, including fibroblasts, osteoblasts, odontoblasts, to secrete their appropriate fibrous protein whether collagen, osteoid or dentin. There is a biochemical failure of hydroxylation of proline in a collagen precursor and Kodicek (1965) suggests that this is due to a microsomal enzyme impairment which also blocks the incorporation of labelled sulphate into glycosaminoglycans.

Gross vitamin deficiency is now a rarity but interest centres on the problem of the detection of latent vitamin C deficiency, both in pre-operative patients and in the elderly on inadequate diets. The laboratory tests available are difficult to interpret and are not entirely reliable.

The vitamin C saturation test depends on the principle that any excess of an administered dose of ascorbic acid is excreted in the urine when the body is fully saturated. However, few healthy people are fully saturated and the renal excretion of the vitamin is dependent on many other unrelated factors. Estimation of ascorbic acid in blood or leucocytes, where the majority is stored, is of more value. The initial signs of scurvy first develop when the plasma ascorbic acid level falls to less than 0.2 mg per 100 ml which corresponds to a leucocyte ascorbic acid level of 15 μg per 10^8 cells. The first characteristic signs are hyperkeratosis of hair follicles and small petechial haemorrhages first visible on the undersurface of the tongue. The extent of latent scurvy in elderly people may be underestimated since many have a dietary intake of less than 10 mg of vitamin C per day and it has been suggested that up to 30% are vitamin deficient. Whether this has any influence on the incidence or healing process of the common fractures in geriatric patients remains to be investigated.

PATHOLOGICAL DISTURBANCES OF MINERAL HOMEOSTASIS

Hyperparathyroidism

Hyperparathyroidism with over-production of parathyroid hormone may be classified as primary, when it is due to an adenoma or other tumour in one or more glands, or secondary when it is associated with hyperplasia of all four glands. Secondary hyperplasia may occur as a compensatory reaction to the low plasma calcium levels associated with chronic renal glomerular failure, steatorrhoea, rickets or osteomalacia. The primary condition is characterized by an elevation of serum calcium above the normal upper limit of 2.6 mmol/l to as high as 5 mmol/l. In some patients the serum calcium is only intermittently increased and it may be necessary to carry out repeated estimations to detect the change. Secondary hyperparathyroidism may be more frequently associated with serum calcium levels which are low or normal. The serum phosphate concentration may be low due to increased urinary excretion but may rise above normal levels if renal failure ensues.

The symptoms of the condition are extremely variable and the patterns of disease have been well described by Dent (1962). The hypercalcaemia and hypercalciuria may result in progressive debility, loss of appetite, nausea, vomiting and sometimes chronic dyspepsia which may be associated with peptic ulceration. The associated polyuria may lead to thirst, dehydration and constipation, while the impaired neuromuscular function results in tiredness, muscle weakness and even heart block. Mild mental symp-

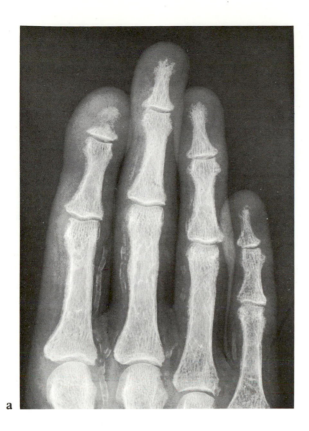

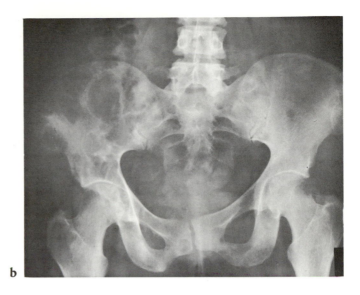

Fig. 15.8a X-ray of hand in hyperparathyroidism to show generalised osteoporosis, sub-periosteal erosions in phalanges, and calcification of the digital vessels; b X-ray of pelvis in hyperparathyroidism showing multiple osteolytic lesions in right ilium.

toms such as loss of concentration and drowsiness may deteriorate to coma and disorientation which can result in referral for psychiatric care.

Radiological changes in bone are very common and characteristic (Fig. 15.8a and b) and are of two main types. There may be a generalized osteoporosis with subperiosteal erosions seen in the phalanges of the hands, or disseminated multiple osteolytic lesions of 'osteitis fibrosa cystica' or Von Recklinghausen's disease. The lytic lesions result from replacement of bone by solid brown tumours containing vascular fibrous tissue and giant cells, or by cystic degenerative lesions containing old blood. The bone disease may present clinically with symptoms of bone pain, progressive deformity, pathological fractures or loosening of the teeth.

Renal manifestations are probably the most common presentation of the disease. They are associated with a widespread deposition of calcium in the tissues resulting in calculi formation or damage to the renal tubular cells. In extreme cases there may be extensive nephrocalcinosis associated with renal failure and deposits may occur in other tissues such as the eye, joint capsule, tendon or sometimes articular cartilage. The renal stones formed as a result of the chronic calcium hypersecretion are of the phosphate or oxalate type. They may obstruct the renal tract producing back pressure effects on the kidney or predispose to recurrent urinary tract infections.

If the diagnosis is suspected, it may be confirmed by the finding of repeatedly elevated serum calcium levels, provided the specimens are collected without a tourniquet as stasis itself produces elevation above the normal level. Further confirmation can be obtained by the cortisone suppression test of Dent in which the patient is given 100 mg of the steroid daily for 1 week. In patients with hypercalcaemia due to excessive skeletal liberation of mineral from metastatic deposits, sarcoidosis or hypervitaminosis D, the serum calcium level will return to normal, but it remains elevated in hyperparathyroidism. Reduction of the dietary calcium intake is normally followed by a fall in urinary calcium output but this does not occur with hyperparathyroidism. A bone biopsy from the iliac crest may confirm the diagnosis if the characteristic features of enlarged bone lacunar spaces and loss of mineralisation are found. Of more recent interest is the use of immunoassays for parathyroid hormone as described by Arnaud et al (1971). Immunology may detect more than one type of circulating hormone or fragment with biological activity and this heterogeneity might explain the differing modes of clinical presentation.

Treatment by removal of any parathyroid tumour leads to a dramatic relief from symptoms, except when these are due to advanced renal failure. Localization of the lesion may be difficult because of the frequency of an aberrant site or number of parathyroid glands. In the first few hours following surgery the serum calcium may fall to subnormal levels and correction of the reactionary hypocalcaemia may be required if it reaches 1.6 mmol/l. The onset of tetany is normally preceded by circumoral numbness and at this stage the hypocalcaemia should be reversed by intravenous infusion of 10% calcium gluconate. If hormone production remains deficient and the hypocalcaemia persists for more than 2 weeks, vitamin D is usually given in a daily dosage of 1000 to 10 000 iu to stimulate intestinal calcium absorption. When no tumour has been found and subtotal resection of hyperplastic gland tissue is undertaken, it is always necessary to leave some normal gland for continued hormone production.

Rickets and osteomalacia

A deficiency of vitamin D in adults results in defective mineralization of the osteoid matrix of bone and is termed osteomalacia. In growing children the failure of calcification in the epiphyseal plates results in the more florid condition of rickets. The classical disease resulted from the defective dietary intake or malabsorption of the vitamin but similar syndromes may arise from other causes of defective vitamin D metabolism. The production of 1,25-$(OH)_2D_3$ may be impaired in renal failure, liver disease and with prolonged anticonvulsant therapy which may affect the liver enzyme conversions. An excellent overall review of the pathophysiology of these disorders is provided by Mankin (1974).

Rickets

The discovery of this classical vitamin deficiency disease and its cure have been well described by Dent (1970). It is only seen when both dietary intake and exposure to ultraviolet light are deficient, a situation once common in the poor areas of industrialized cities. With the improvements in diet and the introduction of smokeless zones it has largely disappeared in Britain, although it may sometimes occur in immigrants from a poor intake of dairy products and an undue reliance on cereal foods.

The clinical features depend on the severity of the deficiency and the age of onset. Under the age of 16 months the infant may present with failure to thrive, restlessness, loss of muscle tone, convulsions or even tetany, but only minimal bone changes. In the rapid spurt of skeletal growth from 6 months to 2 years bone deformities, such as knock-knees and bow-legs, may appear due to bending of the softened bones from muscle action and weight-bearing. In addition the enlarged and widened epiphyses may become palpable and visible at the wrists and ankles, while more rarely, hypertrophy of the costo-chondral junctions results in a 'rickety rosary'. Less frequent manifestations are the skull deformities of frontal and parietal bossing and softening of the ribs at the site of diaphragmatic attachment to produce a Harrison's sulcus.

The diagnosis is confirmed by the finding of an elevated

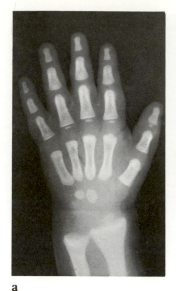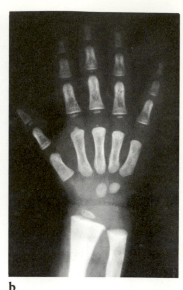

a   b

Fig. 15.9a and b X-rays of wrist and hand of child with rickets, before and 3 months after treatment with vitamin D. The poorly defined epiphysis and irregular 'cupped' metaphysis have become enlarged and normally calcified.

serum alkaline phosphatase level above 30 KA units, frequently reaching 50 or 100 units. This is usually accompanied by depression of the serum calcium or phosphate levels, or sometimes both.

Pathologically, the epiphyseal growth plates show the most dramatic changes with broadening and thickening of the uncalcified pre-osseous cartilage zone resulting from a failure of the normal degeneration of the hypertrophic cells. This seems to be the necessary prerequisite for invasion by the metaphyseal blood vessels which is therefore prevented. In addition, the osteoid laid down on the trabecular bone of the metaphysis fails to calcify with a resultant loss of remodelling.

These bone changes are clearly visible on X-ray (Fig. 15.9a and b) as broad radiolucent 'cupped' epiphyses and irregular porotic metaphyses. Following successful treatment with vitamin D and calcium supplements, in a dosage of 2000–4000 iu daily, these radiological changes show a rapid reversal to normal in the space of a few weeks. Treatment should be monitored by repeated estimations of the serum calcium, phosphate and alkaline phosphatase levels. The bony deformities may improve with normal growth, although severe curves of the longer bones may require later surgical correction by osteotomy, while occasionally distortion of the pelvis may lead to difficulty in childbirth.

Vitamin D-resistant rickets (renal rickets)

When rickets proves resistant to the normal dosage of vitamin D and failure of absorption from steatorrhoea can be excluded, the cause usually lies in the kidney. Renal rickets may be of two types; either a glomerular type associated with chronic renal insufficiency, or a renal tubular lesion with an associated excessive loss of phosphate from the kidney. The glomerular type is diagnosed by the presence of an elevated blood urea and serum inorganic phosphorus level and is assumed to result from a failure of $1,25\text{-}(OH)_2D_3$ production. Conversely, the tubular defects are associated with a normal urea level, hypophosphataemia and usually represent a genetically inherited error of metabolism. Until recently the only treatment available for both types was massive doses of vitamin D of the order of 150 000–500 000 iu daily. The introduction of $1,25\text{-}(OH)_2D_3$, or its cheaper synthetic analogues, for the treatment of all types of renal osteodystrophy has given encouraging early results.

Osteomalacia

After closure of the epiphyses, failure of calcification of bone osteoid is less dramatic in its clinical onset, except in the later stages where it may be associated with pathological fractures. The diagnosis should always be excluded in elderly patients presenting with metaphyseal fractures of the femoral and humeral necks or with Colles fracture of the wrist. Wedge compression fractures of the vertebral bodies may also occur giving rise to symptoms of acute back pain. The features of the disease have been well described by Chalmers et al (1967). The condition is not confined to elderly women with a poor dietary intake but may follow partial or total gastrectomy which can interfere with absorption of the vitamin. Usually the onset of the mild disease is more insidious with loss of appetite and weight, muscle weakness, bone pain and tenderness with progressive deformities of a rounded dorsal spinal kyphosis and bowing of the lower limbs. Radiologically, the extensive loss of bone mineral may be indistinguishable from the more common senile or postmenopausal osteoporosis. One distinguishing feature is the presence of pseudofractures or Looser's zones, best seen around the pelvis and ribs as translucent bands through part or all of the cortex.

The diagnosis is more difficult than rickets since it depends on finding a reduction in the product of serum calcium and serum phosphate with a slight elevation of the alkaline phosphatase level. These changes may be borderline so that if the condition is suspected on clinical grounds it may be necessary to take an iliac crest biopsy to confirm the diagnosis. If osteomalacia is present this will show an excess of unmineralised matrix in undecalcified sections. The urinary calcium excretion is usually reduced compared with osteoporosis and may be less than 75 mg in 24 hours. The treatment of the condition is a simple supplementation of the vitamin D and calcium intake. In frank clinical cases treatment is usually commenced with 50 000 iu daily

reducing to a weekly dosage once the condition is controlled. If it is certain that non-absorption is not the problem and deficiency is purely dietary, a smaller dosage of 4000 iu may be used with calcium supplements of 1 g daily. Treatment should be continued indefinitely but must be monitored with periodic serum biochemistry to avoid over-dosage. Occasional resistant cases due to disorders of vitamin D absorption or metabolism can now be treated with the active metabolites.

Osteoporosis

Osteoporosis is a condition in which there is a deficiency in bone mass which has been attributed to a failure of osteoid production by the osteoblasts. The bone matrix which is present is normally calcified, distinguishing it from that of osteomalacia in undecalcified histological sections. No major disturbance of mineral metabolism has ever been demonstrated in the condition and the serum levels of calcium, phosphate, and alkaline phosphatase are all normal. What has been demonstrated is that the efficiency of intestinal calcium absorption decreases with age and is associated with a 30% reduction in plasma levels of $1,25\text{-}(OH)_2D_3$ (Gallagher et al, 1979).

There is a major difficulty in distinguishing the condition from the normal ageing process since it is known that with advancing age there is a progressive generalised loss of bone mass from the skeleton. The clinical features were well described by Albright et al (1941) who excluded the elderly patient over the age of 65 and described the condition as occurring predominantly in postmenopausal females. He emphasized that the condition mainly affected the spine and pelvis, often presenting with spontaneous fractures of the vertebral bodies following minimal trauma. These were sometimes accompanied by local pain but were also thought to occur asymptomatically leading to a progressive loss in height. The characteristic radiology of the spine (Fig. 15.10) shows bulging discs and biconcave vertebral bodies with little differentiation between the soft tissue and cancellous bone. The appearances are indistinguishable from the osteoporosis associated with steroid overdosage, Cushing's syndrome or hyperthyroidism. There is no clear evidence that there is a separate condition of postmenopausal osteoporosis which can be distinguished from the senile osteoporosis associated with a progressive increase in the incidence of long bone fractures in the elderly patient. These fractures are common in the metaphyseal regions of bones, particularly the neck of the femur, neck of humerus, and the Colles fracture at the lower end of the radius.

The diagnosis cannot be made on radiological appearances alone since any interpretation of bone density must be made against a standard such as an aluminium step wedge included in the same X-ray film. Methods for detection of osteoporosis have been described by comparing the

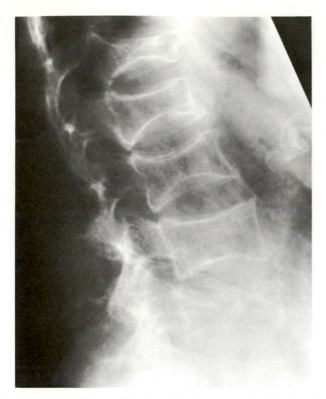

Fig. 15.10 Lateral X-ray of lumbar spine in osteoporosis. The loss of bone density is extreme with 'bulging' of the intervertebral discs and compression fractures of two vertebral bodies.

trials of continued oestrogen supplements to prevent the appearance of osteoporosis. Nordin et al (1980) have suggested that oestrogen supplements are more effective when combined with a small dose of vitamin D metabolite to increase calcium absorption. Other treatment techniques which have been used on an experimental basis include fluoride combined with vitamin D and calcium supplements in an attempt to stabilize bone mineral and thus prevent collagen breakdown.

Osteoporosis is not confined to the elderly or postmenopausal and may occur in a secondary form whenever there is accelerated bone loss due to an imbalance between resorption and formation. Indeed the advent of the era of space flight has presented this medical problem in otherwise fit astronauts. The combination of prolonged weightlessness, reduced exercise and possibly dietary and endocrine disturbances has been reported by Mack and La Chance (1967) to result in losses of up to 20% in bone density during an 8 day flight.

Local osteoporosis in the bones of a limb is a particular surgical problem associated with prolonged immobilization and disuse, denervation, fracture, inflammation or trauma. This may result from the removal of the normal mechanical stimuli on bone formation and the changes in local circulation with increased venostasis. Treatment is designed to limit this effect by encouraging early activity and preserving muscle function.

cortical thickness of the metacarpals or ulna relative to the total diameter of the bone. Other techniques utilize gamma-densitometry to measure photon absorption by the bone. Biopsies can be taken from the cancellous bone of the iliac crest and this will show sparse, but normally calcified, trabeculae in this condition. What remains in contention is whether the histological appearances or radiological density of cancellous bone at one site in the skeleton represents the generalised state in the remainder.

The aetiology of the condition remains in doubt so that all methods of treatment are largely empirical. One theory blames the loss of muscular activity in the elderly which should provide the normal stresses to maintain the bone mass of the skeleton. It is certainly less common in poor and underdeveloped countries where paradoxically the vitamin D, calcium and protein intake in the diet fall far below the levels of sophisticated Western society. The higher incidence in the female suggests some endocrine imbalance possibly related to the menopause and led to

Paget's disease

Paget's disease of bone or osteitis deformans is characterized by localized increases in bone resorption and formation leading to softening and deformities. It has many of the features of a disturbance in the metabolic control of bone turnover but is usually confined to one or two bones at quite different sites in the skeleton. Many theories have been advanced for its aetiology ranging from virus infection to local disturbances in bone blood supply. However, no systemic disturbance has been demonstrated in relation to the disease, except for the marked increase in serum alkaline phosphatase and urinary hydroxyproline excretion from increased bone turnover. Evans and McIntyre (1978) have reported the successful relief of bone pain with small doses of Calcitonin, though larger doses and prolonged therapy are required to stop bone resorption. The diphosphonates have also been used in the treatment of the condition because of their ability to stabilize bone mineral and limit resorption.

REFERENCES

Adams P Jowsey J, Kelly P J, Riggs B L, Kinney V R, Jones J D 1967 Effects of hyperthyroidism on bone and mineral metabolism in man. Quarterly Journal of Medicine 36: 1–15

Albright F, Smith P H, Richardson A M 1941 Post-menopausal osteoporosis. Its clinical features. Journal of American Medical Association 116: 2465–2474

Arnaud C D, Sizemore G W, Oldham S B, Fischer J A, Tsaq H S, Littledike E T 1971 Human parathyroid hormone: glandular and secreted molecular species. American Journal of Medicine 50: 630–638

Atkins D, Zanelli J M, Peacock M, Nordin B E C 1972 The effect of oestrogens on the response of bone to parathyroid hormone in vitro. Journal of Endocrinology 54: 107–117

Bassett C A L 1968 Biologic significance of piezo-electricity. Calcified Tissue Research 1: 252–272

Bauer G C H 1968 The use of radionuclides in orthopaedics IV: Radionuclide scintimetry of the skeleton. Journal of Bone and Joint Surgery 50A: 1681–1709

Belanger L F 1969 Osteocytic osteolysis. Calcified Tissue Research 4: 1–12

Buring K 1975 On the origin of cells in heterotopic bone formation. Orthopaedics and Related Research 110: 293–302

Burwell R G 1969 The fate of bone grafts. In: Apley A G (ed) Recent Advances in Orthopaedics Churchill, London p 115

Chalmers J 1959 Transplantation immunity in bone homografting. Journal of Bone and Joint Surgery 41B: 160–179

Chalmers J, Conacher W D H, Gardner D L, Scott P J 1967 Osteomalacia — a common disease in elderly women. Journal of Bone and Joint Surgery 49B: 403–623

Collip J B 1925 The extraction of a parathyroid hormone which will prevent or control parathyroid tetany and which regulates the level of blood calcium. Journal of Biological Chemistry 63: 395–438

Copp D H 1961 Calcitonin: a second hormone from the parathyroid and its function in regulating blood calcium. In: Gordon ES (ed) The Yearbook of Endocrinology Yearbook Publishers, Chicago p 10–18

Daughadey W H, Salmon W D, Alexander F 1959 Sulphation factor activity of sera from patients with pituitary disorders. Journal of Clinical Endocrinology 19: 743–758

De Luca H F 1975 Calcium metabolism. Acta Orthopaedica Scandinavica, 46: 286–314

Dent C E 1962 Some problems of hyperparathyroidism. British Medical Journal, ii, 1419–1425 and 1495–1500

Dent C E 1970 Rickets and osteomalacia, nutritional and metabolic 1919–1969. Proceedings of the Royal Society of Medicine, 63: 401–408

Evans I M A & McIntyre I 1978 Treatment of Paget's Disease. The Lancet, ii, 213

Follis R H 1943 Effect of mechanical force on the skeletal lesions in acute scurvy in guinea pigs. Archives of Pathology, 35: 579

Gallagher J C, Riggs B L, Eisman J, Hamstra A, Arnaud S B & De Luca H F 1979 Intestinal calcium absorption and serum vitamin D metabolites in normal subjects and osteoporotic patients. Journal of Clinical Investigation, 64: 729–736

Gallie, W E & Robertson D E 1920 The repair of bone. British Journal of Surgery, 7: 211

Hall B K 1970 Cellular differentiation in skeletal tissues. Biological Reviews, 45: 455–484

Ham S W & Harris W R 1971 Repair and transplantation of bone. In:

Bourne G H (ed) The Biochemistry and Physiology of Bone 2nd edn, Vol. 3 338–379. Academic Press, New York Ch 10, p 338–379

Hancox N M 1972 The osteoclast. In: Bourne G H (ed) The Biochemistry and Physiology of Bone, 2nd edn, Vol. 1 Academic Press, New York Ch. 3, p 45–67

Harris W H, Jackson R H & Jowsey J 1962 In vivo distribution of tetracyclines in canine bone. Journal of Bone and Joint Surgery, 44A: 1308–1320

Heppenstall R B, Grislis B A & Hunt T K 1975 Tissue gas tensions and oxygen consumption in healing bone defects. Clinical Orthopaedics and Related Research, 106: 357–365

Horsman A, Gallagher J C, Simpson M & Nordin B E C 1977 Prospective trial of oestrogen and calcium in post-menopausal women. British Medical Journal, ii, 789–792

Jowsey J, Kelly P J, Riggs B L, Bianco A J Jr, Scholz D A, Gershon-Cohen J 1965 Quantitative microradiographic studies of normal and osteoporotic bone. Journal of Bone and Joint Surgery 47A: 785–806

Kaplan M M 1972 Alkaline phosphatase. Gastroenterology, 62: 452–468

Kaplan S L, Abrams C A L, Bell J J, Conte F A & Grumbach M M 1968 Growth and growth hormone. Paediatric Research, 2: 43–63

Kodicek E 1965 The effect of ascorbic acid on biosynthesis of components of connective tissue. In: Fitton Jackson S, Harkness R D, Partridge S M, Tristram G R (eds) Structure and Function of Connective and Skeletal Tissue. Butterworths, London p 307–318

McLean F C 1957 The parathyroid hormone and bone. Clinical Orthopaedics, 9: 46–60

Mack P B & La Chance, P A 1967 Effects of recumbency and space flight on bone density. American Journal of Clinical Nutrition, 20: 1194–1205

Mankin H J 1974 Rickets, osteomalacia, and renal osteodystrophy. Journal of Bone and Joint Surgery, 56A: 101–128 and 352–386

Nordin B E C, Horsman A, Crilly, R G, Marshall D H & Simpson M 1980 Treatment of spinal osteoporosis in post-menopausal women. British Medical Journal, ii: 451–454

Perren S M, Hugglar A, Russenberger M, Allgower M, Mathys R, Schenk R et al 1969 The reaction of cortical bone to compression. Acta Orthopaedica Scandinavica Supplement, 125:17

Potts J T, Keutmann, H T, Niall H D & Tregear G W 1971 The chemistry of parathyroid hormone and the calcitonins. Vitamins and Hormones, 29: 41–93

Pritchard J J 1972 The osteoblast. In: Bourne G H (ed) The Biochemistry and Physiology of Bone, 2nd edn, Vol. 1, Academic Press, New York Ch 2, p 21–43

Prockop D J, Kivirikko, K I, Tuderman L & Guzman N A 1979 The biosynthesis of collagen and its disorders (two parts). New England Journal of Medicine, 301: 13, 17

Rasmussen H, Bordier P 1974 The Physiological and Cellular Basis of Metabolic Bone Disease, Williams and Wilkins, Baltimore p 48

Talmage R V, Whitehurst L A & Anderson J J B 1973 Effect of calcitonin and calcium infusion on plasma phosphate. Endocrinology, 92: 792–798

Stomach

A short account of the anatomy of the stomach, and a note on absorption from the stomach, lead on to the main discussion in which are considered peptic digestion, gastric acid secretion, gastric motor activity and the origin of pain in peptic ulcer.

ANATOMY OF THE STOMACH

The gastric mucosa

The naked-eye appearance of the gastric mucosa during life can be studied at gastroscopy. It is orange-red in colour, and glistens where light is reflected from the covering film of transparent mucus. It is thrown into folds, the thickness of which varies with the degree to which the stomach is distended. These folds are least developed along the lesser curvature, and most prominent along the greater curvature. Here the principal folds are longitudinal, but lesser folds transform the pattern into an irregular honeycomb. This pattern is maintained by the tonic contraction of the underlying muscularis mucosae.

Microscopy under low power shows the surface epithelium to be pockmarked with the minute openings of the gastric pits into which are poured the secretions of the several kinds of tubular glands of the stomach.

Microscopy under higher power shows that throughout the stomach the surface epithelium and the epithelium of the gastric pits consist of a single layer of mucus-secreting cells of uniform appearance, whereas in the different regions of the stomach there are distinctive types of tubular glands opening into the pits. The *cardiac glands* in man occupy a small fringe of gastric mucosa near the orifice of the oesophagus. In these glands the mucus-secreting cell predominates but there are a few oxyntic and peptic cells. The *gastric glands* proper occupy more than two-thirds of the stomach, excluding only the regions of the cardia and pyloric antrum. These glands are parallel sinuous tubes which branch a short distance below the gastric pits. The principal cell types are the oxyntic cells (also called parietal and acid-secreting), and the peptic

cells. The oxyntic cells are large, wedge-shaped, lie against the basement membrane and stain rose pink with eosin. They are distributed throughout the length of the tubule but are more numerous near its neck than in its body, where they are separated from the lumen by the peptic cells. The peptic cells occur only in the body of the gland tubule. They are small, and contain the coarse granules of pepsinogen which tend to disappear after prolonged vagal stimulation but not after stimulation with histamine. The *pyloric glands* occupy the pyloric antrum and pyloric canal. Mucus-secreting cells again predominate, but occasional oxyntic and peptic cells may be found in the junctional area between the body of the stomach and the pyloric antrum. The secretion of the pyloric glands is alkaline at pH 7 to 8. The rate of secretion of the pyloric glands is only 2–2.5 ml/h as against 50–60 ml/h of the gastric glands proper. It has been known for some years that the hormone gastrin is produced by and can be extracted from the pyloric gland mucosa, but it is only recently that its cell of origin has been demonstrated. New techniques have allowed immunofluorescent-stained cells, seen under the light microscope, to be correlated with their electron microscopic appearances. The way is now open to identify the normal distribution and estimate the gastrin cell (G cell) population, and some studies have already been made of the human stomach. Clinicians have repeatedly posed the question as to whether a proportion of patients with chronic duodenal ulcer have G cell hyperplasia (with excessive production of gastrin) as opposed to excessive vagal activity but until now there has been no way of separating patients before operation. This problem now seems nearer to a solution, and this could be of practical importance because patients with G cell hyperplasia would seem to require distal gastrectomy rather than vagotomy as surgical treatment.

Regeneration of the gastric mucosa

Regeneration of the gastric mucosa is a continuous process in the normal stomach. The surface epithelial cells and the mucus-secreting neck cells are labile, show a high mitotic activity and a rapid turnover rate. Cells from the neck of the glands migrate towards the surface of the mucosa, and at the same time mature into surface epithelial cells. These cells are finally sloughed into the lumen of the stomach and it has been calculated that the whole population of surface epithelial cells is renewed every few days. The other epithelial cells forming the glands proper are more stable but there is growing evidence that these cells too are capable of multiplication, although normally at a low rate (Myhre, 1968).

In experimental wounds of the gastric mucosa the specialized cells at the margins lose their characteristics, proliferate and migrate as undifferentiated cells to cover the defect. The surface cells then form pits and glands and finally a new mucosa is formed with the development of parietal and peptic cells. While the physiological regeneration of the gastric mucosa is now well founded, little is yet known about mucosal regeneration in the diseased stomach.

The muscle coat

The muscle coat of the stomach consists of interweaving fibres, but here and there three layers can be distinguished, an inner oblique, a middle circular, and an outer longitudinal. The oblique fibres, a continuation of the circular muscle fibres of the oesophagus, are best developed near the cardia. The circular fibres are abundant in the pyloric region of the stomach and are specially thickened at the pyloric sphincter. The longitudinal fibres are continuous with those of the oesophagus, and are most plentiful along the greater and lesser curvatures.

Blood supply of the stomach

The principal arteries are the right and left gastric, the gastro-epiploics and the short gastrics. These arteries run along the curvatures of the stomach, and their branches pass for a short distance on to the anterior or posterior surface before penetrating obliquely through the muscle coat. They pour their blood into a rich network of large vessels in the submucosa. A finer network lies in the connective tissue around the glands, and arterioles pass from this plexus to individual gland tubules (Fig. 16.1).

It can be seen that the stomach is endowed with a copious blood supply. This is needed to meet the heavy metabolic demands made by its muscular and secretory activity.

The submucosal vascular anastomosis is so free that none of the principal arteries can be said to supply a particular part of the stomach. The lesser curvature and the first part of the duodenum were formerly thought to have a relatively poor blood supply, but radiographic studies have shown that this is not so.

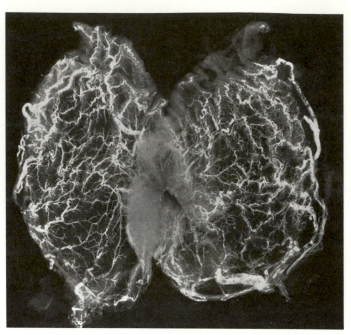

Fig. 16.1 Radiograph of gastrectomy specimen, injected with barium sulphate through the gastro-epiploic artery, and opened along the greater curvature. Note the rich submucosal anastomosis. The anastomosis is partly obliterated around a chronic ulcer on the lesser curvature.

The rich blood supply of the stomach makes for rapid healing after such operations as gastro-enterostomy or gastrectomy. If necessary, three of the principal arteries can be ligated, the remaining artery being sufficient to prevent infarction. The free anastomosis in the submucosal plexus accounts also for the failure of two operations previously practised; a bleeding gastric ulcer cannot be controlled by ligating the nearby vessels, nor can gastric secretion be permanently reduced by the operation of 'physiological gastrectomy' in which 4 of every 5 of the branches of the principal arteries are ligated in the hope of permanently reducing the blood supply.

The veins of the stomach drain chiefly into the portal system, but there is also a small and normally unimportant anastomosis with the oesophageal veins which drain to the azygos system. In portal hypertension (p. 346) the gastric veins share in the hypertension and the oesophageal veins distend and become liable to rupture.

Blood flow in the stomach

Wolf and Wolff (1947) have shown that there is a correlation between the vascularity of the stomach, its acid secretion and its motility. The more blood there is coursing through it, the greater the acid secretion and, in general, the greater the motility. These observations were made on the well-known subject 'Tom', who had a gastrostomy with a cuff of mucosa protruding on to the surface of the abdominal wall. It was noted also that the colour of this protruding mucosa varied with Tom's emotional state, and this suggests that blood flow is under control of the autonomic nervous system.

Surgeons accustomed to operating on the stomach are well aware of differences in its vascularity in different disease states. In patients with duodenal ulcer, the stomach is usually very vascular and is especially so when the ulcer has led to pyloric stenosis and hypertrophy of gastric muscle. In patients with gastric ulcer, the stomach is not engorged with blood, and in patients with atrophy of the gastric mucosa, the stomach is flaccid and pale.

An association between mucosal blood flow and gastric acid secretion has been a matter of controversy for many years. This has been due in large measure to difficulty in obviating the possible effects of anaesthesia and gastric trauma on secretion and flow. Bell and Shelley (1968) made studies in conscious dogs using a thermo-electric technique with simultaneous collection of acid secretion. Histamine regularly caused a rapid increase in mucosal flow which began within 2 minutes of commencing the infusion; a corresponding increase in acid output occurred more slowly. It was notable that a further increase in acid secretion was possible at higher histamine dose rates without any further increase in flow. *Vasopressin* caused a marked reduction in gastric blood flow, a finding which lends support to the use of this agent in the treatment of severe gastric haemorrhage in man. If flow is sufficiently reduced by increasing the dose of vasopressin, secretion cannot continue at its previous level, suggesting that a reduction in blood flow below a critical level will suppress acid secretion. Vagotomy, in the long-term, markedly reduces acid secretion without reduction of mucosal blood flow. It is of interest that Bell and Battersby (1968) showed a transient reduction in mucosal blood flow after truncal vagotomy and it may be that this operation has a place in the treatment of bleeding from acute gastric erosions by producing an immediate reduction in flow lasting for several hours.

In man, similar studies have been made by Demling and Classen (1968). While agreeing that the production of acid by the stomach requires a certain minimal blood flow in the gastric mucosa, they concluded that blood flow and change in acid secretion are basically two independent processes and that there is no clear correlation beyond this level. Histamine, insulin and gastrin affect blood flow as well as acid secretion, but there is no hard evidence that the effects on acid secretion result from blood flow changes. The need for a new and reliable technique for the study of gastric mucosal blood flow in man has been recognized for some time. Jacobson et al (1966) have detailed specifications for the measurement of gastric blood flow which indicate some of the problems involved. These are that the experimental subject should be conscious, that continuous or repeat determinations are preferable, and that the estimations should be expressed in units of flow,

i.e. ml/min. Employing these criteria these workers developed the aminopyrine clearance technique which until recently has proved the most acceptable method of measuring gastric mucosal blood flow in man. A further development has been the use of the isotope $^{99}Tc^m$. The technique is easily carried out and is relatively non-toxic, the dose of isotope being capable of reduction to 100 μCi or less without sacrificing the accuracy of the investigation. Although the results are so far at a preliminary stage, there is good reason to believe that the measurement of pertechnetate clearance is directly related to gastric mucosal blood flow and that it may prove to be a more accurate discriminant in cases of peptic ulceration than the conventional measurement of gastric acid secretion. Taylor and his colleagues (1975) found an overall statistically significant correlation (r = 0.73) between clearance of $^{99}Tc^m$ and acid secretion in a variety of clinical disorders (Fig. 16.2). A high gastric mucosal blood flow was found in patients with duodenal ucler and a low flow in those with chronic gastric ulcer, and this may suggest a relative ischaemia of the mucosa in the latter. With the introduction of this new technique for the study of gastric blood flow the time would seem to be ripe for studying once again the effect of various drugs and of such operations as vagotomy.

Nerve supply of the stomach

Vagotomy has now become one of the standard operations for duodenal ulcer, and the surgeon requires to be familiar with the nerve supply of the stomach and with the nervous control of gastric secretion and motility.

The *parasympathetic supply* reaches the stomach by way

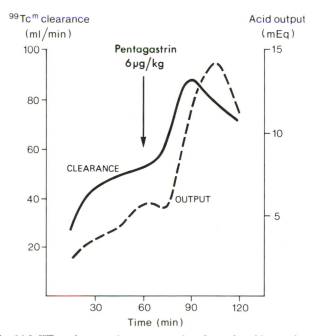

Fig. 16.2 $^{99}Tc^m$ clearance (————) and gastric acid secretion (------------) in response to pentagastrin (Taylor et al. 1975).

of the two vagal trunks which accompany the oesophagus through the diaphragm. The vagi, after forming the posterior pulmonary plexuses, communicate with each other around the thoracic oesophagus and are prolonged downwards as the anterior and posterior vagal trunks. The anterior trunk is derived predominantly from the left vagus and the posterior trunk from the right vagus.

The anterior vagal trunk is closely applied to the front of the lower oesophagus, and, after entering the abdomen, divides into branches which supply the front of the stomach as far distally as the pyloric antrum. In addition, it sends a branch to the porta hepatis and this, in turn, sends a branch downwards to the pylorus and pyloric antrum.

The posterior vagal trunk lies in areolar tissue about 1 cm behind the lower oesophagus. It divides into branches which supply the posterior surface of the stomach, and, in addition, sends a branch to the coeliac plexus.

The vagi are the important secretory nerves of the stomach and are responsible for the nervous phase of gastric secretion (p. 278). Vagal secretion can be evoked in the dog by stimulating the vagus electrically, and in man by inducing insulin hypoglycaemia which stimulates the vagal centres in the brain stem. In both instances, an acid juice rich in pepsin is secreted. The vagi also control gastric motility (p. 284) and, after vagotomy, the stomach becomes flaccid for some time and empties slowly. To avoid distension of the atonic stomach, some form of drainage procedure such as gastrojejunostomy or pyloroplasty is usually added to the vagotomy. Recently, parietal cell vagotomy has gained in popularity; in this operation the acid-secreting cells of the stomach are denervated but the nerve supply to the antrum is retained, gastric emptying is interfered with only slightly, and a drainage procedure is not required. The operation is contraindicated in the presence of significant stenosis.

In contrast to the large number of clinical studies on the effects of vagotomy, there is very little precise information about regeneration of the vagus nerve in man. However, considerable insight into the process of vagal regeneration has emerged from the elegant animal studies of Murray (1969) and, taking into account species variation, the probable changes in vagal nerve fibres following vagal nerve section may now be predicted with considerable confidence. If the nerve is crushed, most of the axons succeed in bridging the lesion and grow down the distal stump. If the nerve is divided and the severed ends left in close apposition, a relatively large number of branches may succeed in growing into the distal tubes. If a segment is removed from the nerve to ensure wide separation of the ends, only a small number may reach the peripheral tubes, but gaps of 2–3 cm have been successfully breached and this may occur at any time between 6 months and several years later. These observations could have an important

bearing on the late development of recurrent ulceration after vagotomy although it should be noted that only about 10–20% of fibres in the vagus nerves are efferent (motor) whereas 80–90% are afferent (sensory); the odds against regeneration of motor fibres are clearly in favour of the surgeon.

The *sympathetic supply* of the stomach is derived from the sixth to ninth thoracic segments of the spinal cord. From these segments, preganglionic fibres pass by way of the ganglionated chains and splanchnic nerves to the coeliac ganglia. Postganglionic fibres pass thence to the stomach mainly in company with the arteries, but some accompany the branches of the vagi.

Preganglionic sympathectomy does not appear to damage the gastric mucosa, but postganglionic sympathectomy may lead to ulcer formation in both the stomach and duodenum. There is some evidence to suggest that this results from ischaemia consequent upon spasm of the blood vessels which have become hypersensitive to circulating adrenaline.

Afferent nerve fibres from the stomach are believed to accompany both the sympathetic and parasympathetic pathways. The fibres run an unbroken course from the stomach to the central nervous system, without any peripheral synaptic relay. Fibres subserving pain run chiefly with the sympathetic nerves. Thoracolumbar sympathectomy was formerly used in the treatment of hypertension and it was notable that ulcer patients became exempt from pain and some indeed perforated or had bleeding without any preliminary pain to warn them that the ulcer continued to exist. On the other hand, vagotomy does not prevent a patient from experiencing gastric pain if he happens to develop a recurrent ulcer.

ABSORPTION FROM THE STOMACH

The stomach, unlike the small intestine, plays only a minor role in the absorption of food. It can absorb water and electrolytes, but is most often engaged in secreting them into its lumen.

Absorption by the stomach is difficult to measure in the intact animal because some of the gastric contents are continually being discharged through the pylorus. Measurements are most often made after ligating the cardia and pylorus, when the rate of disappearance of a test substance from the lumen of the stomach is a measure of its absorption.

Fats are not absorbed. Polypeptides are absorbed only slightly. Sugars are absorbed to an extent which varies with the sugar and its concentration. Galactose is the most readily absorbed, followed by glucose, lactose, fructose and finally, sucrose. Even with glucose, the rate of absorption is slow if the concentration is less than 10%. Ethyl alcohol is absorbed fairly rapidly.

The absorption of water has been studied, using D_2O (heavy water), which behaves like ordinary water. Half the amount of heavy water introduced into the isolated stomach is absorbed in about 20 minutes.

Some poisons, notably hydrocyanic acid and strychnine, are so rapidly absorbed that they are instantly fatal.

PEPTIC DIGESTION

Peptic digestion initiates the digestion of proteins by hydrolysing them to peptones, which are later hydrolysed to polypeptides and amino acids in the small intestine. The whole process of protein digestion can, however, be carried out by the small intestine, and there is no impairment of digestion in those who happen to be achlorhydric.

The secretion of pepsin and the secretion of hydrochloric acid are here described separately, but are to be regarded as complementary. Peptic digestion cannot result from pepsin without acid, nor from acid without pepsin. The activity of pepsin is maximal at pH 1.8, considerable at pH 3, slight at pH 4 and zero at pH 5 or more.

The secretion of pepsin

Less is known about the secretion of pepsin than about the secretion of hydrochloric acid.

Pepsin is formed, not as the active enzyme, but as the inactive precursor pepsinogen. The formation of pepsinogen is a continuous process in the peptic cells of the tubular glands which occupy the fundus and body of the stomach. In the absence of active secretion, granules of pepsinogen accumulate in the peptic cells, especially towards the free end of the cells abutting on the gland lumen. During active secretion the granules are discharged into the tubules, perhaps with a small amount of water and electrolytes, but their transport from the tubules to the stomach depends mainly on the stream of acid from the oxyntic cells. Pepsinogen, on being mixed with acid, is converted to active pepsin by an autocatalytic reaction which liberates also a substance with the character of a pepsin inhibitor.

The secretion of pepsin is mainly under the control of the vagus. Direct stimulation of the vagus electrically, reflex stimulation by sham feeding or by inducing insulin hypoglycaemia, and the administration of parasympathomimetic drugs such as acetylcholine, all lead to the secretion of an acid juice rich in pepsin. Vagotomy in man significantly depresses pepsin secretion, although pepsin secretion induced by histamine stimulation is reduced to a lesser extent by vagal section than is histamine stimulated acid secretion.

Both histamine and gastrin increase pepsinogen output, the latter to a lesser extent; it is of interest that pentagastrin appears to behave more like histamine than gastrin in this respect.

Pepsin secretion in health and disease

Some pepsin secretion occurs in all normal stomachs since synthesis, normally an independent and continuous process, fills the peptic cells with granules and overflow secretion takes place by discharge of the granules to accommodate newly synthesized pepsin. Synthesis may not occur in adrenal or pituitary insufficiency and, at one time, the measurement of gastric pepsin was used as a test of adrenal function. Pepsin and hydrochloric acid are both lacking from the gastric juice in Addisonian pernicious anaemia in which there is total atrophy of the gastric mucosa.

Patients with duodenal ulcer secrete on average about one and a half times more pepsinogen than do normal controls; the composition of the juice differs little and the difference is largely one of volume increase resulting from the enlarged gastric mucosal mass. Hirschowitz (1967) found little difference in the output of pepsin in patients with gastric ulcer as compared with normal controls.

Gastric pepsin or pepsinogen outputs have not gained favour as routine tests of gastric function. Test meals have been of little value because of wide variations in the volume of gastric juice. Again, the use of insulin hypoglycaemia suffers from the disadvantages of uncertain blood sugar response and short-lived stimulation; the use of 2 deoxy-D-glucose has fared no better.

Serum and urine pepsins

Most of the pepsinogen formed in the peptic cells is secreted into the lumen of the stomach, but a small fraction is absorbed into the blood stream and excreted in the urine. The mechanisms of the leak from the cell to the blood are unknown but a steep increase occurs in blood pepsinogen following gastric mucosal damage by surgery, irradiation, very high doses of histamine or toxic doses of cincophen; this evidence suggests that it may normally derive from disintegrating cells. Foods and other stimulants of pepsinogen secretion do not increase blood pepsinogen which is, however, increased by the administration of ACTH or glucocorticoids (Fig. 16.3).

Uropepsin excretion is fairly constant from day to day in the same subject and is lower in females than in males. Mean values for uropepsin in patients with duodenal ulcer are significantly higher than in healthy subjects. Mean values in patients with gastric ulcer tend to be higher than normal although values for lesser curve ulcer are in the normal range. Patients with carcinoma of the stomach have low values, and uropepsin is absent from the urine of patients with total gastric atrophy and after total gastrectomy. It is perhaps surprising that more use has not been

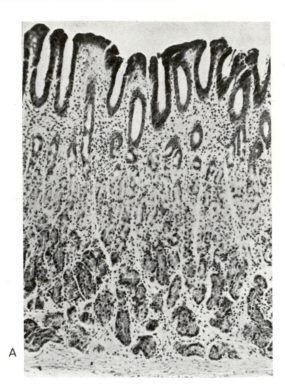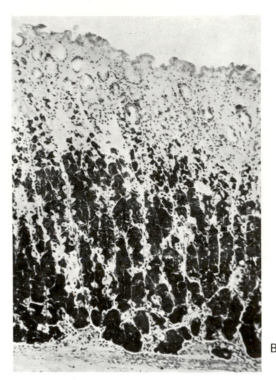

Fig. 16.3 Photomicrographs of human gastric mucosa obtained by biopsy. (A) Fasting, showing dense accumulations of pepsinogen granules. (B) After stimulation by a meal of meat, showing most of the granules discharged.

made of this method of investigation of gastric function since the collection and analysis of specimens is simple and non-invasive. Resuscitation of their use in clinical practice is now unlikely owing to the advent of reliable fibreoptic endoscopy.

SECRETION OF HYDROCHLORIC ACID

The intimate mechanism by which hydrochloric acid is secreted by the parietal cells is still incompletely resolved. Stimulation and inhibition of secretion may be regulated intracellularly by cyclic GMP (guanosine monophosphate) and cyclic AMP (adenosine monophosphate), respectively, the ultimate effect depending on the relative amounts of the two. Hydrogen ion and chloride ion are actively transported into the gastric lumen by separate pumps which are coupled (Fig. 16.4). A negative electrical potential on the mucosal surface is generated by the chloride transport mechanism. The hydrogen ion can be regarded as a product of the dissociation of H_2O. Carbonic acid is formed from the hydration of CO_2, a reaction which is facilitated by the large amounts of carbonic anhydrase in these cells. The carbonic acid dissociates, and the resulting bicarbonate is excreted into the blood stream. Water enters the gastric lumen passively following the actively transported ions, and the secretion is isotonic or nearly so. Acid

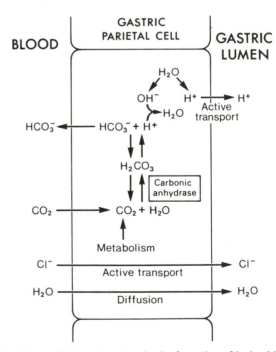

Fig. 16.4 Intracellular mechanisms in the formation of hydrochloric acid by the parietal cells.

secretion, which occurs in a concentration of 165 mmol/l, requires a high rate of blood flow in order to supply hydrogen and chloride ions, to supply nutrients whose combustion provides energy, and to remove bicarbonate.

HISTAMINE AND ACID SECRETION

Histamine is among the most powerful of all known stimuli of acid secretion, but whether it serves as a mediator of normal secretion has long been controversial although recent evidence gives strength to this postulate.

Histamine, injected intravenously, stimulates acid secretion not only from the intact stomach but also from gastric pouches which have been wholly denervated by transplanting them to distant sites, and this suggests that histamine acts directly on the parietal cells.

Histamine released from the tissues can also stimulate acid secretion. In patients with dermatographia, acid secretion can be brought about by inducing whealing of the sensitive skin; similarly, the injection of histamine liberators brings about a striking secretory response. This response is probably the result of histamine carried to the stomach from distant sites by the blood, for the stores of histamine in the skin and muscles are known to be much more labile than the histamine in the stomach itself. The stomach contains a large store of histamine, the concentration being highest in the fundus and body, and localized particularly around the gastric glands. It is therefore hardly surprising that some of it escapes into the gastric juice. Small amounts of histamine are invariably present in acid gastric juice, irrespective of whether the juice is secreted in response to nervous or hormonal stimulation, and this has been adduced as evidence that histamine is the final mediator in stimulating the oxyntic cells. However, it is well known that the antihistamine group of drugs gives protection against the systemic effects of histamine without inhibiting the effect of histamine on gastric secretion, and it is this phenomenon which made possible the 'augmented histamine test' in man.

A major breakthrough came from the work of Black and his colleagues (1972) who have provided evidence of the existence of two types of histamine receptor: at H_1 receptors, conventional antihistamines compete with histamine but, as has been noted, have no effect on acid secretion; H_2 receptors are not affected by the conventional antihistamines, but mediate the secretagogue actions of histamine on the gastric parietal cells. The first H_2 receptor antagonist which became available for physiological and preliminary clinical evaluation was metiamide and it was shown to inhibit not only histamine-stimulated acid secretion but all other forms of acid secretion including that stimulated by food (Black et al, 1973). This provided strong evidence for a physiological role for histamine, but just how it participates remains uncertain. An occasional side effect of metiamide was leucopaenia and this prevented its general use in the clinical management of ulcer patients. However, its successor, cimetidine, became available for clinical use in 1976, is free from significant side effects and has already found its place as an important therapeutic agent for the conservative management of duodenal ulceration. Numerous clinical trials have demonstrated healing of chronic ulcers on treatment with cimetidine or ranitidine, and even ulceration associated with the Zollinger-Ellison syndrome can be brought under control.

GASTRIN AND ACID SECRETION

Gastrin is a gastrointestinal hormone, present chiefly in the mucosa of the pyloric antrum. When meat extracts are brought into contact with the antral mucosa, or when the antrum is distended, gastrin is released into the blood stream, and carried to the mucosa of the body of the stomach where it induces a copious flow of juice. This juice contains much acid, little pepsin, and virtually no mucus.

The history of gastrin is a chequered one. Gastrin was first prepared in 1905 by Edkins. He was careful to point out that his purified preparations, given intravenously, did not depress the blood pressure. Nevertheless, the activity of his preparation came to be attributed to histamine, present as a contaminant. However, Komarov (1942) was able to make potent preparations of gastrin which were beyond doubt free from histamine. A greatly improved method of preparing gastrin from hog antral mucosa was described by Gregory and Tracy (1961), and in 1964 the same workers published a full account of the method of preparation and properties of the hormone. The gastrin molecule is a 17-amino acid polypeptide and exists in non-sulphated and sulphated forms, designated gastrin I and gastrin II respectively. The molecular weight of gastrin I is 2098 and that of gastrin II 2178. The portion of the molecular structure to which physiological importance is attached is the C-terminal tetrapeptide sequence—TRY.MET.ASP.PHE.—and NH_2. The entire range of physiological activity of natural gastrin is displayed by this tetrapeptide although it is less potent than the larger molecule.

Further research has shown that several molecular forms of gastrin occur in the serum as well as in extracts of gastric mucosa and in gastrinomas (Yalow & Berson, 1970). Three major molecular forms of gastrin have been isolated. They share an identical C-terminal portion but differ in their chain length. They have been designated gastrin 14, gastrin 17 and gastrin 34 and each occurs in a sulphated and non-sulphated form. Gastrin 17 is the predominant form of gastrin in tissue whereas gastrin 34, 'big' gastrin, is predominant in the circulation. The 17-amino acid 'little' gastrin can be generated from 'big' gastrin by the action of proteolytic enzymes. A further major advance in the study of gastrin was the precise measurement of serum gastrin levels by radioimmunoassay methods (McGuigan & Trudeau, 1968, 1970; Yalow & Berson, 1970). This has permitted the investigation of serum gastrin levels in normal subjects and in diseased states, studies of the half-life of the various gastrins, and the determination of the metabolic pathways of the hormone. The existence of a 'big big' gastrin has been postulated but it is now generally regarded as an artefact resulting in a spurious gastrin-like reading in the radio-immunoassay system.

In 1966 the synthetic gastrin-like pentapeptide, penta-gastrin, became available commercially and is now in common use in the routine testing of gastric acid secretion in clinical practice.

Basal and stimulated serum gastrin concentrations

Normal fasting concentrations of gastrin immunoreactivity vary among laboratories but usually average between 30 and 80 pg (10^{-12} g) per ml when gastrin I is used as the standard. After a protein meal the values normally increase approximately two-fold with a peak at 15–45 minutes after the meal. Insulin hypoglycaemia produces similar increases, with peak values at 30–60 minutes after injection, but only if gastric contents are maintained at a neutral pH. Acidification below pH 2 strongly inhibits gastrin release by food or insulin. There is little evidence that neutralisation by itself releases gastrin; however when a stimulant for gastrin release such as food, distension, or vagal stimulation is present neutralisation counteracts the inhibition caused by acid. Calcium ions appear to have a direct gastrin releasing action. The gastrin is released from the G-cells in the pyloric gland mucosa but, in man, there is evidence that significant amounts of gastrin are also released from the duodenal mucosa and it is well recog-nized that small but detectable levels of gastrin may be present after total gastrectomy. It is not certain if the pancreas contains gastrin; if so, the amount is very small and not likely to contribute to changes in serum levels.

Serum gastrin in peptic ulcer disease

Patients with duodenal ulcer usually have serum gastrin concentrations which fall in the normal range, but there is some evidence that they release more gastrin than do normal subjects in response to a standard stimulus. There is also evidence that gastrin released by food is inhibited less at pH 2.5 in duodenal ulcer patients than in normal subjects. A small proportion of duodenal ulcer patients have serum gastrin concentrations which are moderately increased (2–4 times normal) in the fasting state but mark-edly elevated in response to a meal. These may be patients with 'antral hyperactivity' in whom normal mechanisms for inhibition of gastrin release are defective, or they may have hyperplasia of G-cells in the pyloric gland mucosa. As has been noted earlier, these patients would seem to require resection of the antrum as part of surgical treat-ment of the duodenal ulcer.

Patients with gastric ulcer have serum gastrin concen-trations which average about twice that of normal subjects both in the fasting and stimulated state.

Serum gastrin is raised in patients who have low gastric acidity but who have an intact antrum. Pernicious anaemia is the best known example, but hypergastrinaemia is also found typically in patients with parietal-cell-antibody-positive atrophic gastritis; these patients have hyperplasia of the pyloric glands which includes hyperplasia of the G-cells.

The major clinical usefulness of serum gastrin measure-ment at the present time is for the evaluation of patients thought to have a gastrinoma (Zollinger-Ellison tumour). In addition, gastrin measurements have occasionally been helpful in establishing the presence of retained antral tissue in patients having recurrent ulceration after partial gastrec-tomy.

THE NEURAL CONTROL OF GASTRIC SECRETION

Gastric secretion continues at a slow rate in the fasting and resting animal and is greatly augmented on feeding. The response to feeding, following the great pioneer work of Pavlov (1910), is customarily described in three phases. The first, the cephalic or appetite phase is of vagal origin; the second or gastric phase is of humoral origin; and the third or intestinal phase is also of humoral origin. It is now appreciated that the secretion of acid by the parietal cells cannot be so sharply demarcated and that it is regulated by the interplay of stimulation and inhibition. The normal stimulus to acid secretion is eating a meal; then all three phases are excited simultaneously but separation into phases is of value for descriptive purposes.

Cephalic phase

For his critical experiments, Pavlov prepared dogs with an innervated gastric pouch (Fig. 16.5), with an oesophageal fistula so that swallowed food was discharged from the stoma, and with a gastrostomy of the main stomach for feeding. Sham feeding these dogs with attractive food led to the gastric pouch pouring out a juice rich in acid and pepsin, but inedible substances placed in the mouth were not followed by secretion. The actual contact of food with the mouth was not essential, and secretion could be evoked as a conditioned reflex by sight or sounds usually associ-ated with feeding. The response was abolished by vagotomy, indicating that the flow of appetite juice is of nervous origin. Equivalent information has since been obtained in man. The vagal stimuli act on the parietal cells directly to increase acid output and, in addition, impulses passing to the antrum release gastrin and thereby indirectly cause acid secretion: the direct parietal cell stimulation is quantitatively more important.

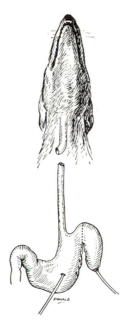

Fig. 16.5 Diagram of a Pavlov pouch. The pouch is separated from the main stomach by a partition constructed from the mucous membrane, but retains its nerve supply. The pouch and main stomach are intubated to allow sampling (Illingworth, 1953).

Gastric phase

The arrival of food in the stomach, through both mechanical and chemical stimulation of the antrum, releases gastrin: distension is the major mechanical stimulus; products of protein digestion liberate gastrin by contact with the antral mucosa.

In addition, the presence of food in the stomach excites long vagal reflexes producing impulses which pass to the central nervous system by way of vagal afferents and return to stimulate the parietal cells.

Finally, distension of the body of the stomach sensitises the parietal cells to gastrin, a mechanism which is probably mediated through local intramural cholinergic reflexes.

Intestinal phase

Contact of food with the lining of the intestine and distension of the intestine also stimulate a modest flow of gastric juice by a humoral mechanism. The hormone concerned may be gastrin itself, cholecystokinin (CCK) which is known to stimulate gastric acid secretion, or another similar as yet unidentified substance.

Physiological inhibition of acid secretion

Mechanisms of stimulation of acid secretion have been outlined above but, as has been noted, the full regulation occurs by the interplay of stimulation and inhibition.

When the pH of the gastric content bathing the antral mucosa reaches 2 or less, all mechanisms of release of gastrin are suppressed. Acid acts directly on the G-cell to inhibit gastrin release and a nervous mechanism is not involved.

Inhibition also occurs from an intestinal source. Acid, fat and hypertonic solutions in the intestine inhibit acid secretion. This inhibition is at least in part hormonally mediated because some aspects of it persist after all nerves between the intestine and stomach have been cut. With extensive intestinal acidification under experimental conditions inhibition is mediated in part by secretin. However, it is doubtful whether enough secretin is released under normal conditions to have such an effect. It seems likely that gastric inhibitory peptide (GIP) plays an important role. GIP is a 43-amino acid peptide belonging to the family of peptides consisting of secretin, glucagon, GIP and VIP (vasoactive intestinal peptide). The highest concentrations of GIP are found in the upper small intestine, especially in the jejunum; the cell responsible for the production of this hormone is the K-cell. The hormone is released by meals and, in particular, by the action of carbohydrates and fat. In addition to its action as an inhibitor of gastric acid secretion, GIP has as its most important property its ability to release insulin from the beta cells.

Interplay between stimulation and inhibition

The parietal cell is unique among effector cells in terms of the degree to which different stimulants and inhibitors interact. For example, blockade of acetylcholine receptors by atropine inhibits responses not only to cholinergic stimuli but also to gastrin and histamine. Similarly, blockade of histamine receptors by H_2 blocking agents inhibits responses not only to histamine but also to gastrin and cholinergics.

Vagotomy reduces the response to high doses of gastrin or histamine by about 70% but this can be restored to the prevagotomy level by giving cholinergic drugs to replace the cholinergic tone lost by vagotomy. This indicates that division of the vagus nerves does not reduce the capacity of the parietal cells to secrete acid but depresses their responsiveness to stimuli.

Antrectomy, by removing the major source of gastrin, decreases the response to large doses of histamine by about 50%. The response to histamine cannot be restored to preoperative levels by giving a background of gastrin, cholinergic drugs, or both.

THE GASTRIC MUCOSAL BARRIER

The integrity of the gastric mucosa depends upon the balance between attack and defence. Acid and pepsin are so obviously capable of attack that for far too long they have been regarded as the almost exclusive subjects for research. One instance in which attack by acid is in itself responsible for ulceration is in the Zollinger-Ellison syndrome in which excessive secretion of acid overwhelms defence; it is unlikely that acid alone is the cause of ulceration in any other situation.

Defence against acid is a function of the gastric mucosal barrier which may be defined as that property of the gastric mucosa which impedes diffusion of acid from the lumen of the stomach into the mucosa, and impedes diffusion of sodium ions from the mucosal interstitial space into the lumen. In the last decade attention has been turned to the gastric barrier and it has been shown to have an important role in protecting the stomach from injury, and that its function can be impaired in many circumstances. When the barrier is broken, acid readily diffuses back into the mucosa and this back diffusion causes pathophysiological responses which go a long way to explain some common clinical conditions.

Substances which directly attack the gastric mucosal barrier include detergents of all kinds, natural and artificial: among the most significant are bile salts and lysolecithin, both of which as constituents of duodenal content can be regurgitated into the stomach where they break the barrier (Davenport, 1968; 1970). Cytotoxic substances which penetrate the barrier include ethanol, eugenol and the salicylates: these cause desquamation of surface epithelial cells.

Once the gastric defences have been breached the acid which diffuses into the mucosa has several injurious effects. Gastric motility is strongly stimulated, probably by increased cholinergic activity of gastric intrinsic plexuses, and the resulting contractions may be accompanied by pain. Histamine is released from the mucosal stores and at the same time histamine forming capacity is greatly increased: the consequence is that histamine reaches a high concentration within gastric interstitial fluid where it causes vasodilatation, increased mucosal blood flow, and increased capillary permeability. These changes result in mucosal oedema, and fluid containing plasma, inorganic and organic constituents is forced through the mucosa into the lumen. In some forms of injury the rate at which plasma proteins are shed by the mucosa may be so high as to cause a protein-losing gastropathy of clinical significance. Bleeding occurs when acid destroys dilated capillaries and venules and it is particularly likely to occur when there is concurrent cholinergic stimulation, a fact which may in part explain the occasional efficacy of vagotomy.

There is growing support for the view that some gastric ulcers result from a disturbance of motility across the pylorus which permits reflux of duodenal content into the stomach, and that the gastric mucosa is then damaged and becomes more susceptible to ulceration (Fig. 16.6). As has been noted above, bile salts and lysolecithn are present in duodenal fluid and both compounds have the ability to

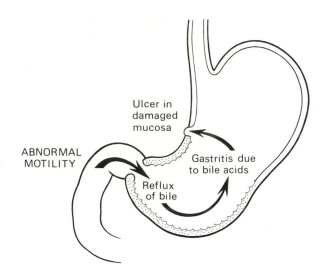

Fig. 16.6 The sequence of events in the pathogenesis of gastric ulcer in patients who reflux bile into the stomach: ulceration occurs adjacent to acid secreting mucosa.

break the gastric mucosal barrier. Several studies have now shown that reflux of bile into the stomach is common in gastric ulcer, but unusual in normal subjects (DuPlessis, 1965; Rhodes, 1972). The presence of a gastric ulcer is regularly associated with a diffuse mucosal lesion (gastritis) and it is a matter of particular interest that the ulcer itself regularly occurs at the junction of mucosa bearing parietal cells and the more distal gastric mucosa which shows an absence of these cells. The starting point of this hypothesis is an abnormality in the pyloric region but it must be conceded that the nature of this defect which leads to reflux has not been elucidated.

THERAPEUTIC CONTROL OF GASTRIC SECRETION

The common aim of the many different ways of treating peptic ulcer is to put a stop to peptic digestion, either by reducing the output of pepsin itself, or more often by preventing the gastric contents from becoming sufficiently acid for the pepsin to be activated. There can be no doubt that exposure to peptic digestion is an essential condition for the development and persistence of peptic ulcers, which occur only in the stomach itself, in the nearby duodenum and oesophagus, and in the jejunum at a gastrojejunostomy stoma, or rarely beside islets of heterotopic gastric mucosa in the intestine. It is recognised that there are other contributory factors, but peptic digestion is the one factor which can be recognised as essential.

The therapeutic control of pepsin secretion has so far been less rewarding than the control of acid secretion and so the following discussion refers almost entirely to the latter, which continues to be the standby of both medical and surgical treatment of peptic ulceration. Maintenance of the gastric acidity at pH 4.5 or more is sufficient to arrest peptic digestion.

Frequent feeding, although it stimulates the hormonal phase of gastric acid secretion, neutralizes the acid by the continual presence of food and also reduces the volume stimulus.

Antacid therapy aims at neutralizing or removing the acid secreted. In the basal state, antacids are effective for only 20–40 minutes and must therefore be taken at least hourly to sustain adequate reduction of gastric acidity in duodenal ulcer patients; doubling the dose of antacids does not enhance appreciably the duration of neutralization since the rate of emptying determines duration of action. Antacids are more effective when taken after a meal and this prolonged effect is due to delayed emptying of the antacid, and also because of reconstitution of acidified meal protein as a buffer. Finally, not only does the response of individual patients to antacids vary widely but vast amounts would be required to maintain continuous neutralisation of hydrochloric acid.

Gastrojejunostomy, although it does not reduce the secretion of acid by the stomach, allows the ready efflux of the acid juice from the stomach and the equally ready reflux of the alkaline juices (containing pancreatic bicarbonate) from the upper jejunum.

Truncal vagotomy abolishes the nervous phase of acid secretion, reduces the hormonal phase and reduces also the basal secretion. This operation regularly cuts down the maximal acid output of the stomach by some 60–70%. Selective vagotomy and parietal cell vagotomy, more recent modifications of the original operation, have each been shown to reduce maximal acid output by a similar amount.

Partial gastrectomy removes some of the acid secreting mucosa and removes also the gastrin-secreting mucosa of the antrum. The latter is probably the more important and it is now recognised that failure to excise the entire antral mucosa frequently results in stomal ulceration, which heals after removal of the antral remnant.

Antrectomy with vagotomy removes both the nervous drive and the hormonal drive on the acid secreting cells and has been shown to reduce maximal acid output by at least 90%. It is therefore not surprising that recurrent ulceration is quite rare after this operation.

Total gastrectomy, by removing the entire acid-secreting mucosa, would give complete control of acid secretion but it is too dangerous for routine use, is accompanied by unpleasant sequelae in the majority of patients, and is reserved as the surgical treatment for some patients with the Zollinger-Ellison syndrome.

Among several approaches which are being investigated for the control of acid secretion, the use of H_2 antagonists has already been mentioned (p. 277). Two others have been chosen for discussion here: gastrointestinal hormones and prostaglandins.

Gastrointestinal hormones

There is growing evidence from experimental studies that acidification of the duodenal mucosa powerfully inhibits the secretion of gastric acid in response to many stimuli, and that this inhibition is mediated humorally. Since it is also known that duodenal acidification is a potent stimulus to the release of both secretin and the single substance which possesses both cholecystokinin and pancreozymin activity (CCK), interest has arisen in the possibility of using either of these substances to control acid secretion. Under experimental conditions in the dog, it has been shown that both will inhibit pouch acid responses to gastrin stimulation. The dose of secretin required to exert good inhibition of acid secretion causes a slight increase in pepsin secretion; the inhibitor dose of CCK is effective against both acid and pepsin secretion and therefore may be the favoured candidate for trial. However, more recent evidence from experimental work suggests that the two substances acting together may potentiate each other, and also the action of GIP, in the inhibition of gastric acid secretion.

Prostaglandins

The inhibitory effects of prostaglandins (PG) on gastric acid secretion have been well documented in animals, but information in man is still scanty. Observations on the effect of intravenous PGF_2 or PGE_2 on gastric acid secretion have been made in patients suffering from peptic ulceration and a significant suppression of basal and stimulated acid output by PGE_2 demonstrated. Analogues of PGE_2 have been shown to inhibit acid production when given by mouth and may therefore be worthy of clinical trial.

Although interest will continue in the use of gastrointestinal hormones and the prostaglandins, drugs capable of blocking the H_2 receptors would seem to offer the greatest promise of an exciting and effective conservative management of the ulcer problem; perhaps the use of these in combination merits exploration.

GASTRIC ANALYSIS

Formerly, the carrying out of a test meal, usually after giving gruel, had a place in the routine investigation of dyspepsia. The major defect of these early methods, however, was their lack of reproducibility. This defect was overcome by the development of the augmented histamine test which provides a measure of the maximal acid output of which a stomach is capable (Kay, 1953).

The use of reliable tests of gastric acid secretion, particularly before and after planned surgery, has added greatly to our understanding of human gastric physiology.

On the other hand the place of these tests in clinical practice, until recently claimed to be important, has now been evaluated on the basis of careful clinical studies and shown to be limited.

The three types of secretory test to be described here are the augmented histamine test, the pentagastrin test, and the insulin test.

The augmented histamine test

This test makes use of the fact that the antihistamine drugs give protection against the systemic effects of histamine without blocking the action of histamine on the stomach. For example, 2 ml of a 2.5% solution of mepyramine maleate (Anthisan) is enough to give protection against the systemic effects of each 1 mg of histamine acid phosphate. Half an hour after giving the antihistamine, enough histamine can safely be given to produce a maximum secretory stimulus. This dose has been found by trial to be 0.04 mg histamine acid phosphate per kilogram body weight which, in the patient of average size, is a little more than 2 mg.

The augmented histamine test can be employed qualitatively to discover if the stomach can secrete at all, but it can also be used quantitatively and has the advantage that replicate tests in one individual yield consistently the same acid response: this is due to the fact that a maximal stimulus is applied to the whole population of parietal cells present in the stomach. That the results of the test do in fact correlate closely with the total number of parietal cells computed on the basis of laborious histological methods has been shown in excellent papers by Marks (1956) and Card and Marks (1960). The response to the test can therefore be legitimately used as an index of the parietal cell population.

The quantitative test is carried out by aspirating the stomach continuously, collecting all the juice secreted in the hour after the injection of histamine, measuring the volume and acid concentration, and expressing the result in millimoles of hydrochloric acid. Three methods of expressing the results of the augmented histamine test remain in use. Kay used the output during the 30-minute period beginning 15 minutes after histamine injection; Card and his colleagues used the output during the entire hour beginning immediately after injection; Baron (1963) suggested that the maximal 30-minute secretion occurred at varying times after the histamine injection and found that the most repeatable measurement was the highest 30-minute output (two consecutive 15-minute periods) without regard to when this occurred in relation to the injection and called this the 'peak acid output'. In a consecutive series of 100 tests we have expressed the results in these three different ways and an excellent and uniform correlation between all three measurements was found, both in intact stomachs and after vagotomy (Table

Table 16.1 Correlation coefficients between methods of expressing augmented histamine response

Peak	Mid $\frac{1}{2}$ hr	1 hr
v	v	v
Mid $\frac{1}{2}$ hr	1 hr	Peak
0.925	0.909	0.942

16.1). Even so, by the common consent of workers in the field of gastric secretion, 'peak acid output' (PAO) is now most commonly used.

The pentagastrin test

When the synthetic gastrin-like pentapeptide, pentagastrin, became commercially available several surgical centres in the United Kingdom co-operated to determine whether pentagastrin was a suitable alternative to histamine as a stimulant of maximal acid secretion and, if so, to describe from combined experience how such a test should be performed (Multicentre Study, 1967 and 1969). It was found that gastric acid responses as great as those from maximal doses of histamine could be obtained with pentagastrin in both normal subjects and in duodenal ulcer patients, and that this applied irrespective of whether the pentagastrin was given by single subcutaneous injection or by continuous intravenous infusion. The appropriate dosage for maximal response to pentagastrin is 6 μg/kg by the subcutaneous route and 6 μg per kg per hour by continuous intravenous infusion. A comparison of the overall mean response to pentagastrin was virtually the same as that to histamine acid phosphate and the route of administration did not influence the magnitude of the response. The reproducibility of the pentagastrin test was also confirmed. Patients having both pentagastrin and augmented histamine tests commented that the side effects were less after pentagastrin. Finally, the 60–70% reduction in maximal acid output found on repeating the augmented histamine test after vagotomy was shown to occur when pentagastrin was used as the stimulus.

In view of the lesser side effects after pentagastrin as compared with a large dose of histamine it is not surprising that the pentagastrin test has now replaced its predecessor in clinical practice. In view of the simplicity of administration, the single subcutaneous injection technique is more appropriate for routine clinical use; the continuous intravenous infusion technique possesses some advantages for the clinical investigator.

The value of the above two tests in diagnosis, in planning surgical treatment, and as a surgical discipline is now discussed. Although the assessment is based largely on data obtained from studies using the augmented histamine test, the conclusions apply equally to the pentagastrin test.

Value in diagnosis

The results of augmented histamine tests have been related to proven diagnosis in patients with duodenal ulcer, duodenal ulcer with gastric ulcer, simple gastric ulcer, gastric carcinoma, peptic oesophagitis, and normal controls (Kay, 1967). In accordance with previous experience, patients with duodenal ulcer, either alone or in combination with gastric ulcer, have an acid response on average twice as great as in any other single group (Fig. 16.7). However, the ranges of these values in all groups are such that the response in any one patient is of limited diagnostic value. The result of maximal acid output testing is, however, of very limited assistance in the clinical situation.

The Zollinger-Ellison syndrome is characterised by an unusually high acid output under basal conditions which is increased only slightly by maximal stimulation with histamine or pentagastrin. The routine use of either test can be of value in screening duodenal ulcer patients for this uncommon condition but it is doubtful whether the gain would merit the effort of subjecting all duodenal ulcer patients to gastric acid secretion studies. The availability of serum gastrin estimations facilitates the confident diagnosis of this condition.

Deformity of the stomach, particularly at the site of anastomoses following surgical treatment for duodenal ulcer, restricts the value of radiological examination and, to a lesser extent, of endoscopy in the diagnosis of recurrent ulceration. A high acid response to histamine or pentagastrin gives support to this diagnosis; an absence of response, preferably confirmed by a second test, excludes recurrent ulceration.

Refined and more direct methods for the investigation of anaemia have reduced the importance of establishing the presence of histamine-fast achlorhydria in patients with suspected Addisonian pernicious anaemia.

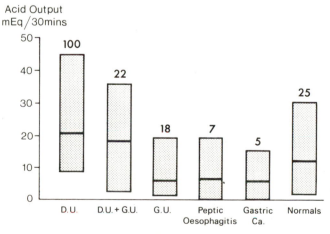

Fig. 16.7 Means and ranges of augmented histamine responses for different disease groups and normal control. Figures above each upper range value are numbers from which means and ranges were derived.

It is worthy of note that the mean and range of values for patients with carcinoma of the stomach are not very different from those in normal subjects and it is important to emphasise that normal acid responses may be obtained in patients with gastric malignancy, and that a histamine-fast achlorhydria occurs with less frequency in this condition than has been claimed in the past.

Finally, the accuracy and reliability of modern endoscopy has greatly reduced the diagnostic value of acid secretion studies.

Value in planning surgical treatment

There have been several attempts to select surgical treatment of duodenal ulcer to meet the requirements of the individual patient. However, since, achlorhydria apart, we do not know the safe level to which acid secretion in the individual patient must be reduced to ensure freedom from recurrent ulceration, the prospect of success by this approach is limited at the present time.

Jejunal interposition, an operation to correct some of the major undesirable sequelae of gastrectomy with gastro-jejunal anastomosis, offers a reasonable prospect of symptomatic relief but carries the risk of ulceration in the interposed segment of jejunum. In our experience this can occur when the gastric remnant continues to secrete even very small amounts of hydrochloric acid. In view of the technical difficulties in achieving satisfactory gastric aspiration after gastrectomy, two pre-operative pentagastrin tests are recommended: if free acid is detected, or if the pH of any specimen falls below 5.0, vagotomy should be added at the time of jejunal interposition.

Value as surgical discipline

The aim of all operations for chronic duodenal ulcer is to reduce the amount of acid produced by the stomach sufficiently to allow the ulcer to heal. It must be admittted that not all surgeons attempt to ascertain that this objective has been achieved. The collection of reliable acid secretion data before and after surgical treatment, and the subsequent correlation with long term clinical results, may influence beneficially the individual surgeon's work and guide future trends in the surgical management of peptic ulceration.

The insulin test

The induction of hypoglycaemia by the administration of insulin is a reliable method of stimulating the vagi (Hollander, 1951), and is the most widely accepted method in use to determine the completeness of surgical vagotomy.

It is important to note that the effective stimulus is hypoglycaemia, and it is essential to verify that the dose of insulin given has reduced the blood sugar concentration to 2.5 mmol/l or less; in man this can usually be achieved with a dose of 20 units of soluble insulin given intravenously. Symptoms of hypoglycaemia (sweating, weakness, disorientation) are usually apparent 30–45 minutes later, and at this time acid is secreted if the vagi are intact or if vagotomy is incomplete. It is now advocated that the dose of insulin should be given according to body weight and it is accepted that this should be 0.02 units per kilogram body weight. At the conclusion of the test a glucose drink is given. Occasionally, severe hypoglycaemia may require to be treated with glucose solution given intravenously.

There continues to be debate on the interpretation of the insulin test and at least four alternatives to Hollander's original criteria have been posed; this subject has been reviewed by Kay (1967). According to Hollander a positive response (incomplete vagotomy) is indicated by an increase in acid concentration of 20 mmol/l over pre-insulin levels in any 15 minute specimen during the 2 hours following insulin injection; a lesser response is interpreted as a negative insulin test (complete vagotomy) provided that the blood sugar has fallen below 2.5 mmol/l. Gillespie et al (1969) have shown that the criteria of Hollander are satisfied within 60 minutes of insulin injection in the majority of subjects with intact vagi. On this basis a positive response after vagotomy has been subdivided into 'early positive' (where the response occurs in the first hour after giving insulin) and a 'late positive' (where the response occurs during the second hour after giving insulin). Patients having an early positive response run a particularly high risk of subsequently developing recurrent ulceration (Table 16.2).

Table 16.2 Relation between insulin status in the immediate postoperative period and subsequent development of recurrent ulceration.

Insulin status	Patients tested	Recurrent ulcer
Early positive	26	6 (23.1%)
Late positive	55	2 (3.6%)
Negative	304	5 (1.6%)

Many patients showing a negative response to an insulin test within ten days of vagotomy subsequently show conversion to a positive response, the time of conversion usually being within 6 months of operation (Gillespie et al, 1970a, b). This finding, which is supported by the work of others, has led to criticism of performing an insulin test before the patient leaves hospital. There are, however, advantages in performing the test at this time: firstly, not all patients are willing to return for insulin testing; secondly, the surgeon is likely to be more careful at the performance of his operation when he is aware that the result of an insulin test will shortly be forthcoming. The data in Table 16.2 show a clear correlation between the existence of a positive insulin test in the immediate postoperative period and the subsequent development of recurrent ulceration, and provide good evidence that the immediate test should continue to be used (Kennedy et al, 1973).

GASTRIC MOTILITY AND GASTRIC EMPTYING

The gastric muscle adapts the capacity of the stomach to the volume of its contents, mixes the food with the gastric juices and discharges the chyme gradually into the duodenum. In order to understand these actions, it is necessary to consider the mechanism of the gastrooesophageal sphincter, the motor activity of the stomach, the receptive relaxation of the stomach in response to distension, the mechanism of gastric emptying, and the overall control of gastric motility.

The gastrooesophageal sphincter

Although food passes freely from the oesophagus to the stomach it does not readily regurgitate. Various mechanisms for preventing regurgitation have been suggested but gastrooesophageal competence is complex and still incompletely understood. The lower 4 cm of the oesophagus serves as a physiological sphincter and here the resting pressure within the lumen usually exceeds intragastric pressure by 15–25 cm water due to tonic contraction of the oesophageal musculature. This pressure is maintained even after excision of the structures around the lower oesophagus and this constitutes important evidence of the existence of a sphincter which can respond to a challenging opening force by increased contraction. Cohen and Lipshutz (1971) have demonstrated that the contraction response is proportional to the basal tone which is in part regulated hormonally by an interaction of gastrin (increases tone) and secretin (decreases tone). When the basal tone of the sphincter falls below a critical level free reflux of gastric contents into the oesophagus may occur. Cholinergic and α-adrenergic stimuli enhance, and β-adrenergic stimuli inhibit, contraction of the sphincter.

Intra-abdominal pressure increases as a result of a variety of normal daily activities. It was formerly thought that the lack of reflux of gastric contents under such circumstances was due to the presence of an intra-abdominal segment of oesophagus which transmitted the pressure increment to the sphincter, thus counterbalancing rises within the stomach. More recent studies have shown that pressure in the sphincter increases in response to induced rises in gastric pressure regardless of the position of the sphincteric segment in relation to the diaphragm. Thus patients with large hiatus herniae, but without symptoms, have an elevation of sphincteric pressure following abdominal compression which is similar to that seen in patients whose sphincter is situated below the diaphragm. In patients with symptoms most operations involve reduction of the hiatus hernia which brings the sphincter back into the abdomen; this is frequently successful in relieving symptoms but it is clearly irrational to believe that this procedure alters the functioning of the sphincter itself.

The intraluminal pressure at various levels in the oesophagus can be studied using a system of multi open-ended tubes of fine calibre. Pressure within the resting oesophagus is uniformly low except for a segment of higher pressure, as noted above, in the lower 4 cm of oesophagus. During swallowing, general intra-oesophageal pressure rises sharply, and the pressure within the sphincter area temporarily falls (Fig. 16.8).

During vomiting, the gastrooesophageal junction rises above the level of the diaphragm, this ascent probably being due to contraction of the longitudinal musculature of the oesophagus. Expulsion of gastric contents by the violent contractions of the gastric antrum and of the abdominal wall then becomes possible. The vomiting episode over, the structures resume their ordinary relationships.

Finally, although it is now generally agreed that the circular fibres at the lower end of the oesophagus serve as a sphincter, it must be conceded that no anatomical structure resembling a true sphincter can be found by exposing the lower oesophagus in life, by dissection or by histological examination.

The motor activity of the stomach

The stomach, considered as a motor unit, consists of two functional areas: a proximal receptacle which is the fundus and body, and a distal pump which is the antrum. Both have three muscle layers which increase in thickness in the antrum, thus accounting for the stronger contractions that can be measured in the distal stomach. The pyloric sphincter was formerly regarded as an independent unit, but all recent studies have shown that it is anatomically and functionally a part of the antral musculature. The muscle of the sphincter, like the muscle of the antrum, is for most of the time relaxed leaving the pylorus open. As each successive wave of contraction reaches it from the antrum, the pylorus briefly closes. The spectacle of a ring of contraction appearing above the mid-point of the stomach and increasing in amplitude as it passes smoothly towards the pylorus is familiar to every gastroscopist. As ring after ring of contraction pass along the antrum, the contents are thoroughly kneaded and mixed. In addition to churning the gastric contents, the forceful contractions of the antrum deliver the gastric chyme into the duodenum in small quantities at a time; most of the gastric contents which are pushed into the antral funnel are propelled backwards as the pylorus closes for further mixing and at this time the pressure rises within the lumen of the antrum. About 5–15 ml enters the duodenum with each gastric peristaltic wave.

Adaptive relaxation of the stomach

Adaptive relaxation is a property of the musculature of the proximal part of the stomach rather than of the pyloric antrum. The volume of the empty gastric lumen is only about 50 ml but by this process of receptive relaxation the stomach can accommodate as much as 1000 ml before the pressure within its lumen begins to rise. Receptive relaxation is an active process mediated by vagal reflexes and abolished by vagotomy. The different behaviour of the proximal and distal musculature is not easily demonstrated in the intact human stomach, but is clearly seen after some kinds of operation. After partial gastrectomy, in which the pyloric antrum is removed, motility records show tonus waves and only rarely slight peristalsis. After resection of the proximal two-thirds of the stomach with anastomosis of the oesophagus to the antrum, the tracings in the antrum show powerful waves of peristalsis. It is the ability of the intact stomach to maintain a continuous state of tone which allows the body of the stomach to accommodate to increases or decreases in gastric content without appreciable change in intragastric pressure.

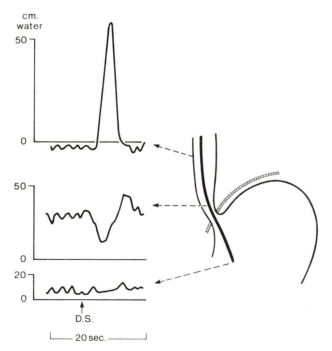

Fig. 16.8 Simultaneous record of pressures from lower oesophagus, cardia, and gastric fundus obtained by using a three-channelled tube. The arrow marked DS signifies *a dry swallow*. Note that the cardia behaves differently from the lower oesophagus. It relaxes during swallowing whereas the lower oesophagus contracts, and its resting tone is high (Atkinson et al, 1957).

The regulation of gastric motor activity

The concept of a pacemaker in the stomach, analogous to the pacemaker of the heart, was first proposed by Alvarez (1948) who observed that strips of longitudinal muscle taken from different parts of the stomach had different spontaneous rates of contraction, the higher rates being found in muscle strips taken from near the cardia. He suggested that at the proximal end of the stomach there was a gastric pacemaker, and more recent studies indicate that this is situated in the fundal musculature near the greater curvature (Weber & Kohatsu, 1970). Regular electrical impulses (pacesetter potential or basic electrical rhythm) arise from this area and move towards the pylorus with progressive acceleration and increase in amplitude. The rate of discharge is about 3 per minute in man. Each impulse is not necessarily followed by a peristaltic muscular contraction, but the impulses determine the maximal peristaltic rate.

A study by Duthie and his colleagues (1971) indicated that, in man, the 3 per minute rhythm extends from the antrum into the proximal 10 cm of the duodenum. These data were obtained by implanting silver electrodes in the stomach and duodenum of patients undergoing cholecystectomy, the implants being removed through the drainage site some days after operation. Thus the antrum, pylorus and duodenum of man appear to act as an electrically coordinated unit. The exact route of conduction from antrum to duodenum has not been defined but it may be by way of the few longitudinal muscle fibres that continue from the antrum across the pylorus.

The muscle layers of the fundus and antrum have cholinergic excitatory fibres arriving by way of the vagus nerves and adrenergic inhibitory fibres by way of the splanchnic nerves. There is also a third supply, the vagal non-adrenergic inhibitory system which participates in receptive relaxation of the fundus and may also innervate the pylorus. The motor activity of the antrum is controlled not only by neurogenic but also by hormonal mechanisms whereas, as far as is known, the fundus is controlled only by a neurogenic mechanism.

The story of hormonal control of gastric motor activity is just beginning to unfold and the present state of knowledge is mentioned in the discussion of gastric emptying.

Gastric emptying

Until quite recently methods of measuring the rate of gastric emptying in man have been either unsuited to clinical investigation or have been unable to provide accurate information.

Clinically, the radiologist provides some information on the emptying of barium from the stomach and has endeavoured to make this examination more physiological by mixing barium intimately with food. However, both barium sulphate and gastrograffin are irritant to the gastric mucosa and therefore may affect the responses of the stomach. Furthermore, to obtain a sufficient number of points with which to plot a mathematical function of emptying would require repeated X-ray exposures and so a high cumulative radiation dose to the patient. Thus, while the ordinary barium meal examination may reveal gross clinical disturbances of emptying, or complete failure of evacuation, it is not satisfactory for accurate quantitative estimates.

Modern techniques rely upon serial dilution of a marker (George, 1968) or upon the clearance of radioactivity from the stomach after the ingestion of a meal labelled with a radioactive marker (Griffith et al, 1968). Each is now described briefly.

In a double sampling test meal the patient drinks a known amount of distilled water containing a marker, usually phenol red. At selected intervals of time (usually 10 minutes) a specimen is withdrawn from the stomach and the concentration of marker determined. A concentrated measure of the same marker is now introduced through a nasogastric tube and vigorous mixing is achieved by rapidly withdrawing and reinserting volumes of gastric content using a syringe. At this time a second sample of the mixed gastric content is withdrawn and its concentration noted. The volume in the stomach is calculated from the concentration of dye in samples of gastric content removed before and after addition of the concentrated measure. The volume of fluid in the stomach on each occasion of sampling can be calculated according to the following formula:

If V_1 = volume to be determined;
  C_1 = initial concentration of dye in V_1;
  V_2 = volume of the measure of dye to be added to V_1;
  C_2 = concentration of the added dye;
  C_3 = final concentration of mixture.

The mass of the dye in V_1 is given by $m_1 = V_1C_1$.
The mass of dye in V_2 is given by $m_2 = V_2C_2$.
The mass of dye in $V_1 + V_2$ is given by $m_3 = (V_1 + V_2)C_3$
since $m_1 + m_2 = m_3$.
Therefore $V_1C_1 + V_2C_2 = (V_1 + V_2)C_3$;

$$\text{Therefore } V_1 = \frac{V_2(C_2 - C_3)}{(C_3 - C_1)}$$

The unknown volume can be estimated at intervals whose length will depend on the nature of the fluid meal and its likely rate of emptying. The procedure of this test is illustrated in Figure 16.9. The characteristics of gastric emptying determined by this test compare well with the classical serial test meal of Hunt (1957) which involves several intubations on different days and is therefore not acceptable for clinical use.

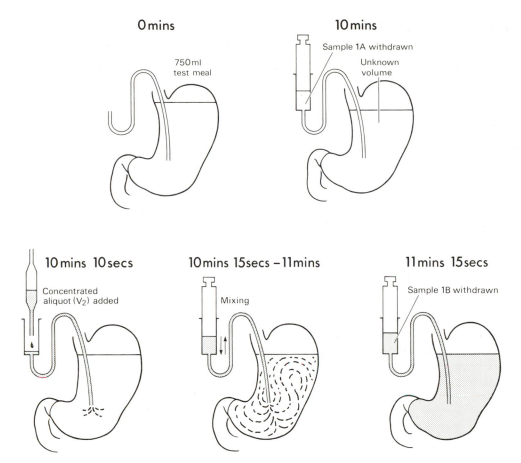

Fig. 16.9 Procedure of the double sampling test meal. 0 min, 750 ml test meal ingested: 10 min, sample withdrawn from stomach; 10 min 10 secs (approx.), concentrated measure of dye added; 10 min 15 secs to 11 min (approx.), mixing of dye in stomach; 11 min 15 secs (approx.), second sample withdrawn from stomach. (From George, 1968)

The use of radioactive markers carries the great advantage that there is no need to pass a nasogastric tube which, by its presence, may influence gastric emptying. After fasting overnight the subject takes a standard breakfast, such as porridge, milk and buttered bread, into which has been incorporated radioactive sodium chromate (200 μCi in 2 ml saline solution), the volume of the meal being kept at approximately 550 ml. After finishing the meal, the subject lies on a couch under the gamma camera which is positioned so that the stomach appears in the centre of the field of an oscilloscope display (Fig. 16.10). One scan is made immediately after the end of the meal and is repeated at half hourly intervals until the stomach is almost empty. The best position for the patient is a matter for further study, but it is customary to have the patient lying supine during the scanning and allow him to walk about or sit in a chair between scans. The information can be fed to a computer which is programmed to print out the total radioactivity count. Background activity can be calculated and subtracted from the total, so that a falling count rate is truly representative of the rate of gastric emptying of the isotopically labelled meal. Emptying rates are usually expressed in terms of the half-life of radioactivity in the stomach area.

At this time it is not possible to predict with any accuracy the place of gastric emptying studies in clinical practice, but it is probable that they will become more useful than estimates of gastric secretion; it is obvious that a true understanding of gastric function is not possible without a knowledge of both motor and secretory information. It is already known that gastric ulceration is commonly associated with delay in emptying whereas the majority of patients with duodenal ulcer empty their stomachs more rapidly than do normal subjects. Perhaps the most likely place for tests of emptying will be in the investigation of patients with symptoms following gastric surgery.

Influence of meal composition on gastric emptying

A wide variety of compounds, including potassium and calcium salts, sulphates and glucose, delay gastric emptying and the delay is related to their osmotic pressure. It is postulated that they exhibit slow penetration into an osmoreceptor, shrink it, and excite a mechanism causing

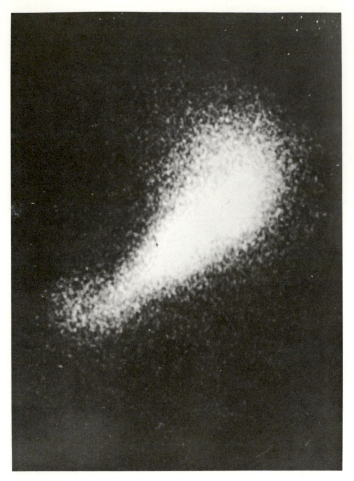

Fig. 16.10 Scan of normal stomach using $^{99}Tc^m$.

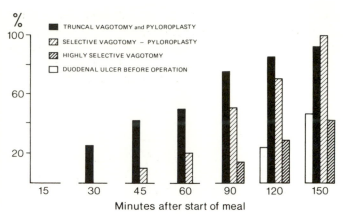

Fig. 16.11 Gastric emptying in patients after various forms of vagotomy and in control patients with duodenal ulcer studied preoperatively. (Wilkinson & Johnston, 1973)

delay. Conversely, substances which penetrate easily such as sodium, urea and glycerol allow accumulation of solute, swell the osmoreceptor and so do not delay emptying.

Acids delay emptying but vary in their ability to do so: thus 45 mM hydrochloric acid is as effective as 121 mM citric acid. Effectiveness is related to the square root of the molecular weight of the acid and this is consistent with the view that anions determine the effectiveness of acid in slowing gastric emptying, possibly due to larger molecules diffusing into the receptor more slowly than smaller molecules. Hydrochloric acid is the only physiological acid and delay in gastric emptying is related to the amount of this acid entering the duodenum.

It has been known for many years that fats are capable of slowing the emptying of the stomach. Fatty acids are more effective than triglycerides and their ability to delay emptying is related to carbon chain length.

Liquids empty more rapidly than solids, but removal of the pylorus or terminal antrum speeds up emptying of solids without having any marked effect on liquids.

One of the substantiated advantages of parietal cell vagotomy as surgical treatment for duodenal ulcer is that, by preserving the innervation of the antrum, there is no need to add a drainage procedure which is a routine accompaniment of truncal vagotomy; the persistence of powerful antral contractions permits adequate gastric emptying provided that there is no distal obstruction at the site of the duodenal ulcer (Fig. 16.11). If this operation is at least as good as others in preventing recurrent ulceration the preservation of the normal emptying mechanism with its lesser risk of postprandial symptoms would constitute a distinct advantage.

SENSATION IN THE STOMACH

The healthy gastric mucosa is quite insensitive to chemical and physical trauma, and the muscular contractions of healthy digestion rarely enter consciousness. Pain does, however, arise from the wall of the stomach when there is an ulcer (p. 289) and the peristalsis that accompanies pyloric stenosis is sometimes appreciated, probably by the movement imparted to the abdominal wall. It can be said that the normal stomach is virtually insensitive, despite the popular belief that the sensations of distension and emptiness have their locus in the stomach itself.

Sense of distension

It is conceded that Wolf and Wolff found that their patient with a gastric fistula had a sense of distension when his stomach was inflated with air, but the distending pressure required to be beyond physiological limits. Patients undergoing gastroscopy, a procedure which necessitates inflating the stomach, rarely experience discomfort. A sensation of repletion and fullness after a heavy meal is familiar to all, but the experiment of Hoelzel (1947) indicated that this sensation may not originate in the stomach. He compounded barium sulphate, cellulose flour, gum and water into a doughy paste and set himself the unenviable task of consuming the mixture until he was replete. At the end of this meal, X-ray examination showed that much of the mixture was in the small intestine and even in the colon. This and other similar observations suggest that the sense of fullness usually attributed to the stomach may arise from fullness of other viscera and of the abdomen as a whole.

Sense of emptiness

A sense of emptiness is commonly combined with a sense of weakness and distress during hunger. This sense of emptiness is a continuous or slowly fluctuating state in most people, but there are a few who experience also brief but intense hunger pangs. These intermittent hunger pangs of the healthy are not to be confused with the continuous, deeply seated, boring hunger pain of duodenal ulcer.

The continuous or slowly fluctuating sense of emptiness, experienced by most, has not been thoroughly investigated.

The hunger pangs, experienced by a few, attracted the attention of Cannon and Washburn as along ago as 1912. They recorded gastric movements by means of a soft rubber balloon in the stomach, attached through a stomach tube to a kymograph, and the subject of the experiment (who was not allowed to watch the tracing) was provided with a signalling device for marking the times of his hunger pangs; Cannon and Washburn found fairly good correlation between powerful gastric contractions and hunger pangs. These findings were confirmed by Carlson (1919) but not by Christensen (1931). Our own experience has been that gastric contractions are only rarely associated with hunger pangs.

THE PAIN OF PEPTIC ULCER

Ulcer pain is usually described as a continuous gnawing ache, rather vaguely located deep in the epigastrium. Severe pain usually radiates through to the back and sometimes upwards to the chest.

The most characteristic feature of ulcer pain is its relationship to meals, for food nearly always gives temporary relief. Most patients, on first being questioned, make the sweeping statement that the pain comes on at some constant time interval after meals, but closer questioning shows that this is seldom so. When their pain is mild, it usually comes on after an interval of 3 or 4 hours, when moderate it comes on after a shorter interval, and when severe it may come on within an hour. Also, pain is not equally common after all meals, but occurs most often after the midday meal and towards the end of the working day. It can be said that mild ulcer pain begins long after one particular meal, is felt in the epigastrium, and rarely disturbs sleep. Severe ulcer pain begins soon after meals,

radiates from the epigastrium to the back and is common by night as well as by day.

The time interval between meals and the onset of pain is reputed to be shorter with gastric than with duodenal ulcer. A survey of our own records does not support this notion.

Ulcer pain can be relieved in a number of ways. It can almost always be relieved by food or a drink of milk, and even a drink of water may suffice to relieve mild pain. Pain can be relieved by taking alkali. Pain is relieved by vomiting irrespective of whether the vomiting is spontaneous or induced, and by emptying the stomach with a stomach tube. It can be seen that these means of relieving ulcer pain have two factors in common: they alter the gastric acidity and they alter the state of gastric distension.

Theories of the cause of ulcer pain

Ulcer pain has been thought to be caused by tension, by exposure to acid, or by a combination of these factors.

In the past tension within the stomach was considered by Hurst as the only stimulus to which the gastric pain receptors are sensitive. He supposed that an abnormally high pressure in the pyloric vestibule could result from powerful contraction waves bearing down on a closed pyloric sphincter. This view is not in accord with the modern conception of the behaviour of the pyloric sphincter. Further, it is rare in radiological experience to observe a relationship between pain and powerful peristalsis.

Evidence that might be held to support Hurst's view was offered by Carlson (1919) and Christensen (1931). Carlson published kymograph tracings, obtained by the intragastric balloon technique, in which the sensation of pain was synchronous with the gastric contractions. Using a similar technique, we have ourselves found an association between pain and high amplitude contractions in only two patients out of a large series, and both patients were later found to have an ulcer situated exactly on the pyloric ring.

Hurst's view that ulcer pain results from gastric contractions is invalidated by the results of introducing hydrochloric acid into the stomach (Fig. 16.12). The instillation of acid usually provokes pain in patients with an active ulcer, but it regularly inhibits gastric contractions; on neutralising the acid with alkali the contractions reappear but the pain is relieved.

The most generally accepted theory of the cause of ulcer pain is the 'acid irritation theory' first put forward by Palmer (1926). He showed that the instillation of 200 ml of 0.5% hydrochloric acid into the stomach would provoke ulcer pain in most ulcer patients, provided that they were in relapse. The acid stimulus was not effective in normal people and only rarely in ulcer patients during remission.

The observations of Palmer have been extended by Bonney and Pickering (1946), who made a detailed study

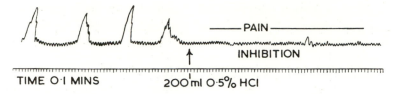

Fig. 16.12 Pain induced by instilling acid in a patient with an active gastric ulcer. Note that in this patient pain happened to be absent during a phase of gastric contractions, and present during muscular quiescence.

of the relationship between the development and subsidence of pain with changes in gastric acidity. Their findings were:

1. Naturally occurring pain is relieved when the gastric contents are aspirated, and recurs when the aspirated material is replaced. Pain does not recur if the aspirated material is neutralised before it is replaced.

2. Naturally occurring pain is closely related to the acidity of the gastric contents (Fig. 16.13). The threshold of acidity required varies from patient to patient and varies even in a single individual according to the state of his dyspepsia.

3. During relapse, but not during remission, the instillation of 200–300 ml of a 50 mmol/l solution of hydrochloric acid brings on pain after a latent period of about 10 minutes. This artificially induced pain and natural pain begin at about the same critical level of gastric acidity.

These observations lend strong support to the theory that ulcer pain results from the action of hydrochloric acid on an ulcerated mucosa. Unfortunately, the theory is felt by many to be unsatisfactory and incomplete: unsatisfactory because it is based on an oversimplification of the facts, and incomplete because it leaves one large question unanswered. It is not clear why pain should be so rare before breakfast when the gastric juice is sometimes strongly acid, nor why in gastric as opposed to duodenal ulcer there can be pain when the gastric content is almost neutral. A more serious objection is that many observers have failed to induce pain by instilling acid. The unanswered question is why an open ulcer should sometimes be symptomless and quite insensitive to exposure to acid.

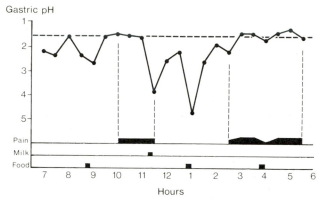

Fig. 16.13 Pain in peptic ulcer. Note that naturally occurring pain is associated with peak levels of gastric acidity (Bonney & Pickering, 1946).

The tension theory of Hurst and the acid irritation theory of Palmer may perhaps be reconciled in the wider generalisation of Kinsella (1948). Kinsella proposed that ulcer pain originates from local increase in tension in the tissues around the ulcer, regardless of whether this results from inflammatory oedema or muscle spasm. According to this view, acid is not the unique cause of pain but merely an added irritant which may increase existing oedema to the point of precipitating local tissue ischaemia. The concept of ulcer pain being due to ischaemia is in full accord with the known occurrence of ischaemic pain in organs which are otherwise insensitive, such as the intestine, the uterus and the heart.

FURTHER READING

Amdrup E, Jensen H E 1970 Selective vagotomy of the parietal cell mass preserving innervation of the undrained antrum. A preliminary report of results in patients with duodenal ulcer. Gastroenterology 59: 522–527

Creamer B 1955 Oesophageal reflux. Lancet i: 279–281

Dragstedt L R, Woodward E R, Harper P V, Storer E H 1948 Mechanism of relief of ulcer distress by gastric vagotomy. Gastroenterology 10: 200–204

Gillespie I E 1959 Influence of antral pH on gastric acid secretion in man. Gastroenterology 37: 164–168

Gillespie I E, Bowen D J 1962 The gastric secretion of pepsin in man. Gut 3: 255–259

Gillespie I E, Clark D H, Kay A W, Tankel H I 1960 Effect of

antrectomy, vagotomy with gastrojejunostomy, and antrectomy with vagotomy, on the spontaneous and maximal gastric acid output in man. Gastroenterology 38: 361–367

Humphrey C S, Wilkinson A R 1972 The value of preserving the pylorus in the surgery of duodenal ulcer. British Journal of Surgery 59: 779–783

Hunt J N, Knox M T 1968 A relation between the chain length of fatty acids and the slowing of gastric emptying. Journal of Physiology (London) 194: 327–336

Isenberg J I, Stening G F, Ward S, Grossman M I 1969 Relation of gastric secretory response in man to dose of insulin. Gastroenterology 57: 395–398

Johnston D, Wilkinson A R, Humphrey C S, Smith R B, Goligher

J C, Kragelund E, Amdrup E 1973 Serial studies of gastric secretion in patients after highly selective (parietal cell) vagotomy without a drainage procedure for duodenal ulcer. Gastroenterology 64: 1–21

Kelly K A, Code C F 1971 Canine gastric pacemaker. American Journal of Physiology 220: 112–118

Kronborg O, Madsen P 1975 A controlled randomized trial of highly selective vagotomy versus selective vagotomy and pyloroplasty in the treatment of duodenal ulcer. Gut 16: 268–271

Madsen P, Kronborg O, Feldt-Rasmussen K 1973 The gastric emptying and small intestinal transit after highly selective vagotomy without drainage and selective vagotomy with pyloroplasty. Scandinavian Journal of Gastroenterology 8: 541–543

Newman A, Prado de Moraes Filho J, Philappakos D, Misiewicz J J

1975 The effect of intravenous infusions of prostaglandins E_2 and F_{2a} on human gastric function. Gut 16: 272–276

Payne R A, Kay A W 1962 The effect of vagotomy on the maximal acid secretory response to histamine in man. Clinical Science 22: 373–382

Samloff I M 1971 Pepsinogens, pepsins and pepsin inhibitors. Gastroenterology 60: 586–604

Smith A N 1959 The distribution and release of histamine in human gastric tissues. Clinical Science 18: 533–541

Zollinger R M, Ellison E H 1955 Primary peptic ulcerations of the jejunum associated with islet-cell tumours of the pancreas. Annals of Surgery 142: 709–728

REFERENCES

Alvarez W C 1948 An introduction in gastroenterology. Hoeber, New York

Atkinson M, Edwards D A W, Honour A J, Rowlands E N 1957 Comparison of cardiac and pyloric sphincter. Lancet ii: 918–922

Baron J H 1963 An assessment of the augmented histamine test in the diagnosis of peptic ulcer. Correlation between gastric secretion, age and sex of patients and site and nature of the ulcer. Gut 4: 243–253

Bell P R F, Battersby C 1968 Effect of vagotomy on gastric mucosal blood flow. Gastroenterology 54: 1032–1037

Bell P R F, Shelley T 1968 Gastric mucosal blood flow and acid secretion in conscious animals measured by heat clearance. American Journal of Digestive Diseases 13: 685–696

Black J W, Duncan W A M, Durant C J, Ganellin C R, Parsons M E 1972 Definition and antagonism of histamine H_2-receptors. Nature 236: 385–390

Black J W, Duncan W A M, Emmett J C, Ganellin C R, Hesselbo T, Parsons M E, Wyllie J H 1973 Metiamide—an orally active histamine H_2-receptor antagonist. Agents and Actions 3: 133–137

Bonney G L, Pickering G W 1946 Observations on mechanism of pain in ulcer of stomach and duodenum. Clinical Science 6: 68–89, 91–111

Cannon W B, Washburn A L 1912 An explanation of hunger. American Journal of Physiology 29: 441–454

Card W I, Marks I N 1960 The relationship between the acid output of the stomach following 'maximal' histamine stimulation and the pariental cell mass. Clinical Science 19: 147–163

Carlson A J 1919 The control of hunger in health and disease. Hoeber, Chicago

Christensen O 1931 Pathophysiology of hunger pains. Acta Medica Scandanavica (Suppl) 37

Cohen S, Lipshutz W 1971 Hormonal regulation of human lower oesophageal sphincter competence. Journal of Clinical Investigation 50: 449–454

Connell A M, McCall J, Misiewicz J J, Rowlands E N 1963 Observation on the clinical use of radio pills. British Medical Journal 771–774

Davenport H W 1968 Destruction of the gastric mucosal barrier by detergents and urea. Gastroenterology 54: 175–181

Davenport H W 1970 Effect of lysolecithin, digitonin and phospholipase A upon the dog's mucosal barrier. Gastroenterology 59: 505–509

Demling L, Classen M 1968 The influence of gastrointestinal hormones on local blood flow and H-ion concentration of the human gastric mucosa. In: Semb L S, Myren J (eds) The physiology of gastric secretion. Williams and Wilkins, Baltimore

Duplessis D J 1965 Pathogenesis of gastric ulceration. Lancet i: 947–978

Duthie H L, Kwong N K, Brown B H, Whittaker G E 1971 Pacesetter potential of the human gastroduodenal junction. Gut 12: 250–256

Edkins J S 1905 On the chemical mechanism of gastric secretion. Proceedings of the Royal Society of London B 76:376

George J D 1968 New clinical method for measuring the rate of gastric emptying: the double sampling test meal. Gut 9: 237–242

Gillespie G, Gillespie I E, Kay A W 1969 Response to insulin of the

intact stomach in patients with duodenal ulcer. Gut 10: 744–748

Gillespie G, Elder J B, Gillespie I E, Kay A W, Campbell E H G 1970a The long term stability of the insulin test. Gastroenterology 58: 625–632

Gillespie G, Elder J B, Gillespie I E, Kay A W, Crean G P 1970b The short term reproducibility of the insulin test in peptic ulcer patients. Gastroenterology 59: 180–187

Gregory R A, Tracy H J 1961 The preparation and properties of gastrin. Journal of Physiology 156: 523–543

Gregory R A, Tracy H J 1964 The constitution and properties of two gastrins extracted from hog antral mucosa. I. The isolation of two gastrins from hog antral mucosa. II. The properties of two gastrins isolated from hog antral mucosa. Gut 5: 103–114

Griffith G H, Owen G M, Campbell H, Shields R 1968 Gastric emptying in health and in gastroduodenal disease. Gastroenterology 54: 1–7

Hertz A F 1911 The sensibility of the alimentary canal in health and disease. Lancet i: 1051–1056, 1119–1124, 1187–1193

Hirschowitz B I 1967 Secretion of pepsinogen. In: Code C F (ed) Handbook of physiology, section 6, volume 2: 889–918 American Physiology Society, Washington

Hoelzel F 1947 The use of non-nutritive materials to satisfy hunger. American Journal of Digestive Diseases 14: 401–404

Hollander F 1951 Insulin-acidity test for determining integrity of vagal influence on the stomach. Methods on Medical Research 4:166

Hunt J N 1957 Inhibition of gastric emptying and secretion in patients with duodenal ulcer. Lancet i: 132–134

Illingworth C F W 1953 Peptic Ulcer. Livingstone, Edinburgh

Jacobson E D, Linford R H, Grossman M I 1966 Gastric secretion in relation to mucosal blood flow studied by a clearance technique. Journal of Clinical Investigation 45: 1–13

Kay A W 1953 Effect of large doses of histamine on gastric secretion of HCl—an augmented histamine test. British Medical Journal ii: 77–80

Kay A W 1967 Memorial lecture: an evaluation of gastric secretion tests. Gastroenterology 53: 834–844

Kennedy F, Mackay C, Bedi B S, Kay A W 1973 Truncal vagotomy and drainage for chronic duodenal ulcer disease: a controlled trial. British Medical Journal ii: 71–75

Kinsella V J 1948 The mechanism of abdominal pain. Australian Medical Publishing Co, Sydney

Komarov S A 1942a Studies on gastrin I. The methods of isolation of a specific gastric secretagogue from the pyloric mucous membrane and its chemical properties. Revue canadienne de biologie I: 191–205

Komarov S A 1942b Studies on gastrin II. Physiological properties of the gastric secretagogue of the pyloric mucous membrane. Revue canadienne de biologie I: 377–401

McGuigan J E, Trudeau W L 1968 Immunochemical measurement of elevated levels of gastrin in the serum of patients with pancreatic tumours of the Zollinger-Ellison variety. New England Journal of Medicine 278: 1308–1313

McGuigan J E, Trudeau W L 1970 Studies with antibodies to gastrin: radioimmunoassay in human serum and physiological studies. Gastroenterology 58: 139–150

Marks I N 1956 The relationship of the acid output to the parietal cell population of the stomach. Scottish Medical Journal 1: 242

Multicentre Pilot Study 1967 Pentagastrin as a stimulant of maximal gastric acid response in man. Lancet i: 291–295

Multicentre Study 1967 The effect of vagotomy on gastric secretion elicited by pentagastrin in man. Lancet ii: 534–539

Multicentre Study 1969 Intramuscular pentagastrin compared with other stimuli as tests of gastric secretion. Lancet i: 341–342

Murray J G 1969 Regeneration of the vagus. In: Williams J A, Cox A G, (eds) After Vagotomy. Butterworth, London

Myhre E 1968 Regeneration of gastric mucosa. In: Semb L S, Myren J (eds) Physiology of Gastric Secretion. Williams and Wilkins, Baltimore

Palmer W L 1926 Mechanism of pain in gastric and duodenal ulcers; achlorhydria. Archives of Internal Medicine 38: 603–611

Pavlov I P 1910 The work of the digestive glands. Griffin, London

Rhodes J 1972 Etiology of gastric ulcer. Gastroenterology 63: 171–182

Taylor T V, Pullan B R, Elder J B, Torrance B 1975 Observations of gastric mucosal blood flow using $^{99}Tc^m$ in rat and man. British Journal of Surgery 62: 788–791

Weber J, Kohatsu S 1970 Pacemaker localization and electrical conduction patterns in the canine stomach. Gastroenterology 59: 717–726

Wilkinson A R, Johnston D 1973 Effect of truncal, selective and highly selective vagotomy on gastric emptying and intestinal transit of food-barium meal in man. Annals of Surgery 178: 190–193

Wolf S, Wolff H G 1947 Human Gastric Function. Oxford University Press, London

Yalow R S, Berson S A 1970 Radioimmunoassay of gastrin. Gastroenterology 58: 1–14

Small intestine

The presence of some functioning small intestine is absolutely essential for life. Whereas reasonably normal health can exist following total removal of either the stomach or the colon, total excision of the small intestine would prove fatal, in view of loss of the all important digestion and absorption of principal foodstuffs, water and electrolytes, and essential substances such as vitamins. In addition, the small intestine elaborates various hormones, and it is the site of production of immune globulins. There are also vital roles for its mucosa to play in the internal economy of both bile salts and vitamin B$_{12}$. The patterns of movement within the muscular wall are responsible for mixing of the intestinal chyme, and its forward propulsion towards the colon.

It is thus a remarkably busy part of the gastrointestinal tract, and disturbances of health can result from removal of segments of the small intestine, or from various diseases which damage these important functions. Of particular surgical interest are the malabsorption syndromes which may follow certain types of gastrointestinal operation, and some of these and other forms of malabsorption are amenable to surgical treatment.

Disorders of motility are common and propulsive movements are temporarily altered by such factors as changes in diet, a wide range of drugs, any irritative process within the abdomen, X-ray and other investigations, nervous influences, etc. It is well known, for example, that intestinal movements are absent following any abdominal laparotomy, although the duration of this 'ileus' may be shorter than previously imagined, even after operations such as vagotomy which divide the extrinsic innervation of the intestine.

The surgeon has a special interest in the disordered physiology which follows acute intestinal obstruction, and this will be discussed separately.

In spite of the very considerable muscular, digestive, absorptive and hormonal activities of this part of the body, and the extremely rapid proliferation and renewal of the small intestine mucosa, it is surprising that many disease processes such as neoplasia so relatively seldom affect the small intestine.

STRUCTURE OF THE SMALL INTESTINE

In the past much discussion has been devoted to the actual length of the small intestine in life. It is generally acknowledged that this is much less than the length which can be measured with the devitalised intestine removed from the body and laid out in a relaxed or stretched fashion along the bench. Various estimates in healthy normal volunteers, using methods such as intubation with tubes or tapes incorporating spaced radio-opaque markers have suggested an approximate length for the small intestine in health of somewhere between 2.5 and 3.5 metres. Disease may alter its length. For example, obstruction or infarction may cause apparent lengthening, due in part to stretching and in part to muscular relaxation. It follows that in these and other conditions estimates of the amount of intestine resected at operation, and more important, of lengths remaining in situ may prove somewhat unreliable.

Mucous membrane

Of much greater physiological importance than the gross overall length of the small intestine is the area of the mucous membrane exposed to the intestinal chyme for the all important actions of digestion and absorption. Simple inspection of the mucous membrane with the naked eye reveals the familiar moist pink smooth glistening appearance, but more detailed examination with the dissecting microscope and electron microscope has revealed a beautiful architecture which results in a very large total surface area being exposed to the luminal content. The first contribution to amplifying area is from the simple mucosal valves (valvulae conniventes), and these are responsible for an approximately three-fold increase in surface area compared to that which would exist if the lining was a simple straight-walled cylinder. Next, projecting from the entire surface of the small intestine are the numerous long finger-like villi ranging in height from 0.2–1.5 mm in length, which increase the surface area by some 20–30 times. Finally, the luminal aspect of each of the columnar epithelial cells covering these villi contains

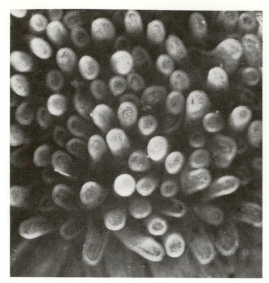

Fig. 17.1 The villi of normal human jejunum photographed through a dissecting microscope. (Courtesy of Professor C C Booth, Postgraduate Medical School, Clinical Research Centre, London.)

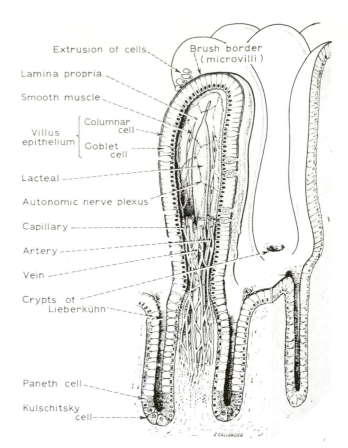

Fig. 17.2 Three-dimensional reconstruction of the intestinal mucous membrane illustrating the structure of a villus and of adjacent crypts of Lieberkühn.

a brush border comprising a further system of microvilli, which in turn increase the total absorptive area by a further 20–40 times. These structural arrangements thus very greatly enhance the capacity of the mucosa of the small intestine to digest and absorb, and in normal health there is thus a considerable reserve of absorptive area.

The majority of villi in healthy Europeans are accurately described as 'finger-like', as illustrated in Figure 17.1. However, some degree of variation from finger shape to more elongated contours, described as 'leaf-like', may occur in otherwise healthy people, and the latter structure is somewhat more frequent in populations of Asia, Africa, Central and Southern America. These population differences should be borne in mind in defining the 'normal' background pattern. Some change in the mucosal architecture from a predominantly leaf-like appearance to finger-like can be seen on moving from one part of the world to another, and a reversion on moving in the opposite direction, which suggests that there is an environmental influence on this particular aspect of structure.

Although the gross appearances indicate a similar overall diameter for the proximal and distal small bowel, the total mucosal surface area is much larger in the duodenum and proximal jejunum than in more distal segments, as a result of the increased density of the folds and villi, so that the mucosal area available for absorption is significantly greater, centimetre for centimetre, at the upper end of the small intestine than at the distal end. This simple physical fact to a large extent accounts for the relatively greater importance of the upper end of the small intestine for normal digestion and absorption.

Examination by the scanning electron microscope reveals further details of the three-dimensional structure

of the villi and the crypts which lie between their bases. The crypts of Lieberkühn, glandular pits, are approximately three in number to each individual villus, and the single layer of columnar epithelium which lines the crypt is continuous with that which covers the surface of the villus (Fig. 17.2). At intervals this single layer of columnar epithelium is interrupted by solitary goblet cells which produce mucus. Connecting the crypts are intervillus ridges which vary in size according to the state of activity and proliferation of the mucosa. The epithelial cells rest on a basement membrane separating them from the connective tissue of the lamina propria which forms the core of the villus, and contains nodules of lymphoid tissue, smooth muscle fibres and blood and lymphatic vessels.

One of the most fascinating features of the small intestine is the life cycle of these columnar epithelial cells, which have been called 'enterocytes' by Booth (1961), on account of their behavioural similarities to other stem cells such as the erythrocytes. The enterocyte is born at the base of an intestinal crypt, it matures as it passes up the wall of the crypt and over the surface of the villus, and dies, being cast off from the tip of the villus into the intestinal lumen. Its life is a mere 3–5 days, and it is thus one of the most rapidly renewed tissues in the body. When one considers the vast number of cells which are shed from the 'zones of extrusion' at the tips of the villi each day, or indeed each hour, this seems basically a somewhat wasteful process. On the other hand, the mucosal cells are extremely industrious throughout their short life, and for proper performance of the intricate series of digestive and absorptive functions, a limited finite life span is probably required. The ill-understood factors which regulate the delicately balanced forces of this very active proliferating tissue, ensuring that production and loss remain constant, must be coordinated in a most precise manner. This is all the more remarkable when one considers the many influences which can be brought to bear on mucosal proliferation, such as various hormones, dietary intake, and other exogenous factors.

It is likely that nourishment of the small bowel mucosa comes both from the blood supply contained in the core of the villus, and also directly from the intestinal lumen. This dual supply of nutrients probably accounts for the relative sparing of the intestinal mucosa from the effects of malnutrition until a fairly advanced stage is reached.

Reference has already been made to the microvillus architecture of the luminal aspect of the mature mucosal cell, and this detail is confined to those cells which cover the villus, being absent from young cells in the crypts of Lieberkühn. This fine brush border (Fig. 17.3), as has been mentioned, greatly increases the total area exposed to the luminal content. It appears that the entire surface of these microvilli is covered with a membrane of three layers, the outer and inner of protein and the centre layer of lipid material. This layer is continuous, spreading from one cell to the next, probably without any interruption or 'pores', and it is attached to the cell surface by a system of fibrils (Fig. 17.4). On the luminal surface of this trilaminar structure is a 'fuzz', a glycoprotein layer containing

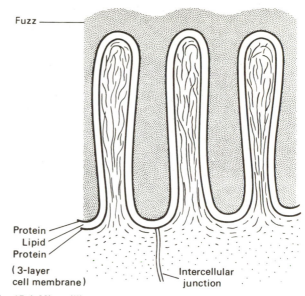

Fig. 17.4 Microvilli.

important enzyme systems such as disaccharidases and dipeptidases, which plays a central role in digestion-absorption. This layer is manufactured within the mucosal cell, travels up through the cell to be extruded at the luminal aspect, and is continually being renewed. Its critical role in digestion-absorption will be discussed later.

A second significant feature of the mucosal cell is also revealed by electron microscopy, and this concerns the relationship between the borders of one cell and its neighbour (Fig. 17.5). Cells are packed closely one to another, and indeed there is fairly firm welding of the 'tight junction' for approximately half of the depth of the cell starting at the mucosal aspect. At this area the cell membranes probably actually fuse together, with a jigsaw configuration. It is not certain whether this tight junction remains permanently in this fixed state, or whether it can open up

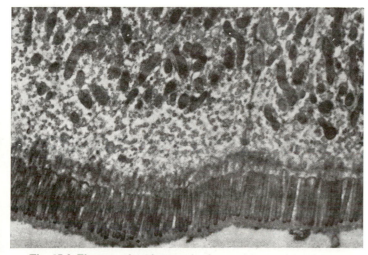

Fig. 17.3 Electron microphotograph of normal human jejunal mucosa, showing apical border of two absorptive cells. Note regularity of length, width and spacing of microvilli. The dark intracellular bodies are mitochondria (Hartman et al 1960 Gastroenterology, 38:506).

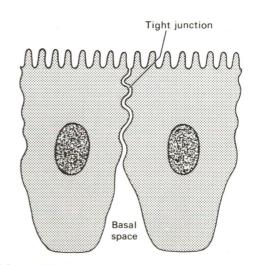

Fig. 17.5 Intercellular junction.

at least partially from time to time. Moving to the more basal aspect of the epithelial cells, the gap between cells is allowed to open up, and the degree of separation increases during the process of absorption.

In addition to the dominant columnar epithelial 'enterocyte', there are three other types of cell interspersed in the mucosal layer.

1. *The goblet cells*, as has already been mentioned, secrete a sulphate-containing mucoprotein. The name of the cell of course reflects its shape on microscopic examination, which also shows the apical part of the cell usually to be distended by secretory material, the precursor of the mucus secretion (Fig. 17.6). Although it has been suggested that intestinal mucus serves to lubricate the passage of the bowel content, this would seem to be unnecessary in the small intestine where the bowel contents are fluid. Goblet cells, of course, occur in a similar situation in the mucosae of other parts of the gastrointestinal tract, where they may have a more important role, but it is not clear as to whether they serve any useful purpose in the small intestine.

2. *Paneth cells*. These occur in small numbers only in the bases of the crypts of Lieberkühn (Fig. 17.7). The histological features strongly suggest a secretory function, the cytoplasm containing easily identified coarse granules, which are glycoprotein material. There is some evidence that they subserve a nutrient function with respect to the neighbouring epithelial cells, but their precise role is as yet uncertain.

3. *Argentaffin cells*. These are also principally located in the crypts of Lieberkühn, and they derive their name from the property displayed by intracellular granules, of reducing ammoniacal silver to metallic silver (see Fig. 17.7). These cells, formerly called Kulchitzky cells, contain 5-hydroxytryptamine (serotonin), and it is likely that this is the tissue which proliferates to excess in carcinoid tumours which produce the carcinoid syndrome. The argentaffin cells may therefore be regarded as endocrine cells, secreting their product directly into the bloodstream. Such cells are distributed throughout the gastrointestinal tract, occurring most frequently in the duodenum and small intestine. They are not particularly concentrated in the ileum.

In the first part of the duodenum, in addition to the normal superficial simple tubular glands present throughout the rest of the small intestine, there are present the deeper tubular glands (Brunner's glands) penetrating deep to the muscularis mucosae, and secreting a mucoid, highly alkaline fluid. Although the material from these Brunner's glands would have the first opportunity to neutralise the acid contents leaving the stomach, and their secretion is stimulated by several hormones of the upper gastrointestinal tract, e.g. secretin, it is likely that they make a relatively small contribution to the overall alkalinisation of the upper small bowel content, when compared to that

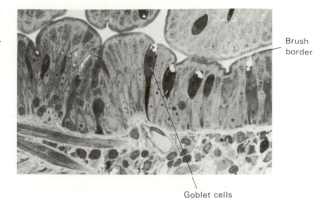

Fig. 17.6 Sagittal section of crypt. (Courtesy of Dr M N Marsh, University of Manchester.)

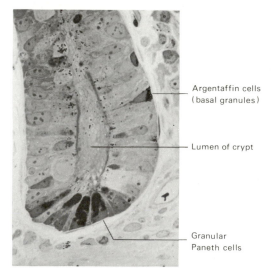

Fig. 17.7 Villous epithelium. (Courtesy of Dr M N Marsh, University of Manchester.)

produced by bile and pancreatic juice. The full physiological role of the Brunner's glands remains uncertain.

In recent years it has become apparent that the epithelial layer of the small intestine mucosa incorporates a liberal sprinkling of specialized actively secreting endocrine cells, some of which have been identified as the source of known hormones of physiological importance. A rapidly increasing number of polypeptides is being extracted from mucosal preparations, and subsequently identified within specific cells, and it remains to be seen how many of these acquire the full status of physiological hormones, and how many prove to be either pharmacological curiosities, or intermediate breakdown products of other hormones. This is certainly a field in which there has been a veritable explosion of knowledge in the past few years. These endocrine cells and their products are discussed in greater detail in a following section.

Underneath the mucosal layer are the many other

important structures concerned with the transport of the products of digestion and absorption, and the integration of these functions and the coordination of motility.

A rich meshwork of capillaries is found closely applied to the basement membrane of the mucosal epithelial layer. There is thus a short distance to travel for the absorbed substances passing through tight junction zones, or extruded into the wider intercellular spaces between the more basal aspects of these cells. Entry of absorbed materials of small molecular size may be facilitated by a number of relatively thin areas, 'fenestrations', on the walls of these sub-mucosal capillaries.

Some absorbed substances, notably products of fat digestion, enter into the lacteals of the lymphatic system, which are more centrally placed in the villi, and the walls of these lacteals are considerably thicker than those of the capillaries. Fenestrations have not been demonstrated in these lymphatic vessels, but somewhat looser junction zones between the endothelial cells comprising the wall may act as pathways for the absorption of chylomicrons and other substances. In addition to this network of lymphatic vessels there are aggregates of lymphoid tissue scattered at intervals throughout the submucosa, with particular concentrations in the terminal ileum.

Also in the fibrous tissue framework supporting this core of vessels and spreading throughout the sub-mucosal layer is a nerve plexus (Meissner's) which is made up of non-myelinated post-ganglionic sympathetic fibres, and para-sympathetic ganglion cells. Enclosing all these structures are the two well-developed layers of smooth muscle fibres, first an inner circular layer, which would be perhaps more correctly described as a gentle spiral rather than truly a transverse encircling one, and secondly an outer longitudinal layer, the fibres of which run more or less in the long axis of the bowel. Between these two muscular layers lies a second nerve plexus (Auerbach's) which contains both unipolar and multipolar ganglion cells, and which is largely responsible for the smooth integration of reflex and other motor responses in the intestine. The outermost coat is the thin but strong layer of visceral peritoneum enveloping the entire circumference apart from the narrow ridge at the mesenteric attachment.

When a surgical anastomosis is made between two pieces of intestine a watertight seal is rapidly achieved by proliferation of this visceral serous coat, but the overall mechanical strength of the union between the two stitched segments depends of course upon the fibrous tissue union derived mainly from the sub-mucosal layers.

THE ENDOCRINE FUNCTION OF THE SMALL INTESTINE

That the mucosa of the small intestine has a widespread endocrine function has only recently attracted attention.

It now appears that this organ may contain the largest mass of endocrine secreting cells in the body. There is perhaps a certain historical justice in this, since the first hormone to be identified by its specific biological actions was secretin (Bayliss & Starling, 1902), and although it took approximately 70 years for the detailed amino acid structure of this hormone to be worked out, and the cells of production confidently identified, the last few years have seen very rapid progress in the isolation of other hormones and polypeptides of less certain status.

Conventional histological techniques do not identify these highly specialised endocrine cells, which on ordinary histological preparation appear indistinguishable from the absorptive mucosal epithelial cells. However, the application of specific immunofluorescence techniques using antibodies raised against the individual hormone or polypeptide material under consideration is capable of picking out these different cell types.

There is a major basic difference in the distribution of these endocrine cells in the small intestine when comparison is made with the other well known endocrine glands. Whereas in the latter the hormone-producing cells are packed together in masses, the endocrine cells of the small intestine mucosa are dispersed widely, often being scattered as single cells at intervals throughout the mucosa. Since many of these hormones are probably primarily concerned with mediating various effects within the gastrointestinal tract itself, this wide dispersion permits distribution of the release and primary actions of these hormones over a considerable length of intestine. It now seems likely that some of the gastrointestinal hormones perform roles other than the traditional endocrine one, i.e. implying the release of the active substance from the cell of origin into the circulation, and the subsequent action on the target tissue at a distant site. Some may have a neurocrine effect, i.e. they may act as neurohumoral transmitter substances. A further role of possible significance is a paracrine effect, i.e. simply acting on cells and tissues immediately adjacent to the hormone-producing cell.

There is some evidence from the work of Pearse et al (1970) that the hormone-producing cells of the small intestine are derived embryologically from the neural crest tissue of the nervous system, the cells travelling to the region of the developing foregut at an early stage, and gradually becoming caught up among the developing mucosal epithelial cells. The principal location of the endocrine cells is within the crypts rather than on the villi, and it is believed that they have a very much more prolonged lifespan than the epithelial cells. Indeed if these are truly of nervous origin one might reasonably expect a failure to regenerate after damage or to hypertrophy in response to increasing physiological demand. It is not known whether changes in the population of such cells are possible during life, although there is increasing evidence that the population of gastrin-producing cells in the pyloric antrum may increase following prolonged physiological stimulation. The application of immunofluorescence reveals that each hormone can be traced to a single specific cell type, and Pearse has hypothesized that all are members of a single family which he has called the 'Apud' ('amine precursor uptake and decarboxylation') series.

The apex of an individual endocrine secreting cell reaches between its neighbouring epithelial cells on either side right up to the lumen; this permits direct contact with the intestinal content, the most important physiological stimulus to such cells being partly digested food materials. In response to stimulation secretory granules form within these cells, and although the direct passage of secreted hormone has not been followed into the sub-mucosal vascular plexus, the base of the cell extends right to the basement membrane, and a secretory pathway from cell to blood vessel is very likely.

Although many biologically-active peptides have been isolated from extracts prepared from mucosa of the small intestine, and although many different cell types have been identified by immunofluorescent techniques, the number of fully substantiated respectable physiological hormones is at present quite small, and the status of a large number of remaining compounds has yet to be substantiated. The precise amino acid sequence contained in at least six peptides is now known, these peptides including gastrin, secretin, the single substance which possesses both cholecystokinin and pancreozymin actions (CCK-PZ), gastric inhibitory peptide (GIP), vasoactive intestinal peptide (VIP), and motilin. Only in the case of the first three, however, can we be absolutely sure that they have a secure role as hormones.

Gastrin

It is known that numerous gastrin-producing cells (G-cells) are distributed in the mucosa of the small intestine especially in the proximal reaches, and these G-cells appear to all intents and purposes identical with those in the main site for gastrin production, the pyloric antrum. The gastrin molecule, mainly released from the small intestine G-cells, is larger, with 34 amino acid components, than that predominantly released by the antral G-cells, which is a 17-amino acid molecule. Both, however, contain the all-important active C-terminal tetrapeptide sequence. It is doubtful whether the mechanisms responsible for the regulation of gastrin release from these intestinal G-cells are the same as obtain in the stomach, but at least the extragastric production of gastrin from such cells might explain among other things the failure of circulating gastrin levels to full to zero after total gastrectomy.

Secretin

It has been known for years that the primary action of this hormone is the stimulation of exocrine pancreatic secretion particularly rich in bicarbonate content. It is not surprising, therefore, that the principal stimulation to secretin release is the presence of acid in the small intestine. Secretin cells are most abundant in the duodenum and proximal jejunum, but they are distributed widely along the remainder of the small intestine. Secretin also stimulates the Brunner's glands to secrete their alkaline product, increases the output of bile secretion and under certain circumstances may inhibit gastric acid secretion. The net result of these various effects is a combined effort to alkalinise the content of the upper gastrointestinal tract after the reduction of pH in the stomach. Further actions of secretin, which can be demonstrated in the experimental laboratory but may not be of such physiological importance, are the stimulation of pepsin secretion and of insulin production.

Cholecystokinin-pancreozymin

It is now known that a single polypeptide structure contains both of these important biological actions, but since the cholecystokinin action was attributed to hormonal action at an earlier date than the stimulation of pancreatic secretion the term cholecystokinin would seem to deserve precedence. Apart from triggering contraction of the gallbladder the other primary action of this material is the stimulation of exocrine pancreatic secretion with a high content of the digestive enzymes. Of interest is the observation that the C-terminal tetrapeptide sequence of CCK is identical with that of gastrin, and this structural similarity suggests that both may have been derived from the same basic family, involving similar production processes.

'Candidate' hormones of the gut

The following is a list of other potent peptides which have either been isolated in relatively pure form from extracts of the mucosa of the small intestine, or which have been identified in specific cells in the intestine. Although many of these have been shown to have potent biological actions, and several are clearly important in pathological states, there is still uncertainty as to whether they possess significant physiological roles.

Gastric inhibitory polypeptide (GIP) has certain structural similarities to both glucagon and secretin. As its name suggests, it is a potent inhibitor of gastric acid secretion, but it also to some extent inhibits gastric motility, increases the secretion from the small intestine, and facilitates the release of insulin.

Motilin. This material, of a structure markedly different from all the other known gastrointestinal hormones, is released into the circulation by the experimental infusion of acid, fat or other substances into the duodenum, and it stimulates an increase in gastric motility. It does not, however, appear to be increased significantly following a normal meal.

Pancreatic polypeptide. Although this material is most abundant in the pancreas itself, some is also identified in the proximal small intestine, and under experimental conditions it displays a wide range of actions on the gastrointestinal tract.

Somatostatin. This hormone which inhibits the release of growth hormone, was first thought to be confined to the brain, but has now been shown to be even more abundant in the intestine, mainly the proximal segments of the small gut. In general, its actions are inhibitory to gastric secretion, gastric emptying, and pancreatic secretion, and it appears to suppress the release of several of the other gastrointestinal hormones.

Bombesin. This fascinating peptide, named after the species of frog in whose skin it was first identified, has now been shown to be present in cells scattered throughout the intestine, with once again the greatest preponderance being in the proximal small bowel. It may facilitate gastrin release in the stomach, and possibly the release of other gastrointestinal hormones, and it may also affect smooth muscle and blood vessel action.

Enteroglucagon. The glucagon material extracted from the small intestine is a larger molecule than the pancreatic hormone, but contains all of the latter's structure within it. Unlike the other gastrointestinal hormones considered so far, it appears that the distribution of enteroglucagon is greatest in the more distal segments of the small intestine. Although it may have several effects on gastrointestinal function, possibly its principal one is to diminish motility and slow transit through the upper portions of the digestive tract.

Substance P. This substance was identified almost 50 years ago, but its structure was discovered only recently. Although present in the gut it is a fairly ubiquitous substance, and in the central nervous system probably acts as a neurohumoral transmitter. It may also have a neurocrine effect in the gastrointestinal tract, and among its actions are stimulation of intestinal motility, suppression of insulin response, and vasodilator changes in various tissues.

Endorphins. These morphine-like substances may also have a predominantly neurocrine action in the gastrointestinal tract as they do in other parts of the body.

Other possible candidates

An inhibitor of gastric acid secretion prepared from extracts of only the most proximal segment of the first part of the duodenum, the duodenal 'bulb', has been given the tentative name of 'bulbogastrone'.

There may also be a specific stimulation of pancreatic exocrine secretion by the action of a peptide released from the distal small bowel, 'pancreatone'.

Even more specific in its action on the pancreas is the postulated 'chymodenin'. This is perhaps the first example of such precise specificity, the substance selectively stimulating chymotrypsin from among the various digestive enzymes of the pancreas. It will be interesting to see whether the further searches being made in the small intestine reveal other examples of enzyme specific effects.

Many years ago it was postulated that the pumping action in the villi of the small intestine could be stimulated by hormonal mechanisms, and relatively pure preparations of a small peptide with such a 'villikinin' action have been reported.

The term enterogastrone was proposed many years ago for the humoral agent released by fat coming in contact with the mucosa of the upper small intestine and which in turn produced inhibition of gastric acid secretion. As time has gone on it has become apparent that not only fat but many other substances in contact with small intestine mucosa brings about a humorally mediated inhibition of the stomach, and therefore the term enterogastrone has tended to refer somewhat loosely to any humoral inhibition of the stomach arising from the small intestine. Perhaps, however, the term should be more specifically reserved for just that inhibition arising from contact with fat. As has already been mentioned, several of the hormones and pure polypeptides extracted from the mucosa of the upper small intestine have been shown to be potent inhibitors of gastric acid secretion, such as secretin, cholecystokinin, GIP and VIP, and whether one or more of these substances might act as an enterogastrone is still uncertain. It is probable, however, that over and above any such action in these substances there is an as yet unidentified additional enterogastrone.

This list of interesting peptides arising from or acting on the intestine goes on at present in an apparently almost endless fashion. Some remain quite enigmatic at the present time, such as 'substance P', and the powerful inhibitor of gastric acid secretion, urogastrone. Although this latter material can now be extracted in pure form from urine, it is not known what tissue is responsible for its manufacture, and there is a hint that this might be located primarily in the salivary glands and in the Brunner's glands in the proximal duodenum.

Probably the principal release of these various hormones of the gastrointestinal tract results from direct contact between various luminal contents and the intestinal mucosa. For example, the products of partial digestion of protein are probably the main stimuli for the release of gastrin and CCK, fat products are the most potent stimuli of the release of CCK and GIP, and carbohydrate products are powerful in the stimulation of glucagon. Acid from the stomach is probably the chief stimulant of secretin release, and bicarbonate of hepatic and pancreatic origin may be the primary stimulants of the release of motilin. In addition, however, nervous activity, principally mediated by the vagus, may initiate or facilitate the release of several of these hormones. The relative significance of the different modes of stimulation remains to be worked out.

Many of the hormones studied to date have been shown to occur in more than one molecular form, the differences between these molecules often being quite small, limited to minor variations in amino acid composition. Each hormone or polypeptide has also been shown to have a wide range of biological actions in the experimental laboratory. Although each has a clearly defined primary action, the range of other effects is often surprisingly wide, and the possibility exists of using some of these actions in a therapeutic manner. One of the interesting secondary effects, of possible physiological and pathological importance, is a trophic action, such as is seen with gastrin in regard to the epithelium of the stomach and the pancreas. Other trophic actions may well come to light.

Interest in the hormones elaborated by the upper gastrointestinal tract also extends to the rare endocrine tumours arising from the appropriate hormone-producing cells. Syndromes analogous to the Zollinger-Ellison syndrome are likely to be encountered by further close search. Already tumours have been identified which are rich in VIP or GIP, both of these presenting clinically as severe and persistent diarrhoea resulting from the over-stimulation of fluid and electrolyte secretion in the small intestine itself. Almost certainly other functioning tumours will come to light with further investigation.

Serotonin

In addition to the numerous polypeptides isolated from the mucosa of the small intestine it has been known for some time that several amines are elaborated in this organ, and serotonin (5-hydroxytryptamine) is perhaps one of the best known. The gastrointestinal mucosa is particularly rich in this substance, although it is widely distributed in many other tissues.

It is not yet certain whether serotonin has a physiological role, but it may well play a part in the mediation of the stimulation of gastrointestinal motility, and influence blood supply to the organ. Interest in serotonin has arisen mainly as a result of its role in the carcinoid syndrome, caused by the release of large quantities of serotonin from argentaffin tumours located mainly in the ileum. Usually the syndrome requires the presence of metastatic deposits in the liver, from which large amounts of the amine are released directly into the systemic circulation through the hepatic veins. Normally the liver itself is responsible for a considerable amount of inactivation of serotonin, and thus deposits of the secreting tumour in the gut itself, draining into the portal vein, would permit a substantial reduction in the amounts of free circulating serotonin in

the systemic circulation, and therefore no obvious systemic clinical feature.

The syndrome is characterized by episodes of cutaneous flushing, alternating with a reddish-blue cyanosis, asthma-like attacks, diarrhoea, and occasional giddiness. In due course valvular lesions of the heart, mainly affecting the pulmonary valve area, may develop.

If clinical suspicion of the syndrome arises the diagnosis can usually be confirmed by the demonstration of grossly elevated levels of urinary 5-hydroxy indoleacetic acid (the inactive excretory product of serotonin).

IMMUNE RESPONSES IN THE SMALL INTESTINE

It is not surprising that the intestine has an extensive role in immunity, since it is presented with large quantities of foreign protein materials swallowed by the individual. It also makes sense for the main concentration of the immune system to be located in that segment of the alimentary tract at which absorption, i.e. entry into the body occurs. The intestine is involved with both cellular and humoral immune responses.

There are prominent collections of lymphoid cellular tissue in the subepithelial layers of the ileum, the so-called Peyer's patches, and closer examination of the remainder of the small bowel shows that there are smaller localized lymph follicles scattered throughout the entire length. Both the T-cells (thymus-dependent) mainly concerned with delayed hypersensitivity, and B-cells (bone marrow) responsible for the production of immunoglobulins, are present in these patches and in addition, large numbers of individual lymphocytes and plasma cells are located predominantly in the lamina propria. These are immunologically competent cells which are absent from the fetus or the germ-free experimental animal, but which start to appear rapidly after the first exposure of the newborn to oral feeding. The evidence is strong, therefore, that these arise directly as a consequence of the introduction of foreign protein to the intestinal wall. It is not certain whether these immunologically-competent cells migrate along with the continuously moving epithelial cells, but some small lymphocytes can be found lying in the spaces between neighbouring mucosal cells, and some migration of both types is probable (Fig. 17.8).

There is considerable production of humoral antibodies, and indeed the small intestine is one of the principal sources of immunoglobulins (Ig), all five known classes being produced (IgA, IgM, IgG, IgP and IgE). The production of IgA greatly predominates over all the others, and most of this immunoglobulin is secreted directly into the gut lumen, attached to a glycoprotein called the 'secretory piece' or 'component', only a small proportion of the IgA finding its way into the plasma. Possibly this material

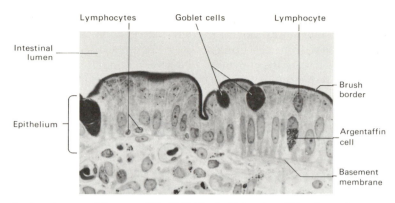

Fig. 17.8 Villous epithelium showing lymphocytes. (Courtesy of Dr M N Marsh, University of Manchester.)

reaches the plasma by being excreted first into the intestinal lumen and subsequently reabsorbed through the absorptive mucosa. This component complex appears to be relatively resistant to the normal proteolytic activity of the intestine.

It seems likely that the most potent stimulus to the further production of IgA by plasma cells in the intestinal wall is the direct presence of a foreign protein, e.g. a bacterial or viral organism, so that the maximal production of the IgA occurs locally in the region of that encounter. Each IgA-secretory piece unit contains four antigen-combining sites. It is therefore a good agglutinating antibody capable of blocking the adherence of bacteria and inhibiting their growth, of inactivating toxins and viruses, of blocking the absorption of proteins and therefore diminishing the opportunity of systemic immunization to food proteins. The role of the IgA secretion is thus seen more as a blocker than as a lytic agent, although some lysis may occur when IgA is in the presence of complement and lysosome. This therefore provides a briskly responsive, locally concentrated, efficient means of attacking a potentially harmful process right at its attempted site of entry into the body.

If there is a major deficiency of IgA, as occurs rarely, another immunoglobulin such as IgM may to some extent substitute in this role of production of anti-bacterial antibodies.

BACTERIAL CONTENT OF THE SMALL INTESTINE

There is interest in the bacterial population of the alimentary tract for several reasons. Firstly, some of the bacteria can be put to good use, e.g. the synthesis of important nutriments such as vitamin K. Secondly, certain bacteria can impair the absorption of fat and perhaps protein, and when they proliferate they may cause symptoms of diarrhoea and/or malabsorption. Thirdly, many of the common gastrointestinal operations may upset the normal pattern of the bacterial population, and this in turn may be responsible for some of the unwanted sequelae.

Normally considerable numbers of organisms are ingested from the air and with food. Perhaps one of the most useful roles of gastric acid is the elimination of a large proportion of these bacteria. So effective is this 'sterilising' effect, that very few organisms can be isolated from samples aspirated from the proximal small intestine. However, as one passes distally the bacterial counts steadily increase, the principal organisms being aerobic ones such as staphylococci, streptococci and lactobacilli. The colon normally has an abundant population of both aerobic and anaerobic organisms such as bacteroides, coliforms and *Streptococcus faecalis*. Some of these organisms, plus increasing amounts of the aerobes normally found in the proximal small intestine, are encountered in the terminal ileum, which in normal health is the only part of the small intestine to have a large bacterial population. After each meal there is a slight proximal extension of the bacterial population from the distal small bowel, but this soon subsides in the hour or so after the meal. Apart from this minor regular fluctuation, the overall pattern of bacterial population along the gastrointestinal tract is kept remarkably constant in normal health. Probably the principal factor keeping the bacteria predominantly at the distal end of the small intestine is the brisk rate of transit of the content which does not allow sufficient time for significant numbers of the organisms to become established. There are, of course, other anti-bacterial factors such as the immune system already discussed, the intraluminal pH changes, the presence of bile, and possibly enzymes, e.g. lysosomes.

Some organisms, particularly anaerobic bacteria, are capable of deconjugating bile salts, thus reducing the effective concentration of these materials and as a consequence interfering with fat absorption. There may also be some interference with amino acid absorption as a result of the presence of these abnormal deconjugates. Furthermore, some dietary proteins may be directly affected by certain coliform bacteria, and a clinical test for the amount of such protein degradation involves the measurement of the output of indoles or the end-product indican in the urine. Since this substance is normally absent from the urine a measurement of indican concentration can thus give an estimate of the population of protein-degrading bacteria. An indirect assessment of the amount of deconjugation of bile salts can be made by measuring ^{14}C carbon dioxide in the expired air, following labelling of the bile salt pool with this isotope.

Direct estimation of the bacterial population of the small intestine has been attempted more frequently in recent years in view of the interest in bacteriology in both surgical and other types of malabsorption syndrome. However, a word of caution should be expressed on placing too much reliance on sampling by intubation of the intestine, since it is possible that a large proportion of the organisms may reside mainly in the mucous layer attached loosely to the mucosa. Sampling from the centre of the bowel lumen may therefore underestimate the total bacterial population.

Disorders in which alterations to the normal pattern of bacterial activity in the gut may have relevance include diverticular disease, 'blind loops', fistulae, and the chronic granulomatous diseases such as Crohn's disease. In each of these, surgical correction of the defect or excision of diseased bowel may correct the malabsorption abnormality resulting from the abnormal bacterial proliferation. The diarrhoea and impaired absorption which may follow various gastric operations which substantially reduce gastric acid secretion may also have a bacterial component, and several studies suggest that significant alterations in the gut bacteria may follow these operations.

It is also known that bacteria may take up vitamin B_{12} within the lumen of the gut, and an increase in such activity may deny the body an adequate supply of this vital haematinic. Megaloblastic anaemia and the other sequelae of vitamin B_{12} deficiency may therefore also complicate the clinical picture due to abnormal bacterial proliferation in the small intestine.

SECRETIONS OF THE SMALL INTESTINE

The greater part of the fluid small bowel chyme arises from ingested material, secretions such as saliva, gastric juice, bile and pancreatic juice, but for years there has been debate as to how much actual secretion from the mucosa of the small intestine contributes to the total volume of this chyme.

Formerly it was thought that this was a large volume of secretion, and the term 'succus entericus' was used to describe it. It is understandable why it was given such prominence in earlier days when the concept of digestion was that enzymes were actually exuded from the lining of the intestine in a liquid phase, the major steps of breakdown of the principal dietary components taking place within the chyme in the lumen, and absorption proceeding only after complete breakdown into individual amino acids, simple sugars and monoglycerides. This view, however, is no longer tenable and it is now clear that enzymatic breakdown and entry into the cells of the intestine take place in a highly co-ordinated fashion at the mucosal aspect of the epithelial cells, chiefly within the fuzzy layer and brush border. It is true that digestive enzyme activity can be demonstrated in samples aspirated from the lumen, but almost certainly these enzymes are simply discarded along with the continuously exfoliated cells from the villi, and they should be regarded as waste material rather than of physiological importance in relation to digestion-absorption. A proportion of this discarded material undergoes normal processes of digestion-absorption, so that much of it is recycled.

With developments in our understanding of digestion within the small bowel interest in the 'succus entericus' as a distinct secretory process waned, and indeed it was disregarded in several physiological texts. However, it does seem clear that in normal health there is a small, fairly constant output of true intestinal secretion throughout the 24 hours, and in certain diseases characterized by massive watery diarrhoea, this secretion may increase to a very large extent. Indeed much of our knowledge of the mechanisms of this secretion is based on the lessons learned in the study of patients with cholera, in which massive outpourings of fluid from the small intestine arise without gross damage to the mucosal cells in the intestine. It seems clear that there is an active secretion through the intact mucosa, although whether this passes directly through the cells or along the junctions between them is not as yet clear. The process is not simply ultrafiltration, and is not just the result of marked diminution in absorptive capacity. It is likely that the bulk of the secretion arises from cells within the crypts rather than on the villi. Both in health and disease affecting the small intestine the tonicity of the fluid remains remarkably constant, and it is almost invariably kept at a neutral pH.

Thus with both absorption and secretion taking place across the mucosa of the small intestine, there is a constant two-way exchange of water and electrolytes, and at any one time the content of the small bowel is the net result of various factors influencing this exchange. There is no evidence of either a nervous or hormonal phase of stimulation of true intestinal secretion. Local irritation of the mucosa does result in an increase in the total volume of intestinal juice, and both the volume and enzyme content are increased in the presence of distal obstruction.

MOTILITY OF THE SMALL INTESTINE

Confusion has reigned in this field for some time, mainly on account of difficulty in correlating observations obtaining by a wide range of different methods. These measurements include changes in electrical potential across the bowel wall, alterations in the gross configuration of bowel content by contrast radiography, estimation of the speed of transit of specific markers along the intestinal lumen, direct observation through endoscopes, and recordings of pressure by a variety of techniques including balloons of different sizes, open-ended tubes, telemetering capsules, etc. However, some progress in our understanding of these complex patterns is emerging, and it seems there is a purposeful dependence between changes in electrical activity and useful muscular action.

Electrical activity

There is an ever-present, inherent slow wave electrical rhythm in the musculature of the entire gastrointestinal tract, and whereas the basic rate of these slow waves in the stomach is approximately three cycles per minute, the rhythm throughout the small intestine is at a more rapid rate. In the duodenum a frequency of twelve cycles per minute is noted, and the wave is propagated distally in a co-ordinated manner at a rate of between 10–20 cm/s. However, as the waves pass distally they diminish both in frequency and in speed of conduction, until in the ileum they may be only 7–8 per minute, and travel at a speed of 0.5–1.0 cm/s. There is thus a very distinct gradient of activity along the course of the intestine. This gradient is probably an important factor in the correct onward transmission of muscle activity, and as a consequence the smooth co-ordination of distal propulsive movements of the intestinal content.

When observable muscle contraction takes place there are superimposed on this basic pattern of electrical rhythm bursts of increased spike discharges, and there appears to be a rough parallel between the frequency and volume of such bursts of activity on the one hand, and the force of muscular contraction on the other. It seems, therefore, that there is a causal link between the increased electrical activity and contraction.

Accepting these basic observations the following further questions arise. First, how does this basic slow wave electrical activity arise? Second, how is it spread from one muscle cell to the next? Third, what is the mechanism underlying the constant distal propagation of this slow wave activity? Fourth, how do factors which alter muscular contraction initiate bursts of high frequency action potentials?

The basic slow wave activity is likely to arise predominantly from inherent cyclical metabolic activity within muscle cells, producing in turn different ionic concentrations both inside the cell and in the neighbouring extracellular fluid. In common with all cells of the body with an active sodium pump there is at rest an electrical gradient across the cell membrane, of approximately 50 mV. This reflects the high concentration of sodium ions in the surrounding extracellular fluid, and the relatively smaller concentration of potassium ions within the cell. However, this membrane potential does not remain static, and during activity of the cell, which appears to occur rhythmically, some influx of sodium ions in return for a somewhat slower leakage of potassium in the opposite direction may occur. The net result of these ion fluxes may bring about temporary alterations in the electrical potential across the cell membrane, the ionic balance being restored as the cell again returns to the resting state. These changes in electrical potential can be detected by suitably sensitive electrodes placed either in the muscle tissue, or simply by the electrodes being closely applied to the mucosal surface.

In the normal, intact small intestine there is an area in the second part of the duodenum near to the opening of the common bile duct which serves as a pacemaker, and it is from this point that the slow waves of the frequency 10–12/min and speed of 10–20 cm/s arise. It has to be admitted that a specific type of tissue comparable to that found in the cardiac muscle has not been identified. Nonetheless, there is sound evidence for the existence of such a pacemaker.

The second question relates to the mechanism by which this basic slow wave electrical activity is propagated from one cell to another. Electron microscopy has identified various points of direct contact or short gap junctions between adjacent smooth muscle cells, occupying approximately 5–10% of the surface area of the cells, and it is likely that these sites represent areas of relatively low electrical resistance across which the electrical slow wave activity would readily pass. The muscle coat, however, does not comprise a true syncytium as in the case of cardiac muscle.

Third is the somewhat more complicated matter of how the electrical activity is regularly and smoothly propagated in a caudad direction. Two hypotheses have been advanced to account for this property. Firstly, some structure running longitudinally in the bowel wall may act as a polarizing 'cable'. Secondly, the passage of slow wave electrical activity from one segment of the intestine to the next might function like a chain of linked relaxation oscillators. It has already been noted that the basic slow wave rhythm of the duodenum is more rapid than that of the ileum, and there appears to be a graded decline in this frequency as one moves distally. Clearly, the more proximal cells will reach peak electrical activity sooner than the more distal ones, and overflow of this activity added to the spontaneous build up in the next distal segment will bring about the discharge within this latter segment at a faster rate than would have occurred if it depended solely upon its own build up of activity. In turn this accelerated rate of discharge would affect the next most distal segment and so on. The overall result of such a mechanism would be the smooth passage of activity only from the segments with higher intrinsic frequencies than the neighbouring segments, and therefore a distally propagated wave. Support for such a mechanism arises from the simple observation that when the small bowel is divided and therefore separated from the influence of the proximal segments, a slower basic slow rhythm is noted than when the intestine is intact. In the normal healthy intestine the linkage hypothesized would explain how activity in the proximal segments can raise the frequency of the more distal slower ones. It is, of course, possible that both the 'cable' mechanism and that of the chain of 'relaxation oscillators' may act in a combined fashion.

The fourth question concerns the possible mechanism by which the bursts of spike potentials associated with gross muscular contraction are initiated. It is known that the local action of acetylcholine and of histamine, both of which increase the depolarization of the cell membrane, result in the appearance of both increased electrical discharges and muscular contraction. It is likely that one or more such humoral agents are involved in the mediation of stimulation to muscular and electrical activity arising from nerve stimulation, local distension, mechanical or chemical stimulation. In addition, acetylcholine may well be important in diffusing the spread of changes in electrical activity from cell to cell along a limited distance.

Although a distinct link in time between these increases in electrical activity and actual muscular contraction has been demonstrated, it is likely that the increase in tension within the contracting muscle cell is related more to the changes in ionic composition which necessarily accompany these electrical events, and it is likely that ionic calcium plays a significant role in this particular property.

Thus in summary, there is always a basic electrical rhythm of slow activity passing distally along the small intestine, having originated from the proximal pacemaker area. The regular distal propagation of this activity may depend on either a 'cable' action of some longitudinal structure in the bowel, or a chain of linked relaxation oscillators. When muscular contraction arises, this is associated with a greatly increased burst of electrical activity superimposed on the background of basic slow wave activity. Although humoral substances such as acetylcholine, histamine and others perhaps liberated in response to local distension or reflex action, can cause increased depolarization of the cell membrane and therefore trigger off bursts of increased potentials, it is not certain whether the increased activity and contraction invariably originate in this fashion. There may well be other initiating factors for these events.

Gross types of contraction

When the cellular events described in the previous paragraphs are translated into gross movements which may be observed with the unaided eye at operation, or during X-ray screening with contrast medium, it is found that the distal propagation of the contraction of a segment of intestine is usually only along a very short distance. By far and away the most frequent type of contraction witnessed is rhythmic segmentation.

Rhythmic segmentation

By this is meant the appearance of two well-defined contraction zones separated by a few centimetres. As a result there is the partial isolation of the segment of intestine between these two contraction rings. Within a few seconds the original contraction rings relax, to be superseded by a further pair of contraction rings situated in the immediately adjoining area. After a further few seconds these secondary contraction rings in turn disappear, to be replaced by either the original ones, or other ones in the adjoining segment. Clearly the prime purpose of such movements is to aid mixing of the intestinal content, and in addition absorption is probably facilitated by the resulting repeated dispersal of the fluid material over the intestinal villi. Furthermore such movements within the intestinal wall may provide a motive force for propelling fluid which has been absorbed into the lymphatic lacteals.

Although the most obvious purpose of these segmental contractions would appear to be to aid mixing and absorption, they probably also contribute to some extent to the forward propulsion of the gut content. It has been observed that the frequency of segmental contractions is greater in the proximal than in the distal small bowel. On occasions episodes of localised segmentation can be seen to pass distally for short distances. A certain amount of 'tonic' increase in intraluminal pressure may result from such contractions, and the greater frequency proximally may thus contribute to a pressure gradient also favouring distal propulsion.

Thus the gradient in basic electrical activity, and differences in frequency, speed and force of contraction passing from proximal to distal reaches of the intestine are probably the main factors ensuring the orderly distal propulsion of the content, rather than any specific pattern of individual contractions.

Peristalsis

This type of movement, which seems beautifully designed and coordinated to achieve distal propulsion, was formerly thought to be the main mechanism by which the small intestine propelled its content in a distal direction. However, true peristalsis is but rarely seen in the small intestine, and when it does occur usually travels over a relatively short distance. Thus its contribution to the normal physiological propulsion in the intestine is probably quite small.

A peristaltic wave has been described as a circumferential contraction proximal to a bolus within the lumen, accompanied by a segment of widening or relaxation distal to this bolus. The bolus is therefore squeezed forward into the distal relaxed segment, and the propagation of this whole pattern in a smooth coordinated manner distally will, of course, carry the bowel content distally.

Although the distal segment of 'relaxation' has been regarded as an important component of the true peristaltic complex, there is a little uncertainty as to whether the dilatation is truly relaxation. An alternative simple explanation is that it merely represents distension by the bowel content distal to the principal segment of contraction.

When peristalsis does occur in the intestine it appears always to be propagated in a caudal direction, and so strongly developed is this property (called the polarity), that when a small segment of intestine is reversed surgically, at least for a while the direction of the peristalsis continues as it was originally, i.e. now against the stream. Truly reversed peristalsis may occur, particularly in the duodenum as a result of nausea and vomiting, but apart from these conditions it appears to be exceptionally rare in health.

Mass contraction

It is doubtful if this type of movement occurs in the small intestine, although it is more important in the colon. These are powerful waves of contraction passing distally over long segments of the intestine, emptying the bowel into the most distal segments.

Nervous and humoral control

Contraction in the small intestine can be influenced by extrinsic innervation, and is to a large extent coordinated by local reflex activity.

The afferent side of the short reflex arcs, triggered off by stretching the mucosal aspect of the intestine, and possibly by direct physical contact between luminal content and mucosa, lie mainly in the basal layer of the mucosal epithelium. The sensory fibres from these receptors travel to cells located in the submucous plexus of Meissner, which contains a large number of both unipolar and bipolar neurones. Their axons in turn connect with multipolar ganglion cells situated in the myenteric plexus of Auerbach. The submucous plexus appears therefore to be mainly sensory, while the myenteric plexus contains mainly the motor neurones innervating the muscle. Such reflex action depends on the integrity of the mucosa, and if this latter is removed, or if a local anaesthetic is applied to it, the reflex is abolished. Humoral transmitter substances such as 5-hydroxytryptamine may play a role in this reflex activity, and certainly increased quantities of this substance stimulate exaggerated contractions including peristalsis.

Extrinsic innervation comes to the small intestine from both parasympathetic and sympathetic sources. Experimentally, increased vagal excitation causes an increase in motor activity in the small intestine, almost certainly acting via the release of acetylcholine in increasing amounts within the wall of the small intestine. However, a pattern of intestinal motility and contraction indistinguishable from normal is seen after total division of the vagal trunks. Although there may be a few days of transient diminution, and disorder of both the electrical and motility pattern after this operation, within about 10 days both patterns are back to normal. The extrinsic vagal innervation, therefore, is not essential for normal motility.

Likewise, sympathectomy has no more than a transient effect on intestinal movements, and normal segmentation and peristalsis can occur in segments of small intestine which have been completely separated from all extrinsic innervation.

Thus while extrinsic autonomic nerve activity may to some extent influence the motility pattern, these are not essential to the normal contractile activity.

Direct damage of the small bowel wall, for example by infection, may bring transport within that segment to a complete standstill, probably as a result of damage to the intrinsic local reflex arcs. A neat illustration of this occurrence in former clinical practice occurred with earlier patterns of ileostomy. Although the advantages of creating a spout ileostomy were early recognized, initially it was felt adequate simply to allow 5 centimetres or so of ileum to protrude from the abdominal wall as a spout, without any additional attempt to cover over the seromuscular coats. However, these outer coats rapidly became infected, and as a result a mechanical obstruction of the small bowel proximal to the ileostomy spout arose (Fig. 17.9). It is now appreciated that this dangerous complication can be avoided by preventing infection of the protruding segment simply by folding over the protruding mucosa and suturing this carefully to the edge of the skin incision through which the ileostomy passes.

In addition to the short intramural reflexes there are one or two well-established distal reflex actions, and at present it is not absolutely certain whether these are mediated entirely by nerves, or whether certain hormones play a part in them. Perhaps the best known is the so-called gastro-colic reflex, which acts on the colon in response to the ingestion of a meal, the afferent impulses supposedly arising within the stomach. However, it is just as likely that the area from which most afferent impulses arise is the proximal small intestine. Again, there is an intestino-intestinal reflex by which mechanical distension of a segment of the small intestine may inhibit contractions in more distal segments. Such reflex action may come into play in the presence of an intestinal obstruction. A third long reflex arises from the rectum, distension of which may bring about increased contractile activity of the ileum. As

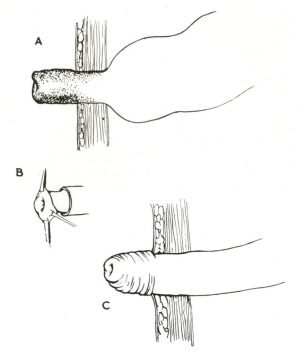

Fig. 17.9 Prevention of intestinal obstruction after ileostomy: in A, the peritoneum of the protruding segment of ileum has been left exposed, and inflammation has led to paralysis and obstruction. In B and C, a cuff of muscle has been removed to allow the mucosa to be sutured to the skin, thus avoiding inflammation and obstruction.

a result there may be an increased rate of emptying of the terminal small bowel into the caecum and ascending colon at the time of defaecation.

RATE OF INTESTINAL TRANSIT

The overall rate of passage of ingested material through the entire gastrointestinal tract can be estimated by adding to the food markers such as insoluble dyes, minute identifiable radio-opaque particles, inert synthetic substances such as polyethylene glycol, or radio-isotopes, and noting either the pattern of distribution at intervals, or the time when the appropriate materials are passed in the faeces. In health, the average time for complete transit is approximately 24 hours, with some degree of individual variation. Of course, many methods do not give an accurate estimate of how much time is spent in the different reaches of the gastrointestinal tract, and passage through the proximal segments might be relatively rapid, with a prolonged period of time being spent in the large bowel. Estimates of the time of transit just through the small intestine have been made by barium meal examinations and the passage of radio-opaque markers, and from such observations it seems likely that an average transit time from duodenum to caecum is in the region of 8 hours. Resection of a segment of intestine results in more rapid transit through

the remaining portion, and since it has been shown that there is more powerful and more frequent contractile activity proximally than distally, it follows that resection of ileum leads to more rapid transit through the residual small intestine than does resection of jejunum. The rate of passage through the entire alimentary tract can be modified by various therapeutic regimes. For example, the use of high residue diets will normally speed up total transit whereas low residue diets will have the opposite effect. However, such dietary factors chiefly affect transit through the colon rather than through the small intestine. Failure of fat digestion-absorption, as occurs in steatorrhea, increases the bulk of the intestinal content, and as a result there may be both an increase in rate of transit and overt diarrhoea.

The diarrhoea which results from a gastrocolic fistula must be noted here, for it is now known to depend upon rapid transit through the small intestine. Most gastrocolic fistulae are quite narrow tracks which allow traffic only from the colon to the stomach. Barium or dyes administered rectally can readily be shown to enter the stomach, but it is the exception to find that barium given by mouth enters the colon by the fistula. This observation suggests that the mechanism of the diarrhoea is the return of faeces to the stomach and small intestine, where the products of putrefaction act as irritants. This furthermore permits colonization of the upper small bowel which in turn may lead to steatorrhoea as a result of alteration in bile salt metabolism. The establishment of a colostomy proximal to the site of the fistula prevents faeces returning to the stomach, and rapidly brings the diarrhoea under control.

INFLUENCE OF DRUGS ON INTESTINAL MOTILITY

Drugs inhibiting motility

As might be expected, sympathomimetic drugs have a generally inhibitory effect on the smooth muscle of the small intestine. This can be demonstrated experimentally by bathing an excised segment of small intestine in warm Ringer's solution to which is added adrenaline in low concentration. This brings about immediate and prolonged relaxation. In the living animal, however, the inactivation of adrenaline by amine oxidases is rapid, so that the inhibitory effect of adrenaline in the intact animal is quite transient. In man, the effect of sympathetic amines is believed to be biphasic, with a short period of relaxation followed by a rebound phase of increased activity. Ephedrine, which retards the destruction of adrenaline, has no constant effect on motility.

Atropine and belladonna alkaloids reduce the propulsive motility of the small intestine and diminish all forms of intestinal movement in the terminal ileum. Propantheline and quaternary ammonium compounds also produce a decrease in propulsive and total contractions and cause a decrease in intestinal tone.

Morphine and its derivatives have a somewhat more complex action on intestinal smooth muscle, but the net effect is predominantly a retardation of intestinal transit and diminution in muscular activity. Within a few minutes of giving a therapeutic dose of morphine the duodenum contracts and the contraction may be sufficiently powerful to occlude the lumen. Segmental contractions are usually completely abolished, and a similar sequence of changes usually occurs more slowly in the jejunum and ileum. Gradually the pressure within the whole small intestine diminishes, and remains depressed for 4 hours or longer. There might therefore be a dual effect on intestinal transit, this being slowed down first by the spasm, and then by the relative atony. Theoretically, therefore, morphine or one of its analogues would be useful clinically in controlling certain disorders associated with an increased rate of intestinal transit. The derivative codeine, usually as codeine phosphate, is perhaps most widely used for this therapeutic purpose.

Morphine also has distinct actions on the musculature of the colon, which will be discussed in the following chapter.

Drugs stimulating motility

As has been mentioned, acetylcholine, even in low concentration, greatly increases the excitability and vigour of contraction of small intestine smooth muscle. Acetylcholine itself is, however, rapidly destroyed by cholinesterase enzymes in the body, but synthetic stable choline esters such as carbachol and urecholine (carbamyl-β-metacholine) resist the rapid inactivation, and may be used clinically to demonstrate the stimulating effects. Such a substance may therefore be used to stimulate the gastrointestinal tract to greater activity in states of paralysis such as following vagotomy or in paralytic ileus. However, the effectiveness of such stimulation is much less on the small intestine than it is on either the stomach or colon. A much more frequent clinical indication for such stable choline esters is in stimulation of micturition from the bladder in urinary retention not associated with physical obstruction. It is a well-known clinical observation that when these drugs are used for this purpose there is usually urgent defaecation and passage of flatus accompanying emptying of the bladder.

Neostigmine, which retards the destruction of acetylcholine by cholinesterase, produces a moderate increase in the frequency and amplitude of the propagated waves in the small intestine. It will therefore result in an increased rate of propulsion through the small bowel, as can be demonstrated in patients with ileostomies.

The administration of pituitrin is followed by transient stimulation of small bowel peristalsis. Because of this, pituitrin has had a vogue in the treatment of paralytic ileus, but stimulation of movement in the diseased bowel is seldom achieved. There is perhaps a more marked effect of pituitrin on the musculature of the colon, and administration is usually followed by the passage of flatus.

Several of the hormones of the gastrointestinal tract have stimulating effects on the motility of the small intestine itself. Examples are gastrin, GIP, VIP, and motilin. Likewise several of the prostaglandins can be shown under experimental conditions to increase small intestinal motility, and it is possible that they may play a physiological role in the regulation of some motor responses in the gut. Such roles, however, require further clarification.

CLINICAL DISTURBANCES OF MOTILITY

Postoperative 'ileus'

Some degree of suppression of intestinal motility occurs after any abdominal exploration, even that which involves the minimal amount of gentle handling of the intestine and other organs. The inhibition probably arises primarily from sensory stimulation of the peritoneum, or any undue stretching or distension. A less complete and less prolonged inhibition occurs in the small intestine than in the stomach and colon, but even although some small bowel motility may be recorded immediately after the operative interference, this may not be normally propulsive. The period of suppression of motility may be quite short-lived, particularly after expeditiously performed operations involving smooth, well-controlled anaesthesia. The administration of a drug such as prostigmine towards the end of an abdominal operation may further hasten return of normal intestinal activity.

As has been mentioned, the operation of truncal vagotomy for peptic ulcer may increase the period of inhibition of intestinal activity, but there is a gradual return to a completely normal pattern.

Intestinal anastomosis

It might be expected that operations involving either the resection of a segment of small intestine, or the side-to-side anastomosis of other structures to the intestine might cause local and general disorders of small bowel motility. There is often remarkably little disturbance of the normal pattern, apart from that which might be expected in any case from the handling of intra-abdominal organs. However, following gastrectomy or gastrojejunostomy there is often a gradual increase in the diameter of the efferent segment of small intestine to which the stomach or stomach remnant is anastomosed, and this has been attributed to a work hypertrophy resulting from the increased rate of delivery of gastric contents through the stoma into that particular segment of small bowel. Some increase in the diameter and surface area of this efferent loop is therefore regarded as a normal adaptation to such operations.

A short segment of small intestine excised from normal continuity and re-anastomosed both proximally and distally in a reversed direction continues to propel its electrical activity, contraction pattern, and therefore propulsion in a polar way, i.e. against the main pathway of the remaining small intestinal contents. Surgical attempts have therefore been made to use such a mechanism to delay the rate of transit through the small intestine in those patients who, following gastrectomy or other gastric operations, have symptoms such as dumping and diarrhoea on account of this increased intestinal transit. Care is required to select a segment for reversal which is not more than a few centimetres, otherwise there is a risk of causing complete functional obstruction.

Endocrine disorders

Several well known endocrine disorders have diarrhoea as an occasional or dominant symptom. It is not surprising that syndromes characterised by excess production of hormones with a direct action on the small bowel produce diarrhoea. Examples are the excess production of gastrin in the Zollinger-Ellison syndrome with direct motor stimulation by the hormone, and the over-production of GIP and of VIP in the rare tumours which elaborate these specific hormones. Again the carcinoid syndrome, to which reference has already been made, produces excessive quantities of 5-hydroxytryptamine, and when metastases arise in the liver, or the normal mechanism of liver inactivation of the amine is bypassed for one reason or another, the direct effects of this substance on motor activity of the small intestine are apparent. Tumours of the adrenal cortex which produce excess aldosterone also cause diarrhoea, probably mainly as a consequence of the greatly increased rate of loss of potassium from the small bowel mucosa.

Commoner endocrine disorders are thyrotoxicosis and diabetes mellitus, and in each of these conditions there may be disturbance of small bowel motility. Diarrhoea in thyrotoxic patients is associated with rapid transit times, and indeed this may be sufficient to lead to malabsorption. It is likely that the principal effect of the excess thyroid hormone is on the small bowel muscle cells directly increasing their general metabolic rate, just as it does with other tissues. Diarrhoea is also not uncommon in diabetes mellitus, and in this disorder there may be an associated autonomic neuropathy akin to the peripheral neuropathy affecting the central nervous system.

THE ILEOCAECAL VALVE

This specialized area of the terminal small bowel seems able to resist or prevent regurgitation from the caecum in normal health. In addition it may serve as a sphincter acting in the opposite direction, maintaining a slightly greater degree of tone than in the ileum proximal to it, and thus encouraging more prolonged exposure of the absorptive mucosa at this last stage in the passage of content through the small intestine. This would be of particular physiological importance with respect to vitamin B_{12}, bile salts, and possibly other important nutrients. The evidence for such a sphincter-like action is that pressures within the terminal ileum show a gradual increase as one passes distally within the terminal few centimetres. Certainly damage of the terminal ileum by disease such as Crohn's disease, or resection of this segment may result in diarrhoea associated with rapid rates of transit through the small intestine and emptying into the large bowel.

DIGESTION-ABSORPTION BY THE SMALL INTESTINE

These two processes of digestion and absorption are taken together deliberately, as it is now clear that both processes are linked and inter-dependent to a considerable degree. Many of the important steps in both the final breakdown of basic nutrients into absorbable components, and uptake into the cells and other tissues of the small bowel mucosa are so closely interwoven, particularly at the luminal cell membrane area, that one process cannot proceed without the other. It was previously thought that digestion—that is, the breakdown of large molecules of protein, fat and carbohydrate into the smallest units of amino acids, fatty acids and simple sugars—took place within the fluid chyme in the lumen of the small intestine as a result of action of the various digestive enzymes principally of pancreatic origin, and as a second distinct process these simple components were then absorbed across the wall of the small intestine. However, current views indicate that although a certain amount of breakdown of food substances may occur within the lumen, most of the important steps in both breakdown and entry into the body occur at the cell/lumen interface. Indeed the adsorption of exocrine pancreatic enzymes may occur on to the luminal surface of the mucosal cell, and this may be the principal location of their digestive action.

In addition to the digestion-absorption of the principal foodstuffs, a large volume of water and electrolytes is absorbed each day by the small intestine. As well as the relatively small volume of water taken orally, a much larger volume, possibly amounting to some 8–10 litres per day, is secreted into the upper alimentary tract in the saliva, gastric juice, bile and pancreatic juice. Furthermore there is an even greater continual two-way flux of water and electrolytes across the mucosa of the small bowel, and the daily transport from bowel wall into the

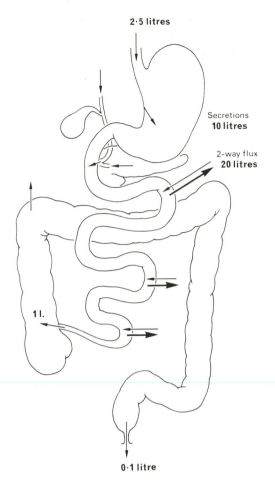

2·5 litres

Secretions
10 litres

2-way flux
20 litres

1 l.

0·1 litre

Fig. 17.10 Water absorption/flux.

expenditure of metabolic energy. There are two principal types of passive transport, the first depending on a difference in the chemical concentration on the two sides of the cell membrane. The molecule simply passes from a region of high concentration across the membrane to the interior of the cell with a lower concentration, and the material is thus said to pass along a concentration gradient. The second type of passive diffusion relates to a gradient of electric charge, and thus it refers to electrolytes. The passage is affected by the electrical charge on either side of the membrane. A potential difference across the cell wall may arise, for example, as a result of the active sodium pump extruding sodium from the interior of the cell, the luminal aspect becoming negative in relation to the serosal side. This electrical gradient may be responsible for transport of charged ions, for example chloride, in a direction which seems to be against the purely chemical concentration gradient.

If the volume of fluid crossing a cell membrane as a result of passive diffusion is sufficiently large this may in itself carry solute across in the same direction, and this process is known as 'solvent drag'. It is also quite passive, requiring no expenditure of energy.

Facilitated diffusion

This process implies that movement of a solute, basically moving along a gradient by passive forces, may be assisted in that same direction of transport by the action of a carrier substance. The total amount of transport of the material may thus be increased above that which would have occurred by passive diffusion unaided.

Active transport

Since some materials require to be transported against either chemical or electrical gradients, these require processes involving the expenditure of metabolic energy. Such transport systems act by involving carriers in the cell membranes. These carriers reside specifically within the cell membranes, shuttling backwards and forwards, taking up the substance to be absorbed at the luminal aspect, carrying it across the membrane, and discharging it free at the intracellular side of the membrane, the carrier in turn going back to the luminal aspect to perform this same task once more. It is likely that most carriers share at least part of the same chemical configuration as the material being transported, and some carrier systems are sodium-dependent, i.e. they require to pick up both the material being absorbed and sodium ions before they are ready to transport both across the membrane, releasing them to the interior of the cell. Carriers are generally specific, accepting solely the appropriate chemical configuration, and since only a certain number of carriers are available this transport mechanism can become saturated.

lumen has been estimated to be from 2–4 times the daily output of gastrointestinal secretions. The bulk of this fluid, from the various sources, is re-absorbed, so that only about 0.5–1.00 litre per day enters the colon through the ileocaecal valve (Fig. 17.10). The small intestine therefore reabsorbs more than 95% of the water presented to its mucosal surface. Further absorption of fluid occurs in the passage of material through the colon.

The end products of digestion-absorption are transferred from the mucosal cells either into the intercellular spaces or directly into the mucosal blood or lymph vessels. The exact mechanisms of transfer of materials from cells to these various compartments are not completely understood. However, there are several distinct mechanisms involved in the absorptive process, namely passive diffusion, facilitated diffusion, and active transport.

Passive diffusion

This refers to the passage of molecules across the cell membrane into its interior, without the accompanying

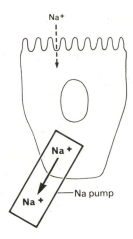

Fig. 17.11 Sodium pump.

Such active transport systems might be regarded in a way as 'pumps' working directly to push the material being absorbed across the membrane. Other active transport systems may act a little more indirectly, e.g. the system for the absorption of sodium. The active sodium pump (Fig. 17.11), to which reference has already been made, acts continuously to expel sodium from the substance of the cell into the surrounding extracellular space. This action appears to be greater in extent at the serosal aspect of the epithelial cell, i.e. the sodium is expelled directly into the lateral spaces between and below the cell. As a consequence the intracellular content of sodium is reduced, and this encourages the further entry of sodium ions into the cell from the luminal aspect. The active process is therefore proceeding at the base of the cell, and the actual entry of sodium from lumen into cell is a secondary, perhaps passive process.

These three processes account for the absorption of most materials from the intestinal lumen. It was formerly thought that pinocytosis, which describes the act of particles being engulfed directly by mucosal cells, was a physiological mechanism for absorption, particularly of fat, but it now seems likely that this is a rare and unimportant phenomenon.

The energy required for the active transport mechanisms is mainly derived from the oxidation of glucose to carbon dioxide and water, with the associated production of energy-rich molecules of adenosine triphosphate.

THE ABSORPTION OF CARBOHYDRATE, FAT, AND PROTEIN

Considerable advances in our understanding of the mechanisms of absorption of these substances have arisen in recent years as the result of direct observation in human subjects, perfusing defined lengths of the intestine with solutions of controlled composition, over definite periods of time, and estimating the rate of disappearance of the material under test from the lumen; the in vitro approach in the animal experimental laboratory, using various preparations of excised segments of small intestine has also been helpful.

Carbohydrate

The bulk of dietary carbohydrate consists of starch, with lesser quantities of polysaccharides, disaccharides, and still less of monosaccharides. The larger carbohydrate molecules are broken down by the action of salivary and pancreatic amylases mainly into disaccharides, although a small quantity of monosaccharides is also released (Fig. 17.12). The disaccharides, such as maltose, maltotriose, α-limit dextrins, lactose, and sucrose are adsorbed on to the brush border of the mucosal cells, where the further breakdown into the component monosaccharides is effected by the disaccharidases which reside in this layer.

The released monosaccharides, the principal one of which is glucose amounting to approximately 80%, are absorbed by active transport into the mucosal cells, by the action of sodium-dependent carrier systems. These may act against a concentration gradient. Although this process of absorption is a rate-limiting process which can be saturated, the amount of carrier in the mucosa of the upper small intestine is more than sufficient for the ingestion of even large amounts of pure carbohydrate solution.

There is some evidence that glucose and galactose share the same carrier system. However, fructose is clearly transported by quite a different mechanism which is probably not saturatable, and does not appear to require metabolic energy on the part of the enterocyte. The rate of transport of this monosaccharide is distinctly slower than that for the others.

As has been discussed, there does not seem to be either a nervous or humoral regulation of the rate of absorption of carbohydrates, and although in diabetes mellitus glucose absorption appears to be more rapid than normal, the underlying mechanism for this altered rate is unknown.

Complete breakdown of disaccharides to their component monosaccharides is essential for absorption, and certain diseases in which disaccharidase action is deficient or absent are characterised by the occurrence of diarrhoea. An example is the congenital absence of the enzyme lactase

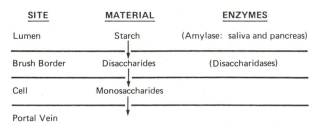

SITE	MATERIAL	ENZYMES
Lumen	Starch	(Amylase: saliva and pancreas)
Brush Border	Disaccharides	(Disaccharidases)
Cell	Monosaccharides	
Portal Vein		

Fig. 17.12 Carbohydrate digestion-absorption.

from the brush border. In this condition the accumulation of lactose in the small intestine has an osmotic effect which increases the volume of the fluid within the lumen. In addition the unsplit lactose on entering the colon may be metabolised by certain bacteria to produce organic acids which have an irritant effect on the colonic mucosa. Both of these mechanisms may therefore contribute to the symptom of diarrhoea. Deficiencies of other disaccharidases also occur, albeit rarely, in clinical practice. Diagnosis of the specific enzyme deficiency can be achieved either by assaying the enzyme in biopsies of the intestinal mucosa, or indirectly by performing absorption studies of the disaccharide, and in turn each of the component monosaccharides.

Fat

An average Western type diet contains between 70–90 g of fat per day, almost all in the form of triglycerides, and in normal health at least 95% of this is digested and absorbed. In addition to the fat ingested there is a considerable output of endogenous fat from discarded cells, bile and bacteria. This total addition of endogenous fat may be around 20–30 g per day and most also undergoes digestion and absorption. Even when fat is totally excluded from the diet there is a minimal daily loss with the faeces of approximately 1–2 g.

Dietary triglycerides are first converted into a finely dispersed emulsion which renders them capable of being approached and initially digested by the water-soluble pancreatic lipase enzymes (Fig. 17.13). The principal action of lipase is to reduce the triglyceride molecules to monoglycerides, maintaining the link between glycerol and the central fatty acid, but releasing the two fatty acid molecules at either end. At this stage in the process a critical concentration of bile salts results in the formation of micelles, which comprise a convenient and efficient mechanism for trapping and transporting both the monoglycerides and free fatty acids. The advantage of micelle formation is that the fatty acids and monoglycerides can be polarised with their fat-soluble ends buried in the depth of the micelle, and their water-soluble ends turned outwards, thus maintaining a relative degree of water solubility in the intestinal chyme. Furthermore, this micellar configuration permits the carriage of cholesterol and fat-soluble vitamins in the lipid core of the micelle, thus ensuring adequate absorption of these important materials along with the main volume of dietary fat. There are two sizes of micelle, the smaller of which requires somewhere in the region of 1–2 mmol/l of bile salts for their formation, but for the carriage of significant added amounts of lipid larger micelles are formed, these latter requiring bile salts in excess of 4 mmol/l.

Micellar configuration is simply a transient arrangement to get the lipid to the luminal aspect of the mucosal cell

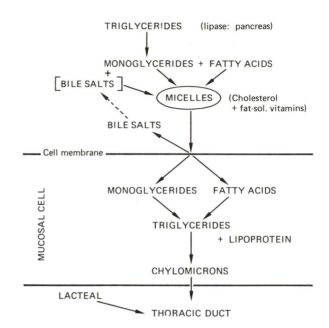

Fig. 17.13 Fat digestion-absorption.

membrane. Once the fatty materials are at this level there is no great problem about transporting them into the interior of the cell, since the cell membrane is largely a lipid structure. The bile salts which are so essential for the formation of micelles almost certainly are separated from the lipid substances at the cell membrane and returned to the intestinal lumen where they may act once more in the capacity of lipid carriers. This is one more example of the body's fine economy with such valuable materials.

The monoglycerides and fatty acids, having crossed the microvillus membrane into the interior of the musocal cells, are mostly reconverted into triglycerides by enzyme action. Particles of reformed triglyceride are then further coated with lipoprotein material to create chylomicrons, large particles of between 500 and 1000 Å (50 and 100 nm). Substantial increases in the number of fat particles and chylomicrons within the mucosal cells can be seen after feeding. In turn the chylomicrons pass to the basal aspects of the mucosal cells, cross the basement membrane and enter the lymphatic lacteals, probably by direct penetration between the endothelial cells. The fatty material then passes along the lymphatic system, up the thoracic duct and thereby enters the systemic circulation. A small proportion of absorbed fat may enter the portal venous system, but the greater proportion travels by the lymphatic route as outlined.

Role of bile salts in fat absorption

Bile salts play a crucial role in micelle formation, and therefore they play an important role in the absorption of fat and fat-soluble substances. In addition bile salts are also useful in the initial stages of fat digestion, in that they facilitate emulsification of dietary triglycerides, and therefore assist the action of pancreatic lipase. Bile salts are so important that the body makes considerable efforts to re-use them by several processes. For example as has already been discussed, bile salts are not absorbed into the mucosa along with the products of fat digestion, but return from the luminal cell surface for re-use. Again, there is very considerable reabsorption of bile salts from the terminal ileum, so that they may return to the liver, and be re-excreted in bile. This arrangement permits the repeated usage of bile salts and when fat absorption should be more or less complete at the lower end of the intestine, they are reclaimed.

However, even when bile salts are totally absent from the small intestine, for example due to blockage of the common bile duct, the breakdown and absorption of 75% or more of dietary fat can still take place. This is a tribute to the great reserve of digestive-absorptive power along the mucosa of the entire small intestine, which can to a large extent cope with a much less efficient breakdown of dietary fat even in the absence of all the valuable assistance normally provided by bile salts.

Absorption of different fatty acids

In health, most of the absorption of dietary fat takes place in the duodenum and jejunum, and only when significant portions of this part of the alimentary tract are excised or damaged by disease is there a significant proportion of digestion-absorption in the ileum. There is, as with most body functions, therefore, a considerable reserve of digestion-absorption capacity.

Some fatty acids are more easily incorporated in micelles and absorbed than others, and as a rule there is a greater capacity for absorption and re-esterification of unsaturated fatty acids than saturated ones. To some extent, also, the length of the fatty acid chain influences the rate and efficiency of absorption. Short and medium chain fatty acids are hydrolysed and absorbed more rapidly than longer chain triglycerides, even when the quantities of lipase and of bile salts are reduced. Indeed medium chain triglycerides may be absorbed satisfactorily without the assistance of bile salts. A higher proportion of these medium chain fatty acids is transported directly across the mucosal cells into the portal venous bloodstream rather than into the lacteals, thus differing from the more usual dietary components.

Cholesterol absorption

There is, of course, cholesterol in a normal Western diet, but in addition some cholesterol enters the lumen of the small intestine in bile, and from exfoliated cells of the intestine itself. Cholesterol is carried mainly dissolved within micelles, although the efficiency of this transport is much less than that for dietary triglycerides. Cholesterol ester must first be converted to free cholesterol by pancreatic enzymes before it is readily available for incorporation in micelles. As with other fatty substances, absorption of cholesterol is maximal in the proximal small bowel, and it is quite dependent upon the presence of bile salts for micelle formation. It passes almost totally into the lymphatic lacteals.

Fat-soluble vitamins

These substances, like cholesterol, require to be transported in micelles and their absorption is much less efficient than that for normal dietary triglycerides, and takes place predominantly in the upper small intestine. Although some enter the portal venous blood, especially vitamin E, it is likely that the principal route of absorption is via the lymphatic system.

In conditions which exclude bile entirely from the alimentary tract, there will of course be reduction in the rate of absorption of all the fat-soluble vitamins. However, the only deficiency of significant clinical importance is that of vitamin K, so essential for the normal formation of prothrombin.

Protein

As with the other main dietary constituents, protein absorption in health is a highly efficient process occurring mainly in the duodenum and proximal jejunum. More than 95% of dietary protein will be absorbed, leaving a very small proportion to be lost in the faeces. In addition to the dietary intake there is a considerable output of protein material from endogenous sources. Perhaps 60–70 g of protein per day may arise in this fashion, which compares with an average daily dietary intake of perhaps 80–100 g. The endogenous protein arises from desquamated cells, and the secretions of the pancreas and other digestive organs. Both dietary and endogenous protein may be regarded as a single protein pool for digestion and absorption.

The minor amount of protein breakdown in the stomach as a result of the action of activated gastric pepsin is quite insignificant, and completely adequate protein breakdown and absorption can take place in the total absence of pepsin, e.g. following total gastrectomy. The principal enzymatic digestion of protein material arises from the action of the proteolytic enzymes from the exocrine pancreas (Fig. 17.14). These are secreted from the pancreatic acinar cells in an inactive form, being rendered active by the presence of enterokinase in the small bowel itself. Enterokinase is produced in the brush border of the mucosa of the small intestine, and its principal action is to activate trypsinogen into the enzyme trypsin. This in turn activates the other inactive precursors of lipase and

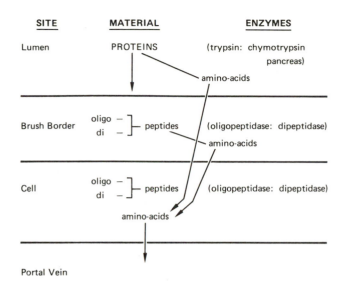

SITE	MATERIAL	ENZYMES
Lumen	PROTEINS	(trypsin: chymotrypsin pancreas)
	amino-acids	
Brush Border	oligo – / di – } peptides	(oligopeptidase: dipeptidase)
	amino-acids	
Cell	oligo – / di – } peptides	(oligopeptidase: dipeptidase)
	amino-acids	
Portal Vein		

Fig. 17.14 Protein digestion-absorption.

amylase; furthermore the presence of active trypsin acts in an autocatalytic fashion to stimulate the activation of still further quantities of trypsinogen. There is thus a highly efficient means of rendering the inactive enzyme precursors fully operational just at the point where their digestive properties are required.

It was formerly believed that the proteolytic enzymes broke down the large protein molecules into their component free amino acids, which in turn were directly absorbed through the mucosal cells. However, it is now known that not only free amino acids are produced as the result of digestive enzyme action, but a significant amount of dipeptides and slightly larger molecules are also liberated. A proportion of the dipeptides are capable of crossing the cell membrane and entering the mucosal cells, and indeed, there are instances where the absorption of dipeptides may be more efficient that that of the two component single amino acids. The larger oligopeptides are further broken down by appropriate oligopeptidases located in the brush border, and it is unlikely that there is appreciable direct penetration of these larger oligopeptides into the cells. Thus the greatest amount of larger oligopeptide breakdown is at the brush border, and the greater amount of breakdown of dipeptides into their component amino acids is intracellular. That these dipeptidase and oligopeptidase activities are important in overall protein digestion-absorption is illustrated by the finding that only approximately 30% of dietary proteins are broken down entirely to free amino acids, the remaining 70% requiring final breakdown at either brush border or intracellular level.

It seems certain that this is the normal mechanism for entry of material of protein origin into the body, but small amounts of certain proteins must also be capable of entering the mucosa, in order to explain the occurrence of allergic reactions to dietary proteins. This entry must be regarded as a pathological process, and although in neonatal life protein materials from colostrum and maternal antibodies may normally enter the small bowel mucosa, in the adult such entry of intact proteins must be regarded as abnormal.

The process by which free amino acids, and possibly dipeptides are transported across the cell membrane, from intestinal lumen to mucosal cell, requires active consumption of energy. Specific carrier mechanisms exist similar to those for glucose, requiring the participation of sodium absorption, and, since several amino acids may share the single carrier system, there is a certain amount of competition among the different amino acids for transport.

From the basal and lateral walls of the intestinal mucosal cells the absorbed amino acids pass directly into the radicals of the portal venous system.

ABSORPTION OF WATER AND ELECTROLYTES

The delicate balance between the oral intake of fluid on the one hand, and the losses mainly through the renal tract, the lungs and the skin on the other hand, is well maintained in health, so that the relationships between the various water and electrolyte contents of the different tissue spaces are kept within very narrow margins of variation. Although the gastrointestinal tract is not regarded as a significant regulator of this fine balance, greater physiological roles being ascribed to the kidney, there is no doubt that major clinical disorders of fluid and electrolyte balance can rapidly occur as the result of even minor changes in the flux of water and electrolytes across the intestinal mucosa. The quantities of water and electrolytes entering and leaving the lumen of the small intestine daily in health are very large. For example, approximately 8–9 l of fluid enter the upper parts of the alimentary tract as secretions of the salivary, gastric and pancreatic glands, and in bile. In addition, there is a continuous two-way flux of water and electrolytes across the mucosa of the small intestine. Since only approximately 1 l of fluid passes daily through the ileocaecal valve into the colon, it follows that many litres per day are reabsorbed in the small intestine itself. There is, of course, further reabsorption of water and some electrolytes in the colon so that the daily loss of fluid in the faeces is only approximately 100 ml.

It is thus apparent that even a small change in the flux of fluid and electrolytes in either direction might result in a profound disturbance of the overall body balance.

The passage of water and the principal electrolytes across the mucosa is known to be rapid. One of the main physiological objectives in the uppermost segments of the small intestine is the achievement of an isosmotic state, the osmotic tension of the usually hypertonic mixture of ingested food plus secretion being rapidly adjusted to that of extracellular fluid. Once this state has been achieved the remaining adjustments can proceed in a slightly more leisurely fashion.

Water

The greater part of the large volume of water absorbed in the small intestine almost certainly is transported as a passive process consequent on the active absorption of the products of carbohydrate and protein digestion, and other solutes such as electrolytes. Since most of the sugars, amino acids and small peptides are absorbed in the proximal small bowel this implies that large quantities of water and ions also enter the bloodstream at this level. In addition, further absorption of water can take place, particularly in the ileum, along with sodium and chloride ions, where the luminal concentration of digestive products is low, but the luminal content is still relatively hypertonic. To some extent the active transport of ions such as sodium would assist the absorption of further amounts of water, but in addition it is possible that other factors assist the transport of additional water across the mucosal cell membranes. One hypothesis to account for this additional transport of water is represented diagrammatically in Figure 17.15. It implies that there is a difference in the permeability between the lumen to cell interface on the one hand, and the base of cell to capillary interface on the other hand. The former membrane, which may be the luminal part of the mucosal cell, or the minute space represented by the tight junction, is a thin membrane with relatively small pores, whereas the second membrane is thicker but with larger gaps. Solutes actively transported across the first membrane would carry water along with them to build up an increased hydrostatic pressure both within the cell substance, and in the lateral intercellular space. This material might also become hypertonic in the process, and as a combination of these forces the larger gaps in the basement membrane capillary interface would easily permit the movement of both solute and water into the capillaries. Solute molecules, however, would find it difficult to pass backwards from the cell and intercellular space towards the lumen, in view of the tightness of the pores separating these from the lumen. Thus the overall effect would be the passage of water from lumen right through to the draining vessels.

Whether this or other mechanisms contribute to water absorption, there can be little doubt that the major influence on water absorption in the small intestine is the transport of the main water soluble nutrients by the intestinal mucosa.

Sodium

The amount of sodium presented to the mucosa of the small intestine by the spontaneous flux across the mucosa is very much greater than the normal daily dietary intake

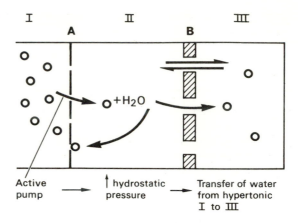

An active solute pump across membrane A causes increased hydrostatic pressure in middle compartment (water being transported along with solute). This increased pressure pushes solute particles plus water in both directions, but more easily to III because of larger pores in membrane B, and small pores in membrane A prevent backward movement of solute particles (plus water). Consequent gross effect is transfer of water from hypertonic I to III.

A = lateral cell membrane (active Na pump)
B = basal membrane and capillary endothelium

Fig. 17.15 Membrane theory for water absorption.

of sodium. Rapid absorption of sodium starts in the proximal small intestine; it is an active process, linked closely with the active absorption of sugars and amino acids. Indeed it has been shown in perfusion studies that monosaccharides (excluding fructose) and some amino acids and peptides introduced into the lumen of the jejunum greatly augment the absorption of sodium (and chloride) and it is likely that the ion transport is principally effected by 'solvent drag' resulting from the large accompanying absorption of water.

However, in addition to this process it is likely that there are additional mechanisms to promote sodium absorption to these predominantly osmotic effects. The well known active sodium pump driving sodium ions from the base and lateral aspects of the mucosal cell is the basis for further intracellular uptake of sodium.

It is also possible that some sodium ion along with water can pass through the so-called 'tight junctions', between the juxtaluminal portions of the mucosal cell.

Potassium

The absorption of potassium is believed to occur primarily as a passive mechanism, probably being more dependent on an electrical gradient than a simple one of chemical concentration. As with water and other ions there is a considerable volume of two-way flux of potassium across the intestinal mucosa, and in addition its transport may be influenced, particularly in the jejunum, simply by large movements of fluid, i.e. 'solvent drag'.

Chloride

Although much of the transport of this ion is almost certainly passive, being linked to the movement of sodium, there are almost certainly additional mechanisms influencing the transport of chloride across the intestinal mucosa. It would appear that the speed of chloride absorption is more rapid than that of sodium, and it may be that a certain amount of exchange of chloride for bicarbonate ions may occur in addition to the sodium-linked transport. Supportive evidence for such an exchange arises from the observation that the normal secretion of bicarbonate into the lumen of the ileum is suppressed if chloride is absent and replaced by another anion, e.g. sulphate.

A similar exchange of chloride for bicarbonate ions occurs, but to a much greater extent, across the mucosa of the colon.

Bicarbonate

There seems to be a difference in the behaviour of the jejunal mucosa from that of the ileum with regard to the handling of bicarbonate ions. Secretions from the pancreas, the liver and the upper small intestine itself are rich in bicarbonate, and it is therefore not surprising that these ions are absorbed swiftly in the upper small intestine. In addition to the absorption of a significant proportion of the bicarbonate ions, it is likely that some also combine with hydrogen ions with the consequent production of water and carbon dioxide within the lumen.

As has been mentioned above, the ileal mucosa normally secretes some bicarbonate, and some of these ions may be exchanged for chloride under physiological conditions.

Calcium

The divalent ions such as calcium are absorbed much more slowly and less efficiently than the monovalent ions already discussed. Although there is a small daily loss into the gastrointestinal tract in the salivary and digestive secretions, there is not a two-way flux as with the other ions, and these secretory components are normally excreted. There is thus a daily dietary requirement for calcium which is in the region of 1 g per day. Only about 50% of the dietary calcium is absorbed.

The absorption of calcium from the small intestine is an active transport mechanism, which can be effective against an electrochemical gradient.

The active absorption of calcium is facilitated by the presence of vitamin D, but there is a delay of several hours after ingestion of vitamin D before a significant effect on calcium absorption is observed. It is likely that time is required for the metabolism of vitamin D in the liver and elsewhere, and the subsequent production of a specific calcium-binding protein in the mucosal cell as a result of the action of a metabolite of vitamin D.

It is also known that parathormone, as well as having other actions in calcium metabolism, aids the absorption of calcium from the intestinal mucosa, and it is probable that it also acts by increasing the production of a similar vitamin D metabolite.

The action of other hormones from the adrenal gland and thyroid may also influence calcium absorption, but the effects of these hormones is probably slight, and the mechanisms by which they act are uncertain.

The efficiency of calcium absorption diminishes with age, and this may be partly due to a decrease in available vitamin D, or other defects.

Magnesium

Although there are considerable quantities of magnesium in the body, and, indeed, it is the fourth most abundant cation after calcium, sodium and potassium, much less is understood about the mechanisms of absorption and metabolism than for other minerals. There is less evidence for an active transport mechanism in the absorption of magnesium, and the rate of absorption appears to be distinctly slower than that of calcium. Although both vitamin D and parathormone have been demonstrated to increase the rate of magnesium absorption, this does not necessarily imply that they are absorbed by a common mechanism. Probably only about 25% of the dietary intake of magnesium is normally absorbed.

Other metals

Zinc and cobalt may be absorbed by a mechanism allied to, or closely similar to that involved in iron absorption, since they are absorbed more rapidly and completely from the intestine in iron-deficient subjects. Probably a different mechanism is concerned with the absorption of copper, though detailed information on this subject is lacking.

The gastrointestinal tract also clearly has a role in the excretion of these metals, copper being most abundant in bile, and zinc and cobalt in the small intestine itself.

Absorption of haematinics

Three vital requirements for the normal production of red blood corpuscles are all absorbed through the mucosa of the small intestine, namely iron, folic acid, and vitamin B_{12}. Details of the mechanisms of absorption and metabolism are given in Chapter 11. Iron absorption takes place mainly in the duodenum and proximal jejunum, and there is possibly a carrier—gastroferrin, elaborated by the stomach—which facilitates the absorption process. Since excessive uptake of iron into the body would be harmful, there are mechanisms acting within the mucosa of the small intestine which prevent over-absorption. Saturation of the ferritin and apoferritin iron-carrying system within the mucosal cells may prevent the further entry of fresh iron presented for absorption to the brush border. Furthermore, iron trapped within the carrier systems of the mucosal cells will soon be shed into the lumen in the normal process of ageing and rapid desquamation at the tips of the villi. This is thus another route for the elimination of excess unwanted iron.

The precise mechanism of the absorption and carriage of folate is not so clear, but it involves at some stage in the digestion-absorption process splitting of large molecules made up of multiple glutamate residues, down to a monoglutamate size. Whether this breakdown takes place at the cell membrane or within the mucosal cell is not known. Like the other materials discussed so far, most of the folic acid is absorbed in the proximal small bowel.

It is well known that the absorption of vitamin B_{12} requires the interaction with the specific intrinsic factor produced in the acid-secreting portion of the stomach. A reversible complex between the vitamin B_{12} and the intrinsic factor occurs with some rapidity, and the specific receptor sites for this complex are restricted to the terminal ileum. The absorption of vitamin B_{12} in health is therefore restricted to this particular segment of the intestine, and it follows that resection of ileum will lead in due course to vitamin B_{12} deficiency anaemia. This, of course, may take some months or even years to become apparent, in view of the considerable stores of vitamin B_{12} in the liver and elsewhere in the body. Once the complex of vitamin B_{12} and intrinsic factor is attached to the cell receptor at the brush border it is fairly certain that the intrinsic factor is split off, and only the vitamin B_{12} enters the mucosal cell. A carrier protein is probably responsible for the further transport of the vitamin B_{12} into the portal venous blood.

Absorption of drugs

Although some drugs may be absorbed through the buccal or gastric mucosa, the principal site of entry of most drugs is certainly the small intestine. The majority of drugs are either weak acids or weak bases, and most are absorbed through the intestinal mucosa by passive diffusion. Factors which influence the rate of absorption include the molecular weight of the drug, the degree of ionization within the lumen, and the solubility in either water or lipid.

Although, theoretically, water-soluble ionized forms of drugs could pass through the aqueous channel represented by 'pores' in the mucosa the molecular weight of many drugs in their ionized forms appears to be somewhat larger than would normally be allowed simple passage through these channels. However, the more lipid-soluble, non-ionic forms of many drugs will have less difficulty in traversing the essentially lipid cell membrane, and it is likely that such a method of diffusion is a major route of drug absorption.

Other factors influencing the efficiency of absorption of drugs include the rate of gastric emptying, of transit through the intestine itself, the pK of the individual drugs, and the pH at the site of absorption.

In addition, the gastrointestinal tract is a major route for the excretion of many drugs, some being conjugated within the liver with glucuronic acid or sulphate and excreted in the bile, others being eliminated directly through the intestinal mucosa. The latter process almost certainly involves active transport mechanisms.

CLINICAL MALABSORPTION

It follows from a consideration of the previous sections that patients may develop clinically obvious malabsorption as a result of various different disorders. These might be classified simply, along the following lines, as suggested by Booth.

1. Disorders of gastric function

Deficiency of the production of intrinsic factor will lead to the typical vitamin B_{12} deficient megaloblastic anaemia.

Following partial gastrectomy a few patients, possibly up to 10%, will develop some degree of steatorrhoea. There are probably several factors which could be partly responsible for this outcome, such as impaired mixing of bile and pancreatic secretions with the chyme, and alteration in the bacterial flora as a result of the reduced gastric acid secretion, an alteration in the motility pattern of the upper gastrointestinal tract, alterations in the liberation of hormones such as secretin and CCK-PZ, perhaps reduced efficiency of gallbladder contraction, etc. If careful controlled measurements of daily faecal fat output are made in postgastrectomy patients, higher than normal fat losses in the stools will usually be demonstrated. However, there is often surprisingly little correlation between the absolute amounts of faecal fat loss and clinical symptoms, so that factors other than simply the proportion of fat digested and absorbed are clearly significant from the clinical viewpoint.

Some of the physiological derangements outlined above, which follow a partial gastrectomy of the Polya pattern (i.e. anastomosing the gastric remnant to a loop of jejunum), can be ameliorated by converting this to a gastroduodenal anastomosis of the Billroth I type. Alternatively, operations which involve the incorporation of a short segment of small intestine interposed between the gastric remnant and duodenum may be of benefit, by providing a more normal mixing of food and digestive secretions, and reducing transit through the small intestine.

2. Defects of digestion

Clearly in disorders in which bile is excluded from entering the small intestine, such as from obstruction due to either a gallstone or tumour in the common bile duct, the digestion and absorption of fat will be impaired. Also in diseases which impair the functioning of the exocrine pancreas, such as cystic fibrosis, pancreatitis, tumours, and following pancreatic resection, there will be a reduction in the capacity to break down and absorb the products of digestion of all major diet constituents.

3. Defects of intestinal absorption

Obviously resection of a portion of the small intestine will reduce its reserves of digestion-absorption function, and if the segment excised is sufficiently large this may lead to a clinically apparent degree of malabsorption with weight loss, diarrhoea, steatorrhoea, and perhaps anaemia and specific ion deficiencies. The clinical picture will vary depending on whether it is proximal or distal small bowel which is removed, the latter of course leading to specific defects of vitamin B_{12} and bile salt absorption.

The proliferation of an abnormal bacterial flora proximally in the small intestine will also result in steatorrhoea and macrocytic anaemia. Such an abnormal bacterial proliferation occurs in any condition which allows significant stasis in segments of the small intestine, such as diverticula, strictures due to granulomatous or other disorders, blind loops of small intestine bypassed by surgical operations, and fistulae between different parts of the alimentary tract. When stagnation occurs, the bacterial flora in the upper intestine is altered, bacteria normally suppressed or confined to the colon proliferate, and many of these are capable of altering bile salt metabolism and metabolising vitamin B_{12}. That these abnormally proliferating bacteria are primarily responsible for the malabsorption picture can be neatly demonstrated by the temporary alleviation of symptoms following the administration of broad spectrum antibiotics. Of course, a more lasting cure of the malabsorption can be obtained by the surgical removal of diverticula or strictures, correction of fistulae, or excision or undoing of redundant blind loops.

Some unfortunate patients have a mixture of lesions all of which contribute to the picture of malabsorption, such as those with Crohn's disease of the small intestine. They may have strictures, blind loops created by fistulae, they may have undergone previous resection, and each of these factors may contribute to malabsorption. In these patients the correction of even one abnormality by surgical or other means may make a worthwhile clinical improvement.

The digestion-absorption function of the small bowel can be impaired by ischaemia from occlusion of the mesenteric arteries, from drugs such as some of the antibiotics, and by the infestation with certain parasites such as *Dibothriocephalus latus* or giardiasis.

Finally, a group of diseases may impair the efficiency of the intestinal mucosa itself. Acute inflammation of the jejunum or ileum by bacterial or other irritative processes occasionally occurs, and a short-lived outpouring of fluid and electrolyte may result. More chronic impairment of mucosal function arises in such conditions as coeliac disease, tropical sprue, and other rare disorders characterised by specific deficiency of one or other enzyme or transport mechanism.

OBSTRUCTION OF THE SMALL INTESTINE

The causes of complete acute obstruction of the small intestine are many and varied, including incarceration of a loop of intestine in a hernial sac, snaring of a loop under a post-operative adhesion, volvulus, intussusception, impaction of a swallowed indigestible bolus, tumour or granulomatous disease in the bowel wall, and a few other rarer disorders; regardless of the mechanism of obstruction there are several distinct features common to all episodes. These include pain, initially of a colicky nature, vomiting which is often copious and repeated, and abdominal distension. Furthermore, the symptoms and clinical features usually appear in that sequence, although this is to some extent influenced by the level at which the obstruction occurs, there being perhaps little distension but early vomiting with a high jejunal obstruction on the one hand, and a prolonged period of colicky pain and perhaps no vomiting until quite a late stage with a distal colonic obstruction.

Complete blockage to the small intestine is a serious, life-threatening condition, and if untreated the patient inevitably sooner or later becomes seriously ill from peripheral circulatory failure, and death occurs as a result of either the severe losses of fluid and electrolytes and metabolic disturbance, or absorption of toxins from the damaged segment, or a combination of both factors. When a loop of bowel is not only obstructed but also has its blood supply occluded, the involved segment is said to be strangulated, and the resultant severe damage to this segment accelerates the metabolic disturbances, adds to them significant losses of blood and plasma, and greatly increases the opportunity for the absorption of dangerous toxins. The occurrence of strangulation, therefore, is of sinister significance, and demands urgent remedial measures.

Paralytic or adynamic ileus is also in many respects a form of 'obstruction', although there may be no obvious physical block to the passage of contents along the bowel lumen. This condition, which has a basically reflex origin from infection, retroperitoneal irritation, mechanical or chemical irritation within the abdomen, or which may be the result of the action of various drugs, is characterized by a local segment of the small bowel which is paralysed, and therefore acts as a functional bar to the propagation of propulsive movement. As a result there is usually reflex cessation of all other motility in the gastrointestinal tract, and a characteristically painless distension due to functional obstruction of the intestine proximal to the irritated segment.

Mechanism of the pain

The first evidence of small bowel obstruction is most often pain of a characteristic kind, severe, cramping, rhythmically intermitting colic. It is not sharply localized but experienced across the abdomen about the level of the umbilicus, since the entire small bowel from about the level of the ampulla of Vater is derived from the embryological midgut. Initially there is usually complete relief between spasms, unless the blood supply to the obstructed segment is also damaged, i.e. by strangulation.

The pain is clearly related to vigorous muscular contraction of the bowel, the result of a local reflex attempt to propel the obstructing agent. It is likely that the factor responsible for the pain is transient ischaemia due to temporary occlusion of the supplying blood vessels by the forceful muscular contraction itself. The nerves carrying the pain impulses pass centrally with the splanchnic sympathetic nerves.

If the obstruction is not relieved, sooner or later the vigorous contractions subside, and the colic may thus diminish or disappear. However, by this time damage to the obstructed segment of bowel is often severe enough to cause more localised continuous pain due to irritation, and in addition localised tenderness or 'rebound tenderness' may be apparent on clinical examination.

Vomiting and distension

The severity of these two features depends to a large extent on the level of the obstruction within the small intestine. A high jejunal obstruction prevents a large quantity of fluid from the stomach and duodenum from reaching the absorptive areas of the small intestine, vomiting tends to be early and copious, and abdominal distension therefore slight. On the other hand, a low ileal obstruction leaves virtually all of the small intestine at least for a while available for absorption, fluid accumulates in it more slowly, and vomiting is usually (but by no means always) delayed in onset; moreover since the stomach and much of the small intestine become loaded with fluid, there may be considerable abdominal distension.

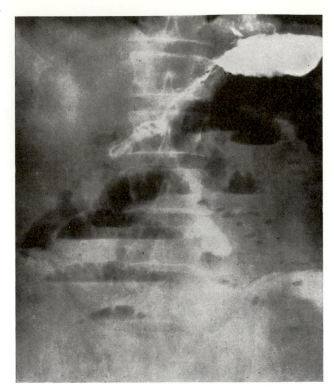

Fig. 17.16 X-ray film of the abdomen, taken with the patient erect, showing the gas shadows and fluid levels characteristic of obstructed small intestine. (Courtesy of Dr S. D. Scott Park.)

The distension of the bowel is due to the accumulation of both liquid and gas proximal to the obstruction. The gas, which rapidly equilibrates with the blood gases, is derived mainly from air which is swallowed, but in addition there are small amounts of methane and hydrogen disulphide which are produced in the intestine itself. These greatly increased pockets of gas, which float upwards above pools of liquid in the various loops of obstructed intestine, give rise to the characteristic 'fluid levels' on straight X-ray of the abdomen with the patient in the erect position (Fig. 17.16). The presence of such multiple fluid levels gives a confident diagnosis of complete intestinal obstruction, and furthermore the distribution of them may give a significant clue as to the location of the obstruction.

As can be imagined, the accumulation of gas and liquid above the site of obstruction causes a significant increase in the pressure within the obstructed bowel. This is normally in the region of 2–4 cm of water, but in obstruction pressure may rise to as high as 15 or even 25 cm of water. Since tension within the wall is related both to diameter and intraluminal pressure, there may thus develop an extreme degree of tension within the bowel wall which affects tissue blood flow and therefore vitality of the muscle and other tissues in the organ.

Fluid and electrolyte disturbance in small bowel obstruction

In simple mechanical obstruction the principal loss is partly of ingested liquids but mainly of gastrointestinal secretions and the water and electrolytes normally taking part in the two-way flux across the intestinal mucosa. The losses are principally of water, sodium and potassium, but when in addition there is strangulation of a segment of intestine there is also a significant loss of both red blood cells and plasma.

Several factors contribute to the overall loss which is chiefly from the extracellular fluid compartment. Firstly, there is the obvious loss by vomiting, and since this symptom is usually present, there is at the same time, secondly, a cessation of further dietary intake. Thirdly, in addition to the liquid expelled by vomiting, a considerable quantity of the secretions and other liquids may lie sequestered in the lumen of the small intestine proximal to the site of obstruction, and therefore lost to the tissue spaces. Fourthly, the area of absorptive mucosa distal to the level of obstruction is unavailable for the processes of absorption. Fifthly, it has been shown by the experiments of Shields (1965) that there is an increased loss of fluid and electrolytes from an obstructed segment of bowel, the flux into the lumen across the wall continuing, but being accompanied by a marked reduction of the flux in the opposite direction, i.e. from lumen back into the tissue spaces. Sixthly, if strangulation is present an oedematous exudate occurs into the damaged segment of bowel, and also a considerable amount of this fluid can exude from the serosal aspect. Finally, also in strangulation, there may be the loss of frank blood or plasma from the affected segment.

From these various sources there thus may be the loss of several litres of valuable extracellular fluid from the body, and this may be reflected in obvious clinical signs of peripheral circulatory failure leading to oligaemic shock. Most causes of small bowel obstruction require urgent surgical correction, but a preliminary period of treatment by nasogastric aspiration of the stomach and intravenous fluid replacement are routine preparatory steps. The intravenous administration of isotonic saline solution is usually regarded as the sheet anchor of fluid replacement and in most cases diagnosed reasonably early the administration of 2–3 l of this solution over the first 3–4 hours is usually satisfactory. If more than this volume is required, or if there is any delay in performing operation, potassium may also require to be added to the intravenous fluid regime. The more severe fluid and electrolyte losses will require more elaborate, repeated estimations of replacement requirements, monitoring by measurement of central venous pressure, and serum electrolyte measurements. Under the circumstances it may also be wise to follow urinary output accurately and frequently by continuous collection from the catheterised bladder.

It should be remembered that a considerable loss of total body potassium may arise in intestinal obstruction before there is a significant reduction in the serum potassium concentration, so that there may be a tendency to underestimate the requirements for this ion in the intravenous replacement regime.

Other factors contributing to risk

The loss of fluid and electrolytes in itself may constitute a threat to life in intestinal obstruction. Furthermore there may be an upset of acid-base balance, with the loss of considerable quantities of bicarbonate ions plus a cessation of dietary intake contributing to an acidosis.

Distension of the intestine itself may have reflex effects on motility elsewhere in the alimentary tract, on respiration, and possibly on the vascular responses to the oligaemic shock state.

A major threat to life, however, is the possible absorption of toxins, mainly from Gram-negative organisms, in the presence of damaged bowel, particularly when strangulation is present. There is certainly every opportunity for bacterial proliferation in the obstructed bowel, and the devitalised bowel wall offers little resistance to the further growth and spread of these organisms. It has already been mentioned that in the presence of strangulation there is a serosanguineous exudate from the serosal aspect of the involved bowel, and it has been shown in experimental animals that the injection of this material is highly lethal. Attempts have been made to separate the responsible toxins, which seem to reside in the particulate deposit resulting from centrifugation, and are not present in the clear supernatant. The important clinical lesson from this consideration is the earliest possible surgical correction where strangulation is suspected on clinical grounds, and the need for every effort to remove such potentially harmful exudate at operation and to minimise the chances of its reabsorption.

Clearly if total obstruction remains unrelieved there is a high risk that a damaged segment of bowel will undergo complete necrosis with the free escape of highly contaminated intestinal content into the peritoneum, thus causing a highly dangerous form of faecal peritonitis.

Paralytic or adynamic ileus

As has been mentioned, this condition appears clinically with several of the features of intestinal obstruction, namely abdominal distension and vomiting. There is, however, no pain, since the lack of propulsion of the intestinal contents is due to paralysis of a segment of the bowel wall and further reflex suppression of the normal motility. A transient cessation of intestinal movement is invariable after any abdominal laparatomy, but the period of such suspended activity is usually limited to a few hours after the operation. More prolonged paralysis of a segment of the intestine may result from a variety of factors.

Peritonitis

Certainly widespread general peritonitis is usually characterized by complete paralysis of intestinal movement, and it used to be thought that even a short segment of small intestine lying in contact with a localised collection of pus would remain completely paralysed until the infective process began to resolve. However, this does not always occur, and conversely there may be temporary paralysis of quite long segments of intestine associated with localized areas of the peritonitis, but at some distance from the actual physical contact with the infection.

Retroperitoneal irritation

Paralytic ileus may also occur in association with haematomata in the retroperitoneal area, damage to the kidney, fractures of the thoracolumbar spine, and after direct surgical interference in and around this area. Such ileus is almost certainly reflex in origin.

Drugs

Some degree of paralysis of intestinal movement might be expected after drugs such as atropine and ganglion blocking agents, but in addition this is seen as an occasional sequel to a variety of drugs such as nortryptiline and amytryptiline and various hypotensive agents.

In each of these causes of paralytic ileus it is likely that both local and reflex pathways participate. The direct effects of local irritants may act through the intrinsic nerve plexuses or very short reflex arcs. The longer arcs are probably all concerned with sympathetic pathways in the splanchnic nerves.

Experimentally a form of paralytic ileus can be induced by the artificial induction of potassium deficiency, and it has therefore been argued that potassium depletion may be a factor contributing to clinical paralytic ileus. It is doubtful, however, whether this is a significant factor in most acutely occurring ileus states following operation or resulting from retroperitoneal irritation. There is little evidence to support the use of potassium administration in the treatment of paralytic ileus.

REFERENCES

Adibi S A, Kim Y S 1981 Peptide absorption and hydrolysis. In: Johnson L R, Christensen J, Grossman M I et al (eds) Physiology of the Gastrointestinal Tract, Vol. 2 p 1073–1095

Bayliss W M, Starling E H 1902 The mechanism of pancreatic secretion. Journal of Physiology, London 28: 325–353

Bloom S R, Polak J M 1981 Gut Hormones, 2nd edn. Churchill Livingstone, Edinburgh

Booth C C 1961 The metabolic effects of intestinal resection in man. Postgraduate Medical Journal 37: 725–739

Booth C C 1970 Enterocyte in coeliac disease. British Medical Journal iii: 725N–731

Burland W L, Samuel P D 1972 Transport across the intestine. Churchill Livingstone, Edinburgh

Carey M C, Small D M 1970 The characteristics of mixed micellar solutions with particular reference to bile. American Journal of Medicine 49: 590–608

Cohn I Jr 1962 The toxic factor in closed loop obstruction. American Journal of Surgery 104: 482–489

Crane R K 1968 A concept of the digestive-absorptive surface of the small intestine. In: Code C F (ed) Handbook of physiology. The Williams and Wilkins Co, Maryland, Sect 5, 5: 2535

Creamer B 1967 The turnover of the epithelium of the small intestine. British Medical Bulletin 23: 226–230

Creamer B 1973 Tutorials in postgraduate medicine: the small intestine. Heinemann, London

Donaldson R M Jr 1964 Normal bacterial populations of the intestine and their relation to intestinal function. New England Journal of Medicine, 270: 938–945, 994–1001, 1050–1056

Gallacher N D, Playout M R 1969 Absorption of saturated and unsaturated fatty acids by rat jejunium and ileum. Gastroenterology 57: 9–18

Grace R 1971 The handling of water and electrolytes by the small bowel following the relief of intestinal obstruction. British Journal of Surgery, 58: 760–764

Gray G M, Cooper H L 1971 Protein digestion and absorption. Gastroenterology, 61: 535–544

Grossman M I 1974 Candidate hormones of the gut. Gastroenterology 67: 730–755

Hartman R S, Butterworth C E, Hartman R E, Crosby W H, Shurai A I 1960 An electron microscopic investigation of the jejunal epithelium in sprue. Gastroenterology 38: 506–516

Hermon-Taylor J, Code C F 1971 Localisations of the duodenal pacemaker and its role in the organisation of duodenal myoelectric activity. Gut 12: 40–47

Hofmann A F, Borgstrom B 1964 The intraluminal phase of fat digestion in man: the lipid content of the micellar and oil phases of intestinal content obtained during fat digestion and absorption. Journal of Clinical Investigation 43: 247–257

Lipkin M 1965 Cell replication in the gastrointestinal tract of man. Gastroenterology 48: 616–624

Losowsky M S 1974 Malabsorption in Clinical Practice. Churchill Livingstone, Edinburgh

Love A H G, Mitchell T G, Phillips R A 1968 Water and sodium absorption in the human intestine. Journal of Physiology 195: 133–140, London

Marsh M N, Swift J A, Williams E D 1968 Studies of small intestinal mucosa with the scanning electron microscope. British Medical Journal iv: 95–96

Pearse A G E, Coulling I, Weavers B, Friesen S 1970 The endocrine polypeptide cells of the human stomach, duodenum and jejunum. Gut 11: 649–658

Peters T J 1970 Intestinal peptidases. Gut 11: 720–725

Schultz S G, Frizzell R A 1972 An overview of intestinal absorptive and secretory processes. Gastroenterology 63: 161–170

Shields R 1965 The absorption of secretion of fluid and electrolytes by the obstructed bowel. British Journal of Surgery 52: 774–779

Shields R 1968 Syndromes of water and electrolyte depletion of intestinal origin. Scottish Medical Journal 13: 122–132

Shields R 1974 The digestion and absorption of food and fluids. In: Wells C, Kyle J, Dunphy J E (eds) Scientific Foundations of Surgery Heinemann, London

Sleisenger M H 1983 Malabsorption and nutritional support. Clinics in Gastroenterology, W B Saunders, London

Tabaqchali S, Booth C C 1970 Bacteria and the small intestine. In: Card W I, Greamer B (eds) Butterworths, London, pp 471–481

Tomasi T B 1972 Secretory immunoglobulins. New England Journal of Medicine, 287: 500–512

Trier J S 1968 Morphology of the epithelium of the small intestine. In: Code C F (ed) Sect 6, III. The Williams and Wilkins Co, Maryland

Ugolev A M 1972 Membrane digestion. Gut 13: 735–747

Colon

The principal roles of the colon are to accept each day approximately 1 l of fluid intestinal content from the small intestine after it has completed its task of digestion-absorption, to reabsorb about 900 ml of the water, plus some sodium and chloride, to add a little potassium, and generally to firm it up and retain it until convenient for a coordinated act of emptying. We are concerned, therefore, mainly with the motility pattern and the further steps in absorption which take place throughout the colon. Since surgeons often require to excise considerable segments of the large bowel for malignant and other diseases, there is interest in the effects which such resections may have on normal function. Furthermore, the colon is an important site for the reabsorption of nitrogenous substances which play a role in the syndrome known as portasystemic encephalopathy complicating liver disease particularly in the presence of significant portacaval shunts. Finally, the colon may be obstructed by cancer or other processes, and this may cause fluid, electrolyte and metabolic problems.

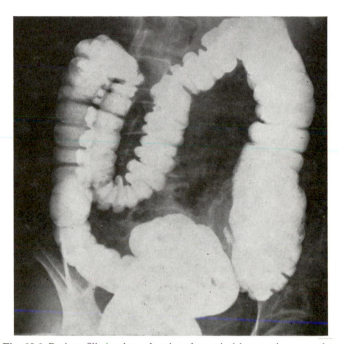

Fig. 18.1 Barium-filled colon, showing the typical haustration caused by the 'principal waves'.

MOTILITY OF THE COLON

The principal motor activity in the colon is basically the same as for the small intestine, namely segmentation. As in the small intestine this is characterized by the appearance of contraction rings separated by a few centimetres, which in turn give way to relaxation at the areas of the original rings, and the subsequent development of new contraction rings in the previously relaxed intervening segments. Repetition of this cycle encourages mixing and dispersion of the bowel content to assist in water absorption. The rate of the segmentation movements in the colon is much slower than in the small intestine, being only 2–4 per minute. They are probably responsible for the normally well developed 'haustration' pattern seen on barium enema examination (Fig. 18.1)

In addition, true peristaltic waves are believed to occur in the colon, but to be relatively infrequent. They are propagated only along short lengths of the bowel wall, and it is unlikely that they are important in the forward propulsion of the bowel content.

The third type of motility sequence, which is important in the distal emptying of the bowel, is mass contraction; this involves vigorous muscular contraction over a considerable length of the colon, passing in a distal direction, expelling the contents into the descending and sigmoid portions of the colon. It seems that regular daily somatic activity is important in stimulating these mass contractions, and when attempts are made to study them in individuals resting in bed, they usually disappear. Following a normally active daily routine it is probable that mass contraction occurs 2 or 3 times throughout the 24-hour period.

In addition to these principal types of movement it is possible that occasionally antiperistalsis, i.e. true peristaltic waves propagated in a proximal direction instead of the usual distal one, may occur.

ELECTRICAL ACTIVITY AND PRESSURE CHANGES

The interpretation of the electrical activity in the colon is much more difficult than in the small bowel, and there is not apparently a regular gradient of uniform slow wave pattern of steadily diminishing frequency passing from the proximal to distal segments. What slow wave activity there is may be intermittent, and possibly there are two basic rhythms of different frequencies and speeds of transit. Superimposed on these are also various other types of electrical activity which again may be of a wider range of types than occurs in small intestine.

Difficulties have also arisen in the interpretation of pressure waves recorded from different segments of the colon and rectum. To some extent the techniques used, i.e. whether recordings are made from balloons of different sizes and tensions, or from open-ended tubes with various rates of perfusion, may be responsible for some of the apparent differences in pressure wave form.

There are obviously difficulties in quantifying changes both in electrical activity and pressure; it is therefore an even more complex matter attempting to correlate precisely changes in pressure with the pattern of electrical activity in the bowel wall, or with radiographic recordings of the change in outline of the bowel.

Analyses of the various pressure wave forms suggest that there may be four distinctly separate types of wave as outlined in Table 18.1 and Figure 18.2. In the colon, Type 1 waves predominate, regardless of the method of recording, but the Type 2 and particularly the Type 4 waves are seen mainly when balloon recordings are made.

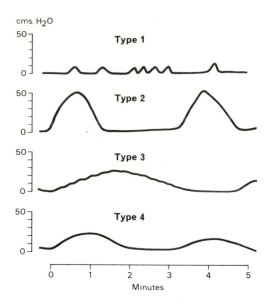

Fig. 18.2 Patterns of pressure wave.

Table 18.1

Type 1	Small monophasic waves lasting from 5–10 seconds, and of low amplitude varying from 5–15 cm of water.
Type 2	Monophasic waves of longer duration — up to 60 seconds, and higher amplitude extending up to 50 cm of water.
Type 3	More prolonged overall increases in baseline pressure above that of resting bowel, with perhaps superimposed waves of either Type 1 or Type 2, the whole complex lasting usually for several minutes before reverting to the resting picture.
Type 4	Waves of intermediate durations, 1–2 minutes, basically a large simple spike wave of 15–20 cm of water.

Overall the various wave forms are much reduced during sleep, and all increase in the morning on resumption of activity and the ingestion of food. It is not possible, however, to relate the wave forms to translation of content along the colon, or other simple physiological changes.

Paradoxically, there is often a diminished pressure wave activity in patients with diarrhoea, and often exaggerated pressure wave activity in those with constipation.

The increase in colonic motility seen to follow soon after the ingestion of a meal, particularly early in the morning, has been partly attributed to a 'gastrocolic reflex'. Whether this is mediated by nervous activity as the word reflex suggests, or by the participation of hormones from the upper gastrointestinal tract, e.g. gastrin, is uncertain. The colonic response, however, occurs quite briskly after the entry of ingested food into the stomach, duodenum and upper jejunum, and it appears to affect the motility in both the small and large intestines. There are both an increased amplitude and frequency of the motility waves, which last for a few minutes and then spontaneously subside.

THE NERVE SUPPLY OF THE COLON

The colon derives a nerve supply from both the sympathetic and parasympathetic outflows of the autonomic system. Largely as deduction from animal experimentation with nerve stimulation or ablation, or pharmacological mimicking of autonomic effects, the view has arisen that in general the sympathetic system acts to inhibit, and the parasympathetic system to stimulate, motility in the colon and rectum. However, it seems more likely that both sets of autonomic fibres are more concerned with alterations in the blood supply to the large bowel than the motility pattern, and it is clear that a completely normal pattern of electrical activity, muscular contraction, and pressure waves can exist following total bilateral sympathectomy.

The pathway by which sensory impulses pass centrally from the colon is in the sympathetic nerve chains, and these are relayed mainly in the first two lumbar sympathetic ganglia on both sides.

In addition to these extrinsic nerves there is an intrinsic plexus amply supplied with ganglion cells, lying in the muscular and submucous coats. It is believed that this intrinsic plexus coordinates the purposeful emptying movements in the colon and rectum, this conclusion being largely based on the well-known clinical finding of obstruction in the condition of congenital megacolon, which is characterized by a total absence of ganglion cells from this plexus over a short distal segment of bowel.

Sympathetic supply

Sympathetic fibres destined for the colon derive from the lower thoracic and upper lumbar segments of the cord, and pass to the lumbar ganglia, from which postganglionic fibres pass in the splanchnic nerves to be distributed to the bowel along with the superior and inferior mesenteric blood vessels. Considerable alterations in the blood flow to the mucosa and other layers of the colon can take place as a result of emotion such as fear, anger or resentment, and in response to changes in skin temperature and other afferent stimuli. Such changes are predominantly mediated by the sympathetic supply. To a large extent the pool of blood in the vessels of the entire intestinal tract, including the colon, constitutes the 'splanchnic reservoir'.

The influence of the sympathetic nerves on colonic movement is not altogether clear, and although short-lived changes in motility pattern can be seen to follow experimental stimulation of segments of the sympathetic outflow, it is doubtful whether there is significant influence of sympathetic discharge to the colon under completely normal conditions. There is experimental evidence that noradrenaline may at the same time cause some degree of relaxation by action on alpha and beta adrenergic receptors, and stimulation by action on alpha adrenergic excitatory fibres.

It has been suggested that retroperitoneal irritation, leading to paralytic ileus, causes this abnormality as the result of direct stimulation of the sympathetic outflow to the colon and small intestine; certainly prolonged stimulation of the sympathetic nerves experimentally can induce a flaccid paralysis. However, depending upon the exact experimental conditions a whole range of motor responses, varying from stimulation to inhibition, can be obtained, and again the influence of sympathetic mediation in paralytic ileus is uncertain.

The parasympathetic supply

Terminal branches of the vagus nerve can be traced anatomically as far distally as about the middle of the transverse colon, but it is not certain whether these colonic fibres serve any physiological function. A second, and possibly more important parasympathetic innervation arises from the sacral outflow of the autonomic system. This arises mainly from the second and third sacral nerves, from which fibres pass forwards through the dense parietal pelvic fascia, giving fibres to the rectum; other fibres on the left side pass proximally along with the middle haemorrhoidal vessels to communicate with the hypogastric plexus and pass across the left common iliac vessels to enter the pelvic mesocolon. From here fibres can be traced proximally to the level of the middle of the descending colon. It is apparent, therefore, that this sacral outflow will be interrupted in operations involving radical resection of the rectum.

INTRINSIC NERVES OF THE COLON

There are two main networks of nerve fibres, one lying within the muscular coat and the other in the sub-mucosal layer. Both plexuses are liberally supplied with ganglion cells, which do not degenerate after section of the extrinsic nerves.

The main function of these plexuses is to coordinate motility responses in the colon in a purposeful way for the onward translation of colonic content. In the condition of true congenital megacolon, with a distal localized segment devoid of these ganglion cells but still liberally supplied with nerve bundles in the plexus areas, the affected segment is still quite capable of contraction and relaxation responses, and therefore it is not in the true sense of the word 'paralysed'. However, mass contractions, segmentations and peristalsis are not conducted across the aganglionic segment, although at more proximal levels the patterns of contraction may be quite normal. There is thus a physiological obstruction at the involved segment.

That reflex action within these intrinsic nerve plexuses has an afferent input from the mucosal aspect of the colon is demonstrated by the effects of local anaesthetic such as cocaine, applied to the mucosa, or the effects of atropine given systemically, on local coordinated muscular contraction in response to mechanical stimulation. Normally, mechanical stimulation of an area of mucosa will lead to local reflex contraction, but this reflex response is abolished by either of these procedures.

EFFECT OF DRUGS ON THE COLON

Morphine

The constipating effect of morphine and its derivatives is in part due to the delayed arrival of chyme from the small intestine, and in part to direct local action on colonic motility.

Within a few minutes of the injection of 15 mg of morphine sulphate there is an increase in the frequency and amplitude of segmentation waves, but peristalsis and other propulsive patterns are usually absent. The changes may not be uniform throughout the length of the colon, with some segments showing increased muscular activity while others remain quiescent. The net effect of these changes is a diminished transport of material along the colon and hence the constipating effect.

Adrenaline

Adrenaline, when given intravenously and occasionally also when given subcutaneously, causes a transient relaxation of the colon.

Atropine

All types of motility are reduced following the subcutaneous injection of 0.6–0.75 mg atropine sulphate, and the effect lasts for 1–2 hours. The inhibiting effect, however, is much more marked in the completely healthy colon than in disease states associated with increased muscular activity.

Neostigmine

The subcutaneous injection of 0.5 mg of neostigmine leads to an increase in background pressure, and also to an increase in the frequency and amplitude of propulsive movements within the colon. This usually leads to the passage of flatus, and often to defecation.

This drug is often administered by the anaesthetist towards the end of a general anaesthetic and the possibility should be borne in mind that the resulting powerful stimulation of colonic motility might put a colonic anastomosis at hazard of disruption.

Posterior pituitary extract

The intramuscular injection of 1 to 2 units is quickly followed (within 2–3 minutes) by an increase in propulsive movements and a diminution in the background of non-propulsive waves. The net result of this is a powerful emptying movement along the colon.

SECRETION IN THE COLON

Virtually the only materials to be secreted into the lumen of the colon from its mucosa are mucus and potassium.

The mucus is the product of the typical goblet cell distributed fairly evenly along the entire mucosa. Since the content of the colon becomes more formed as it passes distally through the organ, a certain amount of lubrication by the secreted mucus is helpful to facilitate passage. An exaggerated mucus production is seen in most disorders which are associated with chemical or mechanical irritation of the colonic mucosa.

To some extent linked with mucus production is the loss of potassium ions into the lumen. As in the small intestine, there is a two-way flux of water and various ions across the mucosa of the large bowel, and where potassium loss exceeds reabsorption, then the net effect may be regarded as a 'secretion' of the ion. The amount of potassium loss, however, is insignificant in physiological terms in health. The loss is greatly magnified, to clinically important levels in association with a villous tumour in the colon or rectum, which may lose very substantial amounts of potassium ion sufficient to render the patient hypokalaemic.

ABSORPTION BY THE COLON

Although it is well known that patients may remain in good health, with satisfactory water and electrolyte balance after total excision of the rectum and colon, there is no doubt that in normal health the colon does contribute to the absorption of water and electrolytes, chiefly of sodium. After panproctocolectomy, e.g. for ulcerative colitis, there is some degree of adaptation within the terminal small bowel to compensate for the loss of the absorptive area of the large bowel which permits the restoration of the satisfactory overall water and electrolyte balance.

As in the small intestine, there is a continual two-way flux of both water and electrolytes across the colonic mucosa, and indeed this traffic is in itself greater than the net absorption, so that small changes in the bi-directional flux can have a considerable influence on net losses or conservation of water and electrolytes.

As has been mentioned, the principal electrolyte absorbed from the normal, healthy colonic mucosa is sodium, and the amount absorbed is significantly greater in the caecum and ascending colon than in the more distal segments. The absorption is an active transport mechanism capable of moving sodium ions against a marked electrochemical gradient. The amount of sodium absorbed under physiological conditions is appreciably less than the maximal capacity, so that there is a considerable reserve for sodium absorption which may be called into action should the need arise from the introduction of an additional sodium load. The active mechanism for sodium transport differs from that in the small intestine, which is facilitated by the presence of sugars and amino acids. These, of course, would not normally be expected to appear in the colonic content to any significant amount, and thus an active mechanism for sodium absorption independent of these materials is required at this site.

Potassium, on the other hand, is absorbed in the large bowel by a purely passive process once the luminal concentration of this ion reaches a certain critical level of approximately 15 mmol/l. As with sodium, a greater amount of potassium absorption occurs in the proximal colon than in the distal reaches.

Chloride is absorbed from the colon by two processes. First, the bulk crosses the mucosa along with the sodium being absorbed, but in addition, the secondary mechanism of ion exchange for bicarbonate, to which reference has already been made in the small intestine chapter, takes place. As a result the overall absorption of chloride is more rapid and larger than that of the sodium.

As has been mentioned approximately 1–1.5 litres of water enter the caecum from the ileum in normal health throughout each 24-hour period, and all but about 100 ml is re-absorbed mainly in the proximal colon. The relatively large amount of water absorbed is the result of secondary passive transfer consequent on the absorption of sodium and chloride ions. However, additional amounts of water are almost certainly absorbed by the mechanism outlined in Chapter 17 dealing with the small bowel handling of water absorption. This invokes the theory of a difference in the permeability of the lumen to mucosa interface as compared to the looser and more permeable interface between the base of the cell and capillary.

As has been mentioned, there is normally a small loss of bicarbonate ions from the colon, and the principal source of these is probably the two-way ion exchange for chloride. Such an exchange involves the action of the enzyme carbonic anhydrase.

There is conflicting evidence about the capacity of the colonic mucosa to absorb glucose and other monosaccharides, but if this occurs it is certainly to a minimal degree, and not physiologically important.

Ammonia and urea

Urea, synthesized in the liver, and excreted in the bile, is broken down by bacteria mainly located within the colon with the subsequent production of ammonia. That the bacteria are the principal producers of this colonic ammonia is demonstrated by the fact that ammonia production virtually ceases following the administration of antibiotics which suppress these bacteria. Little or no urea itself is absorbed across the colonic mucosa, but under normal circumstances the majority of the ammonia ions released by the bacterial breakdown of the urea is absorbed readily by a passive process. Non-ionized NH_3 is more readily absorbed than the ionized NH_4 material, and so the relative proportions of these two ions will to a large extent determine the rate of ammonia absorption. This ratio is, in turn, influenced by the intra-colonic pH, the lower the pH the greater the amount of ionized NH_4. After absorption the ammonia is available to the liver for metabolic conversion, again into urea, and amino acids. It is important to note that although antibiotics may diminish the production of ammonia by colonic bacteria, they will not interfere with the colonic absorption of already formed ammonia within the bowel.

PORTASYSTEMIC ENCEPHALOPATHY

In health the nitrogenous substances formed in the colon by the bacterial digestion are absorbed into the portal blood and passed to the liver where they are further metabolized. In portal hypertension, however, the enlargement of natural portal-systemic anastomoses or the surgical construction of a portacaval shunt allows portal blood to enter the systemic veins directly, bypassing the liver. In such patients the central nervous disorder of portasystemic encephalopathy may arise, largely as a result of the direct entry into the systemic circulation of these metabolic products.

That the harmful toxic substances are of nitrogenous origin is apparent from several clinical observations. For example, the administration of antibiotics which are capable of reducing the bacterial content of the colon often leads to marked clinical improvement. Other measures such as total withdrawal of protein, the administration of enemas and purges, or the surgical removal or bypass of the greater part of the colon, may all improve the encephalopathy, and each of these measures has a place in the clinical management of the condition.

A further therapeutic measure which may help to diminish the absorption of ammonia is the administration of lactulose, a synthetic disaccharide which reduces the pH within the colon, thereby converting an increased proportion of the ammonia to the relatively-insoluble NH_4 form and thus 'trapping' an increased amount of ammonia within the bowel lumen.

Although there is reason to incriminate ammonia as an important aetiological factor in the clinical condition of portasystemic encephalopathy, and it is usual to find elevated blood ammonia levels in this disorder, there is not always a clear linear relationship between the degree of elevation of this ion and the severity of the clinical state; it may well be that other nitrogenous materials contribute to the condition.

OBSTRUCTION OF THE COLON

Obstruction of the large bowel is much commoner than obstruction of the small intestine, and is usually due to either carcinoma or diverticulitis, or more rarely volvulus of a segment, especially the sigmoid colon. Although the basic clinical features are similar to those already described for obstruction of the small intestine, there are some differences in emphasis of the individual components.

Dull lower abdominal pain is usually an early symptom, although it may not have such a clear-cut rhythmic colicky nature as that of the small bowel. Secondly, vomiting may be quite late in making an appearance, there being continual satisfactory absorption in the small intestine for some time after the onset of the colonic obstruction. The abdomen will generally distend, although for a while in distal large bowel obstruction the ileocaecal valve may remain competent, so that the distension by gas and liquid is confined to the large bowel itself, thus producing a predominantly flank distension. Absolute constipation for faeces and flatus is usually early in onset in obstruction of the colon.

It follows that the fluid and electrolyte disturbance and peripheral circulatory failure which are often dominant features in obstruction of the small intestine may not occur for many hours or even days after the onset of large gut obstruction. However, damage to the bowel by the mechanical effects of incarceration, by inflammatory disease, or by the effects of strangulation may also occur in the large bowel, and they may be of very serious consequence in view of the normal high bacterial content of this organ.

With carcinoma of the colon the obstruction may develop gradually, and this is seen particularly with the common type of encircling carcinoma arising in the left side of the colon. As the malignant stricture develops there may be a gradual accumulation of solid faecal material proximal to the lesion, and although the initial complaint may be of constipation, this may be supplemented by a type of 'diarrhoea' which is caused by the escape of the liquid part of the bowel content past this valvular type of obstruction. This so-called 'spurious diarrhoea' may be aggravated by the patient taking laxatives in an attempt to overcome his initial constipation. Eventually obstruction becomes complete by a combination of further growth of the tumour, and impaction by the solid faecal masses. If the obstruction develops gradually in this fashion there may be quite extreme degrees of colonic distension proximal to the carcinoma. A considerable increase in intraluminal pressure up to as much as 40–50 cm of water may occur, and the predominantly gaseous distension imperils the blood supply to the bowel, particularly in the caecal area which may become necrotic and eventually disrupt. A fulminating peritonitis with Gram-negative toxaemia ensues, and this is usually fatal within a few hours.

Most forms of obstruction of the large bowel require urgent surgical correction, apart from volvulus of the sigmoid colon, which can often be alleviated by postural changes and the passage of a flatus tube through a sigmoidoscope. The operation required may either be primary resection of the diseased segment of bowel, or more often some form of colostomy to allow temporary drainage of the obstructed segment, recovery of the patient and the bowel from the effects of the obstruction, and a subsequent planned elective procedure to eradicate disease.

ANORECTAL FUNCTION

Several times each day mass contractions and other propulsive movements in the colon deliver large quantities of faecal material into the most distal segment of the large bowel, which seems well adapted to permit the retention of this material until a time which is socially convenient for the individual. The first prime role of the anorectal region is therefore to maintain continence throughout the greater part of the 24 hours. Secondly, a coordinated mechanism to achieve satisfactory emptying of the distal bowel at the appropriate time is required, and therefore the second role is concerned with the act of defecation. Both of these mechanisms depend on an inflow of sensory information, and each to a large extent involves several types of reflex activity.

Anal continence

Anal continence depends upon the ability to suppress the desire to defecate, which results from the filling and distension of the rectum. Normally such distension of the rectum produces two effects. Firstly, there is a sensation of 'fullness' experienced partly in the perineal region, and partly, although there seems to be some degree of individual variation, low in the hypogastric area. Whether this sensation arises from the wall of the rectum itself, or is the result of the stimulation of afferent fibres in the extrarectal structures, e.g. the puborectalis sling, or the pararectal neurovascular pedicles, is uncertain. Secondly, there is a reflex relaxation of the internal anal sphincter, which in turn permits the descent of faecal material into the upper part of the anal canal. At this level the sensation is of quite a different nature from that within the rectum proper. Whereas the rectum itself is only responsive to distension, the anal canal is sensitive to touch, heat and cold, pain, and there is the capacity to distinguish the physical nature of the luminal content, for example to distinguish between gas and liquid. The interpretation of such information allows the individual the opportunity to decide whether it is socially convenient to permit the escape of contents or remain continent.

At the same time as the reflex inhibition of the internal anal sphincter which follows on distension of the rectum, there is a contraction of the external anal sphincter. The positive pressure in the lower anal canal resulting from a combination of this contraction of the external sphincter plus the residual, although reduced, contraction of the internal anal sphincter is normally sufficient to prevent the escape of anal contents. In addition the voluntary contraction of the muscles of the pelvic floor, and voluntarily exercised increase in the action of the external anal sphincter can reinforce the anal canal pressure, and thus assist continence. Simple physical factors also contribute, such as the normal angle between the rectum and anal canal and the surface tension exerted between apposing surfaces of the closed canal. In health these various mechanisms to ensure complete anal continence do not obtrude significantly into consciousness. The reflex changes in both the internal and external anal sphincter resulting from distension of the rectum probably travel mainly in short nerve pathways either within the bowel wall itself, or involving short sacral arcs. The sensation of fullness appears to be conveyed in the sacral parasympathetic outflow, and the more urgent sensations from stimulation of the sensitive anal canal, chiefly by fluid, are the main ones which rise clearly into consciousness. Thus only when an unusual degree of reinforcement of the continence mechanism is required is the subject made fully aware of the anorectal changes.

Defecation

Where there is no opportunity for the influence of higher cortical control, such as following transection of the spinal cord, a completely automatic reflex coordinated process of defecation can occur. Although there is an initial phase of constipation following a sudden transection of the cord, sooner or later automatic reflex defaecation is established. The prime initiating stimulus to emptying the bowel is distension of the rectum, which, as has been discussed in the previous section on continence, normally leads to relaxation of the internal anal sphincter, and consequent reduction of pressure in the anal canal. Without the influence of higher centres, this will be followed by mass peristaltic movements emptying the proximal colon, further augmentation of intrarectal pressure, a certain amount of 'uptake' of the anal sphincter region, more complete sphincter relaxation, resulting usually in powerful expulsion of the contents. Furthermore, under these circumstances the patient will be unaware of the entire process, and both the bowel and bladder may empty at the same time. Clearly the coordination of the actions leading to this form of defecation are all contained either within the bowel itself, or in short low spinal reflex arcs.

In the healthy intact individual, however, clearly a large number of higher cortical influences are brought to bear on this basic automatic reflex pattern. Although the main stimulus to defecation is probably distension of the rectum, the subsequent series of steps leading to emptying of the bowel is normally suppressed throughout the 24-hour period, unless the distension occurs at a time which is socially convenient for the individual. To a large extent the pattern of normal defecation in the adult has become conditioned by the long-continued suppression of the stimulus to empty over the years, so that this factor in

itself, 'training', may be the dominant one in determining the time of emptying, frequently first thing in the morning, or after the first meal of the day. In many normal people this may be the only time at which the response to rectal distension is the desire to defecate, followed by the act of defecation itself. Yet at other times throughout the 24 hours, as is well known from clinical experience, there may be a considerable amount of faecal material contained within the rectum. It is likely that a number of factors contribute to the actual initiation of the act of defecation.

Firstly, as has been mentioned earlier in this chapter, there is often in health an increase in the frequency and strength of mass emptying movements in the proximal colon in the early morning, and on the resumption of physical activity. Secondly, the assumption of the sitting or squatting posture may considerably reduce the angle between the rectum and anal canal which normally obtains in the erect posture. This straightening of the most distal part of the large bowel may in itself facilitate descent of the rectal contents into the lower more sensitive region. Thirdly, an increase in intra-abdominal pressure brought about by voluntary contraction of the abdominal muscles may add to the hydrostatic forces at work within the bowel itself. Fourthly, a certain degree of voluntary reduction in external anal sphincter contraction, in addition to any reflex changes there might be in the combined sphincters, may be permitted. The contribution of these various factors may vary from individual to individual, and from one community to another, but it seems likely that a summation of these different factors plus the conditioning process of habit are all brought to play on the usual normal pattern of defecation.

Once faecal matter starts its passage through the terminal anal canal there is further fairly complete inhibition of sphincter contraction, and completion of the act of defecation is mainly effected by contractions both in the abdominal wall muscles and in the external sphincter and muscles of the pelvic floor.

In summary, although defecation can be shown to have a basis of coordinated reflex activity, and in lower animals it may arise predominantly from such action, in normal civilised man the pattern of defaecation and the individual factors which influence it are predominantly those arising from cortical activity and voluntary action.

Absorption from the rectum

The only significant absorption which has been shown experimentally to arise from the rectum is that of water and sodium. The degree to which both these materials may be absorbed is clearly much less than that for the more proximal segments of the bowel, and in health it is doubtful if this reaches any significance. At most it seems possible that a small contribution to 'solidifying' the faecal masses may arise at this level.

REFERENCES

Chaudrey N A, Truelove S C 1961 Colonic motility: a critical review of methods and results. American Journal of Medicine 31: 86–106

Connell A M 1961 The motility of the pelvic colon. Gut 2: 175–186

Dinoso V P, Murphy S N S 1981 Characterization of a repetitive motor complex (MC) in the descending colon in man. Gastroenterology 80:1137

Duthie H L 1975 Colonic motility in man. Mayo Clinic Proceedings 50:519

Duthie H L 1984 Physiology of anus, rectum and colon. In: Goligher J (ed.) Surgery of the Anus, Rectum and Colon. Baillière Tindall, London

Duthie H L, Bennett R C 1963 The relation of sensation in the anal canal to the functional anal and sphincter: a possible factor in anal continence. Gut 4: 179–182

Duthie H L, Watts J M 1965 Contribution of the external anal sphincter to the pressure zone in the anal canal. Gut 6: 64–68

Fink S, Friedman G 1960 The differential effect of drugs on the proximal and distal colon. American Journal of Medicine 28: 534–540

Goligher J C, Duthie H L 1984 Surgical anatomy and physiology of the colon, rectum and anus. In: Goligher J C (ed) Surgery of the Anus, Rectum and Colon, Baillière, Tindall and Cassell, London p 1–47

Holdstock D J, Misiewicz J J, Smith T, Rowland E N 1970 Propulsion (mass movements) in the human colon and its relationship to meals and somatic activity. Gut 11:91

Levitan R, Fordtran J S, Burrows B A, Ingelfinger F J 1962 Water and salt absorption in the human colon. Journal of Clinical Investigation 41: 1754–1759

Lipkin M, Almy T, Bell B M 1962 Pressure-volume characteristics of the human colon. Journal of Clinical Investigation 41: 1831–1839

Phillips S F, Edwards D A W 1965 Some aspects of anal continence and defecation. Gut 6: 396–406

Read M G, Read N W 1982 Role of anorectal sensation in preserving continence. Gut 12:350

Ritchie J A, Ardran G M, Truelove S C 1962 Motor activity of the sigmoid colon of humans. A combined study by intraluminal pressure recording and cineradiography. Gastroenterology 43: 642–668

Schuster M M, Hendrix T R, Mindeloff A I 1963 The internal and sphincter response: manometric studies on its normal physiology, neural pathways, and alteration in bowel disorders. Journal of Clinical Investigation 42: 196–207

Todd I P 1959 Discussion on rectal continence. Proceedings of the Royal Society of Medicine 52: 91–93

Liver

INTRODUCTION

The liver has been described in the past as being a large organ about which little is known. There is now much less mystery surrounding the liver's many functions and disorders, but there are still many aspects about which our knowledge remains incomplete.

The remarkably numerous functions of the liver are fundamental to survival. With many of these functions the surgeon requires only a superficial acquaintance, but with some he must be professionally familiar. In order to meet these varying requirements, this chapter deals in a relatively brief manner with the general functions of the liver, while more detailed consideration is reserved for the derangements to hepatic function or circulation which have a direct bearing on surgical practice.

The chapter is arranged in seven main sections:

1. *Structure*: an account of the micro- and macroscopic structure of the liver and its vasculature.

2. *Circulation*: a description of the hepatic blood supply, its clinical measurement and the factors controlling it.

3. *Functions*: an outline of the metabolic functions of the liver, concluding with a description of the non-metabolic functions of biliary secretion and the reticulo-endothelial (mononuclear phagocytic) system.

4. *Portal hypertension*: an account of the causes, effects, investigation and therapy of raised portal pressure.

5. *Hepatocellular failure*: this section explains the causes, effects and treatment of liver failure, with particular emphasis on the pathogenesis of portal-systemic encephalopathy.

6. *Jaundice*: a description of the deranged physiology of jaundice, and an outline of the diagnostic tests used to assess this condition.

7. *Liver regeneration*: an explanation of the current concepts of the mechanisms controlling hepatic regeneration after surgical removal of part of the liver mass, and an outline of the metabolic changes following resection.

STRUCTURE OF THE LIVER

The microscopic structure of the liver has excited comment and conjecture since the 17th century, when Malpighi (1666) first described and named the hepatic lobule. The concept of the lobular structure of the liver was further developed by Kiernan (1833), who described the relationship of one lobule to another and their relation to the vascular system. The lobules are about 1 mm in diameter, and comprise strands of liver cells which appear to converge towards a 'central vein' which is a tributary of the hepatic veins draining into the inferior vena cava. When well developed, the lobules are surrounded by delicate fibrous tissue deriving from the portal tracts. Lobulation of this kind is clearly seen in the liver of the pig, but is indistinct or even lacking in most animals, including man. The fine fibrous tissue framework may become grossly thickened in certain types of liver disease, and this may produce mechanical compression of the sinusoids which results in portal hypertension (see section on portal hypertension).

The liver cells are polyhedral in shape, and approximately 30 μm in diameter, and together comprise about 60% of the liver substance. The life-span of liver cells in the rat has been studied by an autoradiographic technique using tritiated thymidine: the normal life-span varies between approximately 200 and 450 days (MacDonald, 1961). Bile is formed in the hepatic cells, and is secreted into the fine polygonal network of canaliculi, which are minute tubules lying in grooves on the contact face of the liver cells. The canaliculi drain bile into intralobular ductules or cholangioles which in turn drain into larger ducts in the portal tracts. The bile passes to the gallbladder for concentration and storage, before its eventual expulsion into the duodenum (see Ch. 20). There is always hepatic cellular tissue between the canaliculi and the vascular channels, so that normally the blood and the bile are never able to mix. The liver cells are thus well positioned to be

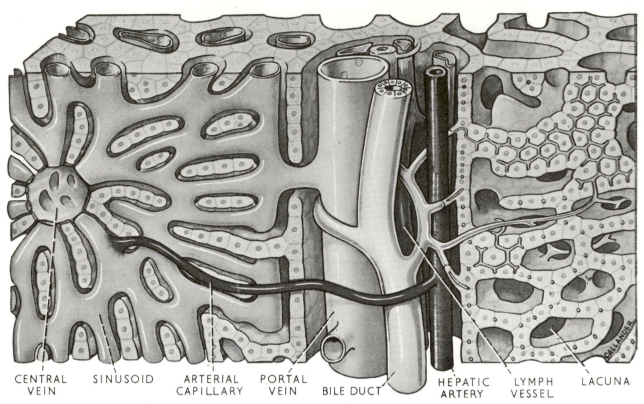

CENTRAL VEIN   SINUSOID   ARTERIAL CAPILLARY   PORTAL VEIN   BILE DUCT   HEPATIC ARTERY   LYMPH VESSEL   LACUNA

Fig. 19.1 Scheme of the structure of the liver. (After Hans Elias, by permission of G D Searle & Co., from Research in the Service of Medicine 37: 26, 1953).

able to transfer materials from the blood into the bile.

A useful representation of the above scheme is illustrated in Figure 19.1, which shows the structure of the vascular and biliary channels in adjacent lobules surrounding a portal tract. The diagram, however, retains the classical idea of the hepatic microstructure in the lobular arrangement around a central hepatic vein. In recent years, there has emerged considerable support for an alternative description in which the functional unit is a group of cells surrounding a terminal branch of the *portal vein*. This 'portal structural unit' was first described by Mall in 1906, and developed by Rappaport et al (1954) who injected coloured gelatin into the portal vein and hepatic artery of rabbits and dogs and observed that the direction of blood flow could be most accurately described as being from the centre to the periphery of the microvascular network and not vice versa. The latter publication also drew attention to the erroneous concept of 'central' necrosis of liver cells around hepatic venous tributaries, pointing out that these cells are really peripherally placed in relation to the portal tracts from which they derive nutriment.

The portal tracts, and not the central veins, should now be regarded as the essential framework of the liver: they supply blood from the hepatic artery and portal vein to, and drain bile and lymph from, aggregations of liver cells

formed in berry-like masses or 'acini' (Rappaport, 1973). These cell masses are closely packed, and the so-called 'central veins' are wedged in the interstices between them (Fig. 19.2).

The foregoing has dealt exclusively with the general microscopic structure of the liver. A more detailed description of the way in which arterial and portal blood are thought to mix in the sinusoids is given in the section on circulation.

The major importance to the surgeon of the orderly structural arrangement of the liver lies at the macroscopic level, where the divisions of the vascular and biliary structures separate the liver into functionally distinct, though anatomically fused, units. The most obvious anatomical marking on the surface of the liver is the deep fissure caused by the insertion of the falciform ligament, the free edge of which contains the ligamentum teres (the remnant of the umbilical vein). This was for long mistakenly believed to mark the division of the liver into its right and left lobes, but this division in fact is found at the porta hepatis, the point of entry of the portal vein and hepatic artery and exit of the common hepatic ducts. While this is clearly seen on the inferior surface of the liver, there is no plane of demarcation visible on the dome of the liver between the right and left lobes; however, during the operation of right hepatic lobectomy, when the right

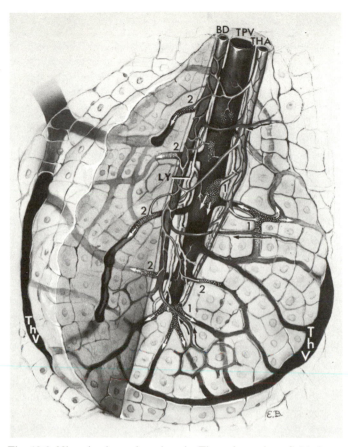

Fig. 19.2 Microcirculatory hepatic unit. The unit consists of: (a) the terminal portal venule (TPV) with the sinusoids branching off it and forming a glomus; (b) the hepatic arteriole (THA) lacing with its branches a plexus around the terminal bile ductule (BD). The THA empties either directly (1) or via the peribiliary plexus (2) into the sinusoids and TPV. The sinusoids run along the outside of cell plates and cords. The glomus of sinusoids is drained by at least two terminal hepatic venules (ThV). LY = lymphatics. (Reproduced from A M. Rappaport; Microvascular Research 6:212, 1973; by kind permission of the author and publisher).

branch of the portal vein and of the hepatic artery have been ligated, a sharp line of demarcation soon begins to appear on the surface of the liver between the ischaemic right lobe and the normally vascularized left. This plane of cleavage between the major right and left lobes runs through the bed of the gallbladder and down to the vena cava as it passes behind the liver inferiorly and emerges superiorly to penetrate the diaphragm high behind the dome of the liver. The branching of the portal vein and hepatic artery takes place outside the liver substance at the hilum. Within the liver substance these vessels divide again to supply an anterior and posterior segment in the right lobe, and a medial and lateral segment in the left. It is in fact at the plane of demarcation between the left medial and the left lateral segments that the falciform ligament cleaves the left lobe of the liver. Further branching then takes place within these four primary segments to form superior and inferior divisions, and then further

successive branching continues down to the level of the liver acini. Tracing the biliary channels in the opposite direction from their origin in the microscopic portal tracts, the anastomosing channels of the progressively larger and larger bile ducts follow approximately the same anatomical course as the hepatic arterial and portal venous branches, the right and left hepatic ducts joining to form the common hepatic duct just anterior to the bifurcation of the portal vein at the hilum. The detailed anatomy of all of these vascular and biliary channels is extremely variable, and knowledge of these variations is essential for safe surgery in this area. A detailed account of the surgical anatomy of the liver and biliary tract is given by Bismuth (1986).

All the hepatic veins drain into the inferior vena cava, and none of them has a long extrahepatic course. The ramifications of these veins within the hepatic parenchyma are different from those of the hepatic arterial, portal and biliary structures. The right hepatic vein lies in a plane between the right anterior and posterior segments and the middle hepatic vein in the plane between the right and left lobes, receiving tributaries from both lobes. The left hepatic vein drains the left lateral segment, usually directly into the vena cava. There are in addition a number of small veins draining from the posterior aspect of the right lobe directly into the inferior vena cava which lies in a groove in the right lobe at this point.

This segmental anatomy is of great importance to the surgeon, since resection of the entire right liver for example may be performed leaving an anatomically and functionally intact left liver vascularized by portal vein and hepatic artery and drained by bile duct and hepatic veins. Furthermore, this operation of right hepatectomy may be extended to include the medial segment of the left lobe, provided the vessels can be left undamaged during this dissection. This 'extended right hepatectomy' or 'trisegmentectomy' may be necessary for curative surgery for tumours arising at the confluence of the hepatic ducts.

HEPATIC CIRCULATION

In 1942, Mann aptly commented that the subject of liver circulation 'is almost buried under its own literature'. Forty years on, the number of publications on the subject has become considerably greater, but a clearer understanding of the hepatic circulation has gradually begun to emerge.

Liver blood supply

The liver derives its blood supply from two sources — the hepatic artery and the portal vein. Blood from these sources intermingles in the sinusoids, which are drained by the hepatic venous system into the inferior vena cava.

Portal vein

The tributaries of the portal vein collect the venous outflow from the whole extent of the intestinal tract from the lower oesophagus to the rectum, and in addition drain the pancreas and spleen. The portal vein itself is short, measuring 6–8 cm from its origin at the union of the superior mesenteric vein and the splenic vein, to its termination at the porta hepatis where it divides into branches for the right and left lobes of the liver. Within the liver the portal veins branch repeatedly and the finest branches become continuous with liver sinusoids. The sinusoids differ from ordinary capillaries in having no endothelium, so that blood is in direct contact with hepatic cells. At intervals along the sinusoids lie the stellate Kupffer cells which belong to the reticulo-endothelial system.

Until quite recently, it has been considered that the portal vein is too short to allow complete mixing of the blood which enters it, and that blood from the splenic vein passes mainly to the left lobe of the liver while blood from the superior mesenteric vein passes mainly to the right lobe. It is now believed that constant portal blood streamlining is most unlikely, but that it may be partly streamlined in certain circumstances; for example, the proportion of splenic blood passing to the right and left lobe can be altered by changing the patient's posture. It is therefore improbable that the pattern of hepatic distribution of portal inflow can explain the localization of blood-borne hepatic lesions seen in some patients (Groszmann et al, 1971).

The portal vein normally carries 70–75% of the total blood flow to the liver, the remainder being supplied by the hepatic artery. Portal venous blood flow in man is usually about 1.0–1.2 l/min. Since portal blood is postcapillary it is already partly deoxygenated, the oxygen content being approximately 16 ml/dl. Despite this degree of deoxygenation, the portal venous blood is able to supply up to 70 per cent of the liver's oxygen requirement because of its large volume flow. The oxygen content of portal venous blood decreases during digestion, but this does not necessarily reduce the delivery of oxygen to the liver by this route since the portal blood flow is significantly increased in the postprandial period. The hepatic oxygen supply may be more at risk when the portal blood flow itself is significantly compromised; in this situation, however, the liver is able to extract oxygen with greater efficiency from the hepatic arterial blood and/or to increase its arterial flow rate, thereby minimizing the effect of the reduced portal supply.

The normal portal venous blood pressure in man is of the order of 7–10 mmHg. The consequences and treatment of portal hypertension are discussed later in this chapter.

Hepatic artery

The hepatic artery supplies the capsule and fibrous septa of the liver and also the bile ducts and gallbladder, as well as the liver parenchyma. The manner in which the hepatic artery terminates in the liver has been the subject of considerable debate, but it is now known that arterial blood mixes with portal venous blood in a number of different ways before leaving the liver through the hepatic venous system. From his transillumination studies in rat livers, Rappaport (1973) has concluded that the hepatic arterioles empty directly or via the peribiliary plexus into the sinusoids and terminal portal venules (Fig. 19.2). Recent scanning electron microscope investigations by Nopanitaya et al (1978) have confirmed the existence of these mixing sites, some examples of which are shown in Figures 19.3 and 19.4. Direct artery to hepatic vein connections do not exist in the normal human liver, but they may arise in some liver diseases such as cirrhosis (see section on portal hypertension).

Many theoretical arguments have been advanced regarding the question of pressure equilibration of arterial and venous blood in the sinusoids. It is probable that the presinusoidal arteriolar resistance (especially that provided by the peribiliary plexus) is sufficiently great to reduce the pressure of arterial blood entering the sinusoids to the same order of magnitude as portal pressure; in addition, intermittent closure of the arterioles provides further shielding of the portal bloodstream from the arterial pressure. Although it has never been measured directly, sinusoidal pressure can be estimated by measuring the wedged hepatic venous pressure which is normally in the region of 5 mmHg. Resistance to flow in the sinusoids may be increased by changes in venous outflow resistance or by direct mechanical compression: the main effect is on the portal rather than the arterial flow, and in some cases of liver disease may lead to portal hypertension (see section on portal hypertension).

The hepatic artery usually provides 25–30% of the total blood flow to the liver, the rate of the arterial flow in man being normally in the region of 300–400 ml/min. Because of this relatively small contribution to the total hepatic blood flow, the hepatic artery may supply as little as 30% of the liver's oxygen requirement, even though the arterial blood is well oxygenated with a content of approximately 19 ml/dl. As explained above, however, the artery has the potential to provide more oxygen to the liver in situations of low portal flow.

Ligation of the hepatic artery in man is not usually fatal, but deaths from infarction of the liver have been recorded. The potential danger of the procedure may be partly related to the position of the ligature: ligation of the artery in its proximal part is harmless since blood flow in the distal part can be maintained by collateral circulation

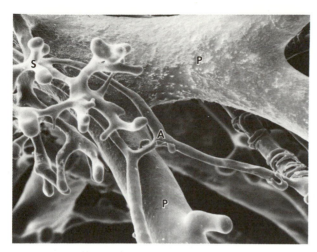

Fig. 19.3 Example of direct hepatic arterial (A) connection with sinusoids (S). The portal vein (P) is also shown.

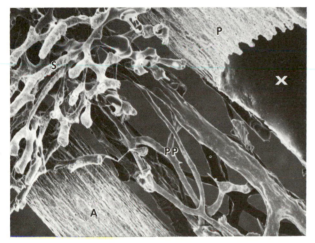

Fig. 19.4 Example of hepatic arterial (A) connection with sinusoids (S) via the peribiliary plexus (PP), which lies between the artery and the portal vein (P). X indicates an incomplete filling of a large portal vein by plastic. (Figs. 19.3 and 19.4 reproduced from W. Nopanitaya et al; Scanning Electron Microscopy, Vol II, SEM Inc., AMF O'Hare, 1978; by kind permission of the authors and publisher).

through the pancreaticoduodenal and gastroduodenal branches. Ligation beyond these branches may be more dangerous, although collateral channels may still be available since vascular anomalies such as duplication of the hepatic artery are fairly common. That the site of interruption of arterial flow has any influence on the incidence of hepatic necrosis has however recently been challenged by Mays (1974).

Even in the absence of any collateral arterial supply, portal venous blood will normally be able to protect the liver from infarction after hepatic arterial ligation — an adequate oxygen supply to the liver is maintained, since portal flow is essentially unaltered by the procedure.

Indeed, it has also been shown that the hepatic oxygen extraction rate from portal blood is slightly increased, thereby minimizing the effect of the loss of arterial perfusion (Andreen & Irestedt, 1976). The liver would probably be seriously compromised, however, if arterial ligation were carried out in conditions of low portal blood flow. Interestingly, the danger of arterial ligation is much more pronounced in the dog, a species in which antibiotic treatment must be provided in order to prevent the growth of anaerobic organisms in the liver.

Hepatic arterial ligation has been recommended as treatment for primary and secondary hepatic tumours, haemangioma, aneurysms, arteriovenous fistula and bleeding from hepatic lacerations after trauma. Hepatic arterial embolization by radiological techniques offers an alternative to surgical ligation in certain cases of liver tumour (Wheeler et al, 1979). Arterial ligation was also used in the 1950s in the treatment of portal hypertension from cirrhosis. This treatment was based on the consideration that the high arterial blood pressure may be transmitted to the portal vein if the normal venous drainage of the liver is impeded. It is now considered that hepatic arterial perfusion is vital to the survival of the liver in portal hypertension, since it not only protects the organ from the diminished portal flow found in many instances but also allows the possibility of further diverting some or all of the portal flow away from the liver by surgical decompression procedures (see section on portal hypertension). It would now be regarded as unjustified and dangerous to ligate the hepatic artery in these patients.

Hepatic veins

The hepatic veins, draining blood from the liver to the inferior vena cava, vary in number from about 5 to 15. In the normal liver, the radicles of the portal vein do not communicate directly with the hepatic veins, but are linked by the sinusoids. In the cirrhotic liver, anastomoses develop between portal and hepatic veins, and blood may bypass the nodules of the regenerating liver cells. The hepatic venous system is the final common pathway of hepatic arterial and portal venous blood after sinusoidal mixing in the normal liver. It is therefore the drainage tract of the entire splanchnic vascular bed, and carries in the region of 1.5 l/min.

In the dog, the liver serves as a blood reservoir. After severe haemorrhage the organ may shrink considerably, discharging the contained blood into the general circulation. Histamine poisoning has the opposite effect and the liver becomes engorged, withdrawing blood from the general circulation; in severe cases, liver congestion can become intense, and results in a marked increase in portal pressure and a decrease in systemic arterial pressure. The mechanism controlling blood volume in the canine liver is thought to be the 'stopcock' action of the hepatic veins, whose muscular walls are thickened like sphincters near their junction with the vena cava. Such sphincters have not been demonstrated in man, in whom neither the liver nor the spleen is an important blood reservoir. This reservoir function in man appears to be served by the capillary network of the intestinal mucosa and by the mesenteric veins. Nonetheless, the hepatic blood volume including that of the large vessels is about 15–20 ml/100 g.

The free pressure in an hepatic vein is about 1–2 mmHg. Wedged hepatic venous pressure measurement is a useful method of estimating sinusoidal pressure, and may also indicate portal venous pressure (Boyer et al, 1977). The hepatic venous blood is normally about two-thirds saturated with oxygen, the oxygen content being approximately 12 ml/dl. Hepatic venous oxygen content may be markedly reduced during periods of low hepatic oxygen delivery, when the liver extracts a larger proportion of the available supply. In normal circumstances, the liver accounts for about 20% of the total oxygen consumption of the body.

The lymphatics of the liver

Lymphatic vessels are present in the portal tracts (Figs. 19.1 and 19.2), but are believed to be absent from the liver parenchyma. The principal route of drainage is to the hepatic lymph nodes in the porta hepatis, but some lymphatics accompany the hepatic veins to nodes around the inferior vena cava.

The equilibrium of fluid exchange across the wall of blood capillaries largely depends on a balance between the hydrostatic pressure in the vessels and the osmotic pressure of the plasma proteins. In the systemic circulation, where hydrostatic pressures are high, the osmotic pressure of the plasma proteins is also high since their influence is virtually unopposed by any protein in the tissue fluid and lymph. In the liver, however, hydrostatic pressures are normally low, and there is free transudation of protein through the highly permeable sinusoidal walls, reducing the osmotic pressure of the protein in the plasma. This situation thus enables a balance of fluid exchange to be achieved in the liver. The extravascular protein enters the lymphatic system by a poorly understood mechanism and returns to the circulation through the thoracic duct. Hepatic lymph has a very high protein content, and actually approximates to that of the plasma. It is probable that over 25% of the thoracic duct lymph flow comes from the hepatic lymphatics.

Trans-sinusoidal fluid filtration is thus highly dependent on the sinusoidal hydrostatic pressure. Obstruction to the venous outflow from the liver produces a striking increase in hepatic lymph flow due to an imbalance of fluid exchange, and may lead to the accumulation of ascites in the abdominal cavity when the hepatic lymphatic system cannot accommodate all the filtrate being produced (Greenway & Lautt, 1970). Ascites formation is discussed more fully later in this chapter (see section on portal hypertension).

Methods of measuring liver blood flow in man

The measurement of the blood flow in any organ presents its own special problems. The liver's dual circulation as well as its relative inaccessibility have provided the major obstacles to its investigation in the past.

The earliest experimental techniques for measuring liver blood flow, such as the intravascular stromuhr or venous outflow collection, could not be applied to the human subject because of their invasive nature, and so it was not until 1945 that hepatic blood flow was estimated for the first time in man using an indirect method based on the Fick principle (Bradley et al, 1945). This important principle allows an estimation of the rate of blood flow through an organ by calculating the quantity of a substance taken up by the organ in unit time divided by the arteriovenous concentration difference of the substance. Bradley's method depended on the fact that intravenously administered Bromsulphalein (BSP) is removed from the bloodstream entirely by the hepatocytes into the bile. The rate of hepatic uptake of BSP was assumed to equal the rate of continuous administration required to maintain a constant peripheral blood concentration of the dye. From the rate of uptake, and the difference between the arterial and hepatic venous concentrations, the liver blood flow was easily calculated. Using this technique, normal total liver blood flow is generally found to be approximately 1.5 l/min. In recent years BSP has tended to be supplanted by other substances which are dependent on hepatocyte extraction, such as ^{131}I-labelled Rose Bengal (Combes, 1960) and indocyanine green (Caesar et al, 1961).

Difficulties with the extraction methods are that none of the dyes is actually removed from the blood entirely by the hepatocytes under normal circumstances, and that there is a variable degree of extrahepatic removal, particularly in cases of liver disease. Another problem which limits their accuracy is the possibility of intra- or extrahepatic shunts allowing the test substance to bypass the liver cells. In addition, the necessity for cannulation of an hepatic vein severely reduces the clinical usefulness of these techniques. Nonetheless, these methods have been widely used for flow measurement, and in liver disease they become increasingly useful as tests of hepatic function rather than flow (see also section on jaundice).

A considerable variety of clinically applicable methods of measuring liver blood flow has been developed in the years since Bradley's original publication, and the most important are outlined below and also listed in Table 19.1.

Two other hepatic clearance techniques have been

Table 19.1 Methods used for liver blood flow measurement in man.

Total flow measurement
  Clearance techniques
    Hepatocyte excretory clearance
      Bromsulphthalein
      Rose Bengal (^{131}I)
      Indocyanine green
    Reticulo-endothelial clearance
      Colloidal gold (^{198}Au)
      Heat-denatured serum albumin (^{131}I)
      Sulphur colloid (^{99m}Tc)
    Hepatic drug extraction
      Lignocaine
      Propranolol
  Indicator dilution technique
    Red blood cells (^{51}Cr)
    Serum albumin (^{131}I)
  Electromagnetic flowmeter technique
    Non-cannulating flow probes
Tissue perfusion measurement
  Inert gas washout techniques
    Krypton (^{85}Kr)
    Xenon (^{133}Xe)

employed: colloidal clearance by the hepatic Kupffer cells (Dobson & Jones, 1952), and hepatocyte removal of highly extracted drugs (George, 1979). Because there is more complete hepatic removal of these substances than those which are excreted into the bile, these methods have the advantage that hepatic vein cannulation is unnecessary in patients with a normal liver, peripheral venous sampling or monitoring being all that is required. Similar problems to those of BSP arise, however, in cases of liver disease.

Total liver blood flow has been successfully measured by indicator dilution since the introduction of the method by Reichman et al (1958). The technique involves the portal venous or hepatic arterial injection of a labelled material which is *not* removed by the liver (red blood cells or serum albumin), and either measuring the changes in hepatic venous concentration by repeated blood sampling or monitoring the hepatic isotope activity with an external detector. It is now possible to determine separately the portal venous flow using a modification of the original method involving portal venous blood sampling after splenic injection (Chiandussi et al, 1968).

A number of other techniques have been introduced which are capable of measuring different aspects of the hepatic circulation. One of the most powerful of these is the electromagnetic flowmeter, as it is able to assess the arterial and portal flow components individually. Its widespread application has been prevented, however, both by the extensive vascular dissection required for placement of the flow probes and by the cost of the equipment involved. Neither the flowmeter nor the indicator dilution technique is specifically dependent on hepatocellular function, but the accuracy of both may be adversely affected by the existence of portal-systemic shunts.

Significant advances have been made in recent years in the application of radioactive inert gas clearance methods

to the hepatic circulation, using either krypton (^{85}Kr) or xenon (^{133}Xe). These methods rely solely on the measurement of the rate of clearance of gas after its injection into the blood supply to the organ (Harper et al, 1974). In their application to the liver circulation, these techniques are *not* affected by the presence of cellular disease or shunts, require no blood sampling and provide a quantitative assessment of the actual tissue perfusion (expressed as ml/min *per gram of tissue*, rather than total flow in ml/min) derived from the combined arterial and venous supplies (Leiberman et al, 1978). The first to use the method for liver blood flow measurement in man were Aronsen and his colleagues in 1966, who recorded the gamma emissions of ^{133}Xe over the liver after the injection of a saline solution of the isotope into the portal vein. Other routes of administration may be employed (umbilical vein, hepatic artery, liver parenchyma, splenic pulp, or gas inhalation), and different types of recording apparatus may be utilized (gamma camera for ^{133}Xe or Geiger-Müller tube for detecting the beta radiation from ^{85}Kr). Normal hepatic tissue perfusion has been found by most investigators to be approximately 100 ml/min per 100 g liver; this result corresponds extremely well to the more widely known normal figures for total flow (1500 ml/min) and liver weight (1500 g). Since the gases are very lipophilic, it is important to take account of the changes in hepatic fat content known to occur in certain conditions (Mathie et al, 1977). It may now become possible to estimate separately the arterial and portal venous contributions to the total perfusion using a relatively simple modification of the ^{133}Xe method, involving injection of the isotope into the thoracic aorta (Holroyd & Peters, 1980).

It is to be hoped that the progress in the methodology of hepatic blood flow measurement achieved in the years since the first publication by Bradley in 1945 will soon be matched by significant advances in the understanding of the human hepatic circulation in both health and disease. The role of such measurement in portal hypertension is discussed in the section on portal hypertension below.

Factors affecting liver blood flow

Most of the available information about the haemodynamics of the normal liver has been derived from investigations in experimental animals rather than in man, human studies having mainly concentrated on hepatic circulatory patterns in disease (see section on portal hypertension and liver regeneration).

The most important aspect about the hepatic circulation is that, while its arterial supply is subject to active control by the normal array of factors influencing peripheral vascular beds, its venous supply is largely controlled *outside* the liver by the resistance vessels of the organs of the digestive tract and spleen. This unique dual circulation also provides the possibility of interaction of the two blood streams within the liver, and many workers have found evidence for an increase in arterial flow after portal flow reduction (e.g. Schenk et al, 1962; Kock et al, 1972; Mathie et al, 1980a), a situation of considerable importance in disorders such as portal hypertension where portal flow is often either spontaneously or surgically shunted away from the liver (see section on portal hypertension). The mechanism controlling the arterial response to portal flow alteration is, in the words of Lautt (1977a), 'at best speculative and at worst completely obscure', and much further work is required on this important topic.

Recent work has revealed the interesting discovery that bile duct pressure may act as a modulator of hepatic artery blood flow after common bile duct obstruction (Nagorney et al, 1982). A dramatic increase in arterial flow was observed after rapidly raising bile duct pressure above 25 mmHg, thus demonstrating a further haemodynamic phenomenon of intrahepatic origin. Neither the mechanism nor possible importance of this haemodynamic response is yet understood.

Despite the crucial importance of the liver for many metabolic processes in the body, surprisingly little is known about the effects of changes in liver metabolism on the hepatic circulation. Indeed, recent evidence (Lautt, 1977a, b) has even challenged the basic assumption that local tissue demands influence hepatic arterial flow, and suggested that this artery is not affected by metabolites or local hypoxia in the same way as many other arterial systems. It is regarded instead as a blood supply which acts as a 'buffer' whereby large irregular changes in total hepatic blood flow are prevented, thus maintaining the clearance rates of blood-borne substances at a more nearly constant level. This concept does not of course imply that the hepatic artery is unimportant in supplying oxygen to the liver — it is vital in situations of low portal flow as mentioned previously — but rather that its blood flow control is not *dependent* on local oxygen demands. It is generally agreed that total liver blood flow is increased after a meal, mainly by a rise in the portal venous component, but recent work has also shown that gastrointestinal hormones such as secretin and pancreozymin can produce a dilatation of the hepatic artery (Richardson & Withrington, 1977).

It is the traditional view that blood flow is diverted away from the splanchnic circulation during exercise in man, but Hopkinson and Schenk (1968) have shown that in dogs there is no change in either arterial or portal venous flow, although these vessels receive a reduced proportion of the elevated cardiac output. The differences between the findings in animals and in man may be due to species variation, the methods employed or the posture of the subject. Change in posture per se undoubtedly affects hepatic haemodynamics, and both Culbertson et al (1951) and Darle et al (1968) found a decrease of about 40% in man on assuming an upright position, presumably due to

splanchnic arterial involvement in a generalized reflex sympathetic vasoconstriction. The position of the liver close to the diaphragm leads to the transmission of the pressure changes of respiration through to the low pressure portal venous system, but while portal pressure undoubtedly changes with the respiratory movements, this would appear not adversely to affect portal blood flow except during extreme degrees of hyperventilation (Hughes et al, 1979a).

Until recently, there had been few carefully controlled studies on the effects of changes in the arterial blood gas tensions on the hepatic circulation, but the experimental work of Hughes et al (1979a, b, c) has done much to clarify the situation. Thus, hypercapnia produces a considerable increase in the portal venous flow and a smaller decrease in hepatic arterial blood flow, while hypocapnia results in a decrease in both inflows to the liver. Systemic hypoxia causes a significant fall in arterial flow but no change in the portal contribution. The underlying mechanisms for these changes are, however, not totally understood.

The nervous control of the hepatic vascular bed has been well summarized by Greenway and Stark (1971): 'Hepatic arterial resistance increases and flow decreases, but this is not maintained and autoregulatory escape occurs. Portal pressure rises but portal flow does not change unless there is a simultaneous change in intestinal or splenic blood flows.' Noradrenaline produces a decreased blood flow in both the hepatic artery and portal vein, the latter probably mainly by mesenteric arterial constriction. The effects of adrenaline are rather more variable, possibly due to the dose-dependency of the reaction, but low doses appear to increase both the arterial and the portal venous flows, while large doses cause a decrease in the two flows. Both α- and β- adrenergic receptors are now known to exist in the hepatic artery, but the question of the distribution of receptors in the portal vein is still not fully resolved, although it is probable that this vascular bed contains α- but not β-receptors. The physiological importance of portal vein receptors for flow control is however doubtful.

Glucagon is a powerful agent for increasing hepatic blood flow: it causes a profound increase in the flow of portal venous blood (as a result of its vasodilatory action on the mesenteric arterial system) and a less pronounced increase in hepatic arterial flow by dilatation of that vessel. Although these results have been obtained in dogs (e.g. Kock et al, 1970; Bashour et al, 1973), Darle and his associates (1968) have also found liver blood flow to increase significantly in man after glucagon injection.

There is rather more limited information about the hepatic circulatory response to other pharmacological agents. The following summarizes the known effects: histamine causes arterial dilatation and, in the dog only, hepatic venous constriction or outflow block; serotonin (5-hydroxytryptamine) produces a decrease in total liver blood flow; angiotensin results in a decrease in both arterial and portal flows; bradykinin increases arterial flow but causes little change in portal flow; vasopressin decreases portal flow and pressure by mesenteric arterial vasoconstriction, but has variable effects on the hepatic artery; prostaglandin El produces an increase in both arterial and portal flows to the liver.

Available information on the effect of general anaesthetic agents on the hepatic circulation is largely confined to investigations of halothane. Early clinical measurements showed that halothane reduced hepatic blood flow in parallel with the blood pressure (Epstein et al, 1966). It has since been shown experimentally that both the hepatic arterial and portal venous blood flows decrease passively in parallel with the cardiac output, with little change in their vascular resistances (Thulin et al, 1975, Hughes et al, 1980). Hepatic oxygen consumption has been found to be relatively unaffected by halothane (Andreen et al, 1975), but in view of the reduced oxygen supply it is clear that the hepatic tissue extraction must have increased markedly to maintain the same consumption rate. The recently available anaesthetic agent enflurane has been the subject of investigation by a number of authors. It was found to produce somewhat similar effects to those of halothane, although there was a significant decrease in hepatic arterial resistance as part of a generalized decrease in peripheral vascular resistance (Hughes et al, 1980). Both cyclopropane and methoxyflurane significantly reduce total liver blood flow, mainly by an increase in the mesenteric vascular resistance (Batchelder & Cooperman, 1975).

Liver blood flow may be further reduced as a result of the surgical trauma of operation, particularly when this involves abdominal organs (Gelman, 1976). A considerable amount of work has been carried out to investigate the influence of haemorrhagic shock on the hepatic circulation, particularly in experimental animals. There is little doubt that total liver blood flow decreases approximately in proportion to the severity of the haemorrhagic hypotension, mainly due to a drop in the portal venous flow. Hepatic arterial flow does not fall until quite severely low pressures are reached, thereby tending to maintain the oxygen supply to the liver. Hepatic oxygen extraction (especially from the hepatic artery) is greatly increased, however, in order to preserve the normal consumption. Hepatic outflow block occurs with retransfusion of the shed blood during or after haemorrhagic hypotension (Greenway & Stark, 1971), but as this phenomenon appears to occur only in the dog, such observations should be interpreted with caution in relation to the problems of shock in man. The hepatic blood flow responses to endotoxin largely resemble those seen after haemorrhage.

It is clear that a multitude of factors may affect hepatic blood flow, some subtly and others more significantly, but there is much that is still not understood about the normal control mechanisms of this complex circulation. A fuller appreciation of the haemodynamic problems of hepatic disease and the most effective methods of their treatment await the outcome of physiological and clinical investigations now in progress.

LIVER FUNCTIONS

Although the liver has been examined by anatomists for many centuries, a knowledge of its function is relatively modern. Claude Bernard was the first to demonstrate its importance in carbohydrate metabolism, and was responsible for the identification and naming of glycogen. In 1922, Mann and his colleagues, by perfecting a technique of experimental total hepatectomy in dogs, were able to give the first full account of liver function, and their series of papers at that time is the foundation of present knowledge.

Within a few hours of total hepatectomy the sugar concentration falls progressively, and as hypoglycaemia develops, there is increasing muscular weakness followed by convulsions, coma and death. When the state first develops, it can immediately be relieved by administering glucose. A few hours later, a somewhat similar state recurs, but accompanied by vomiting, ataxia and apparent loss of sight and hearing. This final state is uninfluenced by giving glucose, and so is not hypoglycaemic in origin. The store of glycogen in muscle decreases only a little even when the animal is dying of hypoglycaemia, and it is concluded that the liver is solely responsible for replenishing the blood sugar.

The importance of the liver in the formation of urea was suspected before experimental hepatectomy became practicable: the liver was known to have a higher urea content than other tissues, and it was known also that fluid perfused through the liver acquired urea in transit. If the liver is removed from an animal, the blood urea concentration falls progressively to almost zero after about 24 hours, but remains stable if the kidneys have also been removed (Fig. 19.5). Furthermore, blood urea rises progressively in animals with an intact liver after bilateral nephrectomy, and it follows that urea formation is dependent on the liver.

Hepatectomized dogs become increasingly jaundiced throughout the period of their survival. The plasma bilirubin begins to rise early, and the yellow colour of the plasma is visible to the naked eye within about 3 hours. The sclerae are jaundiced in dogs which survive about 16 hours, and at post mortem the fat throughout the body is found to be stained. The formation of bilirubin is not prevented by removing all the abdominal viscera including the liver and spleen, and extra bilirubin is still formed after the injection of haemoglobin. It can be concluded that the liver is not essential for bilirubin formation, but is the principal organ of bilirubin excretion.

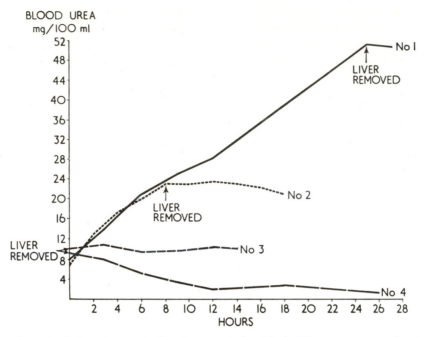

Fig. 19.5 The evidence that urea formation is dependent on the liver. In curves 1, 2 and 3, the kidneys were removed at time zero, and the liver was removed at 24 h, 8 h and at zero respectively. Note that the blood urea concentration remained stable after removal of the liver. In curve 4, the kidneys remained intact and the liver was removed at zero. Note that the blood urea concentration fell to a low level. (Mann & Magath, 1922).

A further account of present knowledge of these and other liver functions is given below.

Carbohydrate metabolism

The liver occupies a key position in carbohydrate metabolism. It stores carbohydrate as glycogen, a condensation product of many molecules of glucose. Glycogen can be formed from dietary monosaccharides in the portal venous blood (glycogenesis), from the glycerol of fat, and from deaminated amino acids (neoglycogenesis). The stored glycogen is converted into glucose (glycogenolysis) as required to maintain the blood glucose concentration at a constant level.

The formation of glycogen and its release as glucose is under the influence of hormones. Insulin favours the laying down of glycogen and retards the liberation of glucose, while the hormones of the anterior pituitary, the adrenal cortex and the thyroid favour the breakdown of glycogen and the liberation of glucose. Glucagon and adrenaline also liberate glucose from glycogen.

Liver glycogen is the only readily available reserve of glucose for maintaining the concentration of the blood sugar; muscle glycogen is not available for this purpose, as shown by the experiments in totally hepatectomized animals where hypoglycaemic death occurred before very much glycogen had disappeared from the muscles.

The average adult liver contains about 100 g of glycogen. This store is exhausted by about 24 hours of starvation, after which time the whole body requirement for glucose must be met by the formation of glucose from body fat and protein. This process, at its normal speed, results in the liberation of small amounts of ketone bodies, and the ketosis of starvation represents the normal process carried to excess. In children, the reserve of liver glycogen is smaller and the metabolic rate higher, and the ketosis of starvation begins correspondingly earlier.

Glycogen, in addition to its fundamental role in carbohydrate metabolism, protects the liver from damage by many poisons, of which chloroform is a classical example.

The liver is also the site of metabolism to glucose of other monosaccharides, such as fructose, and of the lactic, pyruvic and ketoglutaric acids produced by the utilization of glucose in muscle and other tissues.

Amino acid metabolism: formation of urea

The liver is concerned in the breakdown of food and body protein, and particularly in the deamination of amino acids. The amino acids set free by the digestion of protein are absorbed by the small intestine, pass into the portal blood to the liver and some pass through the liver into the systemic blood. The average concentration of amino acids in the blood is 3–5 mg/dl, but this may rise to 10 mg/dl after a meal rich in protein. The absorbed amino acids, together with those released by the breakdown of body proteins, form the 'amino acid pool' which is available for resynthesis into protein or for combustion as a source of energy. The amino acid pool is in a continual state of flux, with amino acids being added, transformed or removed all the time.

Many of the 20 amino acids can be synthesized in the body by transformation from other amino acids, or by the amination of carboyhdrates (notably pyruvic acid); but there is a group of 8 amino acids — valine, leucine, isoleucine, threonine, methionine, phenylalanine, tryptophan and lysine — which cannot be synthesized, and are termed 'essential' since they must be supplied in the diet.

Oxidative deamination occurs principally in the liver. The reaction involves the transformation of an amino acid (e.g. alanine) to the corresponding keto-acid (pyruvic acid) and the liberation of ammonia. The keto-acid can be used for synthesizing other compounds or burned as a source of energy. Most of the ammonia released in the process of deamination is converted to urea and excreted in the urine, and the remainder is used in the synthesis of other amino acids (reamination). Oxidative deamination occurs in tissues other than the liver, but urea formation is probably a hepatic function only. The formation of urea — $CO(NH_2)_2$ — requires the union of carbon dioxide and ammonia with the elimination of water:

$$CO_2 + 2NH_3 \rightarrow CO(NH_2)_2 + H_2O$$

Deamination of an amino acid may also be coupled with the simultaneous amination of a keto-acid (transamination), the enzymes facilitating this reaction being termed aminotransferases (or transaminases). The result is the transference of the NH_2 group from one amino acid, and its use to synthesize another, as in the formation of glutamic acid from alanine facilitated by alanine aminotransferase (ALT):

CH₃		CH₂CH₂COOH			CH₃		CH₂CH₂COOH
CH(NH₂)COOH	+	CO.COOH	⇌ ALT		CO.COOH	+	CH(NH₂)COOH
Alanine		α-Keto-glutaric acid			Pyruvic acid		Glutamic acid

The aminotransferases are intracellular enzymes, but small quantities are normally present in the circulation. When significant cellular damage occurs in an organ, their serum concentration rises, an example of which is the increase in ALT following damage to the liver.

Protein metabolism

The liver manufactures albumin and the proteins concerned with blood clotting (fibrinogen, prothrombin and factors V, VII, IX, and X). Furthermore, the hepatic Kupffer cells are able to synthesise α and β-globulin, and to remove γ-globulin from portal blood.

The evidence that the liver is the major source of plasma albumin is both experimental and clinical. In dogs, after total hepatectomy, there is a slow but progressive fall in the concentration of plasma albumin, suggesting that albumin is being slowly utilized without replacement. In man, the ability to make albumin is reduced in liver failure and hepatic cirrhosis, and the plasma concentration of albumin is often much less than the normal value of 40–50 g/l.

The characteristic change in chronic liver disease is a fall in serum albumin accompanied by a rise in serum γ-globulin. It is therefore necessary to measure both fractions, as the total value may be within the normal range. It should be noted that the serum albumin and γ-globulin concentrations measure different hepatic functions: the albumin is formed in the liver, whereas γ-globulin is formed in the extrahepatic reticulo-endothelial system and removed from the circulation by the hepatic Kupffer cells.

Blood coagulation

As indicated above, the liver is the site of synthesis of the coagulation factors V, VII, IX, and X as well as fibrinogen and prothrombin. The formation of factors VII, IX, and X and of prothrombin is dependent on the presence of vitamin K, and therefore on the absorption of adequate amounts of vitamin K from the intestine. Synthesis of many of the coagulation factors may thus be impaired either by extensive hepatic parenchymatous disease or damage, or by failure to absorb vitamin K from the gut, and may cause the development of a significant bleeding tendency. Lack of the labile factor V occurs rarely with severe liver damage, and never with vitamin K deficiency.

The problem is most often associated with resection for injury, when the bleeding tendency is caused by the transfusion of large quantities of stored blood which is deficient in the factor. The liver is the only site of synthesis of fibrinogen, but impaired formation is rare even in severe hepatic failure. The only common cause of fibrinogen lack is increased fibrinolysis which may occur in all forms of liver disease, and especially in patients with cirrhosis.

Tests for defects in blood clotting include the 'one-stage prothrombin time', and this should be measured in all patients with hepatobiliary disease. A prolonged prothrombin time may indicate deficient vitamin K absorption rather than deficient prothrombin synthesis, especially in the presence of obstructive jaundice. Operation and such procedures as splenic venography or liver biopsy should be postponed until the patient has responded to treatment with the vitamin given parenterally. Failure to respond promptly to parenteral vitamin K may be an index of impaired synthesis, however, reflecting severe hepatocellular dysfunction.

A more general account of the coagulation factors is given elsewhere (Ch. 11).

Fat metabolism

The liver plays an essential role in the metabolism of fat: it is concerned not only in the digestion and absorption of fat by virtue of secreting bile salts into the duodenum, but also in the removal of fat from the bloodstream after absorption has taken place.

The bile salts assist the intestinal absorption of dietary fat by breaking up the fat globules into a fine emulsion, thus allowing greater contact with lipases for hydrolysis and also a reduction in particle size; they also form water-soluble complexes (micelles) with lipids which promotes their absorption (see the section on bile secretion for further details). The products of hydrolysis (free fatty acids, monoglycerides, and to a lesser extent, diglycerides and triglycerides) are probably absorbed as a mixture by the mucosal cells of the intestine. Long-chain fatty acids are converted into triglycerides, enter the lymphatics, and pass by way of the thoracic duct to the systemic veins together with the particulate fat (which gives rise to the cloudy appearance of the blood plasma after a fatty meal). Short-chain fatty acids are water-soluble, enter the portal blood, and pass to the liver; some is metabolized, and some continues to be deposited in the body fat depots.

Fat is removed from the blood by the fat depots as well as by the liver. The depot fat, which is derived not only from food fat but also from carbohydrate sources, is mainly a mixture of triglycerides. The amount of depot fat varies from one individual to another, and is greater in women and children than in men. Even in a lean man, however, the depot fat accounts for about 12% of the body weight. About half of this fat is subcutaneous, and most of the rest lies around the kidneys, in the omentum and mesentery, and in intermuscular planes. This depot fat is a reserve of food, and in addition the subcutaneous fat serves as insulation against heat loss.

The liver receives fat both from body fat depots and from dietary constituents. The fat is converted by hydrolysis into glycerol and fatty acids, the reaction being hastened by liver lipase. The glycerol is utilized through the pathways of carbohydrate metabolism. The fatty acids are either oxidized completely to carbon dioxide and water, or converted into acetoacetic acid by a process termed ketogenesis (acetoacetic acid is a ketone). This acid is converted into β-hydroxybutyric acid and acetone (also ketones), which then diffuse into the systemic circulation because they are unable to be metabolized in the liver. The ketones are thus distributed to the tissues, where they can be completely oxidized to yield carbon dioxide and water with the liberation of energy.

Under normal circumstances, the fat content of the liver varies very little, indicating that the liver normally uses as much fat as is brought to it. Fatty infiltration of the liver can be induced experimentally in animals, and occurs pathologically in man.

In the dog, a particularly severe fatty infiltration of the liver follows total pancreatectomy, even though the diabetes is controlled with insulin. This infiltration can be prevented by feeding the animal choline or precursors of this substance. It is possible that choline produces its lipotropic action by stimulating the transport of fat (as choline-containing phospholipids) from the liver to the tissues or fat depots. In animals given a high neutral fat diet, development of a fatty liver occurs because the uptake of fat for conversion markedly exceeds its rate of despatch.

In man, fatty infiltration of the liver occurs notably in starvation, in chronic alcoholism and in kwashiorkor. In starvation, there is an intensive mobilization of fat from the fat depots without any dietary intake of lipotropic substances. In alcoholism, there may be failure to absorb lipotropic substances through the damaged intestinal mucosa. In kwashiorkor, a deficiency disease of primitive Africans living on a diet devoid of animal protein, there may be a deficiency of lipotropic substances in addition to the very unbalanced diet. Long-continued fatty infiltration may lead to cirrhosis; this is an endemic disease where kwashiorkor is common. Fatty infiltration of the liver can be regarded as a sign of an inadequate diet, and the logical treatment is to provide a diet which is mixed and generous rather than to provide specifically choline or its precursors. Diabetes mellitus also results in an elevated liver fat content, due to impairment of carbohydrate metabolism and consequent increase in fat metabolism necessitating transfer of fat to the liver from the depots. Fatty infiltration also occurs in the early stages of the regenerative process following partial hepatectomy (see also section on liver regeneration).

Fatty infiltration impairs liver function, and (of special interest to the surgeon) interferes with the detoxication of barbiturates, and makes dangerous the administration of fat-soluble anaesthetics such as ether, chloroform, methoxyflurane, enflurane or halothane.

The liver takes up cholesterol absorbed from the food, and also synthesizes the substance from acetyl-CoA. Excess cholesterol is excreted in the bile, where most is kept in solution by the formation of bile salt conjugates, but it may also exist in the free form if there is either an excess of cholesterol or a deficiency of bile salts or phospholipid (see p. 345). The remainder of the cholesterol can enter the circulation, where at least 99% is bound to either high-density lipoprotein (HDL) or very low-density lipoprotein (VLDL), substances also originating mainly in the liver. The concentration of total cholesterol in blood tends to be increased slightly in acute biliary obstruction, but very high concentrations are found in chronic obstruction.

Detoxication

The liver protects the body against many endogenous and exogenous toxic substances. The substances are dealt with by conjugation, by destructive oxidation or by a combination of these processes. The method of dealing with a toxin appears to be fortuitous, depending on the resemblance of the toxin to physiological compounds.

Conjugation may be with amino acids, glucuronic acid, sulphate or acetic acid:

1. The main amino acid involved in this process is glycine, conjugation of cholic acid with glycine giving rise to glycocholic acid which is one of the bile acids; conjugation of benzoic acid with glycine gives rise to hippuric acid which is excreted in the urine.

2. Conjugation with glucuronic acid is the means of disposing of many drugs and hormones containing OH groups (either alcoholic or phenolic) — bilirubin, pregnanediol and other urinary steroids, and morphine are all excreted as glucuronides. This is also one of the major routes of elimination of the hepatotoxic drug paracetamol.

3. Many phenolic compounds such as oestrone and salicylic acid from ingested aspirin are conjugated in the liver with the sulphate from amino acids, and excreted as sulphate esters ('ethereal sulphates').

4. Conjugation with acetic acid is the method of disposing of aromatic amino compounds, e.g. sulphanilamide forms acetylsulphanilamide, which is then excreted.

Oxidative destruction is the method of dealing with many compounds foreign to the body. The alkaloids, strychnine and nicotine, and the short-lasting barbiturates are destroyed in this way. The mild analgesic antipyrine is also eliminated in the same manner, and recent work has shown that measurement of its rate of clearance may be a valuable dynamic test of hepatic metabolic function, even in the presence of jaundice (McPherson et al, 1982). The aminopyrine breath test, in which the excretion in the breath as CO_2 of ^{14}C-labelled aminopyrine administered orally is measured, similarly gives an index of hepatic microsomal enzyme function.

Liver disease or damage may make a patient unduly susceptible to the agents normally conjugated or destroyed in the liver, and this often influences the drug dosage in these conditions.

Reticulo-endothelial function

The hepatic Kupffer cells, which are found lining the sinusoids, are an important part of the reticulo-endothelial (or mononuclear phagocytic) system, the remainder being located in the bone marrow, lymph nodes and spleen. These hepatic cells are able to ingest colloidal particles: their main functions are the ingestion of bacteria and bacterial products such as endotoxin, the removal of γ-globulin, the destruction of erythrocytes, and the extraction of injected colloids from the circulation.

By their ingestion of bacteria, the phagocytic cells are concerned in the defence of the body against infection. In the presence of infection they greatly increase in number, resulting in enlargement of the organs rich in these cells, especially the lymph nodes and spleen. γ-globulin is formed in the extrahepatic phagocytic cells but removed by the hepatic Kupffer cells. The rise in serum γ-globulin in chronic liver disease may be due to a decreased uptake of absorbed intestinal bacterial antigens by the Kupffer cells with consequently increased antigenic stimulation of extrahepatic production. Recent studies have shown that diminished Kupffer cell uptake is largely caused by the bypass of portal blood through portal-systemic shunt channels, rather than by the deterioration of cellular function (Benjamin et al, 1976). The function of these cells is impaired in obstructive jaundice, resulting in decreased removal of endotoxin from the portal circulation, a factor which contributes to the morbidity of surgery in the jaundiced patient (see below) (Ingoldby, 1982). The phagocytic cells throughout the body ingest and destroy erythrocytes, and form and release bilirubin; they also destroy leucocytes and platelets. The uptake of radioactive colloid by the Kupffer cells is the basis of one method of liver blood flow measurement, using ^{198}Au-colloid, ^{131}I-heat-denatured serum albumin or ^{99m}Tc-sulphur colloid (see also section on circulation). This last substance has also been used increasingly in recent years for liver scanning by gamma camera.

Bile secretion

Bile is secreted continuously by the liver but, after concentration and storage in the gallbladder, is discharged intermittently into the duodenum. The normal liver secretes approximately 500 ml of bile daily, the secretion pressure being in the region of 10–15 mmHg. If the common bile duct is obstructed, the liver continues to secrete bile until the pressure in the duct rises to 15–20 mmHg, when secretion ceases.

Bile is a viscous, golden yellow, slightly alkaline fluid. It is a complex solution whose composition varies from time to time, the figures given in Table 19.2 being merely a representative example of the substances normally present in the hepatic duct in man.

The bile salts are the only constituents of the bile which have a useful function to perform in the intestine. The other constituents can be regarded as unwanted substances

Table 19.2 Composition of human liver bile

Component	%
Water	98.0
Bile salts	0.7
Inorganic salts	0.7
Bile pigments	0.2
Fatty acids	0.15
Lecithin	0.1
Cholesterol	0.06

passed to the intestine for excretion. The bile is concentrated in the gallbladder chiefly by the absorption of water and inorganic salts.

Bile salts

The main bile salts are the sodium and potassium salts of glycocholic and taurocholic acid. These acids are formed in the liver as the result of the conjugation of the bile acid cholic acid with the amino acids glycine or taurine. Cholic acid, made in the liver, is the limiting factor on the total output of bile salts. Glycine is abundantly formed in the body; taurine (a derivative of cystine) is derived from food, and the output of taurocholic acid varies with the diet.

Normally about 20 g per day of bile salts are passed with the bile into the intestine, but only 0.2–0.4 g of this represents fresh synthesis by the liver: the remaining proportion of bile salts represents that reabsorbed from the intestine into the portal vein and re-excreted by the liver (enterohepatic circulation). Most of the reabsorption takes place in the terminal ileum by an extremely efficient active transport system, but a small proportion is reabsorbed from the colon as deoxycholate which is formed as a result of bacterial conversion of cholate. The bile salt pool is approximately 3.5 g in total, and recycles repeatedly via the enterohepatic circulation: the cycling frequency of the entire pool is 6–8 times per day, and about twice per meal. The enterohepatic circulation of bile salts is interrupted by external biliary fistula, and after the first day or two the daily loss of bile salts from such a fistula falls to 2–3 g, which may be the maximum rate at which the liver can synthesize them.

There are a number of important properties associated with the bile salts:

1. They reduce surface tension and so help to break the food fat to a fine emulsion. The importance of this fine emulsification is two-fold: firstly, it increases enormously the surface area of the fat globules on which the water-soluble lipases can act, and secondly, it allows particulate fat to be absorbed by the intestinal mucosa if the particle size is sufficiently small.

2. The activation of lipases by the bile salts is not wholly explained by their emulsifying property, for acti-

vation also occurs when lipase acts on water-soluble esters; the bile salts thus have a direct action on the enzyme as well as on the substrate.

3. The bile salts combine with water-insoluble substances, such as long-chain fatty acids, cholesterol and the fat-soluble vitamins (A, D, E and K), to form micelles, which are water-soluble complexes from which the lipids can be more easily absorbed by the gut; this action is called their hydrotropic effect. Loss of the hydrotropic action of the bile salts in obstructive jaundice prevents the absorption of vitamin K and also leads to the appearance in the faeces of as much as 25% of ingested fat (see also section on jaundice).

4. The bile salts are the most potent of the known choleretics. The term choleretic implies the property of inducing the liver to secrete more bile, in contradistinction to the action of cholagogues which stimulate the gallbladder to empty. The output of bile can be greatly increased by giving bile salts by mouth.

Bile pigments

The bile pigments, bilirubin and biliverdin, are the waste products derived mainly from the breakdown of haemoglobin in the reticulo-endothelial system throughout the body. They are excreted exclusively by the liver under normal circumstances. Transfer of bilirubin from the plasma to the bile is a metabolically complex process, in which the hepatocyte must perform a sequence of distinct biochemical operations on the bilirubin molecule and its metabolites. The process can be divided essentially into three phases:

1. The bilirubin molecule is detached from its carrier albumin in the plasma and then attached to a form of binding or transfer protein (ligandin) at the sinusoidal hepatocyte membrane. This carrier molecule transports the bilirubin to the interior of the cell.

2. Bilirubin is then conjugated, principally with glucuronic acid, by the action of glucuronyl transferase located primarily in the smooth endoplasmic reticulum.

3. The conjugated molecule, bilirubin glucuronide, is water-soluble and crosses the epithelium of the bile canaliculus to commence its passage to the larger bile ductules. This substance is responsible for the golden yellow colour of freshly secreted bile. Oxidation to biliverdin gives the characteristic green colour of bile obtained from the gallbladder.

On entering the intestine, the conjugated bilirubin is reconverted to bilirubin which can be absorbed by the mucosa. Some of the unconjugated bilirubin in the intestine is converted by bacterial action to stercobilinogen (synonymous with urobilinogen): most of this, oxidized to stercobilin, is excreted in the faeces giving it the normal brown colour. The remainder of the stercobilinogen is

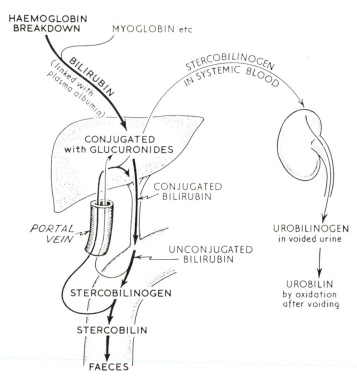

Fig. 19.6 The pathways of bile pigment excretion.

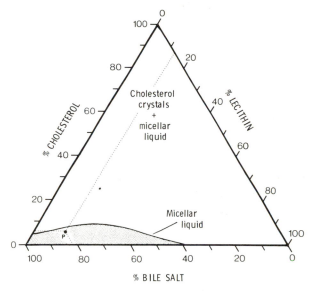

Fig. 19.7 Method of presenting the three major components of bile on triangular co-ordinates. Each component is expressed as percentage moles of total bile salt, lecithin (phospholipid) and cholesterol. The shaded area represents the relative proportions of bile salt and lecithin within which cholesterol remains in micellar solution — the point P represents a mixture having 6 moles of cholesterol, 12 moles of lecithin, and 82 moles of bile salts per 100 total moles. Mixtures having relative proportions outside the shaded area would be expected to separate into two phases: solid cholesterol crystals, and a micellar liquid saturated with cholesterol. (Redrawn from D M. Small 1968 New England Journal of Medicine 279:588).

absorbed into the portal vein, and, together with the re-absorbed bilirubin, is excreted again by the liver (entero-hepatic circulation). Traces of stercobilinogen (urobilinogen) enter the systemic bloodstream, and are excreted by the kidneys (Fig. 19.6).

The patterns of abnormal bile pigment metabolism found in different types of jaundice are discussed in a later section.

Other substances excreted in the bile

Cholesterol is excreted in the bile, and varies with (but is lower than) the concentration in the blood. In the bile, cholesterol is kept in solution by the formation of micelles with bile salts and phospholipids, and tends to precipitate as gallstones if there is an excess of cholesterol or a deficiency of bile salts or phospholipid (Fig. 19.7). Patients with cholesterol gallstones have a reduced bile salt pool (Vlahcevic et al, 1970) and probably a reduced bile salt and phospholipid secretion. The logical consequence of Figure 19.7 is that it should be possible to dissolve cholesterol gallstones by adding extra bile salts to the bile fluid: oral administration of bile acids increased the secretion of bile salts and phospholipids and also reduced cholesterol secretion (Thistle & Hofmann, 1973), and administration via a T-tube has been shown to be useful (Classen & Ossenberg, 1977). While there are a number of complications of oral bile acid treatment (including diarrhoea and

possible hepatotoxicity), the newer synthetic bile acid analogues such as ursodeoxycholic acid may be of value in a few cases. Further reference to gallstones is made in Chapter 20.

The enzyme *alkaline phosphatase* is excreted in the bile. In jaundice, and in parenchymatous disease of the liver with or without jaundice, the serum phosphatase concentration increases. The most significant increase is usually seen when jaundice is due to intra- or extrahepatic obstruction of the bile duct.

Factors influencing bile secretion

The secretion of bile is thought to be only partly under nervous control as it is not arrested by complete denervation of the liver. The most powerful choleretic agents known are the bile salts, but other choleretics include histamine, secretin, salicylates and pilocarpine. There are two components of normal canalicular bile flow, one dependent on the delivery of bile salts to the hepatocyte, and one which is bile salt-independent. The bile salt-dependent fraction accounts for some 70% of bile flow in man, and it is the presence of osmotically-active bile salts excreted into the canaliculi which is the major driving force which generates canalicular flow. In addition to these two components, there may be a degree of ductular secretion into the bile which is bile salt-independent.

Although the metabolism of bile pigments and bile salts are largely independent of one another, there is good evidence that bile salts may stimulate bilirubin excretion at the cellular level (Goresky et al, 1974). In the presence of an external biliary fistula, the drive to bile secretion is diminished and bile volume rapidly decreases. This situation is promptly reversed by oral feeding of bile salts, which stimulates bile salt-dependent canalicular flow and also increases biliary bilirubin excretion (M. H. Lewis et al, unpublished data). Bile flow is increased by a diet of meat and fat, and reduced by sugar. It is also reduced by adrenaline and in starvation. The entry of bile into the duodenum is controlled by the contraction and relaxation of the sphincter of Oddi and the gallbladder, which are influenced by both nervous and humoral factors (see Ch. 20).

PORTAL HYPERTENSION

An account has already been given of the portal circulation and its contribution to the hepatic blood flow (see section on circulation). In normal man, the portal circulation forms a circulatory unit quite distinct from the systemic venous circulation. The pressure within this system is determined by a relatively constant input of blood and the resistance to inflow into the hepatic sinusoids, and rarely exceeds 10 mmHg in normal man. A large number of potential vascular communications between the portal venous and systemic venous circulations exist however, and some of these are in anatomically constant and well-defined sites (see Fig. 19.8). When the pressure in some part of the portal system becomes elevated, these normally collapsed collateral channels open up to form significant routes of blood flow between the two circulations, the so-called portal-systemic anastomoses. Collaterals arising in the abdominal wall from the patent para-umbilical vein, the haemorrhoidal plexus of the rectum from the inferior mesenteric circulation, and the retroperitoneal collaterals between the splenic compartment of the circulation and the systemic venous system are well described; the clinically significant collaterals are, however, those which run to the azygos vein from the short gastric or left gastric (coronary) veins. Large channels develop in a submucosal plexus of veins in the lower oesophagus and upper stomach — oesophageal and gastric varices — and are liable to catastrophic haemorrhage.

In rare cases, the principal contribution to elevated portal venous pressure comes from increased portal blood flow. This may be caused by idiopathic tropical splenomegaly, splenic vascular malformations, and blood dyscrasias. In the majority of cases however, the increased pressure is caused by increased resistance due to obstruction in the portal circulation. The sites of obstruction are conventionally divided into posthepatic (on the systemic side of the hepatic sinusoids), prehepatic (within the vessels of the portal venous system itself), and intrahepatic. The intrahepatic variety may be further divided into sinusoidal or presinusoidal obstruction, although this distinction is more difficult to make. The causes of these varieties of obstruction will be discussed below.

Posthepatic obstruction

Severe right-sided cardiac failure is associated with hepatic venous congestion which may proceed to the formation of

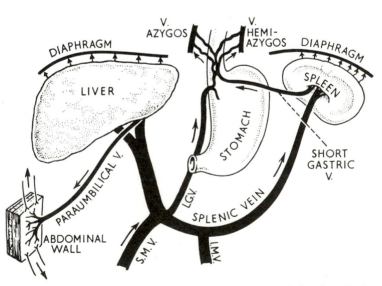

Fig. 19.8 Diagram of the principal anastomoses between the portal and systemic venous systems in intrahepatic obstruction of the portal vein due to cirrhosis of the liver.

fibrous tissue bands between the central veins of the liver, and in rare cases to fully-developed cardiac cirrhosis. Portal hypertension is rare however, except in severe cases such as those associated with constrictive pericarditis. Another rare but important cause of suprahepatic venous obstruction is the formation of a fibrous diaphragm or web across the vena cava at the level of the entrance of the hepatic veins. The Budd-Chiari syndrome and veno-occlusive disease of the liver are due to hepatic venous outflow obstruction arising at sites from the efferent veins of the hepatic lobule to the entry of the inferior vena cava into the right atrium. The syndromes may be produced by thrombosis of the hepatic veins in myeloproliferative disorders, by the oral contraceptive pill, or rarely by ingestion of toxic alkaloids (McGee et al, 1976). Hepatic venous involvement by tumour is another uncommon cause. Catheterization studies of the inferior vena cava and hepatic veins with radiological imaging and pressure measurements may be the only means of diagnosing the Budd-Chiari syndrome which can be distinguished from veno-occlusive disease by needle biopsy of the liver.

Extrahepatic obstruction

The principal cause of this syndrome is portal vein thrombosis. The majority of cases are due to sepsis arising either from the umbilical vein at birth, or from severe suppurative processes within the intestinal tract. In more than half the cases no aetiological factor is ever identified. Thrombosis may also occur as a result of trauma (usually operative), or lymph nodes containing tumour may obstruct the portal vein at the hilum of the liver. A form of segmental hypertension affecting the splenic venous circulation may arise from thrombosis of the splenic vein, sometimes associated with pancreatitis. While the pressures in the portal venous system may be normal in these cases, dilated collaterals in the lower oesophagus may arise from the short gastric veins. Partial nodular transformation of the liver, although due to intrinsic liver disease, may be regarded as a form of extrahepatic obstruction, since the liver nodules found in the hilar region in such cases obstruct the portal venous inflow by compression at the hilum. The importance of these extrahepatic causes of portal hypertension lies in the fact that liver function may be well-preserved, with a consequent improvement in prognosis.

Intrahepatic obstruction

The common cause is cirrhosis. Obstruction is at the level of the hepatic sinusoids, and may be viewed as a strangulation of the sinusoidal blood flow by encroaching fibrous tissue and cirrhotic regenerative nodules. Arteriovenous shunting at the sinusoidal level may also make a small contribution to the elevated pressure. The majority

of cases in the United Kingdom are of the so-called cryptogenic variety, although the incidence of alcoholic cirrhosis is increasing. Chronic active hepatitis and primary biliary cirrhosis are other less frequent causes. Congenital hepatic fibrosis is an uncommon cause of portal hypertension, but is important to distinguish from cirrhosis because of the relatively well preserved liver function and better prognosis. Schistosomiasis is an important cause of portal hypertension in some parts of the world. In this case the obstruction is presinusoidal in origin, and probably related to the inflammatory reaction in the portal zones of the liver.

Effects of increased portal pressure

Opening of collateral circulation

The increase in portal venous pressure due to any of the above conditions is usually gradual. The collateral circulations which have been described open up progressively and may give rise to large channels, individual vessels often being 1 cm or more in calibre. The flow through this collateral bed, however, is insufficient to achieve a significant reduction in the portal pressure, which may be as high as 40–50 mmHg. There is no constant relationship between the degree of portal-systemic shunting and portal pressure. Shunting of blood through the collateral circulation reduces the volume of hepatic blood flow, and in extreme cases there may be no discernible entry of portal blood to the liver sinusoids at all. The exception to this is the case of extrahepatic block due, for example, to portal vein thrombosis. In this situation collaterals may form which re-enter the portal vein in the porta hepatis beyond the block, and maintain hepatic perfusion with portal blood.

Ascites

This accumulation of fluid within the peritoneal cavity is most commonly found in patients with cirrhosis. The mechanism is multifactorial, and may be viewed as a combination of local factors and alterations in renal function. Ascites does not generally occur with extrahepatic blockage of the portal vein, but hepatic venous obstruction may produce ascites as an early phenomenon. An important factor is the failure of the impaired liver to synthesize albumin. The plasma colloid osmotic pressure is largely governed by the plasma albumin concentration, and as this falls to 31 g/l, both ascites and oedema tend to develop. The combined factors of increased hydrostatic pressure and decreased osmotic pressure may in themselves upset the Starling equilibrium sufficiently to produce a transudation of fluid, but this is not the only explanation of the syndrome. This is evident from the fact that in many patients the protein concentration of the ascitic fluid may be higher than that expected in a simple transudate. The protein may in fact be derived largely from hepatic lymph, whose production is increased due to the effect of cirrhosis on the venous outflow from the sinusoids. Distended lymphatics at the hilum of the liver may be seen in cirrhosis, and an increased lymphatic flow through the thoracic duct has been demonstrated.

The second significant factor is that of sodium and water retention. Lieberman and his colleagues (1970) proposed that renal retention of sodium and water is the primary abnormality of cirrhotic ascites, and that the expanded extracellular fluid compartment 'overflows' to the peritoneal cavity if local factors such as portal pressure and hepatic lymph drainage are sufficiently altered to favour this area for fluid accumulation. After reduction of the portal pressure by portacaval shunting ascites may be replaced by peripheral oedema: the retained sodium and fluid is no longer preferentially localised to the peritoneal compartment by the local factors relating to portal hypertension (Cherrick et al, 1960).

The mechanism of sodium and fluid retention is also multifactorial. Cirrhotics with ascites have excessive levels of aldosterone, and the effect of this hormone on the distal tubules probably explains the fluid and sodium retention in cirrhotics with normal renal function. As well as increased levels, there may be an increased renal tubular sensitivity to aldosterone. While some of the hyperaldosteronism is due to failure of hepatic inactivation, increased secretion also appears important, and this may be related to failure of feedback within the renin-angiotensin-aldosterone system. Paradoxically, plasma sodium is frequently reduced in cirrhotic patients with ascites and oedema, but this is most commonly a dilutional hyponatraemia due to excessive fluid retention, and may co-exist with a high total body sodium. An increase in circulating antidiuretic hormone (ADH) may be a factor, but the evidence for this is conflicting (Wilkinson & Williams, 1979).

Many cases of ascites and oedema in cirrhosis are controlled by the use of a low sodium diet, and in addition the aldosterone antagonist, spironolactone, proves effective in the majority of cases.

Hypersplenism

Splenomegaly is common in portal hypertension, but the spleen size bears no relationship to the height of the portal venous pressure (Westaby et al, 1978). Occasionally the size of the spleen may itself contribute to the portal hypertension because of an associated increase in blood flow. Hypersplenism may result in increased destruction of platelets and of leucocytes, but the anaemia of portal hypertension is not significantly due to increased destruction of red cells by the spleen, but to haemorrhage, malnutrition or marrow depression. The deficiency of platelets is rarely severe, the count usually being between 60 000 and 120 000/mm³. Studies using ⁵¹Cr-labelled platelets in congestive splenomegaly indicate that the predominant abnormality is deficient production, although there is also some shortening of platelet life span (Cohen et al, 1961).

Splenectomy is rarely indicated as a primary treatment for the pancytopaenia associated with cirrhosis. Although there is a response in the leucocyte and platelet counts, the effect on portal blood flow is usually insufficient to produce a significant decrease in the portal hypertension, and the opportunity of using the splenic vein for a surgical shunt is usually permanently lost.

Liver failure and portal-systemic encephalopathy

This important consequence of portal hypertension is considered in the section on hepatocellular failure below.

Investigation of portal hypertension

The full investigation of patients with gastrointestinal bleeding due to suspected portal hypertension must of course include careful examination of the blood for haematological disorders and impaired liver function, but the key investigations are those designed to elucidate the anatomy of the abnormal portal venous system. The objectives are to define the level of the block, to demonstrate the extent and direction of the collateral circulation, and when possible, to measure the pressure within the portal venous system. A variety of techniques are in common use.

Splenic venography

By this technique, direct access to the portal venous system is achieved by the passage of a lumbar puncture needle into the pulp of the spleen percutaneously through the eighth or ninth intercostal space on the left side. This technique may demonstrate both the site of obstruction and the nature of the collateral circulation (Figs. 19.9 and 19.10). It is contraindicated in the presence of very gross coagulation disorders or of marked ascites.

In addition, the pressure within the splenic pulp may be measured using the same needle. This technique usually gives a slightly higher estimate of the portal venous pressure than that obtained by catheterization of the portal vein at laparotomy.

Indirect portography

It is often possible to obtain satisfactory radiological pictures of the portal venous system following injection of contrast medium into the coeliac axis following retrograde catheterization of a femoral artery. This 'late phase' technique has several advantages: it may be performed in patients with ascites or severe coagulopathy, allows visual-

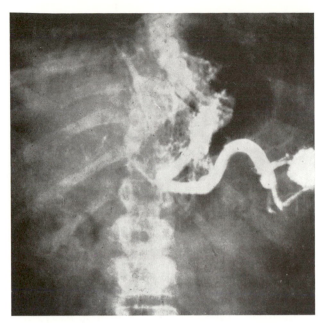

Fig. 19.9 Trans-splenic venogram, showing extrahepatic obstruction of the portal vein and oesophageal varices. (Courtesy of Dr Barnett, Department of Radiology, Western Infirmary, Glasgow.)

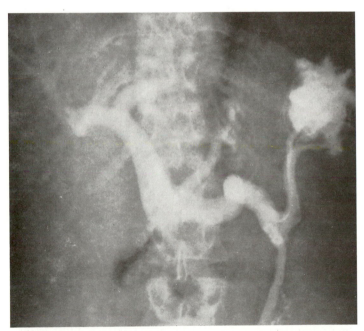

Fig. 19.10 Percutaneous splenic venogram in portal cirrhosis. Note the dilatation of portal, splenic, left gastric, and inferior mesenteric veins: the superior mesenteric vein has not filled.

ization of the hepatic arterial circulation, with occasional detection of hepatocellular carcinoma in cirrhotic patients, and is applicable in patients who have had a splenectomy. Superior mesenteric arterial injection also allows clear visualization of the superior mesenteric vein, which is

rarely achieved by the direct splenic puncture technique. However, portal pressure measurement is not possible by this method.

Trans-hepatic portography

Via a percutaneous trans-hepatic puncture, an intra-hepatic portal venous radicle is catheterized and the catheter is threaded in a retrograde fashion into the main portal vein. The catheter may be further advanced distally into the splenic vein, and even into individual collateral vessels (Boyer et al 1977; Okuda et al, 1977). The method has two main advantages: firstly, direct and accurate portal venous pressure measurement is possible, and secondly, it may be possible to use this route for embolization of bleeding oesophageal varices (Scott et al, 1976).

Hepatic venous catheterization

A catheter may be introduced into the hepatic veins by way of a jugular puncture. The free pressure measured in the hepatic veins is normally equal to that in the inferior vena cava, and it may be possible thus to diagnose cases of the Budd-Chiari syndrome. When the catheter is wedged into the small hepatic veins, the pressure measured (wedged hepatic venous pressure) is equivalent to that in the sinusoids. In patients with portal hypertension of intra-hepatic origin, and in particular in cirrhotic patients, this equates well with the portal venous pressure.

Hepatic blood flow studies

Although radiological examination is the most commonly used method of obtaining information about the portal circulation in portal hypertension, the results obtained are only qualitative and provide little indication about the actual blood flow rate within or around the liver. Most of the previously described quantitative flow measurement techniques (Table 19.1) have been applied to studies of portal hypertension, particularly in cirrhosis. Despite the various shortcomings associated with these methods, there is now a reasonable consensus of opinion regarding the most common haemodynamic patterns in this disease.

From the first report of flow measurement in cirrhosis by Bradley et al (1948), most evidence has indicated that total hepatic flow is significantly decreased in this condition. Information about the relative contributions of the portal vein and hepatic artery has been obtained mainly from studies using the electromagnetic flowmeter, and it would appear that hepatic portal flow is usually considerably reduced (often by more than 50% from the expected normal value) and that the arterial supply provides a greater relative contribution to the total hepatic flow (e.g. Moreno et al, 1967). It is not yet clear however, if the *absolute* hepatic arterial blood flow is actually increased from its resting level in an attempt to compensate for the portal deprivation.

Recently, preliminary investigations have managed to quantify the magnitude of intra- and extrahepatic shunt flow from the portal vein to the systemic venous circulation in small groups of patients. These methods entail the comparison of lung hepatic radioactivity after portal venous injection of labelled serum albumin macro-aggregates. Data from 15 cirrhotics has shown that up to 78% of the portal venous blood flow may bypass the sinusoidal bed in the liver, while evidence from eight patients indicated that up to 49% of the portal flow may circulate through extrahepatic shunt pathways (Okuda et al, 1977). A similar investigation in five cirrhotics has also shown that approximately 10–30% of the hepatic arterial blood may flow through intrahepatic shunt channels to the systemic venous circulation (Groszmann et al, 1977).

Therapy of portal hypertension

The major risk for patients with portal hypertension is that of bleeding from the submucosal plexus of collaterals in the oesophagus or gastric fundus, and the object of therapy is to reduce this risk by either obliterating or decompressing these collateral channels. It must be appreciated that these variceal connections already constitute a pathological portal-systemic shunt, and decompression of the portal system by creation of a surgical shunt simply alters the position of the shunting channels from a vulnerable site to a more protected and perhaps more effective position within the abdomen.

Emergency treatment of variceal haemorrhage

This is usually controlled by inflation of a special balloon catheter passed into the stomach and oesophagus (Sengstaken-Blakemore tube). Use of pitressin (vasopressin) is also effective in the majority of cases. This hormone acts by causing splanchnic vasoconstriction and so reducing the blood flow through the portal circulation. It is active when administered via a peripheral vein, but possibly more effective when infused via a catheter in the superior mesenteric artery. The intense vasospasm may produce intestinal cramps and diarrhoea, but coronary arterial spasm also occurs, and there is a risk of myocardial ischaemia.

Direct attack on varices

Some of the earliest attempts to treat variceal bleeding and portal hypertension were made by ligation of the oesophageal varices from the abdomen or from the chest, with or without total transection of the oesophagus at this level. This form of treatment has more recently been revived by the use of an automatic circular stapling device (Johnston, 1977) or by injection sclerotherapy, i.e. injection of a sclerosing agent into or around the variceal channels by means of an oesophagoscope (Terblanche et al, 1980; MacDougall et al, 1982). The channels may also be obliterated by injection of emboli of sclerosing agents via a trans-hepatic portal catheter (Scott et al, 1977, see above).

Splenectomy

It has already been noted that this treatment is ineffective or even contra-indicated in a majority of cases. One exception to this is the patient with portal hypertension due to splenic vein thrombosis, and such patients may be cured by splenectomy.

Portal-systemic anastomosis

Construction of an anastomosis between the portal vein and the inferior vena cava was first performed experimentally by Eck in 1897 — the so-called 'Eck fistula' (Child, 1953). Its first successful clinical application in portal hypertension was by Whipple in 1945. The procedure is clearly effective in reducing the elevated portal venous pressure, and indeed is the most effective treatment for the prevention of bleeding from oesophageal varices; however, as this form of shunt deprives the liver entirely of inflow from the portal venous system and also enables 'unfiltered' splanchnic venous blood to reach the systemic circulation, liver failure and encephalopathy are common complications in patients subjected to the operation. The liver relies to some extent on portal venous blood for maintenance of its size and function (see below), and so the effect on the liver of sudden portal flow deprivation is likely to be of greatest significance in those patients in whom there is still a large hepatopetal portal blood flow. In patients with a severe or long-standing intrahepatic portal venous block, however, there may already be little significant blood flow from this system, or indeed reversed (or hepatofugal) portal flow. In such cases sudden total portal diversion may have no further harmful effects on the liver. The problems with the total shunt procedure have been highlighted by the results of trials in cirrhotic patients showing that the reduction in mortality from gastrointestinal bleeding is almost completely offset by an increased mortality from hepatocellular failure (Resnick et al, 1974).

These findings have led to the search for alternative shunts which do not compromise the liver in this manner. Side-to-side portacaval shunt, mesocaval shunt and splenorenal shunt (with splenectomy) have all enjoyed varying degrees of clinical popularity, but are essentially based on the same haemodynamic objective of decompressing the central portion of the portal venous system.

The selective distal splenorenal shunt described by Warren and his colleagues in 1967 is based on a different mechanism: the splenic vein is divided and the distal end anastomosed to the side of the left renal vein, while as many as possible of the major collateral vessels from the portal vein to the oesophagogastric region are identified and ligated. Thus the venous blood flow from the intestine and pancreas continues to enter the liver, while the venous drainage of the oesophageal plexus joins that of the spleen and enters the systemic circulation through the shunt, thereby selectively decompressing the variceal region. This promising approach has been reinforced by reports suggesting that the incidence of postoperative hepatic failure and encephalopathy may be decreased in comparison to total or other more conventional shunts (Galambos et al) 1976). Maintenance of hepatic tissue perfusion after the Warren shunt has been recently demonstrated quantitatively (Reichle & Owen, 1979; Mathie et al, 1980b; Rikkers et al, 1981). However, other studies have suggested that a gradual reduction of hepatic perfusion does occur, but that the slow time-course of this reduction may protect the liver from the effects of abrupt portal deprivation (Maillard et al, 1979).

Attempts to correlate liver blood flow with the clinical results of the more established shunt procedures have in general proved somewhat disappointing (e.g. Burchell et al, 1974). Nevertheless, more promising recent work has suggested that the outcome of portal diversion may be better in those patients who show a significant reactive increase in the hepatic arterial flow following the shunt (Burchell et al, 1976). A valuable approach to this question may be intra-operative measurement of hepatic blood flow during *temporary* portal vein occlusion in order to provide an assessment of the changes to be expected in the portal, arterial and total flows immediately after shunt surgery. This method may provide an objective means of helping to determine the most advantageous shunt procedure for individual cases. At present, however, studies of this nature have been limited to a few measurements of changes in tissue perfusion using the ^{85}Kr clearance technique (Leiberman et al, 1978; Mathie et al, 1980 b).

HEPATOCELLULAR FAILURE

Liver failure may be an acute illness caused by fulminating viral hepatitis or precipitated by drugs such as paracetamol, or may represent the end stage of a chronic progressive disease process such as cirrhosis. Either of these processes generally ends in progressive deterioration of neurological function, leading ultimately to coma and death. The pathogenesis of this hepatic encephalopathy is complex and incompletely understood, and this is discussed further below. In acute liver failure, the neurological syndrome dominates the clinical picture, and there may be little time for the other more general manifestations to develop. When liver disease is chronic and

progressive, however, these stigmata are more evident. We shall consider these chronic phenomena first.

General effects of hepatocellular failure

Jaundice. The precise mechanisms of jaundice due to failure of the hepatocytes are discussed in the section on jaundice below. While this is a frequent accompaniment of acute liver failure, it may be absent until a late stage of chronic processes such as cirrhosis, because of the large reserve of the hepatocytes with respect to bilirubin metabolism. A mild degree of elevation of plasma bilirubin occurs with chronic hepatic failure and is an adverse sign.

Serum protein changes. It has already been noted that the liver is the major site of production of albumin, so that hypoalbuminaemia may be a sensitive index of hepatocellular failure. Other factors, however, may be involved, including dilution of the serum albumin due to fluid retention (see above), and a poor dietary intake of protein in the alcoholic cirrhotic. Defects in both synthesis and transport of albumin into the plasma occur in chronic liver disease.

Fibrinogen, prothrombin, and factors V, VII, IX and X are all synthesized by the liver. While the levels of all of these factors may be depressed in chronic liver disease, it is unusual for fibrinogen to be significantly reduced unless there is associated disseminated intravascular coagulation. Reduction in the other factors results in a prolonged one-stage prothrombin time.

Elevated γ-globulin levels are frequently seen in chronic liver disease, and the mechanisms for this are complex. The hepatocytes are neither a significant site of production nor of destruction of γ-globulins, but the Kupffer cells of the liver are responsible for removal of antigenic material from the portal circulation. While these cells may in themselves fail to remove portal antigens, there is experimental evidence to suggest an important role for intrahepatic or extrahepatic portal-systemic shunts in allowing this material to bypass the Kupffer cells and gain access to other sites in the reticulo-endothelial system (Benjamin et al, 1976).

Coagulation disorders. These are due to several factors, all of which have been previously mentioned. The principal of these are (i) failure of synthesis of blood clotting factors, (ii) poor absorption of vitamin K in the jaundiced patient, (iii) platelet deficiency due either to impaired production or increased destruction by the overactive spleen, and (iv) a degree of consumptive coagulopathy, possibly mediated by endotoxaemia.

Fluid and electrolyte imbalance. This has already been described above, and gives rise to the common findings of ascites and oedema in advanced liver disease.

Failure of hormone inactivation. Failure of hepatic degradation of aldosterone has already been mentioned in the context of fluid retention and oedema. Failure to inactivate a wide range of hormones gives rise to numerous valuable clinical signs. Excess circulating levels of oestrogens in males produce gynaecomastia (enlargement of the breasts) and testicular atrophy. Amenorrhoea may occur in females. Spider naevi are common in chronic active hepatitis and alcoholic cirrhosis: these are small vascular malformations confined to the upper part of the body above the nipple line, and are thought to be due to excess oestrogen levels. Palmar erythema (liver palms) may have a similar aetiology.

Portal-systemic encephalopathy (PSE)

This is now the preferred terminology for the neurological syndromes associated with liver failure. The relationship between portal-systemic shunting and PSE is discussed below. The principal component of the syndrome is a disturbance of mental state, ranging from the most subtle changes of behaviour to deep coma from which the patient cannot be aroused (see Table 19.3). Apart from the well-recognized changes in the state of consciousness, subtle changes in intellectual function, personality and behaviour are seen. Changes in intellectual function may be assessed objectively by the use of tests such as the Number Connection Test in which the patient's speed in joining numbers from 1 to 25 in sequence is measured (see Fig. 19.11). Abnormalities of the electroencephalogram are seen, typically slowing of the alpha rhythm. These changes parallel alterations in the metabolism of brain cells which are entirely non-specific, and may also be elicited by decreasing cerebral blood flow, oxygen saturation, or glucose delivery. The degree of slowing of the electro-encephalogram is roughly proportional to the severity of the encephalopathy, and therefore represents a useful tool for semiquantitative serial monitoring of neurological function in these patients.

Asterixis is the characteristic flapping tremor of PSE, and consists of rapid irregular repetitive involuntary flapping movements of the hand while the hand is held in a dorsiflexed position. This sign is again non-specific but is nevertheless clinically valuable.

Constructional apraxia, the inability to carry out purposeful movements in the absence of paralysis or other motor or sensory impairment, is characteristic of PSE. The classic test is that of the ability to copy a five-pointed star. This test is simple and qualitatively useful but difficult to judge objectively.

Foetor hepaticus is a characteristic odour of the breath in patients with PSE and also in some other patients with liver disease. The application of gas liquid chromatographic analysis has revealed that the odour is due to a variety of sulphur-containing compounds (Chen et al, 1970).

The structural lesion of PSE in the central nervous system is not primarily in the neurones but in the astro-

Table 19.3 Assessment of portal-systemic encephalopathy

Grade	Mental State	Number Connection Test (secs)
0	Normal	15–30
1+	Trivial change in behaviour, short attention span	31–50
2+	Obvious change in personality, time disorientation	51–80
3+	Somnolence, advanced confusion, semi-stupor	81–120
4+	Semi-coma, coma	>120 or unable to do test

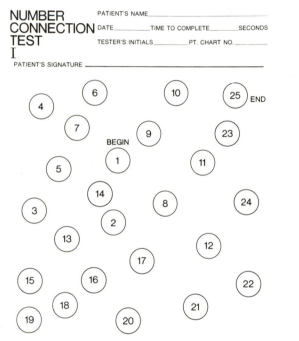

Fig. 19.11 Number connection test. The time taken to connect the numbers in sequence is recorded, and correlates with the clinical status as described in Table 19.3.

cytes, the large star-shaped cells which form the supporting structure of the nervous tissue. These cells subserve an incompletely understood metabolic role in the CNS which probably includes nutritional support for neurones and scavenging and reprocessing of excess neurotransmitters. The so-called Alzheimer Type II change consists of an apparent enlargement and pale staining of the astrocyte nucleus with varying degrees of folding and indentation of the nuclear membrane, and may be seen both in man and in experimental animals (Von Hösslin & Alzheimer, 1912). These changes suggest metabolic hyperactivity, and are irregularly distributed in the brain, being most marked in areas of deep grey matter. Changes in the neurones themselves are relatively late and inconstant.

Pathogenesis of PSE

The PSE syndrome was first recognized in 1893 by Hahn and his colleagues in dogs subjected to Eck fistulae (portacaval shunt). These animals developed neurological symptoms which were described as 'meat intoxication', which proceeded to coma and death if meat feeding continued, but from which the animals made a complete recovery if protein feeding stopped. It was recognized in the 1930s that administration of urea or ammonium chloride caused mental disturbances in cirrhotic patients, and PSE was first described in a patient with a portacaval shunt in 1949 by Adams and Foley.

The belief was long held that PSE was due entirely to direct entry into the systemic circulation of nitrogenous material borne in the portal circulation without first being detoxicated by the liver. This view is supported by the precipitation of PSE in cirrhotic patients by the administration of a high protein diet or by the presence of a large amount of blood in the gastrointestinal tract following bleeding from oesophageal varices. Urea in the gastrointestinal tract is degraded entirely by bacterial action, and results in the absorption of ammonia into the portal blood. If urea is administered to a germ-free animal there is no such rise in blood ammonia, and similarly the nonabsorbable antibiotic neomycin is effective in the treatment of PSE. Once absorbed into the portal circulation ammonia or other nitrogenous waste products are normally detoxicated by the liver, but in patients with liver disease with either intra- or extrahepatic portal-systemic anastomoses this filtration does not take place.

The concentration of ammonia in the plasma shows a good (though not perfect) correlation with the presence and degree of PSE (Stahl, 1963). There are several mechanisms by which ammonia might be toxic to the CNS. Ammonia combines with glutamic acid to form glutamine; the level of glutamine in the brain and in the CSF is high in cirrhotic patients, and very high in the presence of severe PSE. Glutamine or its metabolites may exert a toxic effect in the CNS (Vergara et al, 1974). Depletion of glutamate (an excitatory neurotransmitter) by combination with excess ammonia will also produce nervous depression. Levels of glutamate in the brain and CSF have been shown to be depressed in PSE. It has been suggested that α-ketoglutarate becomes depleted by combination with ammonia to form glutamate, thus slowing down the Krebs cycle, with a consequent decrease in energy metabolism.

More recently it has been suggested that PSE is related to disorders of amino acid balance. In chronic PSE the plasma levels of branched-chain amino acids (valine, leucine, and isoleucine) are reduced, while those of the aromatic amino acids (tyrosine and phenylalanine) are elevated. The failing liver cells are unable to metabolize tyrosine and phenylalanine, while the branched-chain amino acids which are utilized principally in muscle and adipose tissue undergo an increased rate of removal under the influence of elevated levels of insulin found in chronic liver disease (Munro et al, 1975). These two groups of amino acids compete for entry into the CNS via a common carrier-mediated transport mechanism across the blood-brain barrier, a mechanism which is also shared by tryptophan. In the absence of high levels of branched-chain amino acids, the aromatic group and tryptophan gain increased entry to the CNS; this imbalance of substrates may lead to abnormal amine metabolism, with the formation of so called 'false neurotransmitters' such as octopamine and β-phenylethanolamine (Fischer & Baldessarini, 1971). Increased levels of these substances have indeed been found in patients with PSE. Fischer and his colleagues have suggested that restoration of the normal balance of plasma amino acids by the infusion of a solution high in the branched-chain group may produce reversal of neurological changes in patients with chronic liver disease (Fischer et al, 1976). These suggestions have not, however, been widely confirmed, and other substances, such as the inhibitory neurotransmitter γ-aminobutyric acid (GABA) may be of major importance (Schafer & Jones, 1983).

This list of hypotheses for the pathogenesis of PSE is far from complete, and all of the theories remain unproven. It is clear however, that there is a most important relationship between hepatocellular function and portal-systemic shunting in the production of PSE. It is almost certainly true that without some degree of shunting there can be no PSE. Conversely, portal-systemic shunting is less likely to give rise to PSE if the hepatocellular function is near to normal. It is possible to create a model of shunting with near normal liver function in rats by the procedure of portacaval transposition, in which the portal venous blood is diverted to the systemic circulation and the inflow to the portal tracts of the liver is replaced by systemic blood from the vena cava. In this situation liver blood flow is normal (Ryan et al, 1978) and liver function does not deteriorate as it does following creation of standard end-to-side portacaval anastomosis (Benjamin et al, 1984). Rats with a portacaval transposition show a normal plasma amino acid profile, while those with an end-to-side shunt show the characteristic changes in amino acids described above (I. S. Benjamin, unpublished data). Histological changes of PSE are seen in the brains of the rats with portacaval anastomoses, but they occur to a very much lesser extent in rats with a portacaval transposition (Doyle et al, 1978). Thus, despite the presence of total shunting of portal blood into the systemic circulation, the normally functioning liver is able to protect the CNS from metabolic damage.

These findings have an important implication in the selection of patients with chronic liver disease for portal decompression procedures. Those patients who have well maintained liver function, and particularly those with non-cirrhotic liver disease, will usually fare better following portal-systemic shunting than those with severe liver disease. However, the sudden deprivation of a large portal venous inflow from a relatively healthy liver may result in progressive atrophy and deterioration in liver function resulting in severe PSE. It is in these patients that a selective shunting procedure such as the Warren distal spleno-renal shunt may be most indicated (see section on portal hypertension above).

Therapy

Chronic liver failure

Since the treatment of the underlying liver disease is usually expectant, specific therapy is largely restricted to general supportive measures. Nutrition must be maintained, in the face of possible hypoalbuminaemia. Thus the patients require a high carbohydrate intake, coupled with as high a protein level as they can tolerate in the diet. In patients with chronic PSE, it is often impossible to give a high oral protein intake without precipitating neurological changes. A balance must therefore be struck between low and high protein intake. There is some evidence that vegetable protein is less prone to production of PSE than meat protein (Greenberger et al, 1977). Anaemia must be avoided and ascites controlled by the use of salt restriction and diuretics, preferably spironolactone in order to restrict potassium loss which potentiates the toxic effects of ammonia.

Excessive absorption of nitrogenous products from the colon may be avoided by preventing constipation. Reduction of ammonia production in the colon may be achieved by administration of antibiotic agents designed to destroy the intestinal bacteria which are the source of the ammonia-generating enzymes. Administration of antibiotics such as neomycin, however, carries the hazard of toxic side-effects, so that this is not useful as a long-term measure. Acidification of the contents of the colon reduces both the production and absorption of ammonia. Lactulose is a disaccharide which is broken down by bacterial action in the colon to acid metabolites (which in themselves have a valuable laxative effect), and has no known major toxicity. Its chronic use has been shown to improve neurological function and to reduce blood ammonia levels (Conn et al, 1977). In the last resort total colectomy or colonic exclusion with ileosigmoid anastomosis has been performed with good effect, though with high mortality (Resnick et al, 1968), and this procedure is now rarely recommended.

Acute PSE

In the majority of cases, encephalopathy has been precipitated by a gastrointestinal bleed, and in this case the most important treatment is to control the bleeding and thus prevent continuous infusion of protein into the gastro-intestinal tract. Accumulated old blood is removed by enemas and purgation, and neomycin or lactulose may also be effective. Since cirrhotic patients are very susceptible to narcotic drugs, the use of sedatives should be minimal. Electrolyte imbalance may also precipitate coma, and attention to this is important.

Specific measures for the treatment of acute liver failure with deep coma have been extensively investigated, but none is of proven value. The use of amino acid infusions has already been mentioned and this is still under assessment. In some cases of acute liver failure, particularly those due to drugs or to acute hepatitis, there is rapid deterioration of function, but if the patient can be kept alive during the acute illness, liver regeneration may take place with complete recovery.

Unfortunately, there is as yet no machine capable of replacing the functions of the liver. A variety of approaches have been tried:

Charcoal haemoperfusion. The use of activated charcoal as an adsorbent for toxic substances in acute liver failure was initially reported with enthusiasm from the group at King's College Hospital, but the early good results were not substantiated (Williams, 1976). A higher rate of recovery has recently been reported using albumin cellulose nitrate activated charcoal (ACAC) (Chang, 1977). A variety of other adsorbents have been used.

Haemodialysis and peritoneal dialysis. Conventional haemodialysis appears to remove only urea, small amounts of ammonia and other small, water-soluble molecules. However, the use of a large-pore polyacrylonitrile membrane has produced more promising results (Silk et al, 1977).

Exchange transfusion. By this technique, as much of the patient's blood as possible is removed and replaced with fresh donor blood. An exchange of 5.5 l in a 70 kg man replaces 80% of the blood volume; however, this treatment did not prove effective in a controlled trial (Redeker and Yamahiro, 1973). The use of cross-circulation between patients and volunteer subjects has been tried but is fraught with both practical and ethical difficulties.

Extracorporeal liver perfusion. This has been performed using both human cadaver livers and the isolated perfused livers of pigs and baboons (Chalstrey & Parbhoo, 1971). These techniques were also largely unsuccessful, and produced severe coagulation problems in the patients.

Other techniques. Removal of the patient's liver and replacement with a donor organ (orthotopic transplantation) is not a generally applicable technique because of the uncertainty of the prognosis for individual patients in acute hepatic failure. Auxiliary (heterotopic) transplantation, leaving the host organ in situ, has been suggested but remains unproven in practice (Slapak et al, 1970).

The use of cultured hepatocytes in a capillary system to form a synthetic artificial liver has been proposed and is under investigation (Wolf et al, 1978). Further suggestions have been the development of gel-entrapped microsomes or isolated packets of hepatic enzymes to form a 'synthetic' liver (Campbell & Chang, 1975).

The multiplicity of methods proposed for the treatment of acute hepatic failure attests to the lack of efficacy of each.

JAUNDICE

Jaundice or icterus is the name given to the clinical sign of visible yellow pigmentation, due to deposition of bile pigments in the tissues. It is not defined in terms of the level of plasma bilirubin, but usually becomes evident in the skin, mucous membranes and sclerae when the plasma bilirubin exceeds 35 μmol/l (2 mg/dl). It is associated with a variety of distinct pathological syndromes, not all of them surgical, and it is the underlying pathology and not the depth of jaundice which determines prognosis.

The clinical syndromes producing jaundice are classically divided into three groups: (i) haemolytic, or prehepatic, due to an increased bilirubin load; (ii) hepatocellular, due to inability of the liver cells to take up, metabolize or excrete bilirubin, and (iii) obstructive or extrahepatic, due to bilirubin retention secondary to blockage of the major biliary ducts.

These three categories will be described separately, though more than one process may be involved in a single case.

Haemolytic jaundice

The normal liver can readily clear much larger amounts of bile pigment than the body produces. When severe haemolysis occurs, however, due to mismatched blood transfusion, rhesus disease of the newborn or a variety of haematological disorders leading to increased red cell destruction, this reserve may be overwhelmed. Haemolytic jaundice indicates the rapid destruction of blood cells, since the lysis of cells contained in 500 ml of blood is necessary to give rise to mild jaundice lasting one or two days. This is reflected in a marked reticulocytosis, indicating increased production of red cells.

It should be noted that a combination of haemolysis and obstruction may occur in patients with long-standing haemolytic disorders, in whom pigment gallstones form in the bile ducts and may cause ductal obstruction.

The distinction of haemolytic jaundice from other forms is not usually a major clinical problem. The jaundice is generally mild and associated with anaemia and reticulocytosis, and there may be a history of mismatched transfusion, toxic drugs, or haematological disorder in the patient or his relatives. The commonest cause in adults in Western countries is congenital spherocytosis: the spleen may be palpable and haematological tests will make the diagnosis. The stools are heavily pigmented due to excessive stercobilinogen formation and the urine is dark and contains a large amount of urobilinogen when tested. Bilirubin itself is absent from the urine, however, giving rise to the alternative name for this condition, 'acholuric jaundice'.

Hepatocellular jaundice

Several stages of the complex process of transfer of bilirubin from the blood to the bile have already been described (see section on liver functions). The process may fail at any of these stages, giving rise to jaundice of hepatocellular origin. This may be produced by viral or bacterial agents, chemical toxins or drugs. In addition, there is a form of jaundice virtually restricted to newborn infants, in which the glucuronyl transferase enzyme system is insufficiently mature to conjugate a normal load of bilirubin. In this condition the level of unconjugated bilirubin rises and, being lipid soluble, is deposited in the lipid-rich tissues of the central nervous system. This syndrome is termed kernicterus (jaundice of the basal nuclei of the brain) and may produce lethal depression of cellular respiration of the nervous tissues. Phototherapy is effective in stimulating metabolism of the unconjugated bilirubin by means of ultraviolet light.

Probably the commonest cause of hepatocellular jaundice in clinical practice is viral hepatitis. Two principal specific viral agents have been identified: type A ('infectious hepatitis') and type B ('serum hepatitis'). In addition, a third clinical type is presently named by default 'non-A, non-B hepatitis', though the search for a specific causal agent continues.

Type A hepatitis is usually a mild sporadic disease of adolescents or young adults, but severe outbreaks may occur in conditions associated with over-crowding or poor hygiene. Typically, the jaundice succeeds a non-specific prodromal syndrome of nausea, vomiting, lethargy and mental depression and usually fades slowly over 2 weeks or more.

In more severe cases, jaundice persists and may be difficult to distinguish from biliary obstruction, since swelling of the hepatocytes adds an obstructive component to the hepatocellular pathology. Recovery is the rule, though a few cases progress to chronic active hepatitis and posthepatitic cirrhosis, or very rarely to liver failure and death.

The infective agent of type B hepatitis, formerly termed 'homologous serum jaundice', proved much more elusive to investigators, but has now been demonstrated by electron microscopy. Its principal epidemiological marker — the Australia Antigen described by Blumberg in 1967 — is now referred to as hepatitis B surface antigen (HBsAg), and two other antigens ('c' and 'e') have now been described associated with the B virus. The subject is reviewed by Sherlock (1974).

Transmission of hepatitis B is by innoculation with infected material from the plasma or other body fluids of an affected patient or an asymptomatic carrier. The first known outbreak was in Bremen in Germany in 1885, when 199 of 1289 workmen innoculated against smallpox with vaccine prepared from human lymph developed hepatitis. The classical risk is from contaminated needles or syringes, or from infected blood or plasma. The risk from plasma is greatest because this is prepared from the pooled blood of numerous donors. Since the advent of routine screening for HBsAg in donors the hazard is now small, but patients exposed to repeated transfusions of blood or plasma are still at risk. The risk is particularly high in renal dialysis units, and there have been several instances of infection amongst staff or technicians working in such units, some of them fatal. There is also an increased risk amongst drug addicts, and sexual transmission occurs, notably between homosexuals.

Type B hepatitis has a longer incubation period (2–6 months) than type A (2–6 weeks), and runs a much more virulent course, with liver necrosis and a considerable risk of mortality from acute liver failure. Of the survivors, some will go on to develop chronic hepatitis or cirrhosis, and some remain asymptomatic carriers of the antigens.

The principal relevance of hepatocellular jaundice to the surgeon lies in its distinction from obstructive jaundice. This distinction is of more than academic importance: laparotomy as a diagnostic procedure in hepatocellular jaundice carries a high mortality, while prolonged conservative management of obstructive jaundice also increases the hazard of subsequent surgery. The methods applied to making this distinction are described below. Although diagnosis of jaundice using liver function tests and clinical history may be accurate in up to 70% of cases, there remains a group in whom this is more difficult. The standard biochemical tests of liver function are most informative early in the course of the disease, but later, as a mixed pathological and biochemical picture develops, these tests become increasingly unreliable.

There is a heterogeneous group of congenital defects of cellular bilirubin metabolism which cause elevations of plasma levels of no clinical significance. These cases may however cause confusion on routine biochemical testing. They include Gilbert's syndrome (unconjugated bilirubin) and the Dubin-Johnson and Rotor syndromes (conjugated and unconjugated bilirubin).

Obstructive jaundice

The physical and chemical effects of bile duct obstruction are readily predictable. The bile duct above an obstruction increases in calibre under the pressure of continued bile and mucus secretion in the liver and biliary tree. This dilatation occurs also in the intrahepatic biliary radicles, unless the liver is primarily diseased and fibrosis prevents such distension. If this distension is prolonged, back pressure on the hepatic parenchyma and accumulation of bile acids within the hepatocytes ultimately cause hepatocellular damage. The small bile ductules become blocked with inspissated bile, and are stimulated to proliferate. Eventually the liver architecture is distorted by a network of newly-formed bile ducts and fibrous septa infiltrated with periportal inflammatory cells. These changes are particularly marked in the presence of infection in the biliary tree (cholangitis), which may lead to severe progressive liver damage.

For some time the hepatocytes continue to conjugate bilirubin, but cannot secrete this into the obstructed bile duct. Conjugated bilirubin is therefore reabsorbed from the hepatocytes, appears in rising amounts in the plasma and is excreted in the urine. When the obstruction is severe and prolonged, a degree of hepatocellular failure ensues, and unconjugated bilirubin levels also rise, giving a biochemically mixed picture.

Since bilirubin is excluded from the intestine, stercobilinogen is not formed and the stools lose their pigmentation. Urobilinogen is absent from the urine, but conjugated bilirubin is excreted in large amounts, giving rise to the classical picture of 'pale stools and dark urine'. This is in contrast with hepatocellular jaundice, in which neither conjugated bilirubin nor urobilinogen is found in the urine. Intermittent obstruction, such as may occur with bile duct calculi or with tumours of the ampulla of Vater, may not give rise to the completely pigment-free, putty-coloured stools of total obstruction.

In addition to bile pigments, bile salts are excluded from the intestines and retained in the blood stream. The pruritus (itching) which is characteristic of obstructive jaundice may be due to deposition of bile salts in the skin. Exclusion of bile salts from the intestine interferes with the digestion and absorption of fats (leading to steatorrhoea in severe cases) and also fat-soluble vitamins. Deficiency of vitamin K leads in turn to deficient prothrombin synthesis, and to a bleeding tendency. Administration of parenteral vitamin K is thus a routine procedure in obstructive jaundice and the response to this treatment is usually rapid. When hepatocellular disease is severe, however, vitamin K administration may fail to secure a response, since the hepatocytes themselves are incapable of prothrombin synthesis.

A number of other systemic effects of obstructive jaundice are of importance to the surgeon. The absence of bile salts from the intestine is associated with increased absorption of bacterial endotoxin, which may further fail to be filtered by the Kupffer cells (Ingoldby, 1981). The resulting high levels of circulating endotoxin may aggravate abnormalities and have also been held partly responsible for the increased hazard of acute renal failure in the jaundiced patient. Endotoxins produce renal vasoconstriction and are associated with glomerular and peritubular fibrin deposits. The kidneys are particularly susceptible to damage from peroperative and postoperative hypotension in the jaundiced patient, and careful attention to hydration and maintenance of renal blood flow is vital. It is possible that all of these effects are compounded by hypoalbuminaemia, which is common in chronic liver disease, and by sepsis, which is a frequent accompaniment of biliary obstruction. Poor nutritional status may also be a factor in the impaired wound healing which is observed in the jaundiced patient and can be reproduced in the experimental animal. The presence of obstructive jaundice appears to have a specific depressant effect on collagen biosynthesis (Than Than et al, 1977), although the precise mechanism of this is not known. It does not appear to be due to direct toxicity of bilirubin itself.

These various systemic effects of jaundice increase the overall risk of surgery, and many surgeons adopt some form of two-stage approach to operating on such patients. The object of this approach is to avoid carrying out major surgery on the jaundiced patient, and this is achieved by preliminary decompression of the biliary tract, either surgically or by insertion of a catheter percutaneously into the obstructed bile ducts within the liver (Molnar & Stockum, 1974). After a period of drainage of bile and relief of the jaundice, during which attention can be paid to nutritional status and renal function, the patient may be rendered more fit to withstand major surgery.

Causes of obstructive jaundice

The usual causes of obstruction of the extrahepatic bile ducts are calculi which have migrated from the gallbladder to the common bile duct or have formed in a pathological duct (primary common duct stones), tumours compressing the duct in its distal portion, and benign strictures due to inflammatory conditions or to trauma. In neonates, developmental anomalies including total congenital biliary atresia must be added to this list. It may be possible, using a combination of careful clinical history and physical examination, to distinguish between these causes. The jaundice of malignant obstruction, for example, is classically progressive and may be painless: a palpable distended gallbladder is more frequently associated with tumours of the pancreas or distal bile duct than with calculous disease. The more important distinction is that between hepatocellular jaundice (which requires conservative management) and obstruction (which usually requires operative relief). Some of the techniques used to make this distinction are discussed below.

Liver function tests used in the diagnosis of jaundice

Plasma bilirubin. The total plasma bilirubin is of course elevated, and this is essential in monitoring the course of an individual case of jaundice. Fluctuating levels from day to day suggest intermittent calculous obstruction. Determination of the proportions of conjugated and unconjugated bilirubin may be more helpful: older texts use the terms 'direct' and 'indirect', referring to the reaction to the Van den Bergh test for bilirubin. The absence of conjugated bilirubin suggests hepatocellular jaundice, while excessive levels of conjugated bilirubin are suggestive of biliary obstruction. These findings, however, are rarely specific.

Urinary bilirubin and urobilinogen. These tests are unaccountably ignored by surgeons. The persistent absence of urobilinogen from the urine is strong evidence of obstructive jaundice, while marked excess is a feature of haemolysis. Incomplete or intermittent obstruction or hepatocellular jaundice produces intermediate levels in the urine. Bilirubin is usually present in the urine in obstruction, but may be absent with advanced hepatocellular disease.

Serum alkaline phosphatase. This may rise to very high levels in total duct obstruction. More modest elevations are seen in cases of minor partial or intermittent obstruction, and may be a most important biochemical marker in such cases. It may be necessary to distinguish between alkaline phosphatase of hepatic or of skeletal origin, especially when malignant disease is suspected, since bony metastases may produce elevated serum enzyme levels. This can be achieved by separating the alkaline phosphatase into its isoenzymes, which differ with the origin of the enzyme.

Serum aminotransferases. The aminotransferases (or transaminases) are intracellular enzymes of metabolically active tissues, notably liver and muscle, and their appearance in the serum reflects cellular disruption (see section on liver functions). Thus elevated levels are seen in both hepatitis and myocardial infarction. In viral hepatitis the levels of both alanine (ALT) and aspartate (AST) aminotransferases are grossly elevated at an early stage in the disease, with peak levels commonly 7–10 days before the peak elevation of plasma bilirubin. ALT is the more specific of the two enzymes, being more or less confined to liver cells, but in the presence of severe cellular necrosis (for example, in paracetamol poisoning) AST reaches higher levels. While these tests are valuable for the detection of liver damage, they are not specific: they may be elevated late in the course of biliary obstruction, and their principal diagnostic value in hepatitis is in the first few days of the disease. They are useful for monitoring the progress of chronic liver disease such as chronic active hepatitis.

Other enzymes. Gamma glutamyl transferase and 5-nucleotidase are both maximally elevated in obstructive jaundice, but also in hepatocellular disease. They may be useful in elucidating elevations of alkaline phosphatase when bony disease might cause confusion.

Other tests of liver function are even less specific. They are described below for completeness.

Protein electrophoresis. Albumin is frequently reduced and globulins elevated in chronic liver disease, giving a characteristic reversed albumin : globulin ratio. Several tests rely on this phenomenon for their activity. These include thymol turbidity and a variety of 'flocculation tests', but are now seldom used in surgical practice.

Serum cholesterol. This is reduced in chronic liver disease and may be raised in long-standing biliary obstruction.

Bromsulphthalein (BSP). This is a dye which is taken up by the liver, conjugated with glutathione and excreted in the bile. It is thus handled in a similar way to bilirubin, and may give a useful index of this particular facet of liver function. A standard dose is usually given (as an intravenous bolus) which will approach the normal liver's maximum handling capacity, and blood levels are measured at 5 and 45 minutes. This normally results in a retention of less than 5% of the dose at 45 minutes, though the true range in the normal population may be wider. More informative but more elaborate is the information obtained from intravenous infusion of BSP with serial blood sampling, from which values for the relative components of hepatic storage capacity and transport maximum (Tm) may be derived. The Tm for BSP is said to be the best single determinant of hepatic dysfunction and may be valuable in following the course of chronic liver disease or in predicting the outcome of surgery in portal hypertension (Turner et al, 1974). Other dyes, such as indocyanine green and Rose Bengal, have been used in a similar way. These tests are of very limited value in the jaundiced patient, and also depend on the assumption of a near-normal liver blood flow, since delivery of the dye affects its extraction (see also section on circulation).

Non-biochemical tests in the diagnosis of jaundice

Because of the non-specificity of the biochemical tests, more reliable methods are necessary for the important distinction between surgical and non-surgical jaundice in a number of complex cases. The use of ultrasonic scanning of the liver has proved valuable in detecting the presence of dilatation of the intrahepatic bile ducts. Since this is very reliable evidence of the presence of extrahepatic biliary obstruction, the technique is now widely used as a screening procedure for obstructive jaundice. On occasions, it may yield other valuable information, such as the presence of stones in the gallbladder, or evidence of a malignant mass in the pancreas or tumour deposits in the liver.

Orally or intravenously administered contrast media will fail to outline the biliary tract in the jaundiced patient, so that direct means of contrast radiology have to be employed. Contrast may be introduced into the dilated bile ducts by means of a fine, flexible needle passed through the body wall and through liver substance, into the large ducts towards the hilum of the liver. This technique (percutaneous transhepatic cholangiography — PTC) is usually successful, and rarely causes troublesome bleeding or bile leakage. Alternatively, contrast may be injected into the bile duct by way of a plastic cannula introduced through the papilla of Vater using a duodenoscope (endoscopic retrograde choledochography and pancreatography — ERCP). These techniques also allow a precise diagnosis of the level and nature of an obstructing lesion in the majority of cases. The ordering of these diagnostic techniques into a system applicable in most surgical units has been described and is now widely used (Benjamin & Blumgart, 1979).

Histological examination of a percutaneous liver biopsy may provide the distinction between hepatocellular and obstructive jaundice in two-thirds or more of cases, but the performance of this procedure in the presence of obstruction may lead to intraperitoneal bile leakage and biliary peritonitis. Its use is therefore restricted to those patients in whom large duct obstruction has been excluded by the use of one or more of the above techniques.

LIVER REGENERATION

The capacity of the liver to regain its former mass following partial resection has been scientifically documented for almost a century. It has become conventional, however, to attribute the first account of liver regeneration to the Prometheus myth. As punishment for the theft of fire from the gods, Zeus had Prometheus chained to a rock where his liver was eaten each day by a vulture and regenerated each night. This legend does in fact highlight the remarkable phenomenon by which the liver is able to survive numerous (possibly indefinite) successive partial resections, with restoration to physical and functional normality. Clearly this capacity is of great importance in liver surgery, since it permits safe resection of liver substance for tumour or for trauma, in the knowledge that there will be eventual restoration to normal liver function in patients who survive the initial procedure. However, it is of equal importance in medical practice, since the objective of treatment for patients with massive liver necrosis following toxic liver injury or viral hepatitis is the maintenance of vital systems while the residual healthy hepatocytes undergo a proliferative response and restore the liver to normal.

Despite intense research effort into the mechanisms controlling this important phenomenon, the process remains incompletely understood. The liver cells normally form a stable population, in which there is a continuous process of cell death and replacement at the rate of approximately 1 in 20 000 mature cells. Following partial hepatectomy the liver mass is replaced by a process of compensatory hyperplasia of the remaining liver cells, leading to an increase in size of the liver remnant. This process of compensatory hyperplasia of the liver differs from true regeneration from a cut edge of tissue, such as the regrowth of the salamander's limb, in that new liver lobes do not grow but the existing lobes expand. The regenerating remnant moulds to the contours of the abdominal cavity during this process, the direction of growth being determined by the contiguous organs. We have observed a clinical case in which, following a partial hepatectomy, the liver has regenerated to surround the spleen almost completely.

The rate of regeneration varies somewhat from species to species. Because the rat is an economical experimental animal and also has a conveniently lobulated liver, it is in this species that the most detailed information on the process has been obtained. Two-thirds of a rat's liver is easily and rapidly removed (Higgins & Anderson, 1931), and the time course of the restoration of liver mass to normal is shown in Figure 19.12. It can be seen that by 1 week after hepatectomy the liver has achieved 75 per cent of the estimated original weight, and by 21 days it has reached its pre-operative mass. It was formerly believed that 4–6 months were necessary for full restoration of liver mass in man. More recent observations in patients who have undergone resection for trauma or tumour have shown that the process may be much more rapid, and that the majority of this restoration is complete within 10 days to 3 weeks (Blumgart et al, 1971).

The earliest intracellular events following liver resection are seen within a few hours (Bucher, 1967). In the rat the

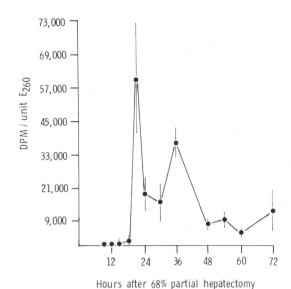

Fig. 19.13 The incorporation of ^{3}H-thymidine (injected 1 hour before sacrifice) into the liver in rats subjected to 68% partial hepatectomy 12–72 hours earlier. (The uptake is expressed as disintegrations/min per unit of extinction at E_{260}.) Note the peaks of uptake at 21 hours and 36 hours, corresponding to activity in hepatic parenchymal and littoral cells of the liver, respectively.

process of cellular replication is best examined by measuring the rate of uptake into nuclear DNA of thymidine labelled with tritium (^{3}H), a radioactive isotope of hydrogen. The kinetics of this process are reliably constant, and consist of a sharp increase in activity at 18 hours, peaking at around 21 hours, with a further sharp fall (Fig. 19.13). A second smaller and less distinct peak is seen at 36 hours. This wave of DNA synthesis is followed in turn by a wave of mitotic activity in the hepatocytes which reaches its maximum at 28–29 hours: the exact timing of these phenomena is related to the extent of the hepatectomy (Weinbren & Woodward, 1964). It is thought that the first peak of mitotic activity occurs in the hepatocytes themselves, and that the second peak is related to division of cells of the supporting structure of the liver, including the vascular and biliary structures and the reticulo-endothelial cells. As the liver cells regenerate, a supporting collagenous 'skeleton' must also be supplied, and an increase in the rate of synthesis of collagen has been demonstrated during the first 4 days after liver resection (Benjamin et al, 1978). Complete maturation of the collagen may require several months (Bucher, 1967).

Control of liver regeneration

The mechanisms which initiate, control, and terminate the hyperplastic response following resection or injury have been extensively investigated, and yet remain unclear. One of the principal areas of debate has concerned the relative importance of liver blood flow and of specific factors

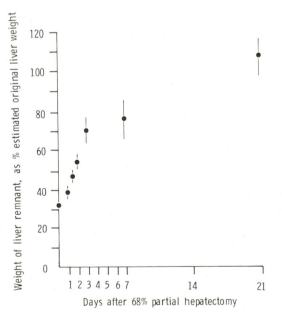

Fig. 19.12 Increase in the liver remnant weight 1 to 21 days following 68% partial hepatectomy in the rat. The remnant weight is expressed as a percentage of the estimated original total liver weight, and shown as mean of 4 rats. Error bars = 1 s.d.

carried in the circulation. This latter group have been named 'hepatotrophic factors', or more specifically 'portal hepatotrophic factors' on the assumption that these are delivered to the hepatocytes by portal venous blood. (This debate is extensively reviewed in a CIBA Foundation Symposium published in 1978.) In 1944 Mann performed an experiment in which an end-to-side portacaval anastomosis was followed by partial liver resection in the dog. He found that liver regeneration was abolished, and concluded that actual portal blood flow through the liver was a necessary stimulus to regeneration. Unfortunately this experiment, and others since that time, failed to take into account the liver atrophy which is produced by diversion of portal blood (see section on portal hypertension). It is now clear that the processes of atrophy/hypertrophy and of regenerative hyperplasia are quite distinct, and to a large degree are independently controlled. This leads to the paradoxical situation in which atrophied hepatocytes retain the capacity to proliferate in response to an appropriate stimulus. Experiments with rats subjected to portacaval transposition, in which the portal venous inflow to the liver is replaced volume for volume by systemic venous blood, highlight this distinction (Guest et al, 1977). After portacaval transposition the liver mass falls slowly in relation to the animal's body weight, presumably due to atrophy consequent upon removal of 'hepatotrophic' substances in the portal blood. If a partial hepatectomy is carried out during the course of this process of atrophy, liver regeneration proceeds as expected, with the cellular kinetics of the process unimpaired by the loss of portal venous inflow. However, the final result of the process of regeneration is not the estimated original liver mass at the time of partial hepatectomy, but the slightly lower liver mass which would have resulted from the continuing atrophy if resection had not taken place. Thus we have simultaneous processes of regenerative hyperplasia and of progressive atrophy proceeding in the same organ.

The nature of the trophic factors in portal venous blood has also been the subject of extensive investigation. Cross-circulation experiments have demonstrated that provided there is an adequate exchange of blood between partners, liver resection in one rat will stimulate regenerative hyperplasia in the liver of the second rat, thus demonstrating the existence of some kind of humoral factor (Bucher, 1967). Elegant experiments by Starzl and his colleagues (1973), in which one lobe of a dog's liver receives blood from the intestines and the other lobe blood principally from the pancreas, have demonstrated atrophy in lobes deprived of pancreatic blood. These workers have suggested that pancreatic hormones, and in particular insulin, are the major determinants of liver cell integrity. Other in vivo and in vitro work has suggested synergism between insulin and glucagon in this respect. The role of nutrients, and specifically of amino acids, carried in portal venous blood has also been investigated. It now seems unlikely that there

is a single 'trophic' substance, but that a combination of portal hormones and substrates, against the metabolic background of non-portal factors including adrenocortical hormones, thyroid hormones and other substances, is important in *permitting* the regenerative hyperplastic response to occur. However, the factors which *initiate* this response, and the mechanism by which it is switched off when regeneration is complete, have yet to be elucidated.

Metabolic changes following resection

A relatively predictable metabolic response occurs following liver resection in both animals and man, and the changes which occur are to a large degree proportional to the extent of liver resected. These changes must be anticipated and managed appropriately in the postoperative period.

Hypoglycaemia

Blood glucose falls rapidly following major hepatic resection, since liver glycogen is the principal short term source of glucose mobilization. Thus postoperative monitoring of blood glucose must be carried out carefully, and replacement with 50% dextrose will prevent attacks of clinical hypoglycaemia.

Hypoalbuminaemia

There is a greater fall in the serum albumin level following major hepatic resection than that expected after non-hepatic surgery of a comparable magnitude. Although the absolute rate of albumin synthesis may in fact be increased in the liver remnant, the total production may fall short of that required to maintain normal serum levels. This hypoalbuminaemia may be markedly refractory to intravenous albumin supplementation (Vajrabukka et al, 1975)

Jaundice

The regenerating liver shows a transient impairment of the ability to conjugate and excrete bilirubin, giving rise to a transient hyperbilirubinaemia mostly of the unconjugated variety. Sometimes there may be a mixed picture (see section on jaundice above) in which there is a high proportion of conjugated bilirubin, due to intrahepatic cholestasis. This usually reflects severe general metabolic problems, often related to postoperative sepsis, and is a serious sign.

Haematological changes

These are diverse and complex, and may pose a real clinical problem. Since the liver is the only site of synthesis of fibrinogen and the major site of synthesis of prothrombin (factor II) and of factors II, V, VII, IX and X, there may be specific defects in these substances. Since the half-life of activity of factors V, VII and IX is short, a deficiency may readily occur if there is severe hepatic impairment. In addition the liver, by virtue of its reticulo-endothelial content, plays a major part in the clearance of activated coagulation factors and also in the prevention of excessive fibrinolysis by production of antiplasmin. Treatment with fresh blood or fresh frozen plasma is the mainstay of therapy in correcting these factors, although some workers have used preparations of concentrated clotting factors (II, VII, IX and X). Clinical coagulation problems are greater following resection for trauma than for tumour, and this in part reflects the general response to severe multiple injuries, possibly aggravated by anoxia and hypovolaemia. Intravascular coagulation may also be a problem in this situation.

Finally, it is worth noting that in patients who have large tumours resected, there may already be a degree of compensatory hyperplasia of the unaffected lobes. In these circumstances the metabolic alterations following resection may be minimal, in contrast to the patient with liver trauma in whom no such compensation has occurred.

Hepatic transplantation

The lack of a satisfactory system for support of the patient with liver failure has already been described (see section on hepatocellular failure). The ultimate solution of total hepatectomy and replacement with a donor organ has been successfully performed since the early 1960s, and more than 250 orthotopic liver transplants have now been performed. The main indications have been primary tumours of the liver, biliary atresia, and end-stage hepatic failure usually due to cirrhosis. The recent British experience has been reviewed by Calne and Williams (1977). There is some evidence to suggest that the liver has less tendency to reject than other organs, although the reason for this is unclear. Nevertheless, following transplantation, patients must be maintained on immuno-suppressant drugs and often on corticosteroids.

The donor procedure requires very careful mobilization of the liver (the kidneys are usually removed at the same time for transplant purposes), and perfusion with cold electrolyte solution. Livers have been successfully transported by road or air having had a total ischaemic time up to 10 hours and have functioned satisfactorily after transplantation. Nevertheless, the donor procedure for this transplant requires great expertise, and this is one of the reasons why liver transplantation has not become more widespread.

The liver transplant is sutured into place by anastomosis of the suprahepatic and infrahepatic vena cava, the hepatic artery and the portal vein. Bile drainage may be established in a number of ways: that used by Calne (Calne & Williams, 1977) consists of placing the gall bladder as a conduit between the donor and the recipient common bile ducts. Because the patient cannot be maintained by an artificial support system such as that available for renal failure, immediate function of the transplanted liver is of great importance. If the liver has not been properly prepared or preserved and has suffered too much ischaemic damage, then the patient suffers progressive hypoglycaemia and deterioration in liver function, and may develop a bleeding diathesis which precedes death without regaining consciousness. Results from the first 100 orthotopic transplants performed by Starzl in Denver (Putnam et al, 1977) showed a 29% one-year survival. In patients who have survived the first year the mortality rate falls markedly, and there are now several five-year survivors of this procedure. Tumour recurrence is not uncommon in patients with primary malignancy of the liver, which limits its usefulness in such cases.

The alternative of heterotopic (auxiliary) liver transplantation is relatively untried. This is in part related to the phenomena discussed above in the section on liver regeneration, since there appears to be functional competition between the host liver and the donor liver for the 'trophic factors' which will maintain hepatic mass and function. Nevertheless, since the host liver is not removed this procedure is not so final as orthotopic transplantation, and if successful techniques become available it might have wider indications for patients with end-stage hepatic failure.

REFERENCES

Adam R D, Foley J M 1949 The neurological changes in the more common types of severe liver disease. Transactions of the American Neurological Association 74: 217–219

Andreen M, Irestedt L 1976 Decrease in oxygen consumption in the dog liver during temporary arterial occlusion. Acta Physiologica Scandinavica 98: 103–109

Andreen M, Irestedt L, Thulin L 1975 The effect of controlled halothane anaesthesia on splanchnic oxygen consumption in the dog. Acta Anaesthesiologica Scandinavica 19: 238–244

Aronsen K F, Ericsson B, Fajgelj A, Lindell S E 1966 The clearance of 133-Xenon from the liver after intraportal injection in man. Nuclear Medicine 5: 241–245

Bashour F A, Geumei A, Nafrawi A G, Downey H F 1973 Glucagon: its effects on the hepatic arterial and portal venous beds in dogs. Pflügers Archiv 344: 83–92

Batchelder B M, Cooperman L H 1975 Effects of anesthetics on splanchnic circulation and metabolism. Surgical Clinics of North America 55: 787–794

Benjamin I S, Blumgart L H 1985 Biliary bypass and reconstructive surgery. In: Wright R (ed) Liver and Biliary Disease:

Pathophysiology, Diagnosis, Management 2nd edn. W B Saunders, London, p 1463–1494

Benjamin I S, Ryan C J, Engelbrecht G H C, Campbell J C, Van Hoorn-Hickman R, Blumgart L H 1984 Portacaval transposition in the rat: definition of a valuable model for hepatic research. Hepatology 4: 704–708

Benjamin I S, Ryan C J, McLay A L C, Horne C H W, Blumgart L H 1976 The effects of portacaval shunting and portacaval transposition on serum IgG levels in the rat. Gastroenterology 70: 661–664

Benjamin I S, Than Than, Ryan S, Rodger M C, McGee J O'D, Blumgart L H 1978 Prolyl hydroxylase and collagen biosynthesis in rat liver following varying degrees of partial hepatectomy. British Journal of Experimental Pathology 59: 333–336

Bismuth H 1986 Surgical anatomy of the liver. In: Bengmark S, Blumgart L H (eds) Liver Surgery. Churchill Livingstone, Edinburgh, p 1–7

Blumberg B S, Gerstley B J S, Hungerford D A, London W T, Sutnick A I 1967 A serum antigen (Australia antigen) in Downs' syndrome, leukaemia, and hepatitis. Annals of Internal Medicine 66: 924–931

Blumgart L H, Leach K G, Karran S J 1971 Observations on liver regeneration after right hepatic lobectomy. Gut 12: 922–928

Boyer T D, Triger D R, Horisawa M, Redeker A G, Reynolds T B 1977 Direct transhepatic measurement of portal vein pressure using a thin needle. Comparison with wedged hepatic vein pressure. Gastroenterology 72: 584–589

Bradley S E, Ingelfinger F J, Bradley G P, Curry J J 1945 The estimation of hepatic blood flow in man. Journal of Clinical Investigation 24: 890–897

Bradley S E, Ingelfinger F J, Groff A E, Bradley G P 1948 Estimated hepatic blood flow and hepatic venous oxygen content in cirrhosis of the liver. Proceedings of the Society for Experimental Biology and Medicine 67: 206–207

Bucher N L R 1967 Experimental aspects of liver regeneration. New England Journal of Medicine 277: 686–696

Burchell A R, Moreno A H, Panke W F, Nealon T F Jr 1974 Hemodynamic variables and prognosis following portacaval shunts. Surgery, Gynecology and Obstetrics 138: 359–369

Burchell A R, Moreno A H, Panke W F, Nealon T F Jr 1976 Hepatic artery flow improvement after portacaval shunt: a single hemodynamic clinical correlate. Annals of Surgery 184: 289–300

Caesar J, Shaldon S, Chiandussi L, Guevara L, Sherlock S 1961 The use of indocyanine green in the measurement of hepatic blood flow and as a test of hepatic function. Clinical Science 21: 43–57

Calne R Y, Williams R 1977 Orthotopic liver transplantation: the first 60 patients. British Medical Journal 1: 471–476

Campbell J, Chang T M S 1975 Enzymatic recycling of coenzymes by a multi-enzyme system immobilized within semipermeable collodion microcapsules. Biochimica et Biophysica Acta (Amsterdam) 397: 101–109

Chalstrey L J, Parbhoo S P 1971 Circuitry and technique of extracorporeal porcine liver perfusion for the treatment of hepatic coma. British Journal of Surgery 58: 522–524

Chang T M S 1977 Albumin-cellulose nitrate coated charcoal (ACAC) hemoperfusion in FHF. American Journal of Gastroenterology 69:378

Chen S, Zieve L, Mahadevan V 1970 Mercaptans and dimethyl sulfide in the breath of patients with cirrhosis of the liver. Journal of Clinical and Laboratory Medicine 75: 628–635

Cherrick G R, Kerr D N S, Read A E, Sherlock S 1960 Colloid osmotic pressure and hydrostatic pressure relationships in the formation of ascites in hepatic cirrhosis. Clinical Science 19: 361–375

Chiandussi L, Greco F, Sardi G, Vaccarino A, Ferraris C M, Curti B 1968 Estimation of hepatic arterial and portal venous blood flow by direct catheterisation of the vena porta through the umbilical cord in man. Acta Hepatosplenologica 15: 166–171

Child C G 1953 Eck's fistula. Surgery, Gynecology and Obstetrics 96: 375–376

Ciba Foundation Symposium 55 1978 Hepatotrophic factors. Elsevier, North Holland

Classen M, Ossenberg F W 1977 Non-surgical removal of common bile duct stones. Gut 18: 760–769

Cohen P, Gardner F H, Barnett G O 1961 Reclassification of the thrombocytopaenias by the ^{51}Cr labelling method for measuring

platelet life span. New England Journal of Medicine 264: 1294–1299, and 1350–1355

Combes B 1960 Estimation of hepatic blood flow in man and in dogs by ^{131}I-labelled rose bengal. Journal of Laboratory and Clinical Medicine 56: 537–543

Conn H O, Leevy C M, Vlahcevic J R et al 1977 Comparison of lactulose and neomycin in the treatment of chronic portal-systemic encephalopathy: a double blind trial. Gastroenterology 72: 573–583

Culbertson J W, Wilkins R W, Ingelfinger F J, Bradley S E 1951 The effect of the upright position upon the hepatic blood flow. Journal of Clinical Investigation 30: 305–311

Darle N, Kock N G, Lewis D H 1968 Liver blood flow in man studied with the Xenon method. Bulletin de la Societe Internationale de Chirurgie 3: 203–207

Dobson E L, Jones H B 1952 The behaviour of intravenously injected particulate material. Its rate of disappearance from the blood stream as a measure of liver blood flow. Acta Medica Scandinavica Supplementum 273: 1–71

Doyle D, Ryan C J, Benjamin I S, Blumgart L H 1978 Changes in the nuclei of astrocytes following portacaval shunting and portacaval transposition in the rat. British Journal of Experimental Pathology 59: 461–466

Epstein R M, Deutsch S, Cooperman L H, Clement A J, Price H L 1966 Splanchnic circulation during halothane anaesthesia and hypercapnia in normal man. Anesthesiology 27: 654–661

Fischer J E, Baldessarïni R J 1971 False neurotransmitters and hepatic failure. Lancet ii: 75–79

Fischer J E, Rosen H M, Ebeid A M, James J H, Keane J M, Soeters P B 1976 The effect of normalization of plasma amino acids on hepatic encephalopathy in man. Surgery 80: 77–91

Galambos J T, Warren W D, Rudman D, Smith R B, Salam A A 1976 Selective and total shunts in the treatment of bleeding varices. A randomized controlled trial. New England Journal of Medicine 295: 1089–1095

Gelman S I 1976 Disturbances in hepatic blood flow during anaesthesia and surgery. Archives of Surgery 111: 881–883

George C F 1979 Drug kinetics and hepatic blood flow. Clinical Pharmacokinetics 4: 433–448

Goresky C A, Haddad H H, Kluger W S, Nedeau B E, Bach G G 1974 The enhancement of maximal bilirubin excretion with taurocholate-induced increments in bile flow. Canadian Journal of Physiology and Pharmacology 52: 389–403

Greenberger N J, Carley J E, Schenker S, Bettinger I, Stammes C, Beyer P 1977 Effect of vegetable and animal protein diets in chronic hepatic encephalopathy. American Journal of Digestive Diseases 22: 845–855

Greenway C V, Lautt W W 1970 Effects of hepatic venous pressure on trans-sinusoidal fluid transfer in the liver of the anesthetized cat. Circulation Research 26: 697–703

Greenway C V, Stark R D 1971 Hepatic vascular bed. Physiological Reviews 51: 23–65

Groszmann R J, Kotelanski B, Cohn J N 1971 Hepatic lobar distribution of splenic and mesenteric blood flow in man. Gastroenterology 60: 1047–1052

Groszmann R J, Kravetz D, Paryson 0 1977 Intrahepatic arteriovenous shunting in cirrhosis of the liver. Gastroenterology 73: 201–204

Guest J, Ryan C J, Benjamin I S, Blumgart L H 1977 Portacaval transposition and subsequent partial hepatectomy in the rat: effects on liver atrophy, hypertrophy and regenerative hyperplasia. British Journal of Experimental Pathology 58: 140–146

Hahn M, Massen O, Nencki M, Pawlow J 1893 Die Eck'sche Fistel zwischen der unteren Hohlvene und der Pfortader und ihre Folgen fuer den Organismus. Archiv für Experimentelle Pathologie und Pharmakologie 32: 161–210

Harper A M, Lorimer A R, Thomas D L 1974 Methods of measuring blood flow. In: Scurr C, Feldman S (eds) Scientific Foundations of Anaesthesia. Heinemann, London, 2nd edn, pp 53–70

Higgins G M, Anderson R M 1931 Experimental pathology of the liver. I. Restoration of the liver of the white rat following partial surgical removal. Archives of Pathology 12: 186–202

Holroyd A M, Peters A M 1980 The measurement of arterial perfusion of the liver in man using the radioisotope xenon-133. British Journal of Surgery 67: 178–180

Hopkinson B R, Schenk W G Jr 1968 The electromagnetic

measurement of liver blood flow and cardiac output in conscious dogs during feeding and exercise. Surgery 63: 970–975

Hughes R L, Mathie R T, Fitch W, Campbell D 1979a Liver blood flow and oxygen consumption during hypocapnia and IPPV in the greyhound. Journal of Applied Physiology 47: 290–295

Hughes R L, Mathie R T, Campbell D, Fitch W 1979b The effect of hypercarbia on hepatic blood flow and oxygen consumption in the greyhound. British Journal of Anaesthesia 51: 289–296

Hughes R L, Mathie R T, Campbell D, Fitch W 1979c Systemic hypoxia and hyperoxia, and liver blood flow and oxygen consumption in the greyhound. Pflügers Archiv 381: 151–157

Hughes R L, Campbell D, Fitch W 1980 Effects of enflurane and halothane on liver blood flow and oxygen consumption in the greyhound. British Journal of Anaesthesia 52: 1079–1086

Ingoldby C J H 1981 Changes in endotoxin handling in obstructive jaundice in rats. British Journal of Surgery 68: 360–361

Johnston G W 1977 Treatment of bleeding varices by oesophageal transection with the SPTU gun. Annals of the Royal College of Surgeons of England 59: 404–408

Kiernan F 1833 The anatomy and physiology of the liver. Philosophical Transactions of the Royal Society of London 123: 711–770

Kock N G, Roding B, Hahnloser P, Tibblin S, Schenk W G Jr 1970 The effect of glucagon on hepatic blood flow. An experimental study in the dog. Archives of Surgery 100: 147–149

Kock N G, Hahnloser P, Roding B, Schenk W G Jr 1972 Interaction between portal venous and hepatic arterial blood flow: an experimental study in the dog. Surgery 72: 414–419

Lautt W W 1977a The hepatic artery: subservient to hepatic metabolism or guardian of normal hepatic clearance rates of humoral substances. General Pharmacology 8: 73–78

Lautt W W 1977b Hepatic vasculature: A conceptual review. Gastroenterology 73: 1163–1169

Leiberman D P, Mathie R T, Harper A M, Blumgart L H 1978 An isotope clearance method for measurement of liver blood flow during portasystemic shunt in man. British Journal of Surgery 65: 578–580

Lieberman F L, Denison E K, Reynolds T B 1970 The relationship of plasma volume, portal hypertension, ascites, and renal sodium retention in cirrhosis. The overflow theory of ascites formation. Annals of the New York Academy of Sciences 170: 202–206

MacDonald R A 1961 'Lifespan' of liver cells. Autoradiographic study using tritiated thymidine in normal, cirrhotic, and partially hepatectomized rats. Archives of Internal Medicine 107: 335–343

MacDougall B R D, Westaby D, Theodossi A, Dawson J L, and Williams R 1982 Increased long term survival in variceal haemorrhage using injection sclerotherapy. Lancet i: 124–127

McGee J O'D, Blumgart L H, Wood C B, Patrick R S 1976 Pathological features of veno-occlusive disease following ingestion of herbal teas. Journal of Clinical Pathology 29: 788–794

McPherson G A D, Benjamin I S, Boobis A R, Brodie M J, Hampden C, Blumgart L H 1982 Antipyrine elimination as a dynamic test of hepatic functional integrity in obstructive jaundice. Gut 23: 734–738

Maillard J-N, Flamant Y M, Hay J M, Chandler J G 1979 Selectivity of the distal splenorenal shunt. Surgery 86: 663–671

Mall F P 1906 A study of the structural unit of the liver. American Journal of Anatomy 5: 227–308

Malpighi M 1666 De Viscerum Structura Exercitatio Anatomica. London

Mann F C 1942 The circulation of the liver. Quarterly Bulletin of the Indiana University Medical Center 4: 43–54

Mann F C 1944 Restoration and pathologic reactions of the liver. Journal of Mount Sinai Hospital 11: 65–74

Mann F C, Magath T B 1922 Studies on the physiology of the liver: II. The effect of the removal of the liver on the blood sugar level. Archives of Internal Medicine 30: 73–84

Mathie R T, Leiberman D P, Harper A M, Blumgart L H 1977 The solubility of ^{85}Krypton in the regenerating liver of the rat. British Journal of Experimental Pathology 58: 231–235

Mathie R T, Lam P H M, Harper A M, and Blumgart L H 1980a The hepatic arterial blood flow response to portal vein occlusion in the dog: The effect of hepatic denervation. Pflügers Archiv 386: 77–83

Mathie R T, Toouli J, Smith A, Harper A M, Blumgart L H 1980b Hepatic tissue perfusion studies during distal splenorenal shunt. American Journal of Surgery 140: 384–386

Mays E T 1974 The hepatic artery. Surgery, Gynecology and Obstetrics 139: 595–596

Molnar W, Stockum A E 1974 Relief of obstructive jaundice through percutaneous transhepatic catheter — a new therapeutic method. American Journal of Roentgenology 122: 356–367

Moreno A H, Burchell A R, Rousselot L M, Panke W F, Slafsky S F, Burke J H 1967 Portal blood flow in cirrhosis of the liver. Journal of Clinical Investigation 46: 436–445

Munro H N, Fernstrom J D, Wurtman R J 1975 Insulin, plasma amino acid imbalance, and hepatic coma. Lancet i: 722–724

Nagorney D M, Mathie R T, Lygidakis N J, Blumgart L H 1982 Bile duct pressure as a modulator of liver blood flow after common bile duct obstruction. Surgical Forum 33: 206–208

Nopanitaya W, Grisham J W, Aghajanian J G, Carson J L 1978 Intrahepatic microcirculation: SEM study of the terminal distribution of the hepatic artery. In: Becker R P and Johari O (eds) Scanning Electron Microscopy Vol II. SEM Inc, AMF O'Hare, Illinois p 837–842

Okuda K, Suzuki K, Musha H, Arimizu N 1977 Percutaneous transhepatic catheterization of the portal vein for the study of portal hemodynamics and shunts. A preliminary report. Gastroenterology 73: 279–284

Putnam C W, Halgrimson C G, Koep L, Starzl T E 1977 Hepatic transplantation. World Journal of Surgery 1: 165–175

Rappaport A M 1973 The microcirculatory hepatic unit. Microvascular Research 6: 212–228

Rappaport A M, Borowy Z J, Lougheed W M, Lotto W N 1954 Subdivision of hexagonal liver lobules into a structural and functional unit. Role in hepatic physiology and pathology. Anatomical Record 119: 11–27

Redeker A G, Yamahiro H S 1973 Controlled trial of exchange-transfusion therapy in fulminant hepatitis. Lancet i: 3–6

Reichle F A, Owen O E 1979 Hemodynamic patterns in human hepatic cirrhosis. A prospective randomized study of the hemodynamic sequelae of distal splenorenal (Warren) and mesocaval shunts. Annals of Surgery 190: 523–534

Reichman S, Davis W D, Storaasli J P, Gorlin R 1958 Measurement of hepatic blood flow by indicator dilution techniques. Journal of Clinical Investigation 37: 1848–1856

Resnick R H, Ishihara A, Chalmers T C, Schimmel E M, and The Boston Inter-Hospital Liver Group 1968 A controlled trial of colon bypass in chronic hepatic encephalopathy. Gastroenterology 54: 1057–1069

Resnick R H, Iber F L, Ishihara A M, Chalmers T C, Zimmerman H, and The Boston Inter-Hospital Liver Group 1974 A controlled study of the therapeutic portacaval shunt. Gastroenterology 67: 843–857

Richardson P D I, Withrington P G 1977 The effects of glucagon, secretin, pancreozymin and pentagastrin on the hepatic arterial vascular bed of the dog. British Journal of Pharmacology 59: 147–156

Rikkers L F, Miller F J, Christian P 1981 Effect of portasystemic shunt operations on hepatic portal perfusion. American Journal of Surgery 141: 169–174

Ryan C J, Guest J, Ryan S, Harper A M, Blumgart L H 1978 Hepatic blood flow studies in the rat before and after portacaval transposition. British Journal of Experimental Pathology 59: 8–12

Schafer D F and Jones A 1983 Potential neural mechanisms in the pathogenesis of hepatic encephalopathy. In: H Popper, F Schaffner (eds) Progress in Liver Diseases, Vol VII, Grune and Stratton, New York. p 615–627

Schenk W G Jr, McDonald J C, McDonald K, Drapanas T 1962 Direct measurement of hepatic blood flow in surgical patients: with related observations on hepatic flow dynamics in experimental animals. Annals of Surgery 156: 463–469

Scott J, Long R, Dick R, Sherlock S 1976 Percutaneous transhepatic obliteration of gastro-oesophageal varices. Lancet ii: 53–55

Sherlock S 1974 Progress report: chronic hepatitis. Gut 15: 581–597

Silk D B A, Hanid M A, Trewby P N et al 1977 Treatment of fulminant hepatic failure by polyacrylonitrile-membrane haemodialysis. Lancet ii: 1–3

Slapak M, Beaudoin J G, Lee H M, Hume D M 1970 Auxiliary liver homotransplantation. A new technique and an evaluation of current techniques. Archives of Surgery 100: 31–41

Stahl J 1963 Studies of the blood ammonia in liver disease. Its diagnostic, prognostic and therapeutic significance. Annals of Internal Medicine 58: 1–24

Starzl T E, Francavilla A, Halgrimson C G et al 1973 The origin, hormonal nature, and action of hepatotrophic substances in portal venous blood. Surgery, Gynecology and Obstetrics 137: 179–199

Terblanche J, Northover J M A, Bornman P 1979 Prospective controlled trial of sclerotherapy in the long term management of patients after oesophageal bleeding. Surgery, Gynecology and Obstetrics 143: 323–333

Than Than, McGee J O'D, Blumgart L H 1977 Prolyl hydroxylase in the skin of patients with obstructive jaundice. Journal of Clinical Pathology 30: 1044–1046

Thistle J L, Hofmann A F 1973 Efficacy and specificity of chenodeoxycholic acid therapy for dissolving gallstones. New England Journal of Medicine 289: 655–659

Thulin L, Andreen M, Irestedt L 1975 Effect of controlled halothane anaesthesia on splanchnic blood flow and cardiac output in the dog. Acta Anaesthesiologica Scandinavica 19: 146–153

Turner J, Cuschieri A, Shields R 1974 The prediction of the outcome of portacaval shunt using BSP: a retrospective aspect. British Journal of Surgery 61: 828–831

Vajrabukka T, Bloom A L, Sussman M, Wood C B, Blumgart L H 1975 Postoperative problems and management after hepatic resection for blunt injury to the liver. British Journal of Surgery 62: 189–200

Vergara F, Plum F, Duffy T E 1974 α-Ketoglutaramate: increased concentration in the cerebrospinal fluid of patients in hepatic coma. Science 183: 81–83

Vlahcevic Z R, Bell C C Jr, Buhac I, Farrar J T, Swell L 1970 Diminished bile acid pool size in patients with gallstones. Gastroenterology 59: 165–173

Von Hösslin C, Alzheimer A 1912 Ein Beitrag zur Klinik und pathologischen Anatomie der Westphal Strumpfell Pseudosklerose. Zeitschrift für Neurologie und Psychiatrie 8: 183–209

Warren W D, Zeppa R, Fomon J J 1967 Selective trans-splenic decompression of gastroesophageal varices by distal splenorenal shunt. Annals of Surgery 166: 437–455

Weinbren H K, Woodward E 1964 Delayed incorporation of ^{32}P from orthophosphate into deoxyribonucleic acid of rat liver after subtotal hepatectomy. British Journal of Experimental Pathology 45: 442–449

Westaby S, Wilkinson S P, Warren R, Williams R 1978 Spleen size and portal hypertension. Digestion 17: 63–68

Wheeler P G, Melia W, Dubbins P et al 1979 Non-operative arterial embolization in primary liver tumours. British Medical Journal 2: 242–244

Whipple A O 1945 The problem of portal hypertension in relation to the hepatosplenopathies. Annals of Surgery 122: 449–475

Wilkinson S P, Williams R 1985 Ascites, electrolyte disorders and renal disorders. In: Wright R et al (eds) Liver and Biliary Disease: Pathophysiology, Diagnosis, Management, W B Saunders and Co Ltd, London, 2nd edn, pp 1341–1365

Williams R 1976 Hepatic failure and development of artificial liver support system. In: Popper H, Schaffner F (ed) Progress in Liver Disease, Vol V, Grune and Stratton, New York, pp 418–435

Wolf C F W, Minick C R, McCoy C H 1978 Morphologic examination of a prototype liver assist device composed of cultured cells and artificial capillaries. International Journal of Artificial Organs 1: 45–51

Gallbladder and bile ducts

INTRODUCTION

The gallbladder and bile ducts are well adapted for the function of storing and discharging bile into the duodenum during digestion. The storage of bile in small bulk is made possible by the concentrating power of the gallbladder. The intermittent discharge of concentrated bile results from co-ordination between the gallbladder and the sphincter of the common bile duct, so that contraction of the gallbladder is accompanied by relaxation of the sphincter. In this chapter the functions of the gallbladder will be considered with an assessment of the tests available to study these functions. Specific conditions affecting the gallbladder, notably gallstone disease, will also be considered together with biliary dyskinesia and pain in the biliary tree.

FUNCTION OF THE GALLBLADDER

Absorption and secretion

It is well known that the gallbladder concentrates bile by removing water and simple solutes. This general fact has been established for man as well as for many animals by direct comparison of bile from the gallbladder with freshly secreted bile from the hepatic duct. Such comparisons have shown that a six-fold to ten-fold concentration is attained. For the details of how this concentration is achieved, it is still necessary to rely on the results of animal experiment because of lack of opportunity to obtain repeated samples from the normal human gallbladder.

A method of obtaining serial samples from the dog's gallbladder was devised many years ago by Ravdin and others (Ravdin et al, 1932). In these now classical studies, they inserted a drainage tube into the common bile duct and passed it along the cystic duct into the gallbladder; the purpose of this retrograde intubation was to avoid injuring the delicate gallbladder wall. The dogs remained in good health for long periods if care was taken to avoid sepsis, and serial samples could be obtained without anaesthesia.

With the gallbladder prepared in this way, natural bile could no longer enter, but by placing various solutions in the empty gallbladder it was possible to measure the rate of absorption of the solutes. Care was taken to distinguish between absorption from the healthy and from the traumatized or infected gallbladder. The healthy gallbladder rapidly absorbed water, sodium, chloride and bicarbonate until the fluid remaining in the gallbladder was isosmotic with blood serum.

The mechanism of this concentrating action of the gallbladder has been studied by Diamond (1965 and 1968). He showed that there was active transport of sodium, chloride and bicarbonate ions. A double carrier mechanism appeared to be involved because neither sodium nor chloride could be carried independently. The absorption of these ions was accompanied by the transport of an isosmotic amount of water. This resulted in a fall in the concentration of chloride and bicarbonate in gallbladder bile and a rise in the concentration of non-absorbable bile salt which then became the main anion. Bile salts, however, are involved in micelle formation and for that reason their osmotic activity is low. This creates a slight osmotic gradient between bile and blood and as a result, some electrolyte free water moves out of the gallbladder. Net water absorption therefore occurs due to two simultaneously occurring processes: water movement associated with active ion transport and water movement due to the osmotic gradient.

The normal gallbladder mucosa is essentially impermeable to bile salts, bile pigments and cholesterol. The diseased gallbladder on the other hand may absorb bile salts; water absorption is decreased and water as well as chloride may then pass into the gallbladder lumen. There is debate as to whether the diseased gallbladder excretes or absorbs cholesterol but on balance the former is probably true. This question of cholesterol transport by the human gallbladder is of special interest in relation to cholesterosis of the gallbladder, which is characterised by extensive deposits of cholesterol in the gallbladder wall. The precise nature of this condition is still unknown.

There is no conclusive evidence as to whether the cholesterol within the gallbladder wall is in process of being absorbed from, or excreted into, gallbladder bile.

Little is known about the regulation of water and electrolyte absorption by the gallbladder in vivo. Svanvik and Jansson (1977) described a technique suitable for studies in animals and showed that intravenous secretin abolished net water absorption from bile in the gallbladder thereby impeding its concentrating mechanism. Intravenous cholecystokinin, on the other hand, was found not to influence net water transport.

Gallbladder absorption is also affected by inflammatory damage to the gallbladder wall. Nahrwold and colleagues (1976) showed that gallstone patients with severe symptoms and marked histological changes in the gallbladder, had poor absorptive function as measured by electrical changes detected on the excised specimen.

Although the main function of the gallbladder is absorptive, gallbladder mucosa also secretes mucous substances variously called mucus, mucins, mucoproteins, mucopolysaccharides and glycoproteins. These substances constitute the 'white bile' found in mucocele of the gallbladder where the cystic duct is blocked by a gallstone. Bouchier and his colleagues (1965) found that bile from pathological gallbladders was more viscous than bile from normal gallbladders largely because of an increase in these mucous substances.

The bile ducts are provided with glands which secrete small quantities of mucus. It is doubtful if the bile ducts have any absorptive function under normal circumstances. It is well known, however, that when the common bile duct is obstructed, the bile is gradually absorbed and replaced by a colourless mucoid secretion. This 'white bile' is the secretion of the mucous glands which continue to function even against a high back pressure. The discovery at operation of 'white bile' in the common duct in a patient suffering from obstructive jaundice indicates that complete obstruction has been present for many days and implies a poor prognosis.

Gallbladder emptying

Gallbladder emptying can be directly studied in animals but only indirectly in man. In the dog, the mechanism of the gallbladder and common duct sphincter was beautifully worked out in the classical experiments of Elman and McMaster (1926). They brought to the surface three drainage tubes, one inserted into the proximal stump of the divided common duct, another inserted into the distal stump and a third inserted into the gallbladder by way of the cystic duct. When these three tubes were connected together outside the body, the bile merely followed a detour on its way from liver to gallbladder, and from gallbladder to duodenum (Fig. 20.1). Provided that sepsis was avoided the dogs lived in health for many weeks and it was

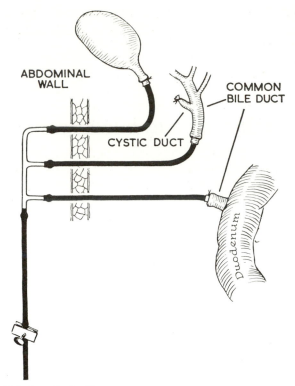

Fig. 20.1 A method of intubating the biliary duct in the dog. During test periods, the various tubes allow collection of bile from the common duct or gallbladder, and measurement of common duct pressure, gallbladder pressure, and sphincter resistance. At other times the clamp is kept closed, and the duct system, though elongated, retains its normal connections. (After Elman & McMaster, 1926)

possible to measure, without an anaesthetic, the pressure in the gallbladder, the resistance offered to the flow of bile into the duodenum, and a maximum pressure against which the liver could continue to secrete bile.

They showed that the liver secreted bile continuously. If the common duct is obstructed, the pressure in it mounts to about 30 cm (measured as a column of bile) and at this pressure, secretion by the liver is arrested. If bile cannot escape to the gallbladder, arrest of hepatic secretion follows rapidly upon obstruction within about 20 minutes. If, however, the bile is free to enter the gallbladder, the extra space, combined with the concentrating activity of the gallbladder, retards the rise of pressure and allows hepatic secretion to continue for many hours. The pressure within the gallbladder is about 10 cm of bile in dogs fasted for 4–12 hours and is not increased as the period of fasting is prolonged. The resistance offered to the passage of bile into the duodenum is about 10–12 cm in dogs fasted for 4–12 hours, and it is much higher (20–25 cm) in dogs fasted for 24–72 hours. At the mere sight of food there is often a marked increase in gallbladder pressure and a simultaneous fall in sphincter resistance. The original pressures are then resumed and for about half an hour after feeding the gallbladder pressure remains at the resting level (10 cm) and the sphincter resistance high

(20 cm or more). Thereafter, while digestion proceeds, there are irregular fluctuations in pressure characterized by a simultaneous increase of gallbladder pressure and a fall of sphincter resistance.

It can be concluded that the liver secretes bile continuously and is capable of maintaining secretion against all pressures normally encountered. During periods of fasting, bile enters the gallbladder to be stored and concentrated, for the pressure in the gallbladder is less than the resistance of the sphincter at the lower end of the common duct. At the sight of food there may be some escape of bile into the duodenum, but the main outpouring of bile begins about half an hour after feeding, and continues at intervals throughout the later phase of digestion. The outpouring of bile is the result of simultaneous gallbladder contraction and sphincter relaxation. This concept of the biliary mechanism is probably applicable to man although here there is no opportunity for measuring changes of pressure within the normal gallbladder and we have to rely on indirect measurement.

It has been shown in the monkey that increased pressure within the common bile duct alters the chemical composition of bile; there is impaired bile salt secretion and synthesis by the liver (Strasberg et al, 1971). It remains to be shown whether or not transitory rises in the pressure within the common bile duct are important for initiating gallstone formation.

The common occurrence of gallbladder disease in multiparous women lends interest to the observation that emptying of the gallbladder is impaired in pregnancy. This was investigated by Gerdes and Boyden (1938) whose method was to compute the volume of bile in the gallbladder from careful measurement of the size of the gallbladder shadow on X-ray films taken during cholecystography. By taking a series of films they were able to estimate the volume of bile discharged within given intervals of time. They first established the normal rate of emptying of the gallbladder after a standard meal in women who were not pregnant. In women examined during the first trimester of pregnancy the rate of emptying was normal, while in women examined during the second

and third trimesters there was marked delay in emptying. Finally, they showed that the impairment of emptying was transient by examining five women towards the end of pregnancy, and again 6–9 weeks after confinement, when the rate of emptying had almost returned to normal. Nilsson and Stattin (1967) studied gallbladder emptying during the normal menstrual cycle and showed that emptying was impaired during the progesterone peak in the menstrual cycle. There is therefore a tendency for stasis within the gallbladder to occur both during pregnancy and during the progesterone phase of the menstrual cycle. This may be partly responsible for the increased prevalence of gallstone disease in females during the reproductive years and is discussed later.

THE SPHINCTER OF THE COMMON BILE DUCT IN MAN

Careful dissection of the lower end of the common duct by a number of anatomists has established beyond doubt that there is a true sphincter distinct from the musculature of the duodenum. Thus, by a special technique that involved maceration and preliminary dissection, followed by hardening and final dissection, Kreilkamp and Boyden (1940) (Fig. 20.2) showed that the sphincter of Oddi comprised the following elements:

1. A sphincter choledochus which ensheathed the lower end of the common duct above its junction with the pancreatic duct
2. A sphincter pancreaticus which formed an annular band round the pancreatic duct just before its junction with the bile duct
3. A sphincter ampullae which began just proximal to the junction of the pancreatic and common duct and continued down as a sheath surrounding the ampulla.

The sphincter choledochus is the only component which is always present and is responsible for guarding the lower end of the common duct. The function of the sphincter choledochus can be investigated by measuring the resist-

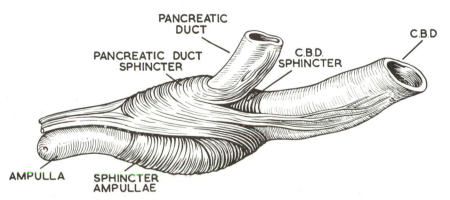

Fig. 20.2 The musculature around the terminations of common bile duct and pancreatic duct. (Redrawn after Kreilkamp & Boyden, 1940)

ance offered to the passage of fluid into the duodenum. This has been done in patients in whom the common duct has been intubated for the purpose of providing biliary drainage. Serial estimations of the sphincter resistance are made by attaching a manometer to the drainage tube and introducing saline solution at a constant rate (e.g. 2 ml/min). It should be borne in mind that observations are almost invariably made on patients whose gallbladders have been removed and whose common duct may recently have been traumatised by the removal of calculi. The possibility must be conceded that the sphincter may not function normally under these adverse conditions of experiment; nevertheless, the results obtained by various workers are in close agreement with the results of animal experiment. Manometry of the biliary tree can also be performed using catheters passed at endoscopic retrograde cholangiopancreatography (ERCP), by percutaneous transhepatic puncture or by direct intra-operative puncture. Although it is possible to test the response of the pressure recording to various drugs and hormones the interpretation of the findings may, however, present difficulties.

While there is no information on the functional importance of the inconstant sphincter pancreaticus, the inconstant sphincter ampullae deserves special notice. It is known that the mode of termination of the pancreatic and common duct is variable; they may enter the duodenum independently, side by side, or by a common ampulla. When they terminate in an ampulla, blockage of its outlet by a calculus or spasm of its sphincter may allow bile to enter the pancreatic duct or pancreatic secretion to enter the bile duct. Furthermore, it is known that when a radio-opaque fluid is injected into the common duct after a dose of morphine, which puts the sphincter into spasm, the opaque fluid passes into the pancreatic duct in about one patient in five — a proportion very similar to the proportion having a well-developed sphincter ampullae.

The determinants of extrahepatic biliary motility are multiple and their integration is complex. The physiology of the sphincter of Oddi remains obscure partly because of species differences, conflicting reports and lack of resolution of a very fundamental concept, i.e. whether 'stimulation' of the sphincter apparatus implies closing the sphincter with less bile flow into the duodenum, or increased pumping action with greater flow.

CONTROL OF THE BILIARY MECHANISM

Gallbladder emptying and sphincter relaxation are under both neural and humoral influences and the two interact to produce control. The biliary mechanism can also be affected by the action of drugs.

Neural effects

The parasympathetic nervous system is clearly involved in the maintenance of gallbladder tone; conversely, gallbladder pressure is decreased after vagotomy. The administration of atropine after vagotomy reduces the resting gallbladder pressure even further suggesting that intramural cholinergic ganglia are also involved in the maintenance of gallbladder tone.

The role of the sympathetic nervous system is less clear. Splanchnic nerve stimulation in the cat does not alter the resting gallbladder pressure but does decrease the pressure response to cholecystokinin. Epinephrine in small doses is variable in its effect. Usually there is no response until unphysiological levels of the drug are administered. Norepinephrine and isoproternol are without effect on the gallbladder.

Histamine has been shown to cause a marked increase in gallbladder pressure in a number of species. Schoetz et al (1978) demonstrated the presence of inhibitory H_2 and stimulatory H_1 receptors in the primate gallbladder but their role is unclear.

Humoral effects

Cholecystokinin (CCK). This hormone was first extracted from the upper intestinal mucosa of the dog by Ivy and Oldberg in 1928. It was isolated in pure form by Jorpes and Mutt (1962) and shown to be a linear polypeptide containing 33 amino acid residues (Jorpes 1968); the activity of CCK residues is in the carboxyl-terminal position of the molecule. Jorpes and Mutt also showed that cholecystokinin (CCK) and pancreozymin (PZ) were one and the same substance.

Cholecystokinin is released from the duodenal mucosa by food, acid, egg yolk and peptone. The release is presumed to be governed by a local nervous mechanism for it is prevented by painting the mucosa with cocaine. Studies from Grossman's laboratory established that essential amino acids were more effective than non-essential amino acids, that only the l and not the d forms were effective and that tryptophan and phenylalanine were most effective in releasing CCK from the duodenal mucosa. Acid in the duodenum released only small amounts of CCK.

Cholecystokinin has a potent stimulant action on the gallbladder muscle and an inhibitory action on the common duct sphincter; it also reduces the sphincter spasm induced by morphine. These actions of CCK on the smooth muscle of the gallbladder and the common duct sphincter are physiological processes and are likely to be direct involving no mediation by nerve although the possibility of H_2 receptor interaction has been raised.

The availability of CCK has led to its use in the clinical situation. Patients suffering from atypical symptoms suggestive of biliary tract disease are sometimes given CCK in an attempt to produce the symptoms — the so-called Cholecystokinin Provocation Test. Patients can also be given CCK following duodenal intubation to obtain bile rich duodenal juice for biochemical analysis.

Secretin. This hormone which was discovered by Bayliss and Starling in 1902 was isolated in pure form by Jorpes and Mutt in 1961. It is a linear polypeptide containing 27 amino acid residues and is released from the duodenal mucosa by acid. Secretin alone does not alter gallbladder pressure but potentiates the action of CCK on the gallbladder and common duct sphincter, the latter role probably being physiological. In addition, secretin increases the flow of bile from the liver.

Gastrin. Gastrin was discovered by Edkins in 1906 and isolated from the dog antral mucosa by Gregory and Tracy in 1963. Gastrin produces contraction of the gallbladder and relaxation of the sphincter in several species but is much less potent than CCK; there is, however, no evidence that gastrin plays anything other than a pharmacological role in the motor function of the biliary tract.

Glucagon. This is a peptide containing 29 amino acid residues. It is similar structurally to secretin and inhibits gallbladder contraction and relaxes the sphincter. It is unlikely that glucagon has a physiological role in the regulation of extrahepatic biliary motor function.

Caerulein. This is a decapeptide isolated from the skin of the Australian frog Hyla caerulea and is structurally akin to CCK and gastrin. It is one of the most potent agents known in producing gallbladder contraction and sphincter relaxation but of course has no physiological role in man.

Drug effects

Morphine (also other opium derivatives, diamorphine or heroin, codeine). All observers are agreed that morphine causes a pronounced increase in sphincter resistance which may last for some hours. Most observers have worked with fasting patients, and it is not sufficiently appreciated that the response is greatly modified by food. The usual response to morphine is mitigated by taking food and when morphine is given in the digestive period it causes only a trifling increase in sphincter resistance. This may well be due to the release of CCK from the duodenum in response to food. There have been many references to the inadvisability of giving morphine to patients suffering biliary pain lest the pressure in the biliary system, already high, should be raised further. It is not clear that these warnings are well founded. Thus, in the majority of patients suffering from acute cholecystitis, the high pressure in the gallbladder is due to occlusion of the cystic duct by a calculus or by oedema and if bile can neither enter nor leave the gallbladder, the condition of the sphincter of the common duct can be of little importance. In those patients who have a calculus impacted at the lower end of the common duct it is, perhaps, undesirable to produce an additional sphincter spasm. There is, however,

no evidence that morphine influences the course of the disease for better or worse and the sympatomatic value of a powerful opiate is beyond dispute. In any event, the spasm induced by morphine can be avoided by giving a preliminary dose of atropine.

Nitrites. Nitrites fail to produce smooth muscle relaxation on isolated gallbladder muscle strips, but the inhalation of amyl nitrite causes a prompt, profound, but short-lived fall in sphincter resistance. Glyceryl trinitrate (0.5 mg under the tongue) causes a less marked but more prolonged fall in resistance.

Magnesium sulphate. Magnesium sulphate was extensively used in the past to promote the evacuation of the gall bladder either as a diagnostic or therapeutic procedure. With the availability of commercially produced CCK, its use as a diagnostic tool has decreased and it is rarely used today as a therapeutic agent to aid gallbladder emptying.

TESTS OF GALLBLADDER FUNCTION

Cholecystography

Cholecystography as a test of gallbladder function depends on the ability of the gallbladder to concentrate the bile which enters it. Radio-opaque compounds, excreted in dilute solution in liver bile, are sufficiently concentrated by the healthy gallbladder to cast a shadow on X-ray examination (Fig. 20.3). The absence of a gallbladder shadow after the administration of a suitable dye, indicates a diseased gallbladder which is no longer capable of absorbing water or, alternatively, obstruction of the cystic duct by a gallstone provided, of course, that the dye

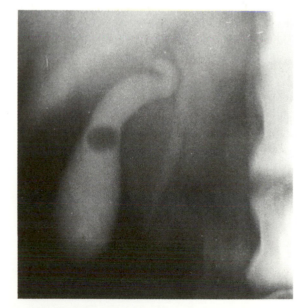

Fig. 20.3 Cholecystogram showing a single radiolucent stone in a functioning gallbladder. (By courtesy of Dr Ramsay Vallance, Gartnavel General Hospital, Glasgow).

administered has been absorbed from the gastrointestinal tract and excreted by the liver. Several kinds of radio-opaque preparations are in use, but all are organic compounds of iodine. These substances are absorbed rapidly from the bowel, then excreted by the liver in high concentration into bile. Maximum contrast is obtained about 10–12 hours after administration. A fatty meal results in the release of cholecystokinin and contraction of the gallbladder can be visualised on the radiograph.

Other organic iodine compounds such as iodipamide and ioglycamide can be administered intravenously. These substances are excreted in bile in much greater concentrations than the oral cholecystographic media and so visualization does not depend on the concentrating ability of the gallbladder mucosa. Their principal use is in outlining the bile ducts when the gallbladder has been removed or is not functioning, but like other iodine compounds they are concentrated by a gallbladder which is functioning. The first film for cholecystography should be taken 30 minutes after the injection. Both gallbladder and bile duct can be visualized on one film usually 60–90 minutes after the administration. In health, such substances are excreted in bile, and only slightly by the kidneys, but where there is liver damage, or even mild obstructive jaundice, most of it is excreted by the kidneys, producing not a cholangiogram but a pyelogram. Various side effects may occur following the intravenous injection of contrast material. For this reason injection should be made slowly and care should be taken especially in patients with hepatic or renal failure or in patients with severe coronary or circulatory insufficiency.

In an attempt to obtain better visualization of the bile ducts, higher doses of contrast material may be injected. While the liver handles a small amount of contrast well, if a large amount is injected rapidly most of it is excreted by the kidneys. If, in addition, there is impairment of hepatic function then 50–90% of the injected dose may be lost via the kidneys. This is the rationale for the infusion cholangiogram in which 40–60 ml of contrast medium is injected in 250 ml of 5% dextrose over a period of about 30 minutes.

Ultrasound

Although radiology remains the most popular method of investigating the biliary tree, it is being replaced increasingly by the use of ultrasound. Ultrasound avoids the hazards of radiation and the discomfort of nasoduodenal intubation. Conventional static grey-scale ultrasonography is an accurate method of diagnosing gallstones (Fig. 20.4) with a detection rate of about 90%. High definition real-time ultrasonic scanning is very rapid and simpler to perform with an even higher detection rate. In addition to detecting gallstones ultrasound can also be used to measure the thickness of the gallbladder wall (Fig. 20.4), increases being indicative of disease. Ultrasound can also be used to measure the calibre of the bile duct but in this area it is less accurate than it is with the gallbladder.

Although the main use of ultrasound is to demonstrate anatomical appearances, real-time scanning can be used to measure gallbladder volume and contraction. Everson et al (1980) concluded that it is a simple, accurate, non-invasive and potentially valuable means of studying gallbladder emptying in man.

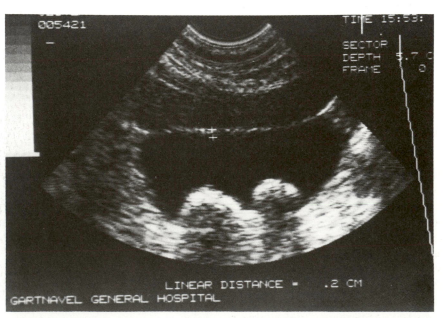

Fig. 20.4 Ultrasound of the gallbladder showing the presence of two gallstones and an assessment of the thickness of the gallbladder wall. (By courtesy of Dr Ramsay Vallance, Gartnavel General Hospital, Glasgow).

Isotope scanning

Gamma-emitting radiopharmaceuticals excreted primarily through the biliary tree are potentially useful for the assessment of hepatobiliary function. This method avoids one of the disadvantages of intravenous cholangiography, viz. reaction to the contrast material and has the added advantage of allowing improved visualization of the biliary system when the serum bilirubin is mildly elevated.

In the past, [131]I Rose Bengal was used for this purpose; it is quickly excreted through the biliary tract and small bowel, but the long residence time in the large bowel and the beta emission of ^{131}I result in a relatively high radiation dosage to the bowel mucosa. Hepatobiliary scintigraphy has been revolutionized by the development of various analogues of iminodiacetic acid. These substances can be labelled with 99m-Technetium as this isotope is excellent for imaging and is readily available in almost all nuclear medical centres. Dimethyl iminodiacetic acid (HIDA) is one of the principal agents. Following intravenous injection in the fasting patient, the patient is scanned by gamma camera with dynamic studies and serial photographs (Fig. 20.5). This assesses patency of the cystic and common bile ducts and the greatest impact has been made in the diagnostic evaluation of suspected acute cholecystitis. This condition is characterised by cystic duct obstruction and so failure of the gallbladder to be visualized is regarded as a positive scan. (Fig. 20.6).

The technique is also of value in the assessment of postoperative problems such as biliary enteric bypass and leakage but is only of limited value in the assessment of chronic cholecystitis and in the presence of clinical jaundice. Other advantages of HIDA and similar preparations include rapid excretion by liver cells, low excretion rates by kidney and a high degree of specificity for localisation in the gallbladder. HIDA scanning can also be used to study gallbladder emptying. Changes in activity can be measured over the liver, bile ducts, gallbladder, small intestine and stomach. CCK can be infused to initiate gallbladder contraction. Quantitative cholescintigraphy offers a new objective means of defining gallbladder function (Shaffer et al, 1980).

SPECIFIC CONDITIONS

Gallstones

Human gallstones can be classified according to their composition into two main categories namely cholesterol stones and pigment stones, substances which are virtually insoluble in water. Pigment stones are so called because they contain appreciable amounts of calcium bilirubinate but in addition a variety of poorly-characterized, amorphous and insoluble compounds. The so-called 'mixed' stones contain both cholesterol and pigment but

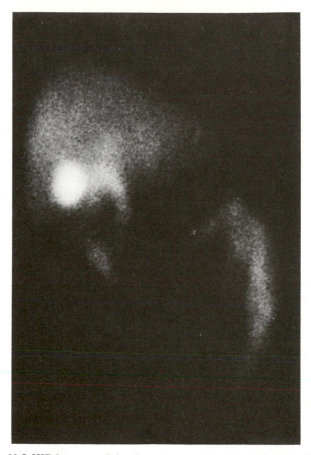

Fig. 20.5 HIDA scan outlining liver, duct system and gallbladder with drainage of isotope into the intestine. (By courtesy of Dr F G Adams, Western Infirmary, Glasgow).

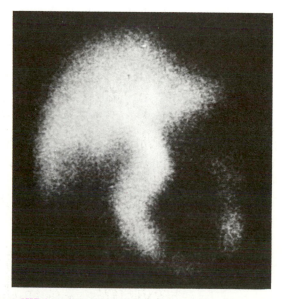

Fig. 20.6 HIDA scan in acute cholecystitis. Liver and duct system are visualized but the gallbladder is not outlined. (By courtesy of Dr F G Adams, Western Infirmary, Glasgow).

usually consist of over 50% cholesterol and may be considered a variant of cholesterol stones.

Cholesterol gallstones are more common in Western countries, the highest prevalence being in the American Indians. These stones, on the other hand, are extremely uncommon in the Masai tribe of Africa. These racial and ethnic variations appear to correspond in a rough way to the relative biliary cholesterol content.

Pigment stones

Little is known about why and how pigment precipitates from bile. Unconjugated bilirubin is largely insoluble in water and so when substantial amounts are present in bile, the bile can be considered to be 'saturated' and precipitation is likely to occur. The origin of this unconjugated bilirubin in bile has been the subject of controversy. It may be secreted in excess by the liver as has been postulated to explain the association of pigment stones and haemolytic anaemia. On the other hand, it could be formed from conjugated bilirubin in the biliary tract by the action of the enzyme glucuronidase; this probably accounts for the high prevalence of this condition in rural Japan where these enzymes are of bacterial origin.

Cholesterol stones

Cholesterol is normally maintained in aqueous solution in bile by the formation of mixed micelles with bile salt and phospholipid. Any factor which increases the amount of cholesterol or reduces the amount of bile salt and/or phospholipid may result in cholesterol precipitation and gallstone formation. The aetiology of cholesterol gallstones is likely to be multifactorial and some of these factors are here considered.

Cholesterol excess. Bile is the major route for excretion of cholesterol from the body. Excessive amounts may be found in bile for several reasons:

1. High secretion rate as is found in obesity
2. High calorie and cholesterol intake
3. The use of blood cholesterol-lowering drugs, e.g. clofibrate
4. Increased activity of hydroxy methylglutaryl coenzyme A reductase (HMG-CoA reductase), the enzyme responsible for controlling the rate of production of cholesterol by the liver

Each of these factors has been reported to be associated with an increased prevalence of gallstones.

Bile salt deficiency. Bile salts are produced from cholesterol in the liver, are secreted into the bile and pass into the intestine where they participate in the digestion and absorption of fat. They are actively absorbed from the terminal ileum, a process which is normally so efficient that only 5% of bile salts are lost per day in the faeces. Bile salts are returned to the liver in the enterohepatic circulation where they regulate bile salt production and are re-excreted into bile.

Bile salt deficiency could result from:

1. Impaired synthesis as occurs in cerebrotendinous xanthomatosis.
2. Increased faecal loss as occurs in severe ileal disease or resection and with the use of bile acid sequestrants such as cholestyramine.
3. Defective feedback regulation

Each of the above conditions has been shown to be associated with an increased prevalence of gallstones.

Phospholipid deficiency. Theoretically, a reduction in phospholipid synthesis and secretion would be expected to be associated with enhanced saturation of bile with cholesterol and an increased prevalence of gallstones but this association remains at the moment unproven and requires further investigation.

Gallbladder factors. Inflammation of the gallbladder leads to impaired water absorption thus rendering gallbladder bile more dilute and less able to hold cholesterol in micellar solution. In addition, inflammation allows the absorption of bile salts but not cholesterol (Andrews et al, 1932). Thus, there is evidence to suggest that inflammation of the gallbladder could produce conditions which would predispose to cholesterol precipitation and gallstone formation.

Impaired gallbladder emptying is another factor which might be expected to predispose to gallstone formation. In this situation of impaired emptying, the bulk of the bile salt pool becomes trapped in the gallbladder, leading to a relative deficiency in the gut, the enterohepatic circulation and in the freshly secreted hepatic bile which will tend to become supersaturated with cholesterol with the risk of its precipitation and stone formation. Gallbladder emptying is said to be impaired in the progesterone phase of the menstrual cycle, in the later stages of pregnancy, with the use of exogenous female sex hormones and after vagotomy. It is interesting to note that there is a higher prevalence of gallstones in females, the difference becoming apparent around the age of puberty and diminishing after the menopause. There is also an association between gallstones and the use of oestrogens either as an oral contraceptive or for post menopausal replacement. In addition vagotomy has been suggested as a factor which predisposes to gallstone formation. Despite this it must be admitted that the evidence to suggest that an alteration in extrahepatic biliary motility plays a pathogenic role in gallstone formation is at best circumstantial.

Biliary dyskinesia

The possibility of a purely functional disorder of the biliary mechanism has been mooted from time to time but the existence of biliary dyskinesia as a disease entity is far from established. It is said that dyskinesia may be either spastic (when the sphincter fails to relax on contraction of the gallbladder) or atonic (when the toneless gallbladder becomes passively dilated). It is postulated, in either variety, that the biliary pressure may become sufficiently high to give rise to distress.

There has been a greater tendency to accept the condition in America and on the Continent than in Britain. The term is often used to account for symptoms which appear to be of biliary origin when careful search fails to reveal any organic lesion. The Cholecystokinin Provocation Test is sometimes of value in assessing such patients.

Pain and disease of the biliary tract

It is a matter of common observation that patients suffering from disease of the biliary tract may experience three varieties of pain:

1. Diffuse pain in the epigastrium or right upper quadrant of the abdomen which may radiate to the interscapular or right subscapular region. The pain varies in severity from an aching discomfort to excruciating agony, and may occasionally be located not on the right side but on the left.
2. Sharp pain accurately localized to the site of the inflamed gallbladder.
3. Aching pain over the top of the right shoulder

The interpretation of these varieties of biliary pain was clarified by the classical studies in man reported many years ago by Zollinger (1933). He studied the effects of distending the gallbladder during operation on patients who were under local anaesthesia, or who were allowed to regain consciousness sufficiently to respond to questioning. Of nine such patients, distension of the gallbladder caused pain in seven. The pain was located deeply in the epigastrium and was not referred to the region of the gallbladder, nor did it radiate to the back. The pain was accompanied by inspiratory distress. When distension was sufficient to bring the gallbladder into contact with the parietal peritoneum, the pain was accurately localized to the gallbladder area. The effect of distension of the common bile duct in patients with a drainage tube in the common duct was investigated by Layne and Bergh (1940). It will be recollected that the normal pressure which the sphincter is capable of withstanding is 12–15 cm of saline. By raising the perfusion pressure suddenly to 50–100 cm they produced pain in 29 of 30 patients, though it is noteworthy that gradually raising the pressure to this level was without effect. The 29 patients all complained of diffuse pain in the epigastrium or right upper quadrant. In addition, 11 of them had pain referred to the right subscapular or interscapular region; the onset of pain in the back was delayed by about 30 seconds. Layne and Bergh were able to make another observation of very great interest. They found that in most cases the tone of the sphincter returned to normal and pain ceased within a minute of removing the distending pressure. In some cases, however, spasm of the sphincter persisted (as evidenced by its ability to withstand pressures as high as 50–60 cm saline). In these cases pain persisted as long as the spasm lasted and was exceptionally severe. A variety of other effects resulted from distension of the common duct. All patients exhibited marked muscular guarding in the right upper quadrant; inspiratory distress and a sensation of epigastric fullness were common while a few of the patients belched when the ducts were distended and a few suffered from nausea or actually vomited.

It is clear from this discussion that the majority of the symptoms of biliary disease, with the exception of shoulder pain, can be produced by distension. Diffuse pain in the epigastrium or right upper quadrant can result from distension either of the gallbladder or the common duct and may radiate to the back. Pain, sharply localized over the gallbladder, on the other hand, indicates that the distended and possibly inflamed gallbladder is in contact with parietal peritoneum. It is noteworthy that muscular guarding and inspiratory distress which are so often attributed to inflammatory irritation of the parietal peritoneum, can readily be produced by simple mechanical distension. Finally, it should be noted that shoulder pain cannot be produced by distension alone and probably requires inflammatory irritation of the phrenic nerve supplying the adjacent diaphragm.

REFERENCES

Andrews E, Schoenheimer R, Hrdina L 1932 Aetiology of gallstones I. Chemical factors and the role of the gallbladder. Archives of Surgery 25: 796–810

Bouchier I A D, Cooperband S R, El Kodsi B M 1965 Mucous substances and viscosity of normal and pathological human bile. Gastroenterology 49: 343–353

Carey M C, O'Donovan M A 1984 Gallstone disease: current concepts in the epidemiology, pathogenesis and management. In: Petersdorf R G et al (eds) Harrison's Principles of Internal Medicine. McGraw Hill, New York

Diamond J M 1965 The concentrating activity of the gallbladder. In: Taylor W (ed) The Biliary System. Blackwell, Oxford. p 495–511

Diamond J M 1968 Transport mechanisms in the gallbladder. In: Code C F (ed) Handbook of Physiology Section 6, Vol. V, American Physiological Society, Washington Ch 115, p 2451–2482

Elman R, McMaster P D 1926a The physiological variations in

resistance to bile flow to the intestine. Journal of Experimental Medicine 44: 151–171

Elman R, McMaster P D 1926b On the expulsion of bile by the gallbladder and a reciprocal relationship with the sphincter activity. Journal of Experimental Medicine 44: 173–198

Everson G T, Braverman D Z, Johnson M L, Kern F 1980 A critical evaluation of real-time ultrasonography for the study of gallbladder volume and contraction. Gastroenterology 79: 40–46

Gerdes M M, Boyden E A 1938 The rate of emptying of the human gallbladder in pregnancy. Surgery, Gynecology and Obstetrics 66: 145–156

Gregory R A, Tracy H J 1963 The constitution and properties of two gastrins extracted from hog antral mucosa. Gut 5: 103–114

Jorpes J E 1968 The isolation and chemistry of secretin and cholecystokinin. Gastroenterology 55: 157–164

Jorpes J E, Mutt V 1961 On the biological activity and amino acid composition of secretin. Acta Chirurgica Scandinavica 15: 1790–1791

Jorpes J E, Mutt V 1962 Exocrine hormones. Ciba Foundation Symposium Churchill, London

Kreilkamp B L, Boyden E A 1940 Variability in composition of the sphincter of Oddi. Anatomical Record 76: 485–497

Layne J A, Bergh G S 1940 An experimental study of pain in the human biliary tract induced by spasm of the sphincter of Oddi. Surgery, Gynaecology and Obstetrics 70: 18–24

LaMorte W W, Schoetz Jr D J, Birkett D H, Williams L F 1979 The role of the gallbladder in the pathogenesis of cholesterol gallstones. Gastroenterology 77: 580–592

Nahrwold D L, Rose R C, Ward S P 1976 Abnormalities in gallbladder morphology and function in patients with cholelithiasis. Annals of Surgery 184: 415–420

Nilsson S, Stattin S 1967 Gallbladder emptying during the normal menstrual cycle. A cholecystographic study. Acta Chirurgica Scandinavica 133: 648–652

Ravdin I S, Johnston C G, Austin J H, Riegel C 1932a Studies of gallbladder function: IV The absorption of chloride from the bile-free gallbladder. American Journal of Physiology 99: 638–647

Ravdin I S, Johnston C G, Riegel C, Wright S L 1932b Studies of gallbladder function: VII. The anion-cation content of hepatic and gallbladder bile. American Journal of Physiology 100: 317–327

Schoetz D J, Wise W E, LaMorte W W et al 1978 Histamine receptors in the primate gallbladder. Gastroenterology 74:1090

Shaffer E A, McOrmond P, Duggan H 1980 Quantitative cholescintigraphy: assessment of gallbladder filling and emptying and duodenogastric reflux. Gastroenterology 79: 899–906

Strasberg S M, Dorn B C, Small D M, Egdahl R H 1971 The effect of biliary tract pressure on bile flow, bile salt secretion and bile salt synthesis in the primate. Surgery 70: 140–146

Svanvik J, Jansson R 1977 An experimental method for studying in vivo gallbladder absorption. Gastroenterology 72: 634–638

Zollinger R 1933 Observations following distension of the gallbladder and common duct in man. Proceedings of the Society for Experimental Biology (New York) 30: 1260–1261

Pancreas

A better understanding of pancreatic disease coupled with advances in pancreatic surgery has brought fresh interest to the study of pancreatic physiology. The internal secretions of the pancreas include insulin, glucagon, gastrin (though this has so far been extracted only from pancreatic tumours) and the recently described neuropeptides somatostatin, substance P and pancreatic polypeptide (PP). The external secretion of the pancreas, the consequences of excluding it from the intestine, and the consequences of a pancreatic fistula are all of practical importance in relation to resection of the pancreas. Several tests of pancreatic function have been described but none is ideal. Pancreatitis still presents many unsolved problems but progress has been made in the laboratory, in the development of diagnostic and prognostic tests, and in the treatment of established acute pancreatitis. The rare insulin-secreting tumours of the pancreas and the equally rare tumours which secrete gastrin or glucagon are of interest as surgical curios. The patterns of referred pancreatic pain have been studied by electrical stimulation after the insertion of electrodes during routine operations.

THE INTERNAL SECRETIONS OF THE PANCREAS

In the embryo the pancreas develops from hollow epithelial buds which grow out from the duodenum as branching pancreatic ducts. Differentiation of epithelium occurs at intervals along the proliferating buds, giving rise either to acinar cells, which become responsible for the external secretions of the pancreas, or to islet cells which become responsible for the internal secretions. The islet cells are arranged in clumps which are divorced from the duct system. These islets of Langerhans contain two main types of cell which can be distinguished by the staining reactions of their granules. There is evidence that 'alpha cells' secrete glucagon and that the 'beta cells' secrete insulin. The recent application of immunocytochemistry to pancreatic tissue has demonstrated other endocrine or APUD cells (amine precursor uptake and decarboxylation) both within and outwith the islets of Langerhans. The neuropeptides somatostatin, substance P and pancreatic polypeptide (PP) have been demonstrated in these cells and are thought to be involved in the neural enteropancreatic and gastropancreatic reflex system. The hormone gastrin has been identified in APUD cell tumours of the pancreas (apudomas) and these gastrin secreting tumours which produce a syndrome characterised by fulminating peptic ulceration, acid hypersecretion and diarrhoea have been termed gastrinomas.

Insulin, glucagon and the neuropeptides are discussed here, and gastrin on page 277.

Insulin

The evidence that insulin is secreted by the beta cells of the islets comes from experiments on alloxan poisoning in animals. Alloxan is known to destroy the beta cells alone and alloxan poisoning results in transient hypoglycaemia attributable to the escape of insulin from the dying cells, followed by permanent diabetes mellitus.

Insulin is a soluble protein, readily obtained in crystalline form and of known structure. Its constituent amino acids and their sequence have been worked out in detail. The most obvious effect of insulin is to reduce the blood concentration of glucose. This results from several actions of insulin on the tissues, which increase the demand for glucose and reduce the endogenous supply. Increased tissue demand for glucose results in increased deposition of glycogen in the liver and muscles, increased conversion of glucose to fatty acids in the liver, and increased oxidation of glucose in the tissues. Reduced supply results from reduced mobilization of glucose from liver glycogen, and from reduced formation of glucose from amino acids.

Classical diabetes mellitus is held to result from deficient secretion of insulin, perhaps in association with excessive secretion of growth hormone from the anterior pituitary; classical diabetes is, however, in the province of the physician and does not call for discussion here. Less often, diabetes results from hyperthyroidism, from Cushing's syndrome and from total pancreatectomy. Total pancreatectomy is followed by diabetes which is relatively mild; it can be controlled with smaller doses of insulin than are required in severe classical diabetes and complications are seen less frequently. This suggests that the effects of lack of insulin, following pancreatectomy, are modified by the concomitant withdrawal of pancreatic glucagon and neuropeptides.

Several hormones, in addition to glucagon, antagonize the effects of insulin.

Growth hormone and crude extracts of anterior pituitary when given to animals over a prolonged period, can lead to permanent diabetes. Similarly pituitary hypersecretion, as in acromegaly, can lead to diabetes in man. Hypophysectomy on the other hand, leads to a state of insulin hypersensitivity, with frequent hypoglycaemia, and this hypersensitivity is alleviated by treatment with preparations of growth hormone. It is difficult to guarantee that preparations of growth hormone are uncontaminated by other pituitary hormones, but it seems almost certain that growth hormone itself is the antagonist of insulin and the diabetogenic factor.

The adrenocorticoids, especially those with a powerful glucocorticoid action, reduce the peripheral utilization of glucose and increase formation of glucose from amino acids in the liver. By these actions they oppose the actions of insulin and induce hyperglycaemia. Reduced glucose tolerance is a usual feature of Cushing's syndrome.

Thyroid hormone can also induce hyperglycaemia and glycosuria. This may, however, result from the need to mobilize glucose to meet the requirements of an increased metabolic rate, rather than from direct antagonism of insulin.

Finally, adrenaline but not noradrenaline, mobilizes glucose from liver glycogen. The secretion of adrenaline can be regarded as one of the defence mechanisms against hypoglycaemia, since hypoglycaemia stimulates the adrenal medulla to discharge, and the discharged adrenaline tends to correct the hypoglycaemia.

Glucagon

Soon after the discovery of insulin (Banting & Best, 1921), it was noted that some extracts of pancreas induced a rise instead of the usual fall in the blood sugar concentration. The name 'glucagon' was given to the hyperglycaemic factor. It has since been found to be a polypeptide and was fully purified in 1953 (Staub et al, 1953).

Glucagon is produced in the alpha cells of the pancreatic islets. Its role in human physiology is still uncertain. The only proven physiological action is to enhance the output of glucose from the liver which it does in conjunction with insulin control of peripheral glucose uptake. Thus insulin and glucagon between them control total glucose turnover.

The control of plasma glucagon level is not as yet fully understood but according to Bloom (1975), of the three possible mechanisms, namely local metabolite concentrations, circulating hormones and the autonomic innervation of the islets, the last may be the most important.

In pharmacological doses glucagon has many varied actions. It releases pituitary hormones and can be used as a test of pituitary function; it releases catecholamines and can also be used as a provocative test for phaeochromocytomas. It has powerful effects on every part of the alimentary tract, namely inhibition of oesophageal, gastric and intestinal motility, inhibition of secretion of gastric and pancreatic juice and the stimulation of bile flow and secretion from Brunner's glands.

Pancreatic neuropeptides

These recently discovered peptides which may have endocrine, paracrine or transmitter functions have been identified in the APUD or clear endocrine cells lying within or around the islets of Langerhans in the pancreas. Somatostatin, substance P and pancreatic polypeptide (PP) have so far been identified in the pancreas. The actions of these neuropeptides are incompletely understood although somatostatin, from the D-cells of the pancreas, is known to reduce gastrin output and acid secretion. Substance P has been found to inhibit the release of insulin while no clear role has yet been described for pancreatic polypeptide. It is thought likely that these neuropeptides contribute to the gastropancreatic and enteropancreatic reflex systems and that their effects are interdependent with the actions of the other upper gastrointestinal hormones, many of which have only been recently identified.

THE EXTERNAL SECRETION OF THE PANCREAS

In experimental animals pancreatic juice can be collected by intubating the pancreatic duct or by exteriorizing the segment of the duodenum containing its orifice. Ideally, pancreatic juice should be collected from an unanaesthetized animal in good health, with the blood supply and nerve supply of the pancreas intact. In practice these conditions are not easily fulfilled; the various techniques employed have been reviewed by Thomas (1959, 1967).

Most of the data on pancreatic function in man have been derived from the collection and analysis of duodenal fluids following pancreatic stimulation. The method originally developed by Agren and Lagerlöf in 1936 continues to be used with only minor modifications. Pancreatic juice, together with the duodenal secretion, is collected through one lumen of a double-barrelled tube passed from the mouth while through the second lumen gastric juice is aspirated and discarded. The model is designed to avoid contamination by gastric juice and to avoid stimulation of pancreatic secretion by acid reaching the duodenum. The major drawback, however, is contamination by bile and intestinal secretions while the effects of a nasogastric tube on the gastropancreatic reflex system have not been elucidated. In addition the recovery of duodenal juice is not complete, an error that can be partially corrected by the use of suitable non-absorbable markers (Lagerlöf et al, 1967). The development of side-viewing fibreoptic duodenoscopes now allows, in sedated humans, cannulation of the ampulla of Vater under direct vision (Oi et al, 1970). This provides the opportunity to cannulate the pancreatic duct and to collect uncontaminated pancreatic juice (Cotton et al, 1974; Cotton & Heap, 1975). This rather sophisticated technique permits biochemical evaluation of pure pancreatic juice as well as cytological screening for pancreatic cancer.

The pancreatic juice is alkaline with a pH of about 8 owing to its high bicarbonate concentration. It is sufficiently alkaline to neutralize the acid in gastric juice about volume for volume. In man, the daily secretion of pancreatic juice is 500–1200 ml. The cations are largely sodium and potassium whose concentrations are similar to those in plasma. The cation concentrations are independent of flow rate unlike those of the anions bicarbonate and chloride. As the flow rate increases so does the concentration of bicarbonate to reach a plateau which may be as high as 150 mmol. The chloride is reciprocally related so that the sum of the concentrations of bicarbonate and chloride is constant and independent of flow rate (Case et al, 1969). Of the other ions present in pancreatic juice, only calcium and magnesium have any practical significance (Scratcherd, 1975).

In addition to water and electrolytes, pancreatic juice contains digestive enzymes which act on protein, starch and fat.

Trypsin and chymotrypsin are the chief proteolytic enzymes. Both are secreted in the form of inactive precursors. Trypsinogen is activated by the enzyme enterokinase present in the mucosa of the duodenum and jejunum; it can also be activated by the products of bacterial growth and by endotoxin. Trypsin itself is the activator of chymotrypsinogen. Chymotrypsin has an action in clotting milk, which trypsin lacks. Both enzymes are endopeptidases, i.e. they hydrolyse peptide bonds along the length of the molecule, at specific sites according to the amino acid make-up of the substrate molecule. In contrast the more specialised enzymes, carboxypeptidase and aminopeptidase, also present in pancreatic juice, attack proteins and peptides only at the ends, splitting off the terminal amino acid which contains either a free carboxyl group or a free amino group and these enzymes are accordingly classified as exopeptidases.

Amylase (diastase) converts all forms of starch to maltose. As amylase is also present in the succus entericus there is seldom any disturbance of starch digestion where the pancreatic secretion is excluded from the intestine.

Lipase secreted largely in the form of an inactive precursor (prolipase), is responsible for the partial hydrolysis of neutral fat. It attacks preferentially the ester bonds in positions one and three of a triglyceride rather than the ester bonds in position two; for this reason the end products of its action, both in the intestine and in vitro, comprise free fatty acid, monoglycerides and di-glycerides but little glycerol. The pancreas is the only important source of lipase in the upper intestine, and exclusion of pancreatic juice leads to steatorrhoea; lipase is also produced by colonic bacteria but the colon cannot absorb the products of fat digestion. Lipase is water-soluble, and acts on fat droplets only at their interface with water. Consequently, the activity of lipase is largely dependent on the fineness of the fat emulsion exposed to its action. Fat is emulsified by the churning action of the stomach and the squirting of chyme through the pylorus into the duodenum. Bile salts also act as emulsifying agents by reducing surface tension. Fat digestion can therefore be impaired following gastrectomy and by exclusion of bile from the intestine as well as by the exclusion of pancreatic juice.

REGULATION OF PANCREATIC SECRETION

Recent advances in the understanding of the APUD system have demonstrated that the regulation of pancreatic secretion is a complex physiological phenomenon which is as yet not fully understood. The regulation of pancreatic secretion involves endocrine, paracrine and nervous mechanisms mediated both by the vagi and by gastropancreatic and enteropancreatic reflex systems. The hormonal mechanism mediated by secretin and cholecystokinin-pancreozymin (CCK-PZ), dominates the response of the pancreas in normal digestion. The actions and interactions of the other mechanisms are as yet less well defined.

The concept of an hormonal phase of pancreatic secretion was first put forward in a classic paper by Bayliss and Starling (1902) in which they showed that the intravenous administration of acid extract of duodenal mucosa induced a copious flow of pancreatic juice. This response was attributed to a hormone which they named secretin. Much later Harper and Raper (1943) isolated from the mucosa of the small intestine a second hormone which induced a scanty flow of enzyme-rich juice and named it pancreozymin. Pancreozymin is now recognized to be the same hormone as cholecystokinin which is related structurally to gastrin.

Secretin has been prepared in crystalline form and is a polypeptide. It is normally present in the mucosa of the duodenum, and to a lesser extent in the mucosa of the upper jejunum. It is liberated from the mucosa, the most important physiological secretin releasing agent being hydrochloric acid which is effective at pH 5 and less. The liberated secretin is absorbed into the portal venous blood and carried to the pancreas by way of the systemic circulation. The action of purified secretin can be studied in man by aspirating the duodenal contents as described previously; secretin must be given intravenously, for it is inactive by mouth. The juice secreted in response to secretin is copious and strongly alkaline owing to a 6-fold increase in the concentration of bicarbonate; its enzyme concentration is low, but because of the large volume of the juice, the total amount of enzyme secreted in a given time is usually increased (Fig 21.1). In animals, stimulation with secretin does not completely discharge the zymogen granules from the pancreatic acinar cells. It will be observed that the secretin mechanism prevents the intestinal contents from becoming too acid, for the entry of acid into the duodenum stimulates the flow of a strongly alkaline pancreatic juice.

CCK-PZ is released from the duodenal and jejunal mucosa by the chemical action of foodstuffs in the lumen of the bowel and its main function is to stimulate the secretion of enzymes from the acinar cells (Harper & MacKay, 1948) together with a small amount of electrolyte (Case et al, 1969). The most important agents which release CCK-PZ are the products of protein and fat digestion, especially the neutral amino acids such as L-phenylalanine and the long chain fatty acids such as palmitic, stearic and oleic acids. Calcium, magnesium and the bile salts are also known to stimulate CCK-PZ release.

Neural stimulation

In animals the exposed vagi can be stimulated directly. In man the vagi can be stimulated indirectly by insulin hypoglycaemia or the effect of vagal stimulation can be mimicked by drugs such as Mecholyl. As with direct vagal stimulation in animals, the pancreatic juice secreted is small in quantity but rich in enzymes. In animals the zymogen granules of the acinar cells are discharged by vagal stimulation. Vagotomy has been found to reduce the response of the pancreas to a meal or infused amino acids and fatty acids and this response has been explained by postulating an interruption of neural reflexes between the stomach, upper small bowel and pancreas. The gut hormones VIP, somatostatin, bombesin, encephalin and substance P have all been observed to have effects on pancreatic secretions which may be mediated through paracrine actions.

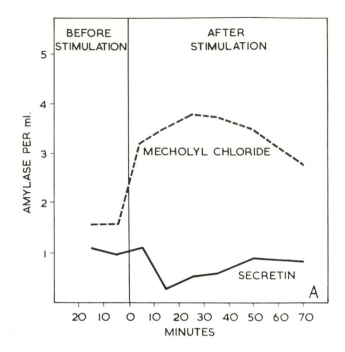

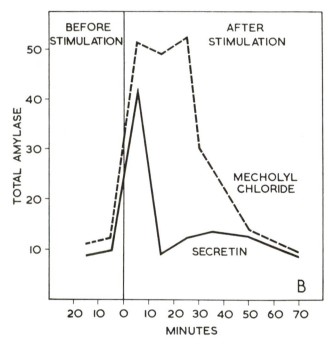

Fig. 21.1 Pancreatic secretion in response to secretin (hormonal stimulation) and Mecholyl chloride (equivalent to vagal stimulation). After secretin, note that despite a fall in concentration of amylase (A) the total output of amylase increases (B), indicating a copious flow of enzyme-poor juice. After Mecholyl chloride, note that the concentration of amylase increases about three-fold (A) and the total output about five-fold (B) indicating a scanty flow of enzyme-rich juice (Comfort & Osterberg, 1940).

TESTS OF PANCREATIC FUNCTION IN MAN

This subject was reviewed by Wormsley in 1972 and Arvanitakis and his colleagues in 1978.

There is still no simple, accurate, physiological method of measuring pancreatic function in man. Exocrine pancreatic function can be assessed, pancreatic enzymes can be measured in body fluids and pancreatic structure can be studied in an attempt to evaluate the function of the gland.

Tests of exocrine pancreatic function

Most tests are based on stimulating the pancreas either directly or indirectly and then analysing the juice secreted into the duodenum. According to Dreiling (1975), few tests have offered any diagnostic advantage over the secretin-pancreozymin test of Lagerlöf involving duodenal intubation and gastric aspiration, stimulation with secretin and CCK-PZ and scrutiny of the aspirates for blood, enzymes, electrolytes and cytology. The limitations of this test are related to poorly-defined normal enzyme secretory responses, overlapping in distribution of enzyme output in normal controls and patients with pancreatic disease, and difficulty in standardization of the dose of pancreozymin which elicits a maximal response.

Indirect stimulation of the pancreas can be carried out using the Lundh test meal (James, 1973) or small intestinal perfusion. The Lundh test meal is the indirect method most widely used to assess pancreatic enzyme secretion. The test involves duodenal intubation, the administration of a test meal by mouth and the aspiration of duodenal contents for analysis at regular intervals. The test is simple to perform and provides a physiological stimulation of pancreatic enzyme secretion which simulates the postprandial state and obviates the administration of exogenous hormones. However, the accuracy of the test is influenced by the periodic sampling of the duodenal contents and stimulation of the pancreas requires structural and functional integrity of the intestinal mucosa which may invalidate the test in cases with mucosal disease. Alterations in gastric emptying may also affect the test and since it does not measure a secretory capacity the test cannot differentiate chronic pancreatitis from pancreatic carcinoma.

A direct infusion of acid into the duodenum and intestine stimulates the endogenous release of secretin which in turn stimulates the secretion of bicarbonate. Similarly Go has shown that duodenal infusion in normal controls with a mixture of amino acids, fatty acids and dextrose produces endogenous release of CCK-PZ and secretion of pancreatic enzymes. These perfusion tests are based on sound physiological principles and a normal response to indirect stimulation by these methods would indicate that the pancreatic tissue is normal.

N-benzoyl-L-tyrosyl-para-aminobenzoic acid (Bz-Ty-PABA) has been used to measure indirectly duodenal chymotrypsin and hence the function of the pancreas. This synthetic peptide is specifically cleaved by the pancreatic endopeptidase chymotrypsin to Bz-Ty and PABA. Accordingly, following oral administration of the peptide, the latter reaches the small intestine where it is hydrolysed by chymotrypsin and liberates para-aminobenzoic acid (PABA). The released PABA is rapidly absorbed from the intestinal mucosa and excreted in the urine. Therefore, the concentration of PABA in the urine reflects intraluminal chymotrypsin activity and the method can be utilised as an indirect test of exocrine pancreatic function.

Pancreatic enzymes in body fluids

Serum amylase is the single biochemical estimation most widely used in the diagnosis of acute pancreatitis throughout the world. Amylase can also be measured in the urine and amylase clearance and the amylase creatinine clearance ratio (ACCR) may be calculated. Amylase may also be estimated in pleural and ascitic fluid and may indicate an exudative effusion associated with pancreatitis, a pancreatic fistula or leaking pseudocyst. Amylase iso-enzymes may be measured in the blood and p-isoamylase, which is believed to arise from the pancreas, may be useful in diagnosing pancreatic hyperamylasaemia. Serum lipase, phospholipase, trypsin and deoxyribonuclease may be of some value in the diagnosis of pancreatic disease but at present the measurement of these enzymes, with the exception of lipase, involves complicated analytical techniques which preclude their widespread use.

STUDIES OF PANCREATIC STRUCTURE

Plain radiology, hypotonic duodenography, angiography, pancreatic scanning, ultrasonography, endoscopic retrograde pancreatography (ERP), computed tomography (CT scanning) nuclear magnetic resonance (NMR) and percutaneous pancreatic biopsy are all techniques which may have a place in the definition of pancreatic structure in man. Angiography, ultrasonography, ERP and computed tomography are most useful in diagnosing pancreatic disease while percutaneous pancreatic biopsy under ultrasound or CT scan control may provide histological information without formal laparotomy. The place of nuclear magnetic resonance in this context awaits definition.

PANCREATIC FISTULA

An external pancreatic fistula may develop after operations on the pancreas, from accidental injury to the pancreatic ducts during gastric resection for penetrating duodenal ulcer or following laparotomy for blunt abdominal trauma when pancreatic duct damage is unrecognised. An internal pancreatic fistula leading to pancreatic ascites may follow blunt abdominal trauma with pancreatic duct rupture or spontaneous rupture of a pseudocyst. An external pancreatic fistula is a serious complication which may lead to dehydration and wound sepsis and occasionally to impairment of digestion through loss of pancreatic enzymes. Loss of fluids from a pancreatic fistula is very variable in quantity and may be as much as 1700 ml daily (Fig 21.2). The loss of water in a patient who is usually gravely ill is itself important, but the concomitant loss of sodium is even more serious. The sodium loss can be assumed (as a first approximation) to be of the order of 100–150 mmol/day but the only satisfactory guide to the

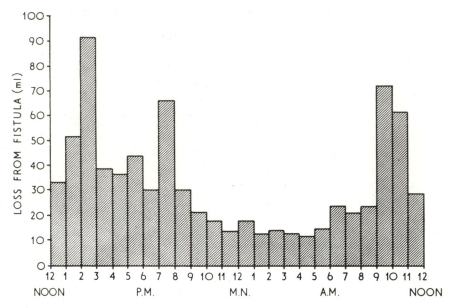

Fig. 21.2 Volume of secretion lost from a pancreatic fistula. Secretion was least during sleep and greatest after meals (Sinclair, 1956).

amount of sodium required for replacement is to measure the amount lost. Sodium bicarbonate can be satisfactorily replaced intravenously. Attempts to control the loss of fluid from a pancreatic fistula by drugs have not been very successful although Sinclair (1956) found a considerable but transient reduction from the use of ephedrine, atropine and ganglion blocking compounds. Diamox which inhibits the action of carbonic anhydrase within the secreting cells, may be effective in some patients (Dreiling et al, 1955). Fortunately the discharge from a pancreatic fistula tends to diminish spontaneously but this process can be accelerated if the pancreas is rested. This can be achieved by using total parenteral nutrition thus avoiding the stimulation of pancreatic secretion produced by food entering the duodenum. If surgery becomes necessary in the management of a pancreatic fistula then the fistula's tract is best outlined preoperatively by endoscopic retrograde pancreatography (ERP).

Infection supervenes when a fistula has been present for a few days, and the bacteria or their products activate the trypsinogen of the pancreatic juice. Under the combined influence of infection and tryptic digestion the wound margins are destroyed, exposing the underlying muscle which is sufficiently vascular to survive. Dehiscence of the wound may follow, but even without this complication the convalescence is slow. Treatment is aimed at keeping trypsin away from the skin. As much as possible of the discharge is carried off by continuous aspiration and the remainder is either taken up by an absorbant powder or prevented from acting on the skin by means of protective dressings and appliances.

Impairment of digestion seldom results from a pancreatic fistula because most fistulae are incomplete. The consequences of complete exclusion of pancreatic juice from the intestine are described below.

RESULTS OF PANCREATIC EXCLUSION

Complete exclusion of pancreatic juice from the intestine is inevitable after total pancreatectomy, and it may follow resection of the head of the pancreas when the attempt to anastomose the remaining pancreas to the intestine fails. It is not a constant feature of carcinoma originating at or near the lower end of the common bile duct (when the accessory pancreatic duct may remain patent) or of fibrocystic disease (where some of the pancreas may escape disorganization). In infants with congenital fibrocystic disease associated with meconium ileus, the exclusion of pancreatic secretion appears often to be complete, though here some of the intestinal dysfunction may result from the generalized disorder of mucus secretion. Total exclusion of pancreatic secretion produces a serious disturbance of digestion which results in the loss of large amounts of fat and protein in the stools. The faeces are light in colour, bulky and soft, but not usually watery.

Fat digestion within the small intestine is grossly impaired by the lack of pancreatic lipase, and an excess of unsplit fat enters the colon. In the colon some of the fat is hydrolysed by the action of bacteria, but as the colon is unable to absorb the products of this hydrolysis both the split and the remaining unsplit·fat are excreted in the faeces. In health the total faecal fat is about 5–7 g/day on any normal diet irrespective of its fat content. In steatorrhoea the faecal fat is not only much increased but varies with dietary fat; in one of our cases the faecal fat was 50 g/day on 100 g intake, but 28 g on a 50 g intake. The excess of fat in the colon may occasionally lead to confusion in the interpretation of a barium enema. The 'fat encrusted colon' as it has been named, may be misdiagnosed radiologically as ulcerative colitis involving the whole colon. This has been demonstrated by Quigley et al (1980) who showed complete resolution of the radiological abnormalities following a fat-free diet.

Protein digestion is also impaired, and the undigested meat fibres can be found in large number in the faeces, where they can readily be identified under the microscope by their characteristic striation. Even more important than the disturbance of protein digestion is the simple loss of protein in the bulky stool. Investigating the importance of the pancreas in digestion in the dog, Coffey and his colleagues (1940) established that after pancreatic exclusion the amount of protein lost in the faeces was unrelated to the protein intake, but varied directly with the bulk of the faeces (possibly being determined by the protein content of the bacteria in the stool). Confirming this observation in man, Bollman and Waugh (1946) showed that if the stools were bulky the nitrogen loss daily in the faeces might be equivalent to as much as 50 g of protein. This observation is of importance in the dietary management of steatorrhoea. It indicates that one of the advantages of reducing the bulk of the stools (by restricting the dietary intake of fat) is the reduced wastage of protein.

Carbohydrate digestion is little affected by lack of pancreatic amylase, and it can be carried through by the enzymes of the succus entericus alone.

In the past the mainstay of the management of patients following pancreatectomy was dietary manipulation by means of a high calorie, high protein, high carbohydrate and limited fat intake. Reliable oral preparations of pancreatic enzymes are now available and these have rendered dietary manipulation less important. It is now appreciated that these preparations are inactivated in an environment with a low pH and it is now recommended that patients receiving pancreatic enzyme preparations orally, should also be given an H_2-receptor antagonist in order to increase the pH of their gastric contents.

ACUTE PANCREATITIS

Acute pancreatitis is regarded as an abdominal emergency and in Great Britain has an overall mortality of 11% (MRC Study, 1977). It has been the subject of much investigation during the past few years and advances have been made in the diagnosis and management of the condition. The pathophysiology underlying acute pancreatitis is still not fully understood and an efficient method of inactivating the inflamed pancreas has still to be described.

Experimental pancreatitis

This subject has been well reviewed by Schiller et al (1974); these authors discuss in detail the various substances and models used to produce experimental pancreatitis.

In experimental animals, pancreatitis can readily be induced by the forceful injection of fluid into the pancreatic ducts at pressures corresponding to, or greater than, the maximum secretory pressure of the pancreas. Many substances can be used including bile, acids, alkalis or duodenal juice and it appears that the cause of the pancreatitis in this model is rupture of the ducts or acini by chemical or physical trauma. A vicious cycle of acinar destruction, pancreatic enzyme release and in situ activation then follows.

In man, Howell and Bergh (1950) induced pancreatitis by an analagous method. In patients whose common bile duct had been intubated for drainage, and in whom cholangiography had previously shown reflux of the opaque fluid into the pancreatic duct, the injection of bile under pressure was followed by mild pancreatitis, as evidenced by a rise of serum amylase. It is now recognized that hyperamylasaemia and indeed acute pancreatitis can follow injection of the pancreatic duct during ERCP.

Another method of inducing pancreatitis in man, by the simultaneous injection of morphine and secretin, had previously been used by Lagerlöf (1945). He was led to try his method by the knowledge that morphine stimulates contraction of the sphincter of Oddi and that secretin evokes a copious secretion of pancreatic juice. Using this method he hoped to induce pancreatitis through the high pressure that must result within the pancreatic ducts. A few of his patients developed the typical features of mild pancreatitis, and the majority had a tell-tale rise of serum amylase and serum lipase.

Aetiology of pancreatitis

Despite extensive work in experimental animals the aetiology of pancreatitis in man remains unknown. There is frequently an association with disease of the biliary tract; although the actual figure varies from series to series, this is the commonest predisposing factor in the United Kingdom, being present in over 50% of cases (Trapnell, 1974; Imrie, 1974). There is also an association with a heavy intake of alcohol in many patients; this is more evident in the United States and France than in the United Kingdom although even here, the association is becoming increasingly common (Imrie, 1975). Rarer causes of acute pancreatitis include abdominal trauma, viruses, hyperparathyroidism, carcinoma of the head of the pancreas, cardiopulmonary bypass and drugs including steroids and thiazide diuretics. Pancreatitis may also occur after a variety of upper abdominal operations, notably cholecystectomy, choledocholithotomy, sphincterotomy and gastrectomy. After thorough investigation it is accepted that no detectable predisposing factor will be discovered in 5–10% of patients and these are labelled 'idiopathic'.

Although the association between biliary tract disease and pancreatitis has been well established, the precise mechanism by which the one leads or predisposes to the other has not been elucidated. It is tempting to suggest that a gallstone becomes impacted at the ampulla of Vater thus permitting reflux of bile into the pancreatic ducts. It has also been suggested that following the passage of a small gallstone into the duodenum the ampulla of Vater may become incompetent for a period of time and thereby allow the reflux of duodenal content into the pancreatic duct.

Reflux of infected bile into the pancreatic duct is possible only when the common bile duct and pancreatic duct terminate in a common ampulla whose orifice into the duodenum can be blocked. The frequency of such an arrangement has been variously estimated on the basis of anatomical studies. An ingeniously direct method was used by Howard and Jones (1947). These workers obtained fresh autopsy specimens comprising the common duct, duodenum and pancreas. They introduced a small gallstone into the common duct and passed it down until it impacted. Coloured fluid was then run into the common duct under moderate pressure and could be recovered from the pancreatic duct near the tail of the pancreas in approximately half the specimens. According to this work, reflux of bile into the pancreatic duct is anatomically possible in about half of the general population but it still remains to be discovered if this half of the population provides all, or even most of the cases of acute pancreatitis.

Further light has been shone on this problem of biliary disease and acute pancreatitis by a study by Acosta and Ledesma (1974). They studied 36 patients with acute pancreatitis and gallstones and a control group of 36 patients with gallstones who were admitted for various complications such as acute cholecystitis, biliary colic, obstructive jaundice, but with no evidence of acute pancreatitis. The stools were collected, diluted and filtered to look for the presence or absence of gallstones. In the pancreatitis group, gallstones were found in the faeces of 34 out of the 36 patients whereas in the control group only three of the 36 patients passed gallstones in their stools. This simple, but most important study shows that pancreatitis seems to be associated with the passage of gallstones through the common duct into the duodenum; the precise mechanism by which pancreatitis results remains to be shown. McMahon et al (1980) studied a group of patients undergoing cholecystectomy and divided them into those with a past history of acute pancreatitis and those with no evidence of acute pancreatitis. It was shown that the patients who had had an attack of acute pancreatitis had smaller gallstones in their gallbladder and a larger cystic duct than those patients with no evidence of acute pancreatitis.

In some patients, however, no mechanical obstruction is demonstrable and it may be that spasm of the sphincter or oedema of the pancreatic duct may be responsible for the acute pancreatitis. Obstruction of exocrine flow with stimulation of pancreatic secretion will result in increased intraductal pressure resulting in increased backflow into the interstitium of the gland. This may partly explain the clinical observation that many attacks of pancreatitis are preceded by excessive ingestion of food or drink or both.

Pathological changes in pancreatitis

Acute pancreatitis is characterized by changes in the pancreas, and by widespread foci of fat necrosis over the surface of the omentum and intestines. Gross oedema of the pancreas, often heavily bile-stained, is the outstanding macroscopic feature of the mild form of the disease, whereas infarction following upon thrombosis or haemorrhage is characteristic of the rarer form which carries a high mortality. It is useful to distinguish these forms of the disease by the terms acute pancreatic 'oedema' and acute pancreatic 'necrosis'. Both forms are believed to result from the escape of pancreatic enzymes into the substance of the gland, the difference between them being of degree rather than time.

Foulis (1980) studied the histological picture in acute pancreatitis and identified three main patterns of necrosis. Periductal necrosis was seen in cases with mild disease and in these patients there was a marked correlation between periductal necrosis, duct inflammation and the presence of eosinophilic proteinaceous concretions within the duct lumen. Duct inflammation was thought to be the initiating lesion in these cases. Perilobular necrosis was also seen in patients with mild to moderate acute pancreatitis. Duct inflammation was seldom seen in these cases whereas venous thrombosis was a common finding. The histological findings supported a primary ischaemic mechanism in this form of pancreatitis. Panlobular necrosis was seen in patients with more severe acute pancreatitis. The histological features were coagulative necrosis, little evidence of inflammatory cell infiltrate within much of the necrotic tissue, and venular and occasionally arterial thrombosis at the junction between necrotic and viable tissue. The likely mechanism here was thought to be destruction and thrombosis of blood vessels exposed to necrotic pancreatic parenchyma, with subsequent infarction, and it was thought that either periductal or perilobular necrosis could progress to panlobular necrosis.

Trypsin is held responsible for initiating the autolysis of the pancreas in acute pancreatitis. The fat necrosis which is one of the characteristic features of acute pancreatitis is attributed to the escape of lipase from the damaged pancreas into the peritoneal cavity. Under the influence of lipase the subserous fat is hydrolysed to glycerol and fatty acids; the fatty acids then combine with calcium to form insoluble calcium soaps.

Diagnosis of acute pancreatitis

The diagnosis of acute pancreatitis is usually suspected on clinical grounds and confirmed by biochemical estimations. A serum amylase level in excess of 1200 iu/dl is regarded as being diagnostic of acute pancreatitis. The diagnostic level of serum amylase for acute pancreatitis is well above the upper limit of normal for this enzyme (300 iu/dl) since hyperamylasaemia may occur in other acute intra-abdominal conditions such as perforated peptic ulcer, acute cholecystitis, ectopic pregnancy, mesenteric vascular occlusion, and ruptured aortic aneurysm. There is no relationship between the magnitude of the rise in serum amylase and the severity of the disease although several authors have stated that a high serum amylase is more likely to be associated with a surgically remediable cause of acute pancreatitis such as cholelithiasis (Adams et al, 1968).

In 5–10% of cases of acute pancreatitis the serum amylase is not significantly elevated on admission to hospital. In the majority of these cases the serum amylase level has fallen rapidly towards normal while in a few cases with severe acute pancreatitis the gland destruction is so complete that hyperamylasaemia does not occur. The amylase creatinine clearance ratio (ACCR) has been suggested as a more reliable discriminative test than serum amylase alone (Levitt & Johnson, 1978). The ACCR is amylase clearance expressed as a percentage of the simultaneous creatinine clearance and is calculated from the amylase and creatinine concentrations of simultaneous venous and urine samples without need of a timed urine collection. The test has been found to be over 90% accurate in the diagnosis of acute pancreatitis with a specificity for pancreatic disease greater than that of serum amylase alone (Murray & MacKay, 1977). It has also been noted that the ACCR returns to normal more slowly in cases of acute pancreatitis than does the serum amylase and this may be useful in patients with delayed presentation to hospital (Fig 21.3). A kit for rapid isoamylase estimation is now available (Pharmacia Diagnostics, Sweden) and this has shown P-isoamylase elevation to be sensitive but not entirely specific for acute pancreatitis. Serum lipase, phospholipase, trypsin and deoxyribonuclease also rise in acute pancreatitis but owing to technical difficulties in their estimation these enzymes are not commonly measured in the acute situation. Some advances have recently been made in the determination of serum lipase which can now be estimated in the acute situation and it may well be that a combination of serum lipase and amylase may improve the diagnostic rate in acute pancreatitis. The ACCR and isoamylase estimations may be helpful in patients with

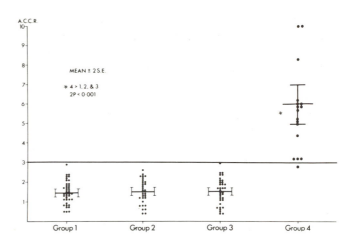

Fig. 21.3 ACCR values in 40 control patients (group 1), 30 patients with chronic non-pancreatic gastrointestinal disease (group 2), 35 patients with acute non-pancreatic abdominal disease (group 3) and 17 patients with acute pancreatitis (group 4) (Murray & MacKay, 1977).

hyperamylasaemia or hyperlipasaemia not in themselves diagnostic of acute pancreatitis.

Treatment of acute pancreatitis

Since the precise pathophysiology of acute pancreatitis is unknown it is not surprising that the treatment is empirical. No reliable mechanism has yet been described to deactivate the inflamed pancreas and at the present time the conservative treatment of acute pancreatitis can be divided into an attempt to inhibit pancreatic activity, general supportive measures and peritoneal lavage in those patients with severe acute pancreatitis.

Inhibition of pancreatic activity

The conventional method of achieving pancreatic inhibition has been by means of discontinuing oral intake of all food and fluids and instituting nasogastric suction. This diminishes the release of secretin and CCK-PZ from the mucosa of the upper small bowel and thus reduces the hormonal and neural drives to pancreatic secretion. Glucagon has been used for this purpose in acute pancreatitis since it inhibits gastric and small bowel motility along with gastric and pancreatic secretion. Unfortunately a multicentre MRC study using this drug showed no benefit in patients with acute pancreatitis. (MRC Trial, 1977, 1980)

Supportive measures

These are designed to replace the fluid and electrolyte loss, to relieve pain, to provide calories intravenously if required and to prevent the recognized complications of acute renal and respiratory failure. In severe cases resuscitation with

Table 21.1 Factors indicating acute pancreatitis (Western Infirmary, Glasgow)

1 White blood count > 15 000/mm³
2 Blood glucose > 10 mmol/l
3 Blood urea > 16 mmol/l and not falling after rehydration
4 Pa_{O_2} < 60 mmHg
5 Serum calcium (corrected) < 2.0 mmol/l
6 Serum albumin < 32 g/l
7 Serum LDH > 600 u/l
8 Serum SGOT or SGPT > 200 u/l

Prognostic factors in acute pancreatitis ≥ 3 positive factors indicates a severe attack.

plasma or even blood may be required and in the older patient central venous pressure monitoring is of value. The pain should be treated with adequate analgesia, usually in the form of pethidine. The urine output should be monitored accurately and an indwelling bladder catheter employed if urinary output is not satisfactory. Blood gases should be estimated early in the course of the disease as a baseline since incipient respiratory failure often does not become apparent until the second or third day of the illness. Both Ranson et al (1974) and Imrie et al (1978) have advocated the use of a prognostic factor score within the first 48 hours of admission to hospital with acute pancreatitis. The presence of three or more prognostic factors within that time period has been shown to indicate the probability of a severe attack of acute pancreatitis (Foulis et al, 1982). At the Western Infirmary, Glasgow any patient with acute pancreatitis who has 3 or more positive factors from the list shown in Table 21.1 within 48 hours of admission is regarded as being at high risk of developing severe acute pancreatitis with a mortality of between 30–40%.

Peritoneal lavage

Ranson (1976) has produced evidence that patients with severe acute pancreatitis, as defined by prognostic factors, may benefit from the use of therapeutic peritoneal lavage. A peritoneal dialysis catheter is introduced into the abdominal cavity and isotonic dialysis fluid is used to wash the peritoneal cavity in hourly cycles. Antibiotics and antiseptic agents have been added to the lavage fluid but the role of these agents awaits full evaluation. Results of a multicentre British study of this technique are awaited but preliminary analysis suggests that lavage only prolongs survival time without reducing mortality.

McMahon et al (1980) has shown that peritoneal lavage may be a useful diagnostic tool in cases suspected of having severe acute pancreatitis. In these cases 'prune juice' fluid should be present within the peritoneal cavity upon introduction of the dialysis catheter. Failure to aspirate dark fluid from the peritoneal cavity at this time should raise doubts about the diagnosis of severe acute pancreatitis.

Early surgical intervention in acute pancreatitis is occasionally indicated where the diagnosis is in doubt, for removal of a calculus at the lower end of the common bile duct, for drainage of a pancreatic abscess or in a deteriorating case of severe acute pancreatitis where pancreatectomy may be required. The place of surgery lies more in the prevention of recurring attacks of acute pancreatitis in patients who have gallstones or in the treatment of an established pseudocyst.

ISLET CELL TUMOURS OF THE PANCREAS

The simple, non-functioning adenomata of the islets of Langerhans are quite common and are of no clinical importance. Tumours of the islets which produce hormones are rare. These can be divided into groups according to their cell of origin. Insulinoma is the commonest and arises from the beta cells. Tumours arising from the G-cells may secrete excessive amounts of gastrin (gastrinoma or Zollinger-Ellison syndrome, page 278) while alpha cell tumours may secrete glucagon (glucagonoma). D-cell tumours may produce somatostatin (somatostatinoma) while H-cell or D_2 cell tumours may secrete VIP leading to the syndrome of watery diarrhoea, hypokalaemia and achlorhydria (WDHA).

Insulin-secreting tumours ('insulinomata')

These tumours are characterized by their ability to secrete insulin. The overwhelming majority develop within the pancreas, usually within the body or tail, but upwards of 2% originate in other sites usually adjacent to the pancreas and presumably in ectopic pancreatic tissue. They are small, seldom more than 1 or 2 cm in diameter, ovoid and grey or pink in colour. Usually they are solitary, encapsulated and benign; occasionally they are locally invasive, and rarely they are frankly malignant and metastasize (Fig 21.4).

Attacks of hypoglycaemia are the chief manifestation of an insulinoma. During an attack the blood sugar is usually less than 3.3 mmol/l and often as low as 1.8 mmol/l. The hallmark of an insulinoma is Whipple's triad, namely clinical features suggestive of hypoglycaemia, the demonstration of hypoglycaemia and the relief of hypoglycaemia by giving glucose. Without treatment the termination of the attacks is gradual but nevertheless spontaneous for the hypoglycaemia stimulates hypothalamic activity as a result of which the medulla and cortex of the adrenal are stimulated to discharge. Adrenaline accelerates the conversion of liver glycogen to glucose, and the adrenal corticoids antagonize the action of insulin on the liver and muscles.

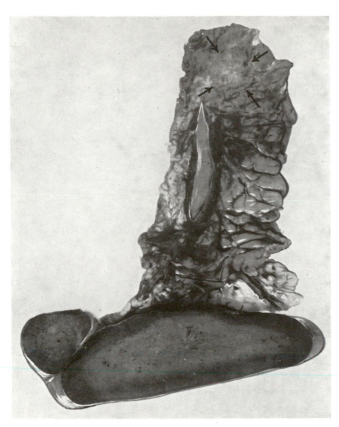

Fig. 21.4 Islet cell tumour situated in the tail of the pancreas, which gave rise to attacks of hypoglycaemia.

The features of the attacks of hypoglycaemia are relatively constant in any one patient but vary widely from one patient to another. The syndrome may include in varying combinations disturbances of the autonomic nervous system (nausea, sweating, pallor, or flushing), of the neuromuscular system (restlessness, muscular twitching, diplopia, convulsions) and of the higher cerebral functions (apprehension, confusion, mania, coma). If attacks of hypoglycaemia are frequent they lead to mental deterioration, and this in conjunction with attacks of coma may erroneously suggest the diagnosis of epilepsy.

Definitive pre-operative diagnosis depends upon the demonstration of inappropriately high plasma insulin levels in the presence of spontaneous fasting hypoglycaemia. The demonstration that hypoglycaemia exists and is the cause of the patient's symptoms, although mundane, is crucial. The next step is to show that the hypoglycaemia develops after a 15-hour overnight fast (Marks & Samols, 1974) and is accompanied by a normal or raised plasma insulin level. Many procedures aimed at facilitating the diagnosis of insulinoma without the necessity of provoking fasting hypoglycaemia have been investigated; most utilise the ability of various agents such as tolbutamide, glucagon, glucose, leucine and arginine to stimulate insulin release

but none has been wholly successful and most become superfluous as plasma insulin radioimmunoassay for the C-peptide of insulin has become more readily available (Buchanan, 1980).

Early surgery is the treatment of choice. The main difficulty is location of the tumour and in this connection, selective arteriography and computed tomography may be helpful. Where the tumour is recognized any operation may be performed so long as the insulinoma is completely removed. When the tumour is occult the most valuable procedure is progressive resection of the pancreas from left to right with immediate histological examination of the resected specimens and intra-operative estimation of the blood sugar. The late results are good where the insulinoma is found (Stefanini et al, 1974).

Glucagonoma and alpha cell hyperplasia

The classic description of the glucagonoma syndrome was published by Mallinson et al (1974). The clinical features include necrolytic migratory erythema, diabetes mellitus, stomatitis and vulvitis, anaemia, psychiatric features and diarrhoea. Of these, the hallmark of the diagnosis is the rash which has a resemblance to that of zinc deficiency. The rash, however, is not always a feature and, when present, probably indicates advanced disease. The perineum and legs are most frequently involved and the rash is painful with necrolysis being the essence of the clinical and histological diagnosis. The diagnosis may be supported by the estimation of plasma glucagon but the ultimate diagnosis depends upon the morphological identification of tumour cells and the extraction from tumour tissue of material with biological and immunological properties of pancreatic glucagon.

Watery diarrhoea, hypokalaemia and achlorhydria syndrome (WDHA)

This syndrome, otherwise known as the Verner-Morrison syndrome, is thought to result from the production of VIP from a tumour involving the H-cell or D_2-cell of the pancreas. The syndrome is characterized by watery diarrhoea, hypokalaemia (potassium levels less than 3.5 mmol/l), absence of peptic ulcer disease and hypochlorhydria or achlorhydria. Flushing and spider naevi, impaired glucose tolerance, hypercalcaemia, tetany and biliary disturbance have also been noted in this syndrome. The major diagnostic step is the finding of an elevated circulating level of VIP and treatment is by local excision where possible (Zollinger & Takeuchi, 1974).

Somatostatinomas

A somatostatinoma has been described (Larrson et al,

1977) and a consistent clinical picture has yet to emerge. Abnormal glucose tolerance, flushing, diarrhoea, and hypochlorhydria can be features. Excessive somatostatin production is thought to be a feature of many pancreatic apudomas and may be more a feature of mixed endocrine tumours than a solitary occurrence. The diagnostic marker for such tumours is the finding of an elevated circulating level of somatostatin.

Pancreatic peptide tumours have not as yet been described as single entities. Pancreatic peptide however appears to be involved in a number of apudomas and elevated circulating levels have been noted in patients with glucagonomas, VIPomas, gastrinomas and insulinomas.

PAIN ORIGINATING IN THE PANCREAS

An interesting study in regard to the localization of the referred pain from pancreatic stimulation was made by Bliss and his colleagues (1950). Tiny insulated electrodes were inserted at various sites in the pancreas at routine laparotomies and observations made during convalescence. Successful stimulation of the head of the pancreas produced pain located to the right of the midline from xiphoid to umbilicus; this pain was mediated by the right splanchnic nerves through the right sympathetic ganglia and corresponded to dermatome segments 6–11 (Fig 21.5a). On stimulation of the body of the pancreas, pain was localized to the mid-epigastrium and was mediated by both right and left splanchnics by way of the same segments (Fig 21.5b). On stimulating the tail of the pancreas, pain was experienced to the left of the midline anteriorly anywhere between the xiphoid and the groin (6th dorsal to 1st lumbar dermatomes) (Fig. 21.5c).

Electrical stimulation, whether of head, body or tail, to the limit of tolerance produced a bandlike pain across the upper abdomen which radiated through to the back. This type of pain also followed simultaneous stimulation by all the electrodes. Patients with previous attacks of acute pancreatitis described this pain as similar to the pain experienced during an attack.

Pain arising in the head of the pancreas can be relieved by right-sided splanchnicectomy; pain arising in the body of the pancreas requires bilateral splanchnicectomy; pain arising from the tail of the pancreas can be relieved by left splanchnicectomy. Some success has been achieved recently in the treatment of chronic back pain resulting from chronic pancreatitis or pancreatic carcinoma; in selected cases the coeliac ganglion has been injected with 50% alcohol with relief of symptoms of up to 9 months duration being achieved in the majority of patients.

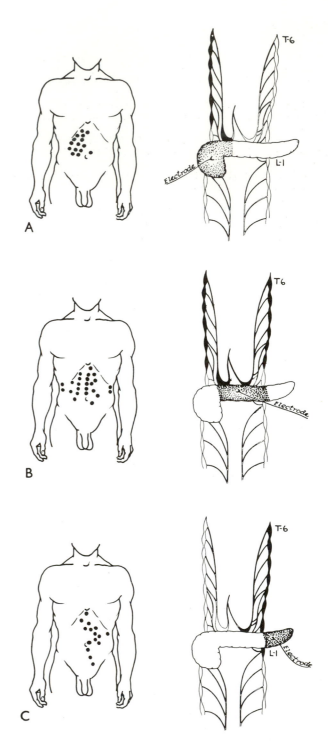

Fig. 21.5 The localization of pain from stimulating (A) the head, (B) the body, (C) the tail of the pancreas by means of electrodes inserted at laparotomy several days before. Afferent nervous impulses are believed to pass through the sympathetic trunks, as indicated (Bliss et al., 1950).

REFERENCES

Acosta J M, Ledesma C L 1974 Gall stone migration as a cause of acute pancreatitis. New England Journal of Medicine 290: 484–487

Adams J T, Libertino T A, Schwartz S I 1968 Significance of an elevated serum amylase. Surgery 63: 877–884

Agren G, Lagerlöf H (1936) Pancreatic secretion in man after intravenous administration of secretin. Acta Medica Scandinavica 90: 1–29

Arvanitakis C, Cooke A R, Greenberger N J 1978 Laboratory aids in the diagnosis of pancreatitis. Medical Clinics of North America 62: 107–128

Banting F G, Best C H 1921 Pancreatic extracts. Journal of Laboratory and Clinical Medicine 7: 464–472

Bayliss W M, Starling E H 1902 The mechanism of pancreatic secretion. Journal of Physiology (London) 28: 325–353

Bliss W R, Burch B, Martin Mary M, Zollinger R M 1950 Localisation of referred pancreatic pain induced by electrical stimulation. Gastroenterology 16: 317–323

Bloom S R 1975 Glucagon. British Journal of Hospital Medicine 13: 150–158

Bollman J L, Waugh J M 1946 Total pancreatectomy; symposium presenting four successful cases and report on metabolic observation. Proceedings of the Staff Meeting at the Mayo Clinic 21: 25–46

Buchanan K D 1980 Gut hormones and gut endocrine tumour syndromes. British Journal of Hospital Medicine 18: 190–197

Case R M, Harper A A, Scratcherd T 1969 The secretion of electrolytes and enzymes by the pancreas of the anaesthetised cat. Journal of Physiology (London) 201: 335–348

Coffey R J, Mann F C, Bollman J L 1940 Influence of pancreas on utilisation of foodstuffs. American Journal of Digestive Diseases 7: 144–149

Cotton P B, Cremer M, Robberecht P, Christophe J 1974 Biochemical studies of pure pancreatic juice obtained by duodenoscopic cannulation of the pancreatic duct in conscious patients. Gut 15:838

Cotton P B, Heap P R 1975 The analysis of pancreatic juice. British Journal of Hospital Medicine 14: 659–666

Dreiling D A (1975) Pancreatic secretory testing in 1974. In: Symposium on Diagnosis of Pancreatic Disease. Gut 16: 653–657

Dreiling D A, Janowitz H D, Halpern M 1955 The effect of a carbonic anhydrase inhibitor diamox on human pancreatic secretion. Gastroenterology, 29: 262–279

Foulis A K 1980 Histological evidence of initiating factors in acute necrotising pancreatitis in man. Journal of Clinical Pathology, 33: 1125–1131

Foulis A K, Murray W R, Galloway D J, McCartney A C, Lang E, Veitch J, Whaley K 1982 Endotoxaemia and complement activation in acute pancreatitis in man. Gut, 23: 656–661

Harper A A, McKay I F S 1948 The effect of pancreozymin and vagal nerve stimulation upon the histological appearance of the pancreas. Journal of Physiology (London), 107: 89–96

Harper A A, Raper A S 1943 Pancreozymin: Stimulant of secretion of pancreatic enzymes in extracts of small intestine. Journal of Physiology, 102: 115–125

Howard J, Jones R 1947 The anatomy of the pancreatic ducts; the aetiology of acute pancreatitis. American Journal of Medical Science, 214: 617–622

Howell C W, Bergh T S 1950 Pancreatic duct filling during cholangiography. Gastroenterology, 16: 309–316

Imrie C W 1974 Observations on acute pancreatitis. British Journal of Surgery, 61: 539–544

Imrie C W, Whyte A S 1975 A prospective study of acute pancreatitis. British Journal of Surgery, 62: 490–494

Imrie C W, Benjamin I S, Ferguson J C, McKay A J, MacKenzie I, O'Neill J, Blumgart L H 1978 A single-centre double-blind trial of Trasylol therapy in primary acute pancreatitis. British Journal of Surgery 65: 337–341

James O 1973 The Lundh Test. Gut, 14: 582–591

Lagerlöf H 1945 Normal esterases and pancreatic lipase in the blood. Acta Medica Scandinavica 120: 407–436

Lagerlöf H O, Schütz H D, & Holmer S 1967 A secretin test with high doses of secretin and correction for incomplete recovery of duodenal juice. Gastroenterology, 52: 67–77

Larsson L I, Holst J J, Kuhl C, Lundqvist G, Hirsch M A, Ingemansson S, Lindkaer Jensen S, Rehfeld J F, Schwartz T W 1977 Pancreatic somatostatinoma. Clinical features and physiological implications. Lancet i: 666–668

Levitt M D, Johnson S G 1978 Is the Cam/Ccr ratio of value for the diagnosis of acute pancreatitis? Gastroenterology, 75: 118–119

Mallinson C N, Bloom S R, Warin A T, Salmon P R, Cox B 1974 A glucagonoma syndrome. Lancet ii: 1–5

Marks V, Samols E 1974 Insulinoma: natural history and diagnosis. Clinics in Gastroenterology 3: 559–573

MRC Working Party on the Treatment of Acute Pancreatitis 1977 Death from acute pancreatitis. Lancet ii: 632–635

MRC Working Party on the Treatment of Acute Pancreatitis 1980 Morbidity of acute pancreatitis: the effect of aprotinin and glucagon. Gut 21: 334–339

Murray W R, MacKay C 1977 Amylase creatinine clearance ratio in acute pancreatitis. British Journal of Surgery 64: 189–191

McMahon M J, Playforth M J, & Pickford I R 1980 A comparative study of methods for the prediction of severity of attacks of acute pancreatitis. British Journal of Surgery 67: 22–25

McMahon M J, Shefta J R 1980 Physical characteristics of gallstones and the calibre of the cystic duct in patients with acute pancreatitis. British Journal of Surgery 67: 6–9

Oi I, Kobayashi S, Kondo T 1970 Endoscopic pancreato-cholangiography. Endoscopy 2:103

Quigley E M M, Mills P R, Cole T P, Girdwood T, Scott-Harden W G, Watkinson G 1980 'The fat-encrusted colon'. A radiological abnormality of colonic mucosa occurring in patients with steatorrhoea. Scandinavian Journal of Gastroenterology 15 841–848

Ranson J H C, Rifkind K M, Roses D F, Fink S D, Eng T, Localio S A. 1974 Objective early identification of severe acute pancreatitis. Surgery, Gynecology & Obstetrics 136: 443–451

Ranson J H C, Rifkind K M, & Turner J W 1976 Prognostic signs and non-operative peritoneal lavage in acute pancreatitis. Surgery, Gynecology & Obstetrics, 143: 209–215

Schiller W R, Suriyapa C, Anderson, Marion C 1974 A review of experimental pancreatitis. Journal of Surgical Research 16: 69–90

Scratcherd T 1975 Pancreatic function tests: the physiological background. In: Symposium of Diagnosis of Pancreatic Disease. Gut 16: 648–663

Sinclair I S R 1956 Observation on a case of external pancreatic fistula in man. British Journal of Surgery 44: 250–262

Staub A, Sinn L, Behrens O K 1953 Purification and crystallisation of hyperglycaemic glycogenolytic factor (HGF). Science 117: 628–629

Stefanini P, Carboni M, Patrassi N 1974 Surgical treatment and prognosis of insulinoma. Clinics in Gastroenterology 3: 697–709

Thomas J E 1959 Methods for collecting pancreatic juice. Gastroenterology 36: 362–367

Thomas J E 1967 Neural regulation of pancreatic secretion. In: Code C F (ed) Handbook of Physiology Vol. II, American Physiological Society, Washington Section 6, p 955–967

Trapnell J E 1974 Acute pancreatitis. British Journal of Hospital Medicine 12: 193–203

Wormsley K G 1972 Pancreatic function tests. Clinics in Gastroenterology 1:1, 27–51

Zollinger R M, Takeuchi A 1974 Surgical treatment of gastrinoma and WDHA syndrome. Clinics in Gastroenterology 3: 685–696

Kidney

The structure and basic physiology of the kidney are dealt with here, but the very important homeostatic functions of the kidney in maintaining water balance, electrolyte balance and acid-base balance are dealt with in other chapters.

The chief topics of clinical importance to the surgeon concern the pathophysiological changes in acute and chronic renal failure, and the formation of renal calculi. The chapter concludes with a survey of the problems involved in renal transplantation.

ANATOMY

The external aspect of the kidney presents a smooth surface covered by the renal capsule. The medial margin is concave, due to the presence of the hilum, in which lie the renal pelvis, vessels and nerves. On cross-section, the cut surface of the kidney shows two distinct regions, the outer cortex and the inner medulla.

Renal circulation

The renal arteries usually arise from the aorta opposite the upper border of the second lumbar vertebra and run towards the hilum. The renal artery divides into branches, the interlobar arteries, which run peripherally between the medullary pyramids; all of these are functionally end-arteries (Fig. 22.1). At the corticomedullary junction, each vessel divides into arcuate branches which pass along the corticomedullary boundary zone parallel to the surface of the organ. From these arches arise the intralobular arteries, which run a short course into the cortex and give off the afferent arterioles to the glomeruli. The subsequent course of the vessels depends on the position of the glomeruli; in the outer part of the cortex, the efferent arterioles from the glomeruli divide again into capillaries which supply adjacent renal tubules. There are, therefore, two capillary beds supplying the nephron — one is the glomerulus and the second the peritubular capillaries. The

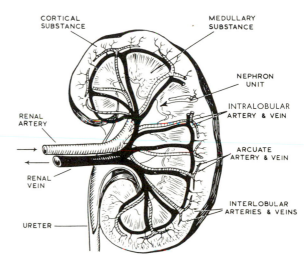

Fig. 22.1 The principal blood vessels of the kidney (schematic). (After Research in Medicine, G. D. Searle & Co.)

glomerular capillary bed receives its blood directly from the afferent arteriole and this bed is separated from the peritubular capillary bed by the efferent arteriole which offers considerable resistance to blood flow. As a result, the glomerular capillary bed is a high pressure bed while the peritubular capillary bed is a low pressure bed. As a result of this arrangement, the glomerulus resembles the usual arteriolar ends of the tissue capillaries with fluid filtering continually out of the glomerulus into Bowman's capsule. On the other hand, the low pressure in the peritubular capillary system causes it to function in much the same way as the venous ends of the tissue capillaries with fluid being absorbed continually into the capillaries. Juxtamedullary glomeruli, in the inner part of the cortex, have efferent arterioles which drain into wide thin-walled veins, the vasa recta, which descend into the medulla surrounding the lower portions of the Loops of Henle. This is a specialized portion of the peritubular capillary system which is intimately concerned in the concentration of urine (q.v.). Trueta et al (1947) claimed that the circulation through the juxtamedullary glomeruli could serve as a vascular shunt between renal artery and vein, bypassing cortical glomeruli. Although this view has been contested (O'Connor, 1962), further evidence has now accumulated to suggest that such a mechanism may be involved in the production of acute renal failure (q.v.).

Abnormalities of the renal vascular supply are not uncommon, and this problem has increased in importance with the advent of renal transplantation. The apical segment of the kidney is usually supplied by a branch from the anterior division of the renal artery, but the branch may also arise direct from the main stem, or from the aorta. Aberrant arteries supplying the lower pole of the kidney are more common and usually arise from the renal artery, aorta or common iliac artery. The surgical problems involved have been discussed by Woodruff et al (1969).

Lymphatics of the kidney

A rich network of lymphatic capillaries is present in the renal cortex, and lymph probably flows centripetally from the cortex alongside the intralobular, arcuate and interlobar arteries to emerge at the hilum and drain to aortic lymph nodes. A fine lymphatic plexus also exists in the renal capsule. Although very little is known of the mechanism of lymph formation within the kidney, it may well be of considerable importance since Mayerson (1963) has demonstrated in dogs an average lymph flow from a single kidney of 400 ml in 24 hours.

Innervation

The nerves which enter the kidney accompany the arteries. They are derived from the plexus which surrounds the renal artery and from the large ganglion which is often present on the posterior surface of the artery. The fibres come from the lower thoracic and upper lumbar segments of the spinal cord and reach the renal plexus through the coeliac ganglia, through the aortic plexus or through the least splanchnic nerve. Afferent fibres from the kidney probably pass through the coeliac plexus, but do not relay until they reach their cell stations in the lower thoracic segments of the spinal cord.

Within the kidney, nerve fibres have been shown to penetrate the basement membrane of the tubules, while other fibres end in the periglomerular area; occasionally, fibres seem to penetrate the glomerular tuft.

The renal nerves appear to be mainly sympathetic in structure and adrenergic in function. The close proximity of the majority of nerve fibres to blood vessels suggests that they have a primary vasomotor function, but this has not yet been defined. Because the renal nerves are intermingled with fibres for the adrenal medulla, attempts to stimulate these nerves are apt to influence the kidney both directly and by discharge of adrenaline. Experiments in animals have produced conflicting evidence on the effect of stimulation of nerves on renal function, but it seems likely that the renal nerves are of little importance in the day-to-day control of urine formation (O'Connor, 1962). This view is supported by the fact that the transplanted (and denervated) kidney seems to function normally in most respects.

The nephron

The functional unit of the kidney is the nephron, and each human kidney contains about 1 million of these. Each nephron consists of a glomerulus and its related tubule. The glomerulus is a richly branched and interconnected capillary network, supplied by the afferent arteriole and occupying Bowman's capsule. The capsule can be regarded as the expanded and thinned blind extremity of the renal tubule, invaginated by the capillary tuft, leaving a narrow sickle-shaped lumen (the urinary space) which drains into the tubule proper (Fig. 22.2). Blood within the capillaries is separated from the lumen of the capsule by the glomerular membrane which is composed of three major layers: (i) the endothelial layer of the capillary itself, (ii) a basement membrane, and (iii) a layer of epithelial cells that line the surfaces of Bowman's capsule. Despite the number of

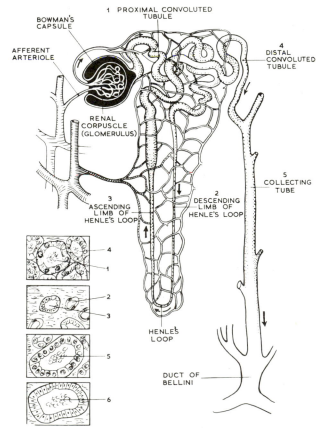

Fig. 22.2 The component parts of a nephron (schematic). (After Research in Medicine, G. D. Searle & Co.)

layers, the permeability of the glomerular membrane is up to 1000 times as great as that of the usual capillary. This is perhaps related to the fact that the capillary endothelial cells lining the glomerulus are perforated by thousands of small holes or fenestrae. Outside of the endothelial cells is a basement membrane composed mainly of a meshwork of mucopolysaccharide fibrillae. The final layer of the glomerular membrane, the epithelial cells, are not continuous but consist mainly of finger-like projections that cover the outer surface of the basement membrane. Just before the afferent arteriole enters the glomerulus, the muscular cells of the media alter in character, and are seen to contain large granules; these, together with nearby cells of renal origin, form the juxta-glomerular apparatus which is the site of renin production.

The renal tubule is about 3 cm in length and 20–60 μm in diameter. It comprises three segments which differ in structure and function (see Fig. 22.2). The lumen of Bowman's capsule is directly continuous with the proximal convoluted tubule, which, like the distal convoluted tubule, lies in the cortex of the kidney. The intervening U-shaped segment, the loop of Henle, lies in the medulla. In all segments the epithelium consists of a single layer of cells set upon a basement membrane. The cells lining the proximal convoluted tubule are cuboidal and have a large number of microvilli projecting into the lumen, providing a vastly increased surface area for reabsorption of substances. The loop of Henle is the narrowest segment, lined by flat cells with few mitochondria. The distal convoluted tubule is again lined by cuboidal cells with short micro-villi, less abundant and coarser than those of the proximal segment.

Tubular urine passes from the distal convoluted tubules into the collecting ducts, which pass down through the medulla. They drain into the ducts of Bellini, and several of these empty into the pelvis of the ureter at the apex of a pyramid. The collecting tubules are lined by cuboidal cells, and the ducts by columnar cells.

RENAL FUNCTION

The process of urine formation is initiated by the separation, across the walls of the glomerular capillaries, of an ultrafiltrate of plasma. Driven by the net filtration pressure, the glomerular filtrate flows through the tubules, where, through the activity of the epithelial lining, the composition of the fluid is drastically altered by both re-absorption and secretion.

Glomerular filtration

The glomerular fluid is an ultrafiltrate of blood, and substances with a molecular weight over 65 000 normally do not pass into the filtrate. This means that the plasma proteins and, of course, all the formed elements in the blood are retained within the capillaries.

The glomerular filtration rate (GFR) is a very important measurement of renal function. Four factors operate in its control: permeability of glomerular capillaries, hydrostatic pressure in glomerular capillaries, hydrostatic pressure in the glomerular space and colloid osmotic pressure of the plasma.

Glomerular permeability

This depends on the area of capillary wall available for filtration; in other words the number of surviving and functioning glomeruli. If the other three variables are static, the glomerular filtration rate is therefore a means of measuring the amount of functioning renal tissue and the best clinical guide in the management of progressive renal disease.

Hydrostatic pressure in glomerular capillaries

This is controlled locally by variation in calibre of the afferent and efferent arterioles, which is probably under neural control. It might be expected that increases in arterial pressure would cause a proportionate increase in all pressures in the nephron and therefore increase the glomerular filtration rate significantly. Similarly, it might be expected that systemic hypotension would reduce GFR markedly. In the intact animal, however, this effect is greatly blunted because of a phenomenon called auto-regulation, as a result of which elevation in the systemic arteriolar pressure automatically produces afferent arteriolar vasoconstriction preventing a major rise in intraglomerular pressure. Similarly, a fall in systemic blood pressure is compensated for locally to a certain extent. Even in the denervated kidney some form of autoregulation of blood flow and GFR exists so that over a considerable range of variation in mean blood pressure GFR remains fairly constant. If the mean blood pressure falls below 70 mmHg, however, a fall in GFR follows.

Hydrostatic pressure in glomerular space

This acts against the hydrostatic pressure in the capillaries, but in normal conditions is very low, and contributes little to the regulation of GFR. In urinary tract obstruction, the pressure in the tubules and glomerular space will rise sharply and progressively, and, if the obstruction is not relieved, will cause glomerular filtration to cease entirely.

Colloid osmotic pressure in the plasma

This is almost entirely due to the plasma proteins, and normally provides a hydrostatic pressure of 25–30 mmHg opposing filtration of fluid. It is usually a stable factor and has little effect on regulation of GFR, in severe dehydration, increased plasma protein levels will contribute to the reduction in GFR.

Clearance concept and measurement of GFR

The kidney handles the excretion of many substances, and a rough guide to the state of renal function may be obtained by measuring the concentration of such substances in the blood. Such levels, however, are also affected by many other factors, particularly the rate of production of the substance. Also, the rate at which the kidneys excrete any substance is dependent upon its concentration in the plasma. Hence, to obtain a more accurate estimate of the kidney's functional ability to excrete any substance, it is useful to relate the rate of excretion of the substance to the plasma level. The rate of excretion is found by multiplying the concentration in the urine (U) by the rate of urine production (V). If U is in mg/ml and V in ml/min, then UV will be the rate of excretion in mg/min. If the concentration in the plasma is P mg/ml, then UV/P is the rate of excretion per unit of concentration in the plasma. This ratio is the renal clearance (C), and provides a numerical value for renal functional ability in relation to the substance measured.

The clearance concept is important principally in that it can be used to measure GFR. Any substance freely filtered at the glomerulus will have the same concentration in the glomerular filtrate as in the blood; if at the same time the substance is not either reabsorbed or secreted by the tubules, it will be excreted exclusively by glomerular filtration. If such a substance, X, had a concentration PX in the plasma, it will enter the glomerular space at a rate F × PX when F is the GFR. Since the substance is unaffected by the tubules, and cannot accumulate, it must be excreted in the urine at the same rate: i.e. U × V = F × PX. Solving this equation for F, F(GFR) = U × V/PX. In other words, the clearance of X is equal to the GFR. As has been stated, substances suitable for measuring GFR must be freely filtered at the glomerulus and neither reabsorbed nor secreted by the tubules. Such substances include inulin, which gives accurate results but has to be infused intravenously and is difficult to estimate. Inulin clearances may be used to measure GFR experimentally, where accuracy is vital, but creatinine clearances are satisfactory for most clinical purposes. Urea clearances are very unreliable because urea is reabsorbed by the tubules at a variable rate depending on urine flow and other factors. Glomerular filtration rate, measured by creatinine clearance, is widely used to assess degree of renal impairment, and serial measurements to determine rate of progression of disease. Serial measurements are also of great importance in monitoring the function of transplanted kidneys and in detecting rejection episodes. The normal GFR is 125 ml.min^{-1}. 1.73 m^{-2} of body surface.

Tubular function

The principal function of the tubules is to reabsorb water and those solutes in the glomerular filtrate which are of value to the body. The extent to which tubular reabsorption modifies the glomerular filtrate is shown in Table 22.1. Reabsorption occurs along the whole length of the tubule, but the distal tubule is also capable of secreting various substances, both endogenous and exogenous, into the tubular urine.

Table 22.1 Comparison of glomerular filtrate with voided urine

Substance	Amount in glomerular filtrate (per 24 h)	Amount in voided urine (per 24 h)
Water	180 litres	1.5 litres
Sodium	600 g	6 g
Potassium	35 g	2 g
Calcium	5 g	0.2 g
Glucose	200 g	none (trace)
Urea	60 g	30 g

Tubular reabsorption

Reabsorption, both active and passive, is the principal function of the proximal tubule. For example, sodium is reabsorbed from the tubular fluid into the blood against the gradient — this is an active, energy-requiring process and is an example of active reabsorption. Water accompanies the sodium, thereby increasing the concentration of other substances remaining in the tubular lumen; for example, the urea concentration is increased above that of the blood. As a result, urea diffuses with the gradient from tubular lumen into blood — passive reabsorption, requiring no energy expenditure. Many other substances are actively reabsorbed by the proximal tubule, resulting in their virtual absence in the final urine produced, including glucose, sulphate, urate and amino acids. All of these substances *will* appear in the urine if their plasma levels are raised, and such rate-limited processes are typical of mechanisms involving a 'carrier'.

Tubular secretion

This is the process whereby substances are transported from blood in the peritubular capillaries into the tubular lumen, and occurs principally in the distal convoluted tubule. Substances secreted by the tubules include the strong monovalent cations (potassium, hydrogen, ammonium), dealt with later, and various organic substances. Although the organic substances vary widely in structure, and few are normal constituents of body fluids, the transport mechanisms seem to be similar, again involving a rate-limited 'carrier' process. These substances include para-amino hippuric acid (PAH), iodopyracet ('Diodrast', used for intravenous pyelography), penicillin and chlorothiazide.

Para-amino hippuric (PAH) acid can be used to measure renal blood flow. If PAH is infused to maintain a constant blood level of around 2 mg/dl, the substance is virtually entirely removed from the blood on one passage through the kidney, both glomerular filtration and tubular excretion being involved. The Fick Principles states:

$$Flow = \frac{Removal\ rate}{A - V\ difference}$$

The removal rate can obviously be determined by multiplying the concentration of PAH in the urine by the urine volume ($U_{PAH} \times V$). The concentration of PAH in the renal vein can be ignored, so that $A - V$ difference is simply the concentration of PAH in blood reaching the kidney. Thus the rate of plasma flow is calculated:

$$Renal\ Plasma\ Flow = \frac{Removal\ rate}{A - V\ difference} = \frac{U_{PAH}\ V}{A_{PAH}}$$
$$= \frac{UV}{P} = C_{PAH}$$

The clearance of PAH is equal to the effective renal plasma flow, and the renal blood flow can then be calculated using the haematocrit:

$$RBF = \frac{RPF}{1 - Hct}$$

Tubular handling of water

Approximately 80% of the water filtered at the glomeruli is reabsorbed in the proximal tubule; this reabsorption is obligatory and passive, being secondary to the active reabsorption of solute, principally sodium. The tubular fluid entering the loop of Henle is isotonic, and in the descending limb water and salt continue to be lost. In the ascending limb, the tubule becomes impermeable to water, but sodium continues to be actively pumped from the lumen into the medulla. This has two effects: the urine entering the distal tubule is now hypotonic, while the tissues of the medulla are hypertonic. The distal tubule is in the cortex, an area of high blood flow, and the tubular fluid is rapidly restored to isotonicity (Fig. 22.3). The concentration and volume of the final urine is then determined as the tubular urine passes through the hypertonic medulla in the collecting ducts, under the control of the antidiuretic hormone of the posterior pituitary gland (ADH). If water needs to be conserved, then small rises in serum osmolarity stimulate production of ADH, which acts by rendering the cells of the collecting ducts permeable to water. Because of the high osmolarity of the medulla through which the ducts are passing, water is withdrawn from the tubular lumen and a small volume of concentrated urine is produced. In conditions of water

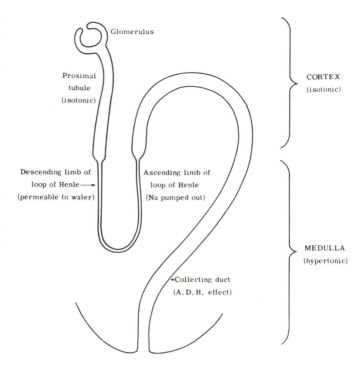

Fig. 22.3 Tubular handling of water.

load, reduction in serum osmolarity inhibits ADH production, the cells of the distal and collecting tubules become impermeable to water and hypotonic urine traverses the hypertonic medulla with relatively little loss of water and the production of large volumes of dilute urine.

The above outline of the mechanism of control of water balance by the kidney is based on the 'counter-current multiplying system' proposed by Wirz (1957, 1961). There are various objections to the relatively simple system described; for example, the cells of the ascending limb of the loop of Henle do not have the histological characteristics of other cells known to be capable of pumping sodium. Against this, the changes in the osmolarity of the tubular fluid are certainly as described, and it is likely that counter-current exchange, medullary hyperosmolarity and ADH are the principal factors in controlling water balance.

Tubular handling of sodium and potassium

Approximately 80% of the filtered sodium is reabsorbed in the proximal tubule, and the process continues as already described in the ascending limb of the loop of Henle. Control of the amount of sodium excreted is achieved in the distal tubule and collecting ducts, under the influence of aldosterone. In sodium depleted states, the production of renin by the juxtaglomerular apparatus is stimulated; this in turn stimulates aldosterone production by the adrenal cortex. Aldosterone increases the reabsorption of sodium from the distal tubule, largely in exchange for hydrogen and potassium (Fig. 22.4).

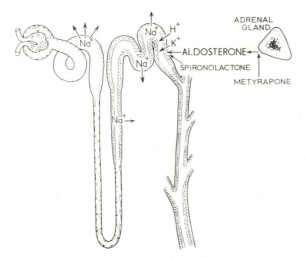

Fig. 22.4 Sites of reabsorption of sodium ions, and excretion of hydrions and potassium ions: and sites of action of aldosterone and aldosterone antagonists. (Redrawn from Wilson 1963)

Potassium is both reabsorbed and secreted by the tubules, reabsorption being an active process occurring in the proximal tubule, and secretion in the distal tubule, in exchange for sodium. Regulation of potassium loss is poorly understood, but seems to involve intracellular potassium levels, delivery of sodium to exchange sites, and factors modifying hydrogen ion excretion.

Acid-base balance

Control of acid-base balance is the final main function of the distal tubule. Waste products of intake and metabolism include a number of acids, the hydrogen ion of which has to be excreted by the kidney to prevent the development of metabolic acidosis. Acids cannot exist free in the body, but are taken up by buffer systems, of which the principal one is the bicarbonate buffer system:

$$H^+A + NaHCO_3 \rightleftharpoons NaA + H_2CO_3 \rightleftharpoons H_2O + CO_2$$
(acid produced
by metabolism)

The carbon dioxide is excreted by the lungs, while the anion must be excreted by the kidneys; if it were to be excreted along with the sodium ion, the net result of the production of one hydrogen ion would be the loss from the body of one molecule of sodium bicarbonate. Depletion of the body stores of sodium and bicarbonate is prevented by the kidney by various means. The principal mechanism involves the formation of carbonic acid within the cells of the distal tubule, from water and carbon dioxide under the influence of carbonic anhydrase. The cell then exchanges hydrogen for sodium in the tubular lumen, and sodium bicarbonate is returned to the blood (Fig. 22.5). Another mechanism for the excretion of hydrogen ion in the urine

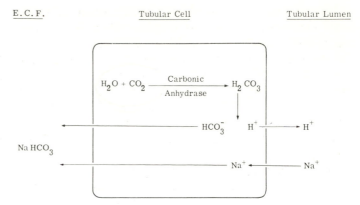

Fig. 22.5 Mechanisms of acidification of urine.

involves the production of ammonia by the cells of the distal tubule. The ammonia ion combines with a hydrogen ion and a chloride ion in the tubular lumen, sodium is reabsorbed in exchange and ammonium chloride is excreted in the urine.

DRUGS AND RENAL FUNCTION

A very large number of drugs have minor effects on various aspects of renal function; only those at present known to be of clinical importance will be discussed.

Anaesthetic agents

Most studies of the effect of anaesthesia on the kidney have failed to separate the effects of the anaesthetic agent and the accompanying surgery. Very little information is available concerning the isolated effect of anaesthetic agents alone. It has been shown that urine formation is diminished in association with a reduction in glomerular filtration rate during the action of cyclopropane, ether and various barbiturates. These effects follow a reduction in renal blood flow and are probably due to renal vasoconstriction (Habif et al, 1951). Many other changes in renal function have been described in association with premedication or the administration of volatile anaesthetic agents but are largely non-specific and probably result from alterations in cardiac output and in renal blood flow and distribution. These in turn lead to secondary effects on glomerular filtration rate and tubular function.

A series of complex and incompletely understood hormonal and vascular responses govern the postoperative excretion of sodium. During and after surgery in adults there is a considerable increase in the secretion of both glucocorticoids and mineralocorticoids; this has been thought to be due to an increase in aldosterone secretion. Sympathetic stimulation accompanying surgery, or a fall in pressure in the renal arterioles, produce an increase in renin production resulting in a redistribution of blood from the superficial to the juxtamedullary cortex and consequent sodium retention. Perhaps most importantly for a variable period postoperatively a considerably increased tubular reabsorption of water can be demonstrated, almost certainly due to enhanced secretion of antidiuretic hormone produced either by the anaesthetic agent or its circulatory effects. Renal function apparently returns to normal soon after termination of anaesthesia although oliguria due to excessive ADH production may persist for 36 hours (Bevan et al, 1973).

There have been many reports of an association between prolonged anaesthesia with methoxyflurane and polyuria with and without renal impairment. It has been suggested that fluoride ions released during metabolism of methoxyflurane are probably responsible for the polyuria by rendering distal tubules and collecting ducts unresponsive to the action of ADH.

Diuretics

Organic mercurial diuretics, effective but potentially toxic, have now been largely replaced by the thiazide diuretics and related compounds such as frusemide and ethacrynic acid. All of these substances act by inhibiting tubular reabsorption of sodium.

The thiazide group of diuretics were developed following the observation that sulphanilamide is a mild diuretic, acting principally as a carbonic anhydrase inhibitor. Such diuretics act by inhibiting the exchange of hydrogen ion for sodium ion in the distal tubule, promote the excretion of bicarbonate and have a short, self-limiting action owing to the development of a metabolic acidosis. Chlorothiazide was the first thiazide compound which was found to be a powerful diuretic, acting principally by increasing the urinary losses of sodium and chloride, and having relatively little carbonic anhydrase inhibiting effect. By various chemical substitutions in the basic molecule, many other thiazide diuretics have been developed. Many of these compounds are more active than the parent substance in inducing natriuresis, and have virtually lost carbonic anhydrase-inhibiting activity; the compound most widely used at present is bendroflumethiazide. This diuretic is well absorbed from the intestine, highly effective and remarkably non-toxic.

Frusemide, although not a thiazide, is chemically related to this group, and also acts by inhibiting tubular reabsorption of sodium and chloride in Henle's loop. It is characterized by an unusually rapid diuretic effect of short duration, and by a maximal natriuretic effect considerably greater than that evoked by maximal doses of the thiazides. Frusemide may be effective in cases of fluid retention where other diuretics have failed, and increasing doses continue to evoke an increased response up to very high levels. The drug is of great value in patients with gross overhydration, pulmonary oedema and congestive cardiac failure, although its use is not entirely free of risk. Lowe et al (1979) reported that in a large series of patients in hospital receiving frusemide 21% had some adverse reaction the most common being hypovolaemia, hyperuricaemia and hypokalaemia. There is also a risk of massive diuresis, severe loss of water and salt, producing shock (Kerr & Robson, 1965). In patients with normal renal function initial dosage of frusemide should not exceed 40 mg daily and should probably begin at 20 mg daily.

Ethacrynic acid is another diuretic which produces a rapid and massive diuresis of sodium, chloride and water. The mode of action within the nephron is probably similar to that of frusemide, and ethacrynic acid does not seem to have any major advantage over that drug. In common with the thiazides and frusemide, ethacrynic acid may induce potassium depletion in the patient. The extent of the potassium depletion depends less upon the diuretic used than on the patient's underlying condition. Potassium excretion increases with repeated administration of a diuretic, and is greatest in those conditions associated with increased levels of aldosterone (Laragh & Kelly, 1964). Potassium depletion in patients on diuretics may easily be overlooked, as the symptoms of fatigue and muscle weakness may be attributed to the underlying disease. A considerable body deficit of potassium may occur before any change in the serum potassium level is manifest, and measurement of urine potassium losses may be necessary. Special care is required in patients on digoxin, as moderate potassium depletion may increase the toxic effects of that drug.

Other diuretics, unrelated to those already described, include various steroid lactones which antagonize the action of aldosterone on the distal tubule. The most commonly used of these, spironolactone, resembles aldosterone in structure, and acts as a competitive inhibitor. Its effects are cumulative, and its full diuretic action develops over a few days. The steroid lactones are not in themselves powerful diuretics, but are valuable adjuvants to other diuretics, particularly in conditions such as the nephrotic syndrome and hepatic cirrhosis, which give rise to secondary hyperaldosteronism.

Nephrotoxic drugs

The kidney is particularly liable to suffer damage from drugs or poisons because of its extremely rich blood supply and because excreted compounds may be concentrated in renal tissue during urine formation. Substances and drugs which are potentially nephrotoxic include heavy metals, organic solvents such as carbon tetrachloride, radiologic contrast media and many antibiotics. The latter two groups deserve special consideration.

As long ago as 1954 reports appeared suggesting that acute renal failure might follow intravenous pyelography

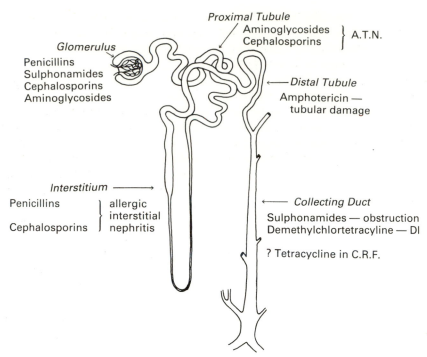

Fig. 22.6 Sites of antibiotic-induced renal damage.

in patients with multiple myeloma (Bartels et al, 1954) but this was thought to be an unusual event related to obstruction of the tubules with the abnormal protein. More recently it has become clear that acute renal failure may follow angiography of various kinds, particularly in diabetics (Weinrauch et al, 1977); a very high percentage of diabetics exposed to intravenous pyelography may develop evidence of renal impairment, particularly if dehydrated prior to the procedure. Despite these reports, the circumstances and frequency of the occurrence of acute renal failure following angiography were not well described until Swartz et al (1978) reported that of 109 patients undergoing angiography over a 6 month period, 14 showed significant deterioration in renal function and in 4 of these the degree of renal failure was relatively severe. It is now clear that the administration of radio-opaque dyes of any kind should be reviewed in the light of their nephrotoxic potential and this is particularly the case in patients with myeloma, in diabetics and in those with pre-existing renal insufficiency, impaired liver function, hypoalbuminaemia or proteinuria. Acute renal failure following angiography is usually reversible and its mechanism is unclear; nevertheless, the development of uraemia and its complications is to be avoided if possible, particularly in the critically ill patient.

Renal damage secondary to the administration of antibiotics may be an even more common cause of acute renal failure in a hospital population. Recent studies have suggested that between 9–20% of all cases of acute renal failure seen may be related to the administration of nephrotoxic antibiotics (Werb & Linton, 1979). Antibiotic induced renal damage is not a single pathological entity; the term encompasses several different pathophysiological mechanisms ranging from acute hypersensitivity reactions producing glomerular damage through acute tubular necrosis to acute or subacute interstitial nephritis. The major sites of renal damage induced by various antibiotics are indicated in Figure 22.6. Some are now largely of historical interest including the proximal tubular damage and Fanconi's syndrome induced by degraded tetracycline and the nephrogenic diabetes insipidus due to demethyl-chlortetracycline. The clinically important syndromes are those produced by antibiotics currently widely used — the aminoglycosides and the penicillin/cephalosporin group. The aminoglycosides, including gentamicin and tobramycin, can probably induce renal damage by several different mechanisms. It has been shown in animals that gentamicin can induce changes in the glomerular capillary permeability resulting in reduction in glomerular filtration rate, a phenomenon which is reversible upon withdrawal of the drug. The aminoglycosides can also, however, induce acute renal failure due to acute tubular necrosis, probably by a direct toxic effect; this renal damage does not reverse immediately following drug withdrawal but does usually recover slowly. Most of the cephalosporins can produce renal impairment as a result of direct tubular toxicity and this damage may be exacerbated by the coincident administration of frusemide (Bailey et al, 1973). Cephalosporin nephrotoxicity particularly tends to occur in the elderly and in those in whom renal function is already impaired. Finally, any of the penicillins or cephalosporins may induce temporary and reversible renal impairment as a result of the development of an acute, allergic, drug-induced interstitial nephritis. It is important to consider this diagnosis in unexplained cases of acute renal failure and it may be supported by the finding of coincident fever, arthralgia, eosinophilia and elevated IgE levels. The importance of diagnosis lies in the fact that the lesion will reverse with drug withdrawal in most instances, but rapid and full recovery may follow the administration of prednisone (Linton et al, 1980).

CHRONIC RENAL FAILURE

Chronic renal failure is the syndrome which results from progressive kidney damage from any cause. The clinical manifestations arise, not from the underlying disease, but from the increasing inadequacy of the damaged kidneys to perform their normal functions. Any renal disease can eventually produce chronic renal failure by continuing destruction of nephrons; the commonest causes of the condition are glomerulonephritis and obstructive uropathy, and among less common causes are included polycystic kidneys, calculous renal disease, collagen vascular disease, hypertension and analgesic nephropathy.

Clinical Course

Because of the considerable functional reserve of renal tissue, chronic renal failure is usually symptomless until renal function is reduced to approximately 40% of normal. With gradual loss of functioning nephrons, the increasing osmotic load on the remainder leads to polyuria and nocturia, two of the earliest symptoms. Once glomerular filtration falls below 40% of normal, a complex biochemical disturbance begins to develop and to produce symptoms. Retention of nitrogenous waste products gives rise to increasing malaise, anorexia, vomiting and diarrhoea. Failure to excrete hydrogen ion results in a metabolic acidosis, and hyperkalaemia may occur. These biochemical abnormalities are probably responsible for the haemorrhagic tendency which appears, and alimentary bleeding is common. Failing production of erythropoietin by the kidney, together with toxic bone marrow depression and increased haemolysis, lead to a refractory anaemia, which does not respond to any available haematinic. Cardiovascular problems arise, including pericarditis, and the problems of hypertension, which is frequently associated with all forms of renal disease. The widespread effects of renal insufficiency also affect the nervous system, in the form of uraemic peripheral neuropathy or tetany. Calcium metabolism is disturbed, with the appearance of various forms of bone disease, and metastatic calcification in blood vessels and other sites. All of these problems increase in severity as renal function deteriorates, and the end-stage is reached with increasing neuro-muscular dysfunction, convulsions and coma.

Treatment of chronic renal failure

Treatment is seldom required until renal function is reduced to levels at which symptoms occur, except that the blood pressure must be controlled with drugs such as methyldopa or propranolol. When malaise and gastrointestinal symptoms appear, much symptomatic benefit can be obtained by restricting protein intake to reduce the accumulation of toxic nitrogenous waste. Many patients can be maintained in good health for long periods by utilizing the dietary principles outlined by Giovannetti and Maggiore (1964). The Giovannetti diet contains reduced amounts of protein (approximately 18 g per day), but all of the protein is given as first-class protein of high biological value, high utilization and yielding only small amounts of waste. Implementation of this diet results in striking relief of symptoms and a rapid fall in blood urea levels, since urea is then re-utilized in the production of non-essential amino acids. Apart from dietary measures, the conservative treatment of chronic renal failure involves control of blood pressure, correction of acidosis and hyperkalaemia, and occasionally blood transfusion if bleeding occurs. It should be remembered that patients in the late stages of renal insufficiency are dependent on a high fluid intake and a large volume of urine of poor concentration; dehydration is an ever-present risk and will produce a sharp rise in blood urea with rapid clinical deterioration. Postoperative care in these patients should involve meticulous care over fluid balance, and a high fluid intake should be maintained.

Regular dialysis treatment

Once renal function is reduced to less than 5% of normal, death will ensue within a short time, often precipitated by intercurrent infection. In 1960 the development of artificial arteriovenous shunts by Quinton made it possible to undertake long-term repetitive haemodialysis, and to maintain alive patients with irreversible, end-stage renal failure (Scribner et al, 1960). Such shunts consist of 'Teflon' tips inserted into the radial artery and an adjacent vein, and connected by inert 'silastic' tubing (Fig. 22.7). The shunt is opened to connect the patients to the artificial kidney, and after dialysis it is reconstituted to allow blood to flow directly from the artery to the vein. Possible sites for insertion of such shunts are limited, and problems of access to the circulation may arise; this difficulty is now being circumvented by the creation of subcutaneous arteriovenous fistulae. Commonly, the radial artery at the wrist is anastomosed end-to-side with an adjacent medium-sized superficial vein. Increased flow dilates the superficial

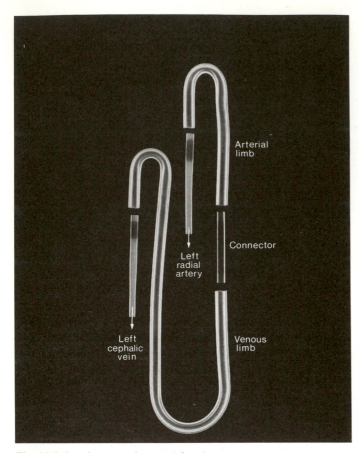

Fig. 22.7 Arteriovenous shunt at left wrist.

venous system in the forearm, and after a few weeks the vein walls become 'arterialized', permitting multiple punctures when required for dialysis.

More recent developments in blood access sites include the use of bovine arterial grafts to create an arteriovenous fistula, and the creation of 'new' arteries by installation of a woven prosthesis. These techniques have largely resolved the problems of inadequate access.

Parallel with the development of regular haemodialysis many attempts have been made to utilize intermittent peritoneal dialysis to maintain patients in end-stage renal disease. In general, intermittent peritoneal dialysis has proved an ineffective method of treatment providing a much poorer quality of life than regular haemodialysis. In 1977, however, Popovich and his colleagues described the technique known as continuous ambulatory peritoneal dialysis (CAPD) which is now being utilized in many areas around the world as an alternative to regular haemodialysis. This technique involves the placement of a permanent peritoneal catheter through which the patient exchanges four or five 1-litre cycles of peritoneal dialysate each day; this can readily be carried out on an ambulatory basis and fitted into a normal daily schedule. It is now clearly established that CAPD can indeed provide a quality

of life for some patients which approximates that produced by regular haemodialysis. A significant number of patients prefer CAPD, usually because it confers freedom from a machine and from extracorporeal blood circulation. It has been claimed that CAPD may even be a more efficient form of dialysis than haemodialysis since the peritoneal membrane clears some larger molecules better than does cuprophane in the artificial kidney. CAPD of course has its individual problems, the most prominent of which is the occurrence of peritonitis which may be either bacterial or chemical. The place of CAPD in the management of end-stage renal disease is not yet finally determined; it is likely that there will be a subset of patients for whom it proves to be the optimal form of treatment but the results of long-term CAPD remain unknown.

Regular dialysis treatment can restore to relatively good health and productive living the majority of adults who would otherwise die of end-stage kidney disease. There remain many problems: selection of patients from the large numbers who are potentially suitable, technical problems with apparatus, shunt difficulties, the increased incidence of hepatitis in dialysis units and, not least, the high cost of this form of treatment. Nevertheless, many patients are happy to accept the limited quality of life it allows, and extension of the principle to the installation of artificial kidneys in patients' homes may well provide at least a partial answer to the problem of chronic renal failure. Of equal importance, regular dialysis treatment for a limited period is necessary for patients awaiting renal transplantation, and adequate pretransplant dialysis allows the operation to be carried out on a healthy patient.

ACUTE RENAL FAILURE

Acute renal failure (ARF) is a condition fraught with difficulties concerning definition, diagnosis, management, specific treatment and prognosis. It is, therefore, appropriate to begin with a simple definition which is broad enough to encompass all possible conditions to be considered in the differential diagnosis. ARF is therefore defined as a temporary (and usually reversible) failure of the kidneys to excrete the waste products of metabolism. This wide definition obviously includes some non-renal causes of uraemia such as that due to hypovolaemia but stretching the definition is justified by the convenience of having a single term to embrace all acute causes of uraemia. With this definition a preliminary diagnosis of ARF can be applied to all cases where there is oliguria accompanied by a rise in blood urea and serum creatinine from whatever cause. Indeed, in a small number of cases even oliguria is not a prerequisite — so-called 'non-oliguric' ARF.

Causes of acute renal failure

Acute renal failure, as defined above, can result from:

1. Pre-renal factors (hypovolaemia, dehydration, electrolyte upset)
2. Renal factors (vasomotor nephropathy, nephrotoxins, glomerulonephritis)
3. Postrenal factors (urinary tract obstruction)

In every patient presenting with oliguria and a rising blood urea, the possibility of postrenal obstruction must be considered. Clues may be found in the history; a story of renal calculi, prostatism, loin pain or a recent abdominal surgical procedure should all raise the question of possible obstruction. Physical findings such as an enlarged prostate or a full bladder would obviously point to a lower tract obstruction. If the patient is totally anuric rather than simply oliguric, obstruction is a commoner underlying cause than intrinsic renal disease. In all cases, if any doubt exists as to the patency of the urinary passages, then cystoscopy and retrograde ureteric catheterization is indicated. The management of urinary tract obstruction is considered elsewhere in this book, but of course consists primarily of removing or bypassing the blockage; thereafter, good urine flow is the rule, although occasionally prolonged obstruction may lead to intrinsic renal damage which may or may not be reversible. Management of such a case is essentially similar to the management of other types of intrinsic acute renal disease, to be described later. One other hazard which may complicate the relief of acute urinary tract obstruction is a very profuse diuresis, which may be so severe as to produce acute dehydration or profound electrolyte deficits. Such a diuresis is a temporary phenomenon, and can be readily corrected with intravenous fluids.

One of the commonest diagnostic problems in the oliguric patient (after obstruction has been excluded) is to decide whether the oliguria is due to renal or prerenal causes. Patients developing uraemia for either reason have usually suffered trauma, surgery or obstetric catastrophe, and variable factors such as blood loss, transfusion and fluid and electrolyte imbalance render the usual indices of dehydration unreliable. Perhaps the most useful clinical guide to the differentiation of renal and prerenal causes of uraemia is based upon renal concentrating ability. In the patient with prerenal uraemia, with normal kidneys, the urine produced will be highly concentrated; on the other hand the patient with oliguria due to renal damage will produce urine of low concentration. Urinary concentration can be measured by several methods. Specific gravity of the urine is still often quoted, but is a poor method of assessing concentration, since it is affected by many substances which may be present in the urine but are not related to concentrating power, such as protein.

Measurement of urine osmolality is the most direct method of assessing the abilities of the kidneys to concentrate the urine. In the oliguric patient who is simply dehydrated the urine osmolality will significantly exceed that of plasma, usually in a ratio greater than 2:1. The measured urine osmolality will normally be greater than 600 mosm/kg. In contrast, patients who are oliguric because of a renal lesion will produce urine which is approximately isosmolar with plasma. Additional information may be gained by measuring the urinary sodium levels; the patient who is dehydrated and hypovolaemic will be retaining sodium avidly and the urinary sodium level will usually be less than 10 mmol/litre. In contrast, when an intrinsic renal lesion exists urinary sodium levels will usually exceed 40 mmol/litre. Separation of the group of patients whose oliguria is pre-renal, i.e. due to dehydration or hypovolaemia, allows these patients to be rapidly and safely treated with intravenous fluids and will normally result in restoration of urine flow.

This simple diagnostic process will provide the answer in the vast majority of cases. In the critical care situation, however, patients are sometimes seen in whom these procedures either give no clear answer or provide confusing results. This may occur, for example, with the administration of diuretics, with hypokalaemia, with coincident or associated liver or cardiac failure, or when renal concentrating power has been reduced prior to the insult by chronic renal disease or old age. The situation may be further confused by the fact that factors producing hypovolaemia, if allowed to continue, may eventually produce vasomotor nephropathy. One may, therefore, see a patient progress from oliguria due to hypovolaemia to full-blown vasomotor nephropathy. Diagnosis in these difficult cases may call for extensive haemodynamic assessment.

The diagnostic procedures in acute renal failure can be summarized as shown in Table 22.2.

The management of dehydration, hypovolaemia and electrolyte disturbances are dealt with elsewhere. The remainder of this section deals only with the commonest renal cause of acute renal failure, vasomotor nephropathy ('acute tubular necrosis').

RENAL CAUSES OF ACUTE RENAL FAILURE

Sudden onset of oliguria and uraemia may occur in many types of parenchymal renal disease, including many varieties of glomerulonephritis, systemic lupus erythematosus, polyarteritis and many others. Diagnosis in such cases usually rests upon findings of associated hypertension, the presence of red cell casts in the urine, immunological studies and renal biopsy. The only renal condition which need be considered here is acute reversible renal failure secondary to trauma or shock, and hitherto usually

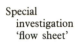

Table 22.2.

Problem: Oliguria and rising blood urea

Minimal
  routine
  investigations
	Full history (recent surgery, trauma, hypotension, toxins, previous renal disease, drugs)
	Physical examination (especially hydration state, external genitalia, bladder, rectal and vaginal examination)
	CBC, electrolytes, creatinine, BUN, serum osmolality
	Urine: Vol/hour (i.e. catheterise)
	      Micro, culture
	      Osmolality and Na$^+$

Special
  investigation
  'flow sheet'

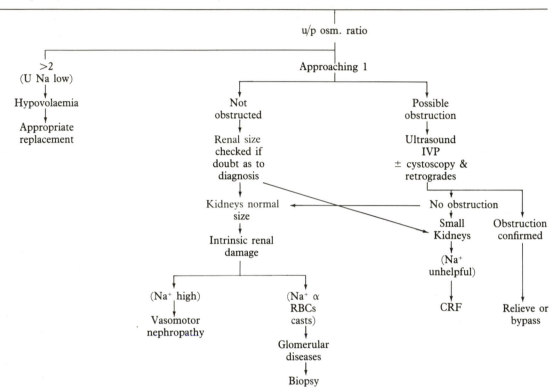

referred to as 'acute tubular necrosis'. For reasons which will become obvious, this title is misleading, and the condition would better be known 'vasomotor nephropathy'.

Vasomotor nephropathy or acute reversible intrinsic renal failure may follow any episode of hypotension or shock or the administration of nephrotoxic drugs. It was long thought that the preceding insult damaged tubular cells causing sloughing and consequent tubular obstruction (hence 'acute tubular necrosis'). It has now been clearly established that the clinical syndrome of vasomotor nephropathy may occur without the pathological lesion of tubular necrosis, and vice versa (Sevitt, 1959). However, the renal pathophysiology of the condition remains uncertain (Linton, 1974). It is not possible here to discuss the mass of conflicting evidence relating to the precise pathophysiology of vasomotor nephropathy. Two major points of view have emerged, one emphasizing necrosis of tubular cells and/or back diffusion of filtrate and the other focussing on preglomerular vasoconstriction as the prin-

cipal cause of the oliguria and uraemia. The fact that the condition almost always presents with oliguria, despite convincing evidence of continuing renal blood flow, defied explanation for some time since patients with chronic renal failure and similar renal blood flow normally exhibit a diuresis. Some change in glomerular dynamics, therefore, had to be postulated and it has been shown that glomerular filtration rate can virtually stop despite continuing renal blood flow when there is vasoconstriction of the afferent arteriole to the glomerulus (Fig. 22.8).

While it is likely that a reduction in renal cortical blood flow and preglomerular vasoconstriction constitute part of the pathophysiological disturbance in this type of renal failure, it is still uncertain how this change is brought about. Circumstantial evidence exists to implicate the renin angiotensin system in the genesis of vasomotor nephropathy. Renin, produced at the juxtaglomerular apparatus, would be admirably sited to regulate directly the preglomerular arteriolar calibre; at a clinical level, plasma renin

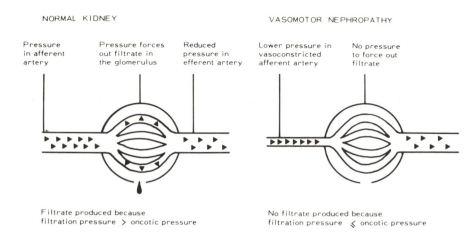

NORMAL KIDNEY   VASOMOTOR NEPHROPATHY

Pressure   Pressure forces   Reduced   Lower pressure in   No pressure
in afferent   out filtrate in   pressure in   vasoconstricted   to force out
artery   the glomerulus   efferent artery   afferent artery   filtrate

Filtrate produced because   No filtrate produced because
filtration pressure > oncotic pressure   filtration pressure ≤ oncotic pressure

Fig. 22.8 Possible mechanism in vasomotor nephropathy

levels are raised during the early stages of the condition, both in animals and man (Brown et al, 1970). Salt loading, which depresses renin, protects against vasomotor nephropathy, while salt depletion, which stimulates renin, renders animals and man more susceptible. On the other hand, immunization against renin or angiotensin II has produced conflicting results in experimental renal failure, so the hypothesis remains not proven. Even if angiotensin or another vasoactive substance can be identified as the cause of the original haemodynamic disturbance, it is difficult to envisage any such substance maintaining preglomerular vasoconstriction for the period of days or weeks that may elapse before the diuretic phase ensues. Despite a large volume of research on this subject the pathogenesis of vasomotor nephropathy remains unresolved and it may be that in man it is not a homogeneous condition but rather one in which vasoconstriction, tubular damage and even direct damage to glomerular capillaries all participate to a variable degree.

Clinical course of vasomotor nephropathy

The condition has three phases, the onset or functional phase (48 hours), the established oliguric phase and the diuretic phase. In the functional phase there are no symptoms attributable to the condition, and the problems are those of diagnosis and prevention. There is some evidence to suggest that the administration of mannitol, 100 ml of 20% solution, may abort the condition if given within 48 hours of the precipitating insult; there is also better evidence that mannitol given during operation on 'high risk' cases such as operations on the abdominal aorta will greatly reduce the incidence of acute tubular necrosis (Luke et al, 1965).

In the past few years many authors have published anecdotal information relating to the use of frusemide in high doses in the onset and early phases of vasomotor nephropathy. The only two of these studies which adopted rigid criteria of diagnosis and attempted to utilize control groups showed that frusemide had no benefit either in the early or established phases of the condition and indeed there are theoretical reasons for supposing it might be dangerous (Muth, 1973).

In the early days of the established oliguric phase symptoms are also few until the various biochemical abnormalities have developed. Blood urea rises at a variable rate, depending upon the rate of catabolism, which may of course be high in the patient after extensive trauma. Although the height of the blood urea is often taken as a guide to the stage of the illness, there is little evidence that urea is itself responsible for many of the symptoms of uraemia. It is probable that increasing retention of other nitrogenous waste products produce anorexia, nausea, vomiting, diarrhoea and neurological disturbances which comprise the syndrome of uraemia. Many of the symptoms which develop in acute reversible intrinsic renal failure are due to excessive fluid intake in face of negligible urine output. If the need to restrict fluid is not appreciated early, then expansion of extracellular fluid may progress to oedema and pulmonary congestion. Reduced serum sodium levels are often seen in renal shutdown and are almost always due to dilution with excess water; sodium deficit is seldom present. Failure of renal excretion of hydrogen ion leads to a metabolic acidosis producing acidotic respiration and clinical deterioration. Accumulation of potassium occurs also because of fall in renal excretion, and because of destruction of tissue and shift of potassium from the intracellular space as a result of the acidosis. Hyperkalaemia causes increasing muscular weakness and eventually cardiac arrest.

The established phase of vasomotor nephropathy may last for up to 3 months before the diuretic or recovery phase ensues. Renal concentrating power does not return at once, so that the daily urine volume usually has to exceed 1 litre a day before the blood urea level begins to fall. The twin hazards in the diuretic phase are dehydration, after massive diuresis, and hypokalaemia, due to the loss of large amounts of potassium in the urine.

Management of vasomotor nephropathy

Despite the availability of various dialysis procedures, the development of renal impairment particularly in critically ill patients identifies a group in which the eventual mortality is between 50 and 80%. Since the basic pathophysiology is unknown, vasomotor nephropathy cannot usually be reversed and has to run its natural course; the correct management, therefore, must focus first of all upon prevention of the condition. It is probable that a significant number of cases of acute renal failure develop either because of failure to observe proper precautions or as a result of the administration of known nephrotoxic agents. In the area of treatment of trauma and shock, there is ample evidence to indicate that rapid and complete replacement of fluids, electrolytes or blood as indicated will significantly reduce the incidence of vasomotor nephropathy. The recognition that many cases of renal failure are iatrogenic and follow the administration of nephrotoxic drugs is not well enough known. As mentioned earlier, drugs which should be exhibited only with care include nephrotoxic antibiotics, iodinated contrast media and potent diuretics. In some surgical situations prophylactic measures can be taken. In a patient scheduled for any of the major surgical procedures which are known to be associated with a high incidence of postoperative renal failure (e.g. major aortic surgery or operations on the gallbladder and bile ducts) good evidence exists to suggest that preoperative sodium loading has a prophylactic effect in preventing subsequent renal damage. A third aspect of prevention relates to the possibility of reversing vasomotor nephropathy at the early stages with mannitol as mentioned previously. This of course depends upon early diagnosis which in turn hinges upon careful monitoring of volume and electrolyte status of postoperative and critically ill patients.

The conservative management is aimed at minimizing the biochemical disturbances in order to allow time for the patient's kidneys to recover. During the oliguric phase, fluid intake is restricted to 400 ml per day plus a volume equal to the previous day's urine output. This may have to be modified if overhydration already exists, or if vomiting or diarrhoea complicate the picture; the success of fluid control can be gauged by daily weighing, aiming at a weight loss of 0.2 kg per day. Protein in the diet is usually restricted to 20 g per day, while the calorie content is kept as high as possible with carbohydrate. If vomiting necessitates intravenous feeding, the same principles are observed. In the past few years there has been a significant change in orientation with regard to management, particularly in the critically ill patient. It is increasingly recognized that these patients require adequate nutrition if they

are to survive their underlying illness or injury. In the majority of patients with renal failure, therefore, the conservative management now consists of attempts to provide at least the essential amino acids in adequate amounts from the outset. Studies have suggested that oral or intravenous feeding which provides these amino acids improve nitrogen balance and produce symptomatic relief (Abel et al, 1973). Furthermore, the provision of sufficient calories to meet the metabolic expenditure spares endogenous protein with further benefit. Acidosis may require treatment with bicarbonate, although the concurrent administration of sodium ions is undesirable. Potassium should be excluded from the diet, but hyperkalaemia often demands treatment with cation exchange resins such as sodium polystyrene sulphonate (Resonium A).

Although these conservative measures will maintain the patient for a few days in reasonable condition, death will soon ensue unless some form of dialytic treatment is employed. The use of haemodialysis or peritoneal dialysis in vasomotor nephropathy is to remove toxins and correct electrolyte disturbances in order to allow more time for the patient's kidneys to recover. Such measures are no substitute for early diagnosis and good conservative care, but their use has undoubtedly reduced considerably the mortality in this condition. Dialysis is urgently indicated when the blood urea level exceeds 350 mg/dl, or the serum potassium exceeds 7 mmol/l despite the use of resins; it is always better to dialyse early rather than late, and clinical deterioration of the patient now constitutes the overriding indication for dialysis. Again in an attempt to reduce mortality, early, frequent dialysis is now being used in patients with severe trauma or infection, often in association with intravenous protein feeding. There is still only marginal evidence that this regimen is beneficial (Kleinknecht et al, 1972).

The artificial kidney

The basic principle of dialysis is that most of the toxic substances in uraemia can be removed from the blood if it is brought in contact with a dialysing fluid, separated from it only by a semi-permeable membrane. The principle was first used by Abel and his colleagues (1914), and all modern artificial kidneys are modifications of the simple apparatus first used therapeutically by Kolff (1947). This consisted of a large drum revolving on a horizontal axis and carrying a long, spirally-wound cellophane tube which dipped under the surface of a water bath containing the dialysing fluid (Fig. 22.9). Blood from the patient's radial artery was led to the cellophane tube, and returned by a pump to a vein. The principal improvements on this technique include the use of semi-permanent, arteriovenous shunts to provide access to the arterial tree, and the use of more compact and disposable coils for the process of dialysis. Reduction in the length of cellophane tubing

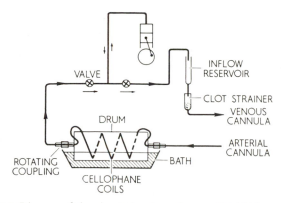

Fig. 22.9 Diagram of the circulation through an artificial kidney. (After Kolff, 1947).

required reduced the volume of the extracorporeal circulation, and has obviated the need to prime the circuit with blood. The dialysing fluid is a simple solution of various electrolytes in concentrations approximating those in body fluids. The composition can be varied to meet the needs of individual patients, and the fluid does not need to be sterile, since the cellophane membrane is impermeable to bacteria and most bacterial products.

Peritoneal dialysis

This procedure is based on exactly the same principle as haemodialysis, using the peritoneum as the semi-permeable membrane. Sterile dialysing fluid is instilled into the peritoneal cavity via a catheter inserted through the anterior abdominal wall. The fluid is then in direct contact with the blood in the capillary plexus beneath the peritoneum, and dialysis takes place. Repeated infusion and removal of 1 or 2 litre volumes of dialysis fluid ('cycles') may be continued for long periods, and, although the process is less efficient than haemodialysis, the same end-result is achieved. The value of peritoneal dialysis is that, in an emergency, it can be employed in any hospital where biochemical facilities are available.

Complications of vasomotor nephropathy

Anaemia of moderate degree develops rapidly as a result of marrow depression and increased haemolysis; it seldom necessitates transfusion, and recovers spontaneously with return of renal function. Infection is the commonest cause of death in acute renal failure. Both uraemia and malnutrition interfere with resistance to infection and wound healing, and bacteraemia and septicaemia occur readily. Prophylactic antibiotics have been shown to be ineffective, but antibiotics should be given rapidly in effective dosage once infection is diagnosed. It should be remembered, however, that antibiotics normally excreted by the kidney will accumulate in renal failure, and therapeutic blood levels can be achieved by reduced doses.

With the introduction of dialysis techniques capable of maintaining life in patients with no renal function, it was widely felt that the problem of acute reversible renal failure had been resolved. More recently, however, there has been a growing suspicion that somehow dialysis has failed to make its expected impact on mortality from this condition. Review of the literature reveals that the mortality rate in patients suffering vasomotor nephropathy after trauma or surgery remains around 50% which is not significantly lower than 20 years ago (Stott et al, 1972). Studies during the Vietnam conflict revealed that, despite the excellent results of improved overall management of combat casualties, the onset of vasomotor nephropathy was a grave prognostic sign. Attempts to identify the cause of the persistingly high mortality have produced some information. There seems little doubt that there has been a shift in the spectrum of patients referred to renal units in that patients who might previously have developed mild degrees of the condition are now saved from this by better management, while many critically ill patients are now kept alive long enough to develop renal failure. As examples, patients referred with acute renal failure in 1960 were often young adults in whom the condition was due to obstetric causes or following trauma; now the typical patient seems to be over 60 years of age, to have developed renal failure following heroic vascular surgery and to have many complications, particularly cardiovascular and infective. Adverse risk factors which have been identified include infection and gastrointestinal complications. Modifications in the treatment referred to above have produced only minimal advances and it seems improbable that much further benefit will accrue until identification of the pathophysiology allows prophylactic measures to be undertaken.

RENAL TRANSPLANTATION

Renal transplantation can now be regarded as an established method of treatment for chronic renal failure. This view is supported by recent improvements in survival rates, particularly those from the larger units. World figures are difficult to assess because of varying standards and techniques, but even these indicate that the 2-year graft survival after cadaveric renal transplant approaches 50% while with live related donors up to 90% may be functioning at 2 years. Despite improved results, however, many basic problems remain unsolved and of course the most important of these is the 'homograft reaction' which gives rise to rejection and necessitates the use of toxic drugs to prevent this. The nature of the homograft reaction, and the importance of lymphoid tissue in bringing it about, are discussed elsewhere (p. 467).

Histocompatibility testing

The severity and intensity of rejection of tissue allografts is dependent upon many factors, the most important of which is the degree of histocompatibility between the graft donor and recipient. At the present time, however, methods of determining histocompatibility remain fairly primitive and although the determination of maximal histocompatibility may improve clinical results of transplantation in homogeneous populations, it has not so far been shown to do so in populations of multiple racial origin. This observation applies in particular to definition of the HLA-A and HLA-B antigen systems which have been widely used over the past 15 years. HLA typing is now performed by cytotoxicity methods and to a small extent by complement fixation. Target lymphocytes are incubated with an anti-serum and complement. If the lymphocytes carry a cell surface antigen recognized by antibodies in the antiserum the cell walls of the lymphocytes are lysed; the development of microcytotoxicity techniques conserves the precious monospecific sera which measure only a single HLA antigen. Since rejection of an allograft is thought to involve lymphocyte-mediated immune responses against non-self antigens, several additional tests have been designed that use the biological response of lymphocytes to form antigens as a measure of histocompatibility. The most important of these is the MLC test. The discovery by Yunis and Amos (1971) of the locus HLA-D has opened another avenue which may eventually lead to better matching of recipient and donor. Studies using skin grafts have indicated that HLA-D incompatibilities are of considerable importance in rejection; evidence is accumulating that this is also the case in respect to kidney grafts. It should also be noted that despite the problems associated with HLA-A and HLA-B matching in cadaver transplantation, it is quite clear that with regard to living related donors, four antigen identity is associated with a very high success rate and with a very low incidence of rejection reactions and minimal immunosuppressive requirements.

Selection and preparation of recipients

Clinical practice in transplantation varies widely from centre to centre but the overall tendency is to liberalize the criteria for selection of transplant recipients just as it has been for selection of patients for regular dialysis treatment. Although patients of virtually all ages from a few months to 80 years have received transplants, in most cases transplantation is confined to those between the ages of 3 and 50. In general, patients over 50 years of age do less well following transplantation and, it seems, may do very well indeed on regular dialysis treatment. The presence of major extrarenal systemic disease must always be considered and relative contraindications include chronic infections such as tuberculosis, advanced myocardial disease, severe vessel calcification, chronic peptic ulcer or irreversible disease of the lower urinary tract; none of these individually, however, is a complete contraindication. Diabetes mellitus was once regarded as a complete contraindication although now virtually all units transplant diabetics from time to time although in most cases with rather poor results. Extrarenal disseminated malignancy is probably one of the few complete contraindications to transplantation.

Patients with end-stage renal disease who are potential transplant recipients require extensive preparation both in terms of adequate dialysis to improve their clinical condition and to assess their suitability for subsequent transplantation. Preparation includes complete haematological assessment, definition of the underlying renal disease and the state of the lower urinary tract, assessment of the stomach and duodenum with particular reference to possible peptic ulceration, immunological studies to define any possible adverse immunologic effect on the graft, pulmonary and cardiac function studies and careful cultures to determine the presence of unsuspected infection. Psychiatric and social service evaluation are of considerable importance and of course ABO and HLA typing are performed routinely. Once the patient is accepted for the transplant list, cytotoxic antibody screening is commonly done monthly. Recent evidence suggests that pretransplant blood transfusions may improve cadaveric allograft survival and this is now increasingly forming a part of the preparation of the patient (Williams et al, 1980). Finally, nephrectomy may be required prior to transplantation although this is now performed less frequently than previously. One of the few indications for nephrectomy is the presence of large polycystic kidneys which might later present operative or infective problems.

Selection of cadaver donors

The ideal cadaver donor is one who can be defined as 'brain dead' while being maintained with live support systems. Such patients are commonly those with cerebral trauma, vascular lesions or brain death from respiratory or cardiac arrest. It is important to establish guidelines for declaring a patient clinically dead and indeed this has provided a focus of considerable public interest recently. Donor procurement programmes generally exclude patients over 70 and those with a history of significant hypertension. Obviously pre-existing renal disease, diabetes, the presence of significant infection or a history of malignant disease constitute other exclusions. If the cadaver is brain dead, maintained on the respirator with an adequate circulation and urine output, bilateral donor nephrectomy can be performed as an elective operation by the transperitoneal route. After removal, the kidneys are promptly cooled by perfusion with iced crystalloid solutions usually including heparin and methylprednisolone; the kidneys may be further preserved prior to use by hypothermic preservation by pulsatile perfusion or simply by non-pulsatile perfusion and storage in ice. Improved preservation methods now allow kidneys to be stored for up to at least 48 hours prior to transplantation. The surgical techniques involved in removal of donor organs and the operation of renal transplantation are well described by Calne (1963).

Immunosuppressive therapy

However good the recipient/donor match be on tissue typing, virtually all transplantation centres use prophylactic immunosuppressive therapy commonly prescribing azathioprine and prednisone. The tendency over the past few years has been to reduce the dosage of prednisone given routinely and indeed, after the early postoperative period, to move to alternate day therapy. Acute rejection episodes are frequently treated by high dose intravenous methylprednisolone. The production of anti-lymphocyte globulin seemed to offer the possibility of considerable improvement in prevention of rejection but many problems have emerged in relation to this. Quality control of the material has proved difficult, thrombocytopenia has often limited therapy and clinical evidence of benefit has been variable. Other immunosuppressive procedures including local graft irradiation, splenectomy and prophylactic thoracic duct drainage have not proved to confer significant benefit.

The most exciting new development in organ transplantation and the prevention of rejection has been the appearance of cyclosporin A. In a screening programme searching for new antifungal agents, cyclosporin A was isolated from the fungus *Trichoderma polysporum*. This substance was found to impair cell-mediated cytolysis in an assay in which spleen cells were taken from mice sensitized with allogeneic neoplastic cells. The compound does not appear to be toxic to bone marrow and in this respect is different from most other immunosuppressive agents. It seems to be most effective given in the sensitization phase affecting T-cells at an early stage in transformation. In animal studies cyclosporin A has been found to prolong survival of renal grafts in dogs receiving kidneys from unrelated donors; similar effects have been demonstrated with heart grafts and skin grafts (Calne et al, 1981).

The value of cyclosporin A in human renal transplantation is not yet finally identified. Early experience suggests that the drug may have some direct nephrotoxicity and of considerable concern have been reports suggesting an increased incidence of neoplasm, particularly lymphoma, in patients treated with it. Abnormalities of liver function occur in most patients but are reversible.

URINARY CALCULI

The two major constituents of renal stones are (i) substances of low molecular weight ('crystalloids'), which form the bulk of most stones and (ii) mixtures of higher molecular weight substances which form the matrix in which the low molecular weight components deposit and crystallize. The commonest low molecular weight substance found in renal calculi is calcium, but others include uric acid and cystine. The incidence of urinary calculi in Britain and North America is approximately 1/1000 population and analysis of stones shows that 50–60% are calcium (oxalate, phosphate or mixed); 25–30% are 'infective' (magnesium, ammonium phosphate); 5–15% are uric acid and 2% are cystine.

Aetiology of calculus formation

When a solid dissolves in a liquid the maximum concentration of the substance that can be held in solution is defined as the *solubility* and is governed by a variety of factors including the properties of the solid, the nature and properties of the liquid, the pH, temperature and ionic strength. In the case of 'crystalloids' the solubility is most correctly expressed as the product of the concentrations of the constituent ions. This is called the 'solubility product'. At solute concentrations below this product the solution is undersaturated, but if the solubility product is exceeded the solution is supersaturated or 'metastable'. In this 'metastable' state precipitation does not occur spontaneously but may be induced by bacteria or other debris (e.g. matrix) and preformed crystals will grow larger. If the ionic concentrations are raised further, a 'formation product' is eventually reached and spontaneous precipitation occurs. This consideration of physical chemistry forms a logical basis for understanding calculus formation.

Calcium stones

Renal calculi most commonly consist of calcium oxalate frequently admixed with calcium phosphate. In approximately 75% of such patients an underlying metabolic abnormality will be detected and may be susceptible to treatment. In one series of 759 patients with calcium nephrolithiasis, 32% of the patients were found to have idiopathic hypercalciuria, 17% had hyperuricosuria, 15% had both hypercalciuria and hyperuricosuria. 7% of the patients were found to have primary hyperparathyroidism and another 4% had miscellaneous disorders including hereditary distal renal tubular acidosis (Coe & Favus, 1980).

The commonest underlying metabolic disorder is that defined as normocalcemic hypercalciuria of unknown aetiology. This excludes known causes of hypercalciuria including sarcoidosis, renal tubular acidosis, immobilization, neoplasms, glucocorticoid excess, hyperthyroidism and vitamin D excess. There appear to be at least two forms of idiopathic hypercalciuria, one the absorptive variety in which calcium enters the blood at an abnormally rapid rate after each meal, and the other the renal form in which hypercalciuria occurs because of defective tubular calcium reabsorption. In the absorptive type, PTH secretion is suppressed while in hypercalciuria due to a renal leak PTH secretion is stimulated. At least in theory, it might be important to distinguish between these two varieties of idiopathic hypercalciuria since, while it might be expected that the absorptive variety would be corrected by a low calcium diet or by the administration of phosphate, it is possible that these measures, if applied in the renal leak situation, might further stimulate PTH and eventually produce autonomous hyperparathyroidism. It is now clear, however, that whatever the pathogenesis of idiopathic hypercalciuria, it can be satisfactorily treated using thiazide diuretic agents. If serum PTH is initially elevated it will gradually fall to normal, while if the hypercalciuria has been due to increased absorption from the gut the PTH level will not be significantly altered. It can be demonstrated that urinary supersaturation with calcium oxalate falls quickly to the normal range during thiazide treatment and calcium stone recurrence falls to 10% or less of the pretreatment rate. The mechanism of thiazide hypocalciuria involves action at two sites. First, because it is a diuretic the drug causes depletion of extracellular fluid which stimulates the renal proximal tubules to reabsorb sodium chloride, water and calcium. Second, the drug also stimulates calcium reabsorption by the distal tubule, probably by direct action.

More recently many investigators have observed that renal calcium stones may be associated with uric acid disorders. There is a high frequency of calcium oxalate stones in patients who have gout and even without this hyperuricosuria is frequent among patients with calcium oxalate nephrolithiasis. Study of such patients has provided evidence which links the hyperuricosuria to calcium stone formation and setting them apart from other calcium stones formers. The evidence includes an atypical natural history of stone disease, in vitro evidence for heterogeneous nucleation of calcium oxalate crystallization by seed crystals of sodium hydrogen urate or uric acid, and a dramatic effect of allopurinol in reducing new stone formation. The basic investigation of recurrent stone formers therefore must include assessment of renal function, measurement of urinary calcium excretion and estimation of urinary urate excretion. If hypercalciuria is found then a thiazide diuretic is the indicated treatment. If urinary urate excretion is found to exceed 800 mg per day in men or 750 mg per day in women then treatment with allopurinol seems to reduce the formation of stones to about 10% of the expected (Coe, 1978).

Primary hyperparathyroidism is a less common but important cause of recurrent calcium nephrolithiasis. The main clinical problem it poses is that of recognition because hypercalcaemia may be slight. The diagnosis should be suspected when serum calcium levels exceed 10.1 mg per 100 ml and may be aided by serum PTH levels although it should be noted that these estimations are frequently unreliable. Distal (type 1) hereditary renal tubular acidosis usually produces calcium phosphate stones or nephrocalcinosis. Other forms of RTA produce stones only occasionally. The basic defect in this condition is an inability to lower the pH of the final urine much below that of the blood so that acid excretion is inadequate and metabolic acidosis develops. The acidosis is accompanied by hyperchloraemia and the diagnosis is confirmed by demonstrating a urine pH above 5.5 during the 6 hours after an oral load of ammonium chloride.

In about 20% of patients with recurrent calcium stone formation no metabolic cause can be found. In these patients it has been suggested that recurrent stone formation can be reduced by a low calcium diet but not with diet and oral phosphate; the reason for this apparently adverse effect of phosphate is not clear. Other workers have suggested that the treatment of such patients with thiazides is effective although not so effective as in those patients with hypercalciuria.

Uric acid stones

Uric acid stones have a structure similar to calcium stones in that they consist of an accumulation chiefly of uric acid on a framework of matrix. They may be pure stones or mixed, containing calcium oxalate or phosphate as well as uric acid. All causes of uric acid stones produce a low urine pH, hyperuricosuria or both. The common causes of a low urine pH are gout, familial uric acid lithiasis (a hereditary trait), a hot dry climate and disorders causing increased intestinal fluid loss such as ileostomy, colostomy or persistent diarrhoea. Hyperuricosuria may be dietary or due to over-production as in some forms of gout, myeloproliferative disease and subsequent to the treatment of lymphoma or leukemia. In all cases treatment must raise urine pH if it is reduced and also attempts to reduce the total uric acid excretion. In some cases the simple administration of one or two sodium bicarbonate tablets three or four times a day will be effective but in severe cases allopurinol should be utilized.

Cystine stones

Cystinuria is an inherited defect in tubular transport of four amino acids — cystine, arginine, lysine and ornithine. This results in their excretion in the urine in abnormally high concentrations and cystine, the least soluble, precipitates to form stones. Lithiasis occurs almost entirely in homozygotes of the recessive form, and is often manifested first in childhood. Treatment primarily hinges on the administration of enough water to maintain excreted cystine in solution. Since excretion is constant, urine flow must be kept at the proper level at night as well as in the daytime and usually two to three litres of urine daily is the volume needed. Supplemental alkali can be used but solubility of cystine does not increase until the urine pH exceeds 7; for this reason large doses of bicarbonate are required and alkalinization is usually reserved for patients in whom fluid treatment alone is unsuccessful. If cystine stones persist in recurring despite water and alkali, D-penicillamine can be used but this drug carries considerable hazards (Crawhall et al, 1964).

SYMPTOMS AND EFFECTS OF URINARY CALCULI

Calculi in the urinary tract tend to give rise to pain, bleeding, obstruction and infection in various combinations depending on whether the stone is in the kidney, ureter or bladder.

Renal calculi

A calculus impacted in a calyx of the renal pelvis is often symptomless. If the stone is free in the pelvis, it often causes bouts of pain probably due to temporary obstruction and dilatation of the pelvis. The pain is usually described as a gnawing ache in the loin, much less clamant than that induced by a stone in the ureter or bladder.

Bleeding from injury to the lining membrane may be profuse, but is usually detected only by microscopy. Urinary obstruction tends to be episodic, and seldom leads to hydronephrosis. A renal calculus is frequently complicated by infection, which may progress to established pyelonephritis, pyonephrosis and extensive destruction of renal tissue. Finally, the long-continued presence of a renal calculus in the renal pelvis can lead to epidermoid metaplasia of the transitional epithelium and to epidermoid carcinoma.

Ureteric calculi

Ureteric calculi originate in the kidney, and in their passage from the ureter tend to impact at the sites where the ureter is narrow. The three common sites of impaction are near the outlet of the ureter, at the pelvi-ureteric junction, and at the brim of the pelvis. The pain that results from impaction of a calculus in the ureter can be excruciatingly severe. Its properties and the neurological mechanism of its radiation are discussed on page 412.

Haematuria, either gross or microscopic, is the rule. Not all patients with 'renal colic' have a demonstrable lesion of the renal tract (p. 413), but the occurrence of haematuria indicates that a urinary tract lesion is indeed present. It is for this reason that a search for red blood cells in the urine should be made routinely as soon as possible after the episode of pain.

Urinary obstruction, with slight dilatation of the renal pelvis and ureter above the level of an impacted calculus, is common. A small hydronephrosis is not necessarily important, but progressive enlargement of the hydronephrosis over the course of a few weeks is an indication that the calculus should be removed surgically. In most patients, however, the hydronephrosis does not enlarge, and it is permissible to wait (sometimes for several weeks) till the calculus is voided spontaneously. Rarely an impacted calculus obstructs the ureter completely, and the kidney ceases to function — recent renal colic in conjunction with a calculus in the ureter and a non-functioning kidney is an indication for immediate operation.

Infection is a rare complication of ureteric calculus. The calculi which are capable of entering the ureter from the renal pelvis are necessarily small, and such calculi do not develop in kidneys which are already infected.

Vesical calculi

Urate calculi in the bladder usually develop by accretion on a nucleus which has descended from one or other kidney. Calcium phosphate calculi more often originate in the bladder in the presence of infection and bladder-neck obstruction, and are therefore commoner in the male. The pain of a vesical calculus can be extremely severe, especially towards the end of micturition, when the contracting bladder compresses the calculus against the sensitive trigone.

Bleeding is common, and also tends to occur towards the end of the act of micturition. Infection is particularly common, either as a cause or as a result of the calculus. It commonly leads to an intractable cystitis, to fibrous contraction of the bladder, and eventually to infection of the dilated ureters and renal pelves, and death from renal failure.

Carcinoma of the bladder is no longer regarded a common sequel of vesical calculus.

TREATMENT OF RENAL CALCULI

The treatment of renal calculi falls into two parts: the surgical measures necessary to remove existing calculi, and medical treatment aimed at preventing recurrence or occasionally to dissolve stones already present.

Most calculi lying in the renal pelvis must be removed, although occasionally a symptomless calculus wedged in a calyx may be left. Pre-operative assessment should include thorough radiologic examination to determine the number and positions of stones and the presence or absence of hydronephrosis. Infection should be suppressed with antibiotics and renal function measured and reviewed. The surgical procedure used should aim to remove as many of the calculi as possible with minimal damage to renal tissue, and pyelolithotomy is commonly used. In most difficult cases partial nephrectomy may be required while staghorn calculi usually lead to nephrectomy, particularly if there is superimposed infection.

In all cases it is vital that the content of the stone be determined. In all cases persisting infection must be sought for and treated as required. Subsequent treatment aimed at the prevention of further stone formation obviously depends upon the metabolic abnormality determined; the indicated treatment has been discussed above in relation to each type of renal stone.

REFERENCES

Abel J J, Rowntree L B, Turner B B 1914 On removal of diffusable substances by dialysis. Journal of Pharmacology and Experimental Therapeutics 5: 275–280

Abel R M, Beck C H Jr, Abbott W M, Ryan J A Jr, Barnett G O, Fisher J E 1973 Improved survival from acute renal failure after treatment with intravenous essential L-amino acids and glucose. New England Journal of Medicine 288: 695–699

Bartels E D, Brun G C, Gammeltoft A et al 1954 Acute anuria following intravenous pyelography in a patient with myelomatosis. Acta Medica Scandinavia 150: 297–302

Bailey R R, Natale R, Turnbull D I, Linton A L 1973 Protective effect of frusemide in acute tubular necrosis and acute renal failure. Clinical Science and Molecular Medicine 45: 1–17

Bevar D R, Dudley H A, Horsey P J 1973 Renal function during and after anaesthesia and surgery: significance for water and electrolyte management. British Journal of Anaesthesia 45: 968–972

Brown J J, Gleadle R I, Lawson D H, Lever A F, Linton A L, MacAdam R F et al 1970 Renin and acute renal failure: Studies in man. British Medical Journal 1: 253–258

Calne R Y 1963 Renal Transplantation. Arnold, London

Calne R Y, Rolles K, White D J G, Thiru S, Evans D B, McMaster P et al 1981 Cyclosporin A in organ transplantation. In: Hamburger, Crosnier, Grunfeld and Maxwell (eds) Advances in Nephrology, Year Book Medical Publishers, Chicago 10: 335–347

Coe F L 1978 Hyperuricosuric calcium oxalate nephrolithiasis. Kidney International 13: 418–426

Coe F L, Favus M J 1980 Treatment of renal calculi. In: Stollerman G H (ed) Advances in Internal Medicine, Year Book Medical Publishers, Chicago 26: 373–392

Crawhall J C, Scowen E F, Watts R W E 1964 Further observations on use of D-penicillamine in cystinuria. British Medical Journal 1: 1411–1414

Giovannetti S, Maggiore Q 1964 A low nitrogen diet with proteins of high biological value for severe chronic uraemia. Lancet i: 1000–1002

Habif D V, Papper E M, Fitzpatrick H F, Lowrance P, Smythe C M, Bradley S E 1951 The renal and hepatic blood flow, glomerular filtration rate and urinary output of electrolytes during cyclopropane, ether and thiopental anaesthesia, operation and the immediate post-operative period. Surgery 30: 241–247

Kerr D N S, Robson A O 1965 Frusemide. Lancet 1: 655–657

Kleinknecht D, Jungers P, Chanard J, Barbanel C, Ganeval D 1972 Uremic and non-uremic complications in acute renal failure: Evaluation of early and frequent dialysis on prognosis. Kidney International 1: 190–196

Kolff W F 1947 New Ways of Treating Uraemia. Churchill, London

Laragh J H, Kelly W G 1964 Aldosterone: its biochemistry and physiology. In: Advances in Metabolic Disease. Academic Press, London. 1:217

Linton A L 1974 Acute renal failure. A review article. Canadian Medical Association Journal 110: 949–951

Linton A L, Clark W F, Driedger A A, Turnbull D I, Lindsay R M 1980 Acute interstitial nephritis due to drugs. Annals of Internal Medicine 93: 735–741

Lowe J, Gray J, Henry D A, Lawson D H 1979 Adverse reactions to frusemide in hospital inpatients. British Medical Journal 2: 360–365

Luke R G, Linton A L, Briggs J D, Kennedy A C 1965 Mannitol therapy in acute renal failure. Lancet 1: 980–982

Mayerson H S 1963 The lymphatic system with particular reference to the kidney. Surgery, Gynaecology and Obstetrics 116: 259–262

Muth R G 1973 Furosemide in acute renal failure. In: Friedman E L, Eliahou H E (eds) Proceedings, Conference on Acute Renal Failure. DHEW Publication No. (NIH)74–608: 245–253

O'Connor W J 1962 Renal Function. Arnold, London

Popovich R P, Moncrieff J W, Nolph K D 1977 Continuous ambulatory peritoneal dialysis. Abstracts, American Society of Nephrology 10:35a

Scribner B H, Buri R, Caner J E Z, Hegstrom R, Burnell J M 1960 The treatment of chronic uraemia by means of intermittent haemodialysis. Transactions of the American Society for Artificial Internal Organs 6: 114

Sevitt S 1959 Pathogenesis of traumatic uraemia. A revised concept. Lancet ii: 135–137

Stott R B, Cameron J S, Ogg C S, Bewick M 1972 Why the persistently high mortality in acute renal failure? Lancet II: 75–79

Swartz R D, Rubin J E, Leeming B W, Silva P 1979 Renal failure following major angiography. The American Journal of Medicine 65: 31–37

Trueta J, Barclay A E, Daniel P M, Franklin K J, Prichard M M L 1947 Studies of the Renal Circulation. Blackwell, Oxford

Weinrauch L A, Healy R W, Leland O S Jr, Goldstein H H, Kassissieh S D, Libertino J A et al 1977 Coronary angiography and acute renal failure in diabetic azotemic nephropathy. Annals of Internal Medicine 86: 56–59

Werb R, Linton A L 1979 Aetiology, diagnosis, treatment and prognosis of acute renal failure in an intensive care unit. Resuscitation 7: 95–100

Williams K A, Ting A, French M E, Oliver D 1980 Preoperative blood transfusions improve cadaveric renal allograft survival in nontransfused recipients. Lancet i: 1104–1106

Wirz H 1957 The location of antidiuretic effect in the mammalian kidney. In: Heller H (ed) The Nephrohypophysis. Butterworth, London. p 157

Woodruff M F A, Nolan B, Robson J S, MacDonald M K 1969 Renal transplantation in man. Lancet 1: 6–8

Yunis E J, Amos D B 1971 Three closely linked genetic systems relevant to transplantation. Proceedings, National Academy of Science 78:3031

Ureter

The structure and innervation of the ureter are briefly described as a preliminary to a discussion of the movements of the ureter and the transport of urine.

The muscle of the ureter is strikingly unaffected by the drugs which are commonly prescribed with the aim of relaxing it.

Severe pain with a characteristic pattern of distribution can arise from obstruction of the ureter — 'ureteric colic'. The view is put forward that similar pain often arises from structures outwith the urinary tract.

Transplantation of the ureters into intact and isolated bowel can be carried out with results which are satisfactory for several years but marred by late complications. The mechanism of the latter is discussed in some detail.

STRUCTURE OF THE URETER

The wall of the ureter comprises a mucosal lining, a middle coat of muscle, and an outer coat of connective tissue.

The mucosa, like the mucosa throughout the urinary tract, is a transitional stratified epithelium, 4 or 5 cells deep. It is thrown into longitudinal folds when the ureter is empty, but is smooth when the ureter is filled. The submucosa contains a plexus of lymphatic vessels which may provide a path for the spread of infection, not only downwards from kidney to bladder in renal tuberculosis but upwards from bladder to kidney in chronic cystitis.

The muscle coat has only two layers in the upper part of the ureter, but three lower down. An inner longitudinal layer is surrounded by a circular layer, and this in turn (in the lowest third of the ureter) by another longitudinal layer. These layers become slightly thicker as they are traced downwards, and they cease to be distinct from each other as they merge into the thick muscle of the bladder. Elastic collagen fibres are interspersed with the unstriated muscle. The elasticity of the ureter diminishes with advancing age, but there is no obvious histological change in the appearance of either the elastic or the muscle fibres.

The connective tissue coat carries the nerve supply and the blood supply of the ureter: a few lymphatics are present also, but most of the lymphatics lie in the submucosa. The nerve supply is dealt with below. The arteries to the ureters are branches of the renal, spermatic, superior vesical and inferior vesical arteries, but their arrangement is variable and indeed often asymmetrical (Daniel, 1961). They usually anastomose freely, and the ureter can be mobilized with little risk of infarction.

The lumen of the ureter, which has an average diameter of 3 mm, is slightly constricted at the pelvi-ureteric junction, at the level where it crosses the psoas, and at the entry to the bladder. A ureteric calculus is liable to impact at one of the constrictions, and on X-ray films is most often found near the tip of the transverse process of the second or third lumbar vertebra, superimposed on the sacro-iliac joint, or just medial to the ischial spine.

Dilatation of the ureters and renal pelves is usual in pregnancy and dates from about the 10th week. The early onset suggests that the dilatation can hardly be due to mechanical obstruction by the enlarging uterus. The dilatation may be the result of the relaxation of the muscle of the ureter in response to increased amounts of circulating progesterone. Progesterone, unlike oestrogen, is known to decrease the tone of the ureteric muscle in vitro (Kumar, 1962).

The innervation of the ureter

The source of the autonomic nerve supply of the ureter remains controversial, but most of the extrinsic fibres appear to be derived from the renal plexus and the hypogastric plexus. Whatever their source, the nerves form a network along the whole length of the ureter under the connective tissue coat. From this network nerve fibres pass into the muscular coat, and some can be seen to pass through into the mucosa. Most observers believe that specialized end-organs are lacking.

Ganglionic nerve cells are present in quite large numbers at the lower end of the ureter, in smaller numbers at the upper end, and are sparse in the segment between. In two cases of idiopathic mega-ureter, Milton and Robb (1954) found that the lower and undilated segment of the ureter lacked ganglion cells, and did not respond to mechanical or electrical stimulation. This finding indicates that the aetiology of at least some forms of mega-ureter conforms with that of idiopathic megacolon (p. 325). In other cases studied by Leibowitz and Bodian (1963), however, the ganglion cell status of the terminal segment of ureter was found to be normal.

The nerve supply of the ureter is doubtless derived from both the sympathetic and parasympathetic systems, for the motor activity of the ureter can be modified by both sympathomimetic and parasympathomimetic drugs. The functional importance of the extrinsic nerve supply is not clear. The idea that the sympathetic influences the motility of the upper ureter, and the parasympathetic the lower ureter, is no longer tenable: this idea was based on some old observations now believed to be faulty. Satani (1919) claimed that adrenaline increased the motility of the upper ureter, and pilocarpine increased the motility of the lower ureter, but modern research has shown that the effect of these drugs on ureteral tone increases progressively from above down (p. 411). There is no antagonism between adrenergic and cholinergic drugs, both of which bring about an increase of tone without any effect on peristalsis. As peristalsis appears to be the chief form of motor activity, the functional importance of the extrinsic nerves is probably small.

The presence of both α- and β-adrenergic receptors in the lower third of human ureter has been demonstrated by Malin and his colleagues (1970). The dominant α-receptors are motor, whereas the recessive β-receptors are inhibitory, and Deane (1967) postulated that enhancement of the latter activity could predispose to lower ureteric dilatation, stasis, and even ureteric reflux. Obviously this concept deserves further study.

MOVEMENTS OF THE URETER

The first reliable account of peristalsis in the ureter was given in 1869 by Engelman, who made careful observations on the ureters of anaesthetized animals. He noted that peristalsis continued after the ureters had been denervated and must therefore be independent of the extrinsic nerve supply — an observation which has been amply confirmed.

Peristaltic activity in the ureter is closely related to the rate of urine excretion by the kidney. This relationship was first clearly pointed out by Lapides (1948), who made his observations on the intact ureter in man. He measured the pressure in one ureter by means of a whistle-tipped catheter inserted into its lowest third, and as a guide to the rate of urine flow from the kidney, he measured the output

from a freely draining catheter inserted into the opposite renal pelvis.

The ureter is almost quiescent when little urine is being excreted by the kidney. The entry of urine initiates peristaltic activity which is propagated down the ureter. If the renal output of urine increases there is an increase in ureteral tone and peristalsis, and if the renal output diminishes, ureteral activity diminishes also.

Ureteral tone and peristalsis increase, even though the renal output of urine remains constant, if the emptying of the ureter is impeded. This is most clearly seen under experimental conditions when the resistance to outflow from the ureter can be controlled artificially. Under natural conditions the resistance to emptying of the ureter is the pressure within the bladder. As the bladder pressure increases markedly only when micturition is imminent, back-pressure cannot be an important stimulus to normal ureteral activity.

The relationship between the rate of urine excretion, renal pelvic pressure, and ureteral peristaltic activity has been elegantly demonstrated by Rosenkilde Olsen (1981), working with dogs. Diuresis was produced with intravenous frusemide or mannitol, and resulted in a simultaneous rise in pelvic pressure and frequency of ureteral peristalsis. When diuresis ceased, the changes were reversed, and Rosenkilde Olsen claimed that his findings supported the views of Weiss and his co-workers (1979) that the renal pelvis governs ureteral activity in pacemaker fashion, probably independent of neuromuscular transmission.

Ureteral tone and peristalsis also increase in response to an increase of intra-abdominal pressure (Fig. 23.1). The frequent changes in intra-abdominal pressure that occur during bodily activity must influence the behaviour of the ureter.

The importance of distinguishing between tone and peristalsis has been stressed by Gould et al (1955a). In experiments upon the ureter of the water buffalo, in which segments from the upper end, the middle and the lower end were mounted in the same water bath under identical conditions, they found that tone, sensitivity to electrical stimulation, and also muscle mass increased progressively from above down (Fig. 23.2). Tone was increased, especially at the lower end of the ureter, by both adrenaline and acetylcholine, but these drugs were without effect on peristalsis. They concluded that tone is under the influence of the extrinsic nerves, but that peristalsis is not under neural control. They were able to show, like Rosenkilde Olsen later, that peristalsis is governed by the pressure within the ureter, and they agreed with Satani (1919) that peristaltic waves are propagated mechanically. Since then, however, Deane (1967), Malin et al (1970), and Struthers (1973) have conclusively demonstrated increased peristaltic activity in pig and human ureter in response to adrenaline and acetycholine. The precise significance of

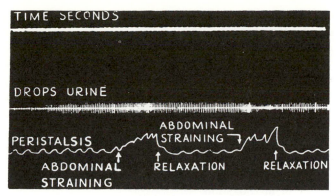

Fig. 23.1 Below, ureteral peristalsis is recorded from a catheter in one ureter. Above, urine flow is simultaneously recorded, drop by drop, from a catheter in the other ureter. Note that voluntary abdominal straining increases both peristalsis and rate of flow. (Lapides, 1948)

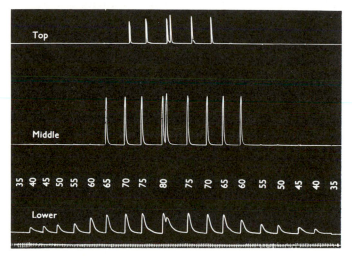

Fig. 23.2 Effect of graded electrical stimulation of sections from the upper, middle, and lower portions of the ureter of the water buffalo. Numerals indicate strength of stimulus. Note that the sensitivity of the ureter increases progressively from above down. (Gould et al, 1955a)

these various, apparently contradictory, observations is not yet clear.

Two types of flow through the ureter, *continuous* and *segmental*, have been described (Gould et al 1955b). In the dog, simultaneous pressure records from each third of the ureter were obtained from string-gauge manometers attached to suitably placed hypodermic needles which did not interfere with the flow of urine. At low rates of urine flow through the ureter the flow was continuous. At high rates, the flow was segmental with the formation of pools of urine along the course of the ureter, each pool receiving urine from above and discharging it downwards when filled. Pooling appeared to increase the vigour of peristalsis, and occurred not only during diuresis but also when the bladder pressure was raised. Further, an increase in bladder pressure did not necessarily lead to an increase in pressure in the upper ureter, for pooling occurred and a

constriction might be maintained between a quiescent upper pool and a vigorously contracting lower pool; such a mechanism may be of value in protecting the kidney from the effects of back-pressure.

In man, Murnaghan (1957) reports that perfusion of the isolated ureter may similarly yield either continuous or segmental flow. He adds that when the ureter is overdistended the entire musculature becomes lax, but the lowest segment is the last to stop contracting. Again, the outline of the ureter on intravenous pyelography is often cystoid, suggesting a segmental type of flow, and cineradiography with the aid of an image intensifier has confirmed this interpretation.

EFFECT OF DRUGS ON URETERAL ACTIVITY

Much work has been done on the effect of drugs on isolated rings of ureter and a few observations have been made on the effect of drugs on the intact ureter in animals, but comparatively little is known of the effect of drugs on the healthy ureter in man. It can be said that ureteral activity is strikingly unaffected by most drugs with the exception of adrenaline and acetylcholine. In particular, morphine and atropine, which are still often given to patients with ureteric colic, have very little effect on the ureter, although Ross and his colleagues (1973) did record a variable, usually slight, inhibitory effect on activity in the intact ureter in response to intravenous atropine.

Obviously drugs which affect the rate of urine production will have an indirect influence on ureteral activity via the pelvic pacemaker mechanism discussed above. In a study of patients with ureteral colic, Kubacz and Catchpole (1972) used the α-adrenergic blocking agent, phentolamine, to reduce blood pressure and hence the pelvi-ureteral pressure, with consequent relief of pain. Prostaglandin E_2 improves renal blood flow, increases urine output, and may thus raise the intrapelvic pressure in obstructed ureters. This pressure rise may initiate a vicious circle, as Olsen et al (1976) demonstrated that an acute rise in pressure within the renal pelvis stimulates the synthesis of prostaglandin E_2 in the kidney. Drugs which inhibit prostaglandin synthesis, such as indomethacin, may therefore have a part to play in the management of ureteral colic (Sjödin & Holmlund, 1982; Flannigan et al 1983).

Isolated rings of ureter

Adrenaline and noradrenaline increase ureteric tone and contractions; their action can be inhibited by piperoxane. Acetylcholine also increases tone and contractions; its action is completely abolished by atropine. Pilocarpine was reported by Satani (1919) to increase the activity of the ureter, especially in its lowest third, but was found by Gould et al (1955a) to be inactive. Recent studies by

Abrams and Feneley (1975) on the prostaglandins show that those of the F series cause increased tone and contractions whilst those of the E series are inhibitory. This action appears to be direct rather than transmitted by acetylcholine.

The intact ureter in dogs

In anaesthetised dogs, Abrahams and Pickford (1956) perfused the ureter in situ with saline solutions, inferring changes in ureteral activity from changes in the rate of flow of the saline. Adrenaline and noradrenaline, given intramuscularly, brought about a temporary cessation of transureteral flow during the same period that the arterial pressure was increased (Fig. 23.3). This cessation of flow was attributed to contraction of the ureteric muscle.

Intravenous 5-hydroxytryptamine, by causing spasm of the ureter, completely arrested the flow of saline through the ureter for 1–2 minutes, and slowed the flow for a further 1–2 minutes.

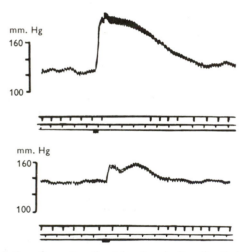

Fig. 23.3 Action of noradrenaline (above) and adrenaline (below) on systolic blood pressure and rate of urine flow through the dog's ureter. In each chart, the top line records systolic blood pressure, the second line rate of urine flow, the third line time in 10-second intervals, and the bottom line the signal for 5 micrograms of the drug intravenously. Note that urine flow is arrested for a longer period after noradrenaline than after adrenaline. (Abrahams & Pickford, 1956)

The intact ureter in man

As stated earlier, Lapides (1948) pioneered the concept that the normal stimulus to ureteral activity is the urinary flow. In accordance with this view, he considered that adrenaline and acetylcholine influence the ureter only indirectly by their influence on renal excretion; this belief is not substantiated by the later work of Abraham and Pickford (described above) who were able to demonstrate a direct effect upon the ureter perfused with saline. Lapides also found that atropine did not relieve spasm, and had no effect on ureteric peristalsis, but the studies

of Ross et al (1973) would indicate a minor antispasmodic effect. Morphine has an inconstant effect, but usually reduces ureteral activity by reducing renal excretion. Atropine and morphine are commonly prescribed together for the relief of ureteral colic, but the beneficial effect appears to depend wholly on the central action of the morphine. Probanthine, given intravenously, leads to a transient diminution of ureteral peristalsis (Weinberg & Maletta, 1961).

Further information on the activity of the intact ureter is becoming available with the development of newer techniques of investigation.

Electro-ureterography was first shown to be practicable in man by Hanley (1953). Its chief advantage is that it provides a record of muscular activity which is independent of urine flow. Its technical disadvantage is the necessary presence of an indwelling catheter to carry the electrical leads.

Percutaneous pressure-flow perfusion studies have been used by Whitaker (1973, 1976) to elucidate patients with suspected upper urinary tract obstruction, but the invasive nature of this investigation has inhibited its use as a routine procedure.

Diuresis renography (O'Reilly et al 1978), has become widely accepted as a reliable and practical investigation in the evaluation of upper urinary tract dynamics. The standard isotope renogram is modified by giving an intravenous injection of frusemide after the initial renogram and recording the 'wash-out' response of the individual pelviureteric systems utilizing paired gamma cameras linked to a computer. The technique is particularly valuable in the differentiation of the obstructed and non-obstructed dilated upper urinary tracts (O'Reilly et al, 1981).

PAIN ARISING IN THE URETER

The ureter, like the intestine, can give rise to severe pain if it is obstructed, but is believed to be insensitive to physical stimuli such as cutting or burning. It is conceded that incising the orifice of the ureter with a diathermy knife can cause pain, but this probably results from heating the overlying peritoneum.

Ureteral pain most often results from intermittent obstruction by a foreign body, commonly a calculus but also blood clot or even tuberculous debris from the kidney. The pain is excruciating and has a characteristic pattern of distribution. Above the obstruction the rise in urine pressure creates an increase in the tension of the wall of the upper urinary tract, especially in the renal pelvis, and this produces the typical severe pain of ureteric colic (Kiil, 1957). Mention has already been made of the findings of Olsen et al (1976) that an acute rise in pressure within the obstructed renal pelvis stimulates prostaglandin E_2 synthesis in the kidney, and this in turn improves renal blood flow (Allen et al 1978) and increases diuresis (Feigen et al 1976), thus producing a further rise in intrapelvic pressure. The possible role of hypotensive agents (phentolamine) and prostaglandin inhibitors (indomethacin) in the management of ureteral pain has already been indicated.

Pain of similar severity and distribution can result from stimulation of the first lumbar supraspinous ligament, and doubtless from other structures innervated by the lumbar segmental nerves.

The term 'renal colic' is loosely applied to any severe pain of the typical segmental pattern irrespective of the source of the painful stimuli. Rather less than 50% of the patients who present with renal colic can be shown to have a lesion of the urinary tract; the source of pain in the remainder has so far eluded recognition.

Pain from ureteric calculus

Migration of a calculus down the ureter leads to agonizing pain, various reflex symptoms and usually haematuria. A stationary calculus in the ureter may also, from time to time, obstruct the ureter and give rise to pain, but as the obstruction is often incomplete the pain is usually less severe.

Pain usually begins abruptly, lasts for a few hours, and passes off in the course of a few minutes. During the attack the pain is liable to excruciating exacerbations, but these do not wax and wane with the clockwork rhythm of intestinal colic. Pain begins behind in the renal angle, spreads forwards round the flank and down towards the external inguinal ring. When the pain is extremely severe it may radiate farther down to the scrotum or labium majus and to the front of the thigh. The pain is usually most severe at the uppermost limit of the painful area, and the level of severest pain often corresponds in a general way with the level of impaction of the calculus. The sensory nerves from the ureter enter the spinal segments D11, 12 and L1, and the distribution of pain corresponds with the dermatomes of these segments. Radiation of pain below the inguinal ligament corresponds with the territory of the genitofemoral nerve which arises from segments L1 and 2, and passes to the front of the thigh and to the tunica vaginalis of the testicle in the male and to the round ligament in the female. Hyperaesthesia is usually present in the area of referred pain above the inguinal ligament, but is absent from the skin of the scrotum which is innervated from the sacral segments of the spinal cord.

Various reflex symptoms may occur. These include pallor, sweating, a thready and rapid pulse, nausea and vomiting: such effects commonly accompany severe pain of any kind. In addition, there may be frequent and urgent micturition, especially if a calculus is impacted near the lower end of the ureter. Anuria is rare, but may occur if the opposite kidney is absent or destroyed by disease: examples of anuria when the opposite kidney is healthy are extremely rare and probably result from a fall in blood-pressure.

Haematuria from abrasion of the lining of the ureter may be either gross or microscopic. Haematuria should be diligently sought in all patients who present with 'renal colic', for it is strong evidence of a lesion of the urinary tract. When haematuria is absent, the source of the pain very often eludes recognition.

'Renal colic' without a lesion of the urinary tract

In rather more than 50% of patients who present with pain of the severity and pattern of ureteral obstruction, no lesion of the urinary tract can be found. There is no shadow of a calculus to be seen in X-ray films, even though with modern apparatus nearly all calculi that occur can be demonstrated. The easy passage of a ureteric catheter to the kidney excludes any inflammatory or other obstruction. Pyelograms fail to show any lesion of the kidney. Cystoscopy excludes the possibility of any foreign body lurking in the bladder after extrusion from the ureter. In such patients the pain is commonly attributed to a small calculus which has been voided, to crystalluria, or even to 'spastic ureteritis' though none of these diagnoses can be made with any confidence. The work of Kellgren and Lewis, described below, suggests that the source of the pain may well lie outside the urinary tract.

Pain from stimulation of the first lumbar supraspinous ligament

The distribution of pain arising in the first lumbar segment can be demonstrated by injecting a few drops of strongly hypertonic saline into the tough supraspinous ligament between the first and second lumbar vertebrae a little lateral to the midline. By this technique, Kellgren (1938) showed that the induced pain had exactly the same pattern as the pain of renal colic, and could be extremely severe (Fig. 23.4). In further studies, Lewis and Kellgren (1939) confirmed the earlier findings, and observed that as the induced pain reached its greatest intensity it was accompanied by retraction of the testicle and by muscular guarding in the lower quadrant of the abdomen. Doubtless the same pattern of pain can arise from other extra-renal sites innervated from the spinal segment L1, and the identification of these sites remains as a challenge to future clinical investigation.

TRANSPLANTATION OF THE URETERS INTO THE INTESTINE

The operation of transplanting the ureters into the intact colon was first performed more than 100 years ago by John

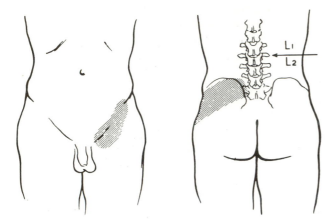

Fig. 23.4 The location of pain from injecting hypertonic saline into the first lumbar supraspinous ligament is the same as in renal colic (After Kellgren, 1938)

Simon, but until the 1940s the operative mortality from peritonitis, renal infection and renal failure was prohibitive. With the advent of antibiotics, and with improvements in technique, the operation became relatively safe and was performed for such various conditions as ectopia vesicae, irreparable vesicovaginal fistula, extensive carcinoma of the bladder, and the shrunken fibrotic bladder of tuberculosis.

In the early postoperative period, oliguria and paralytic ileus are common. Anuria probably results from transient oedema of the ureterocolic anastomosis and rarely lasts for more than 24–36 hours. Ileus of some degree occurs in virtually all cases. Despite these early complications the immediate postoperative mortality has been greatly reduced, and more attention has been devoted to the late complications, renal failure and electrolyte disturbance.

Renal failure after uretero-sigmoidostomy

The ureters can be transplanted from the bladder to the intestine in a number of ways. Transplantation into the intact sigmoid colon is the classical operation, and the late results are now known in large series of patients. Dissatisfaction with the considerable late incidence of renal failure has led to the development of other types of uretero-enterostomy, and these will be discussed later.

Transplantation of the ureters into the intact colon can only be carried out in patients who have a competent anal sphincter, and although the rectosigmoid now becomes a cloaca, accidental soiling is surprisingly infrequent, but the social restrictions imposed by the need for frequent bowel emptying may well be underestimated (McConnell & Stewart, 1975). The urine is heavily infected and strongly alkaline, but seldom causes proctitis or pruritis. For many years the patient can lead an active and useful life, but in a large proportion of cases recurring attacks of pyelonephritis due to ascending infection develop, and consideration may then have to be given to converting the form of urinary diversion to an isolated intestinal conduit (see below). Failure to do so may well lead to progressive chronic pyelonephritis, stone formation, and eventual renal failure. The average period of survival has improved with more careful follow-up and timely surgical intervention where necessary, and many patients remain in good health over 40 years after operation.

In an attempt to reduce the risks of ascending infection, operations have been devised to prevent faecal contamination of the transplanted ureters. These include transplantation of the ureters to an isolated loop of ileum (Bricker, 1950), to an isolated loop of terminal ileum and caecum (Merricks, 1954), to the isolated recto-sigmoid from which faeces are diverted by a permanent colostomy (Pyrah, 1954), to an isolated loop of sigmoid colon (Mogg, 1965), or to an isolated loop of ileum discharging per urethram (Pyrah, 1956). In all of these procedures except the last, the patient has to cope with a discharging stoma on the anterior abdominal wall and an appropriate collecting appliance, but the reduced incidence of renal complications and electrolyte upset is often well worth the inconvenience. Late results in animals are satisfactory.

Comparison of various methods of uretero-enterostomy in the dog

In dogs, Irvine et al (1956) transplanted the ureters into the intact colon, into the colon from which faeces were excluded by a proximal colostomy, or into a loop of ileum draining freely through an ileostomy (Fig. 23.5). In order to avoid any possibility of cicatricial narrowing of the anastomoses, the whole bladder base bearing the ureteral orifices was excised and used for the transplant.

After transplantation of the ureters into the intact colon the dogs' health deteriorated and they lost weight. In most, ureteral reflux could be demonstrated by X-ray films taken after instilling radio-opaque fluid into the rectum at a pressure of 20 mmHg. In some, excretion pyelograms showed minor abnormalities. At autopsy 9 months after operation, evidence of pyelonephritis was nearly always found.

After transplantation into the colon from which faeces were diverted by a colostomy, and after transplantation into an isolated loop of ileum, the dogs maintained their health and weight. Ureteral reflux did not occur, and excretion pyelograms remained normal. At autopsy at 9 months, evidence of pyelonephritis was found only occasionally and the structural damage was slight.

It can be concluded that in the dog the risk of late renal damage can be greatly reduced by using a form of uretero-enterostomy that avoids the mingling of urine and faeces in a common cloaca.

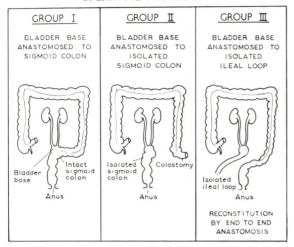

DIAGRAMATIC REPRESENTATION OF
OPERATIVE PROCEDURES

Fig. 23.5 Diagram of methods of uretero-enterostomy used in the dog. (Irvine et al, 1956)

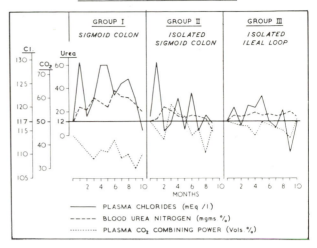

COMPARISON OF BIOCHEMICAL FINDINGS IN
TYPICAL DOGS OF GROUPS I, II & III

Fig. 23.6 Comparison of the biochemical findings after different types of uretero-enterostomy (see Fig. 23.5). Note that hyperchloraemic acidosis developed only after the ureters were transplanted to the sigmoid colon without faecal exclusion. (Irvine et al, 1956)

Electrolyte imbalance after ureterosigmoidostomy

In a report from the Mayo Clinic on the blood chemistry of 141 patients after ureterosigmoidostomy, Ferris and Odel (1950) recorded that 80 per cent showed hyperchloraemia and a reduction of plasma bicarbonate; most of these patients were free from symptoms, but suffered from thirst, fatigue and a salt taste in the mouth. A systematic search for hyperchloraemic acidosis began to be made at other clinics, and some widely differing estimates of its incidence were published. The condition is now known to be present intermittently, but in nearly all patients can be found at one time or another if the blood is examined repeatedly.

Hyperchloraemic acidosis is believed to result mainly from the combination of selective reabsorption of chloride from the colon, and renal failure, although Wrong (1970) favours colonic secretion of bicarbonate as a more important factor. The selective reabsorption of chloride in preference to sodium has been demonstrated experimentally on administering urine as an enema (Parsons et al 1952) and also on perfusing the colon with a solution of sodium chloride. If renal function is good there is compensatory excretion of chloride by the kidney, but if renal function is impaired, as by pyelonephritis, homeostasis fails and hyperchloraemic acidosis develops. Hypokalaemia may also occur, though not invariably: if it does, it is usually preceded by acidosis.

In dogs, Irvine et al (1956) found that hyperchloraemic acidosis was common after transplantation of the ureters into the intact colon, occurred in transient episodes after transplantation into the colon from which faeces were excluded, and was absent after transplantation into an isolated loop of ileum (Fig. 23.6). He noted that the severity of the acidosis varied in proportion to the area of colonic mucosa in contact with urine, a finding confirmed by Hopewell (1959).

After ureterosigmoidostomy in man, the extent of the colon that becomes a receptacle for urine is variable. Early studies following excretion urography showed that the entire colon might contain contrast medium, and this led Stamey (1956) to advise that the ureters should be transplanted not to the intact sigmoid but only to an isolated rectosigmoid loop. However, Daniel (1961) noted that the volume of mingled urine and faeces voided at any one time varied from 60–360 ml, but was usually 120–180 ml, and this suggested that urine usually occupied only the distal colon. In later studies, using barium enemas of constant volume, he showed there was marked individual variation in the distribution of the barium: in some patients it was confined to the rectum and lower sigmoid, but in others it was distributed as far proximally as the hepatic flexure (Fig. 23.7). Such variations in the area of colonic mucosa exposed to urine may well explain the variable liability to hyperchloraemic acidosis.

Awareness of the late complications should not be allowed to obscure the practical merits of simple transplantation of the ureter into the intact colon. This remains the operation of choice in elderly patients and in patients suffering from incurable disease. In such patients the risk of renal failure in the remote future can be ignored, and hyperchloraemic acidosis can be prevented by giving alkali by mouth, restricting the intake of salt, and encouraging

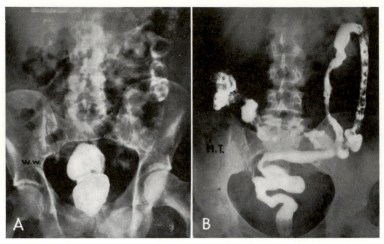

Fig. 23.7 Radiographs after administering a 150 ml barium enema. In patient A the barium remains in the lower bowel. In patient B the barium spreads throughout the colon, and ureterocolic anastomosis might result in excessive reabsorption of urinary constituents. (Courtesy of Mr O. Daniel, Royal Alexandra Hospital, Rhyl.)

the patient to empty his colonic bladder frequently so as to reduce the reabsorption of chloride (Pyrah, 1961). The ileal or colonic conduit methods of urinary diversion are technically more complicated and time-consuming, and are probably justifiable only in patients whose condition is compatible with many years' survival.

REFERENCES

Abrahams V C, Pickford M 1956 Action of drugs on the ureter. British Journal of Pharmacology 11:44

Abrams P H, Feneley R C L 1975 The actions of prostaglandins on the smooth muscle of the human urinary tract in vitro. British Journal of Urology 47: 909–915

Allen J T, Vaughan D E Jr, Gillenwater J Y 1978 The effect of indomethacin on renal blood flow and ureteral pressure in unilateral ureteral obstruction in awake dogs. Investigative Urology 15:324

Bricker E M 1950 Bladder substitution after pelvic evisceration. Surgical Clinics of North America 30: 1511–1521

Daniel O 1961 The complications which follow diversion of the urinary stream. Annals of the Royal College of Surgeons of England 29:205

Deane R F 1967 Functional studies of the ureter. British Journal of Urology 39: 31–37

Feigen L P, Klainer E, Chapnick B M, Kadowitz P J 1976 The effect of indomethacin on renal function in pentobarbital anaesthetised dogs. Journal of Pharmacology and Experimental Therapeutics 198:457

Ferris D, Odel H 1950 The electrolyte pattern of the blood after bilateral ureterosigmoidostomy. Journal of the American Medical Association 142:634

Flannigan G M, Clifford R P C, Carver R A, Yule A G, Madden N P, Towler J M 1983. Indomethacin — an alternative to pethidine in renal colic. British Journal of Urology 55: 6–9

Gould D W, Hsieh A C L, Tinckler L F 1955a The behaviour of the isolated water-buffalo ureter. Journal of Physiology 129:425

Gould D W, Hsieh A C L & Tinckler L F 1955b The behaviour of the intact ureter in dogs, rabbits and cats. Journal of Physiology 129:436

Hanley H G 1953 The electro-ureterogram. British Journal of Urology 25:358

Hopewell J 1959 The hazards of uretero-intestinal anastomosis. Annals of the Royal College of Surgeons of England 24:159

Irvine W T, Allan C M & Webster D R 1956. Prevention of the late complications of uretero-colostomy by methods of faecal exclusion. British Journal of Surgery 43:650

Kellgren J H 1938 Observations on referred pain arising from muscle. Clinical Science 3:185

Kiil F 1957 The response of the upper urinary tract to distension and obstruction. In: The function of the ureter and pelvis. Oslo University Press, Oslo, Ch 7 p 122–131

Kubacz G J and Catchpole B N 1972 The role of adrenergic blockage in the treatment of ureteral colic. Journal of Urology 107:949

Kumar D 1962 In vitro effects of steroids on human female ureter. American Journal of Obstetrics and Gynecology 83:978

Lapides J 1948 The physiology of the intact human ureter. Journal of Urology 59:501

Leibowitz S & Bodian M 1963. A study of vesical ganglia in children. Journal of Clinical Pathology 16: 342–350

Lewis T & Kellgren J H 1939 Observations relating to referred pain, visceromotor reflexes and other associated phenomena. Clinical Science 4:47

McConnell J B, Stewart W K 1975 The long-term management and social consequences of ureterosigmoid anastomosis. British Journal of Urology 47: 607–612

Malin J M Jr, Deane R F & Boyarsky S 1970 Characterisation of adrenergic receptors in human ureter. British Journal of Urology 42: 171–174

Merricks J W & Gilchrist R K 1954 The ileocaecal segment as a substitute bladder: a review of 18 cases. Journal of Urology 71:591

Milton G W & Robb W A T 1954 Electrical studies in hydro-ureter: report of two cases. British Journal of Urology 26:274

Mogg R A 1965 The treatment of neurogenic urinary incontinence using the colonic conduit. British Journal of Urology 37: 681–686

Murnaghan G F 1957 Experimental investigation of the dynamics of the normal and dilated ureter. British Journal of Urology 29:403

Olsen U B, Magnussen M P and Eilertssen E 1976 Prostaglandins, a link between renal hydro- and haemodynamics in dogs. Acta Physiologica Scandinavica 97:364

O'Reilly P H, Testa H J, Lawson R S, Farrar D J and Charlton Edwards E 1978 Diuresis renography in equivocal upper urinary tract obstruction. British Journal of Urology 50: 76–80

O'Reilly P H, Lupton E W, Testa H J, Sheilds R A Carroll R N P, and Charlton Edwards E 1981 The dilated non-obstructed renal pelvis. British Journal of Urology 53: 205–209

Parsons F M, Pyrah L N, Powell F J N, Reed G & Speirs F W 1952 Chemical imbalance following ureterocolic anastomosis. British Journal of Urology 24:317

Pyrah L N 1954 Ureterocolic anastomosis. Annals of the Royal College of Surgeons of England 14:169

Pyrah L N 1956 Some uses of the ileum in urology. British Medical Journal 1:135

Pyrah L N 1961 Transplantation of the ureters. In: Smith R (ed) 'Progress in Clinical Surgery'. Churchill, London

Rosenkilde Olsen P 1981 The renal pelvis and ureteral peristalsis II. The pelvic pressure and its relation to the frequency of ureteral peristalsis. Scandinavian Journal of Urology and Nephrology 15: 53–58

Ross J A, Edmond P & Griffiths J M T 1973 The action of drugs on the intact human ureter. British Journal of Urology 39: 26–30

Satani Y 1919 Experimental studies of the ureter. American Journal of Physiology 49:474

Satani Y 1919 Experimental studies on the ureter: the cause of ureteral contractions. American Journal of Physiology 50:342

Sjödin J G, and Holmlund D 1982 Indomethacin by intravenous infusion in ureteral colic. A multicentre study. Scandinavian Journal of Urology and Nephrology 16: 221–226

Stamey T A 1956 The pathogenesis and implications of the electrolyte imbalance in uretero-sigmoidostomy. Surgical Gynecology and Obstetrics 103:736

Struthers N W 1973 An experimental model for evaluating drug effects on the ureter. British Journal of Urology 45: 23–27

Weinberg S R & Maletta T J 1961 Measurement of peristalsis of the ureter and its relation to drugs. Journal of the American Medical Association 175:15

Weiss R M, Basset A L, Hoffman B F 1979 Clinical implications of ureteral physiology. Journal of Urology 121:401

Whitaker R H 1973 Diagnosis of obstruction in dilated ureters. Annals of the Royal College of Surgeons of England 53: 153–166

Whitaker R H 1976 Equivocal pelviureteric obstruction. British Journal of Urology 47: 771–779

Wrong O M 1970 Effects of diversion of urine into the alimentary tract. In: Thompson R H S, Wootton E D P (eds) Biochemical Disorders in Human Disease', 3rd edn, Churchill, London p 680–682

Bladder and urethra

The bladder and urethra provide the means by which urine can be stored until voiding is convenient and socially acceptable. The lining of the bladder and urethra is waterproof, preventing absorption of urine. The bladder wall is capable of holding an increasing volume of urine with minimal increase in intravesical pressure. The behaviour of bladder and urethra during the storing and voiding phases is mediated by spinal reflexes which are controlled by the higher centres. Disorders of micturition are common and their causes multitudinous. Disorders may affect either or both the motor or sensory components of the bladder and urethra which may become over or under active. Functionally the bladder and urethra normally behave as a unit, but for the purposes of description will be dealt with separately.

Neurological conditions commonly affect micturition and indeed may first come to light when the patient reports variation in frequency, voiding pattern and control. Multiple sclerosis is a good example, bladder function varying as the condition waxes and wanes. Correct interpretation leads to effective management, relieving or minimizing the upset in micturition and control.

Adequate voiding is necessary for the protection of the upper urinary tract against back pressure and subsequent infection. Poor voiding may result from obstruction, commonly due to benign prostatic hypertrophy in men over 50, or may result from a defect of innervation of bladder or urethra, or both. Adequate control over micturition is necessary for the preservation of hygiene, social acceptance and independence. Incontinence has become less of a taboo as a result of the explosion of interest in recent years, but negative attitudes persist among doctors, nurses and the public. The cost to the individual and the community is high with an estimated 2 million individuals in this country suffering from intractable incontinence, probably 50% of all women wetting at some time in their lives, and innumerable teenage and child bed wetters. Surgeons should be aware that pelvic surgery such as proctocoloctomy, commonly damages the innervation of the bladder and urethra. As a result bladder emptying may be poor or the patient may become incontinent. In addition, sexual function in the male may be damaged, with poor or absent erection and ejaculation. It is necessary for surgeons to take an intelligent interest in this aspect of their patients well-being, but unfortunately this is by no means universal. There are basic misunderstandings about innervation, and the reader is advised to keep an open mind in order to benefit from current work in the field of surgical anatomy and physiology. For example, most surgeons still believe that the motor nerve supply to the muscles of continence lies below the pelvic floor, and that dissection above the pelvic floor can be carried-out without risk of permanent incontinence. This is not entirely accurate and a fuller description will be given later.

THE BLADDER MUSCLE: DETRUSOR

The muscle of the bladder is called the detrusor and a simple estimate of its function can be obtained by recording the frequency of voiding and volume voided. The motor and sensory component in patients with apparently normal innervation can also be assessed by specific questions (Table 24.1). While this is largely subjective, a reasonably accurate initial assessment can be made by the clinician experienced in urodynamics, without recourse to instrumentation. Urologists have long employed these questions in the diagnosis of prostatism in the male, the condition in which prostatic hypertrophy obstructs the flow of urine. The prevailing attitude to incontinence has been less enlightened, particularly when dealing with women in whom incontinence has been almost synonymous with the need for gynaecological surgery. Current interest in urodynamics is gradually producing an awareness that the presence of urgent micturition, urge incontinence, and increased frequency are contra-indications to immediate routine gynaecological surgery. Surgeons and gynaecologists in training can now benefit from rotation to a urodynamic specialist referral centre. The clinician can then develop an awareness of the wide spectrum of bladder

Table 24.1 Routine questions about bladder and urethral function should cover at least these aspects of bladder and urethral function.

Frequency of micturition by day and night.
Degree of urgency
Urge incontinence
Stress incontinence due to movement or coughing etc.
Water trigger effect: working with water or hearing the noise of
  running water can provoke extreme urgency and may lead to
  incontinence
Hesitancy in starting flow
Strength of flow and whether it is interrrupted
Slow flow
Terminal dribbling: that is, dribbling continuing after the voluntary act
  of micturition
Constant dribbling with or without awareness
Flooding with or without sensation
Bed wetting
Painful micturition
Known precipitating factors including treatment, e.g. diuretic
Known predisposing disease, e.g. diabetes
Male: ability to achieve erection and ejaculation

Table 24.2 Urodynamic investigations: degree of sophistication.

Observation of voiding characteristics
  Simple Observation: Although this can be useful, many individuals
  are unable to void on demand in public and direct observation is
  virtually impossible in the female.
  Flowmeter Recording: All measuring devices require calibration to
  avoid artefact. Flowmeters are mostly simple and the average
  clinician can soon learn the technique.
  Flowmeter combined with voiding pressure measurements: Complexity
  increases, involving the measurement of intravesical and intra-
  abdominal pressures as well as measuring flow characteristics. Close
  liaison with a bio-engineer or physicist is now required to avoid
  artefact and malfunction of the apparatus.
  Micturating cystourethrography ± the above: Ideally a special commode
  should be used to enable females and disabled males to void in a
  familiar posture. The special equipment is expensive, especially when
  combined with pressure flow studies. Radiological expertise is now
  desirable.
Cystometry:
  Equipment ranges from an inexpensive and simple water manometer,
  to tranducers, pen-recorders and electronic subtraction to determine
  detrusor pressure by subtracting intra-abdominal pressure from
  intravesical pressure. Again physicist help is advisable.
Urethral closure pressure profile measurement
  This requires simultaneous measurement of intravesical pressure. It
  is sometimes combined with electromyography. A catheter
  withdrawal platform is advisable. Physicist help is indicated.

and urethral dysfunction, resulting in more accurate clinical assessment.

A description now of basic investigation and classification of nomenclature will facilitate clearer understanding of the subsequent account of bladder and urethral mechanisms.

URODYNAMICS

Urodynamics encompasses the morphological, physiological, biochemical and hydrodynamic aspects of urine transport from kidney to the exterior. A multidisciplinary approach has produced a range of valuable investigations for the lower urinary tract, and old concepts on anatomy and physiology are being challenged. Clinicians, engineers, mathematicians, physiologists and anatomists are all active in the field and the bibliography is extensive. The upper urinary tract is less accessible and progress has been slower there.

The investigation of bladder and urethral function will now be described and the main abnormalities defined. The degree of sophistication required is outlined in Table 24.2. The International Continence Society's Committee for Standardisation of Terminology, has defined terms and procedures for several urodynamic investigations. This account conforms to ICS recommendations, exceptions being clearly described.

Cystometry

This is the method by which the pressure/volume relationship of the bladder is measured. It is the most useful single indicator of bladder function. It is easy to perform, requiring in its simplest form a single catheter connecting bladder to a water manometer. First described by Mosso

and Pellacini in 1882, cystometry was neglected until 1927 when Rose demonstrated its value in the investigation of bladder function. Recording apparatus was then somewhat clumsy, and cystometry has only come to the forefront with the development of the transducer, an electromanometer that converts pressure changes into electrical signals which are amplified and displayed on a suitable recorder. Transducers are necessary for the measurement of dynamic changes such as those occurring during voiding or coughing. Due to the innertia of the water system, the simple water manometer is only accurate for the measurement of resting intravesical pressure. Zero reference for pressure calibration is the level of the superior edge of the symphysis pubis. Cystometry is normally performed without anaesthesia although this is not always possible in children. In the absence of anaesthesia, an estimate can be made of the sensory and motor characteristics of the bladder with the minimum of intervention. Usually a urethral catheter is used, 8FG being suitable. For the passage of the catheter, a little local anaesthetic gel can be used. However, most gels are water-miscible rather than soluble and may interfere with transmission of pressure if the gel enters the lumen of the measuring cannula. As an alternative to a urethral catheter, a fine suprapubic cannula can readily be inserted through the skin, without irritating urethra or bladder neck.

Residual urine should be measured before filling starts but it should be recognized that an isolated result is of limited value. Residual urine is defined as that volume of fluid remaining in the bladder immediately after the completion of micturition. The effect of environment, anxiety and other factors must be considered. Measurement of residual urine is an integral part of the study of micturition and may be roughly assessed by palpation, but more accurately by withdrawal of urine by means of a catheter or cystoscope. Some bladders are very thin-walled and flop into all the corners of the pelvis. This type of bladder may contain 2 litres and more without being readily detectable by palpation or percussion particularly in the obese.

Residual urine may also be measured by radiography, but then it must be realised that the opaque medium will coat the surface of the mucosa and interpretation is not always easy. Ultrasound is not sufficiently accurate when residual volume is small. The use of radio-isotopes for the measurement of residual volume is uncommon but can be very accurate. False residual urine is produced when urine drains down the ureters following micturition in the condition of vesico-ureteric reflux, or when bladder diverticula drain into the main bladder reservoir following voiding.

Residual urine may result from:

1. Detrusor insufficiency
2. Infravesical obstruction
3. Psychological inhibition
4. Artefact
   a. Urine draining from ureters following vesico-ureteric reflux
   b. Diverticula

When infravesical obstruction exists, the connection between the presence or absence of residual urine and abnormalities in pressure/flow relationships is variable and poorly understood. The residual urine in a high pressure bladder system is more dangerous since reflux into ureters and subsequent damage to the kidneys is more likely.

Storage phase

The normal bladder is capable of storing an increasing volume of fluid with minimal increase in pressure, provided filling is continuous and no faster than about 50 ml/min, well above normal physiological levels. Incremental and fast filling produce sharp rises of pressure settling after each flow of fluid as the bladder relaxes to accommodate the new volume. Compliance is the name given to the change in volume for a change in pressure, and is defined by the formula $C = \Delta V / \Delta P$, where ΔV is the volume increment and ΔP is the change in pressure associated with the volume increment. Compliance is usually considered to be equivalent to accommodation but differences may occur since accommodation is nerve mediated.

Clinicians often refer to bladder tone. The word 'tone' is imprecise in common usage. It does not distinguish between detrusor activity and the viscoelastic properties of the bladder. For example, bladder capacity may be reduced by detrusor overactivity which is an active state,

or by the passive condition of fibrosis following radiation or chronic infection. The fibrosed bladder produces a high pressure rise during filling, demonstrating low compliance.

Rate of bladder filling can affect bladder response and it is useful to perform cystometry at two filling rates for comparison. Individual bladders react in different ways and the functioning capacity may differ with the rate of filling. Similarly mental state affects functioning capacity, common knowledge to candidates at interview or examination. Overactivity of the detrusor may be provoked in some and suppressed in others by rapid filling, defined as over 100 ml/min. This rate of filling is usually regarded as provocative, inducing contraction in the so-called unstable bladder. Whether this is significant for the diagnostic and clinical management of the patient is not always clear, but there seems reasonable correlation in most. However, in some individuals, rapid filling actually depresses overactivity. On the whole it is preferable to keep initial investigations as near to physiological normal as is possible. A filling rate of about 20 ml/min is a suitable compromise between normal urine production rate and the time available in the urodynamic clinic. Some workers prefer to fill the bladder by forced diuresis, using a fluid load with or without a diuretic. Urine production rate is variable, and the technique is hardly more physiological. Since a catheter is required for pressure measurement it is easier for the patient and staff alike for it to be used also for bladder filling. An estimate of urine production rate during filling can be made by subtracting from the volume voided at the end of cystometry that volume which has been run into the bladder. This measurement however will be inaccurate if voiding is incomplete, if diverticula exist or if vesico-ureteric reflux occurs. Diverticula and reflux may lead to the need for double emptying. These conditions can be detected by the X-ray procedure of voiding cystourethrography which is often nowadays combined with bladder pressure recording and flowrate measurement. When voiding is again necessary shortly after the initial micturition, the term encores is employed.

Cystourethroscopy

The bladder and urethra can be visualized by cystourethroscopy using a telescope passed along the urethra, employing either local or general anaesthesia. Although this is not considered a urodynamic procedure, it is invaluable for the detection of local physical abnormalities such as urethral stricture, infection of the bladder, bladder tumour etc. An estimate of functioning capacity is also possible but can be erroneous in the fully anaesthetized individual, or in nervous patients upset by the procedure when only local anaesthesia is used. Cystoscopy can combine a visual inspection of the bladder and urethra with a form of cystometry. Some gynaecologists favour the American system of cystourethroscopy using CO_2 gas as a filling medium, subsequently coupling the cystoscope to a recorder to obtain cystometry. CO_2 has the advantage of being a dry medium providing fast filling but it has major disadvantages. It is compressible, leading to inaccuracies in recording and it dries the mucosa producing a non-physiological state. It may actually cause pain. Following the discussion at the ICS Annual Conference in Los Angeles in 1980, few can believe that gas is a suitable filling medium for cystometry.

TERMINOLOGY

Terminology has been plagued by the use of poorly-defined terms such as the unstable bladder. Bio-engineers and physicists have contributed greatly to the development of precise terminology. Even so, the ICS Standardisation Committee has had difficulty reconciling the use of some words, particularly when those words have different meanings in different disciplines. The committee's reports are required reading for any clinician or scientist proposing to work in the field of urodynamics. Most of the following definitions are taken from the ICS Fourth Report, which attempts to rationalize nomenclature in the difficult field of neurological disorders.

Classification of detrusor function

The following simple classification can be applied both to motor and sensory function:

1. Normal
2. Overactive
3. Underactive

Sensation cannot accurately be evaluated but should be assessed as best as possible. Current methods are largely subjective but improvement in monitoring can be expected. The normal individual can usually contain 150–350 ml of urine in comfort before developing an awareness of fullness, but this varies with conditions. If socially convenient, micturition will follow the first desire to void. With 500 ml or more in the bladder, pain may develop and is felt in the lower abdomen, perineum or urethra. Respiratory and pulse rates increase. The sensory nerves detect pain, touch, temperature, and stretch which is important for the proprioception of continence and micturition.

Detrusor activity can be interpreted from measurement of changes in intravesical (Pves) or detrusor pressure (Pdet) during filling and voiding. Pves is the pressure within the bladder with reference to atmospheric pressure. Pdet is that component of intravesical pressure created by passive and active forces in the bladder wall itself. Detrusor pressure equals intravesical pressure minus intra-abdominal pressure:

$$Pdet = Pves - Pabd$$

Intra-abdominal pressure is taken to be the pressure surrounding the bladder. It is usually estimated by measuring intrarectal pressure. A small, water-filled balloon is placed in the rectum and is connected by a water filled cannula to a transducer, the zero line being the upper edge of the symphysis pubis.

Calculation of Pdet is necessary to distinguish between the pressure changes produced by detrusor activity and those caused by coughing, abdominal straining and postural changes. Detrusor resting pressure ranges will usually be at or near 0–10 cm of water. It is convenient to subtract intra-abdominal pressure electronically as described by Bates et al (1970).

Normal detrusor

During filling the normal bladder responds to increasing volume with an insignificant increase in pressure. There are no involuntary contractions despite provocation. Normal voiding is produced by voluntarily initiated, sustained detrusor contraction that can be suppressed voluntarily. The complex system of innervation is described later (Fig. 24.1). Of course, if filling is continued without the opportunity to micturate, control is eventually overcome.

Overactive detrusor

In this type of bladder, involuntary contractions occur spontaneously or as a result of provocation, and cannot be suppressed by the individual (Fig. 24.2). Provocation includes activities like alteration of posture, coughing and jumping. Rapid filling of the bladder is commonly considered a provocative action but may in fact depress bladder activity. Involuntary contractions may or may not lead to voiding. The detrusor is also considered overactive if voluntary contractions leading to voiding cannot voluntarily be suppressed. The term overactive detrusor includes that type of bladder previously called unstable by some workers. Detrusor hyper-reflexia is defined as the state of overactivity resulting from disturbance of the nervous control mechanisms. This term should only be used when there is objective evidence of a neurological disorder. Popular but imprecise clinical terms such as hypertonic, uninhibited or automatic should be abandoned.

Underactive detrusor

There are no contractions during filling. Voiding may be produced by increasing intra-abdominal pressure, detrusor contractions being absent or inadequately sustained. If the detrusor is unable to contract under any circumstances it is called non-contractile. When an abnormality of nervous control causes complete absence of centrally co-ordinated

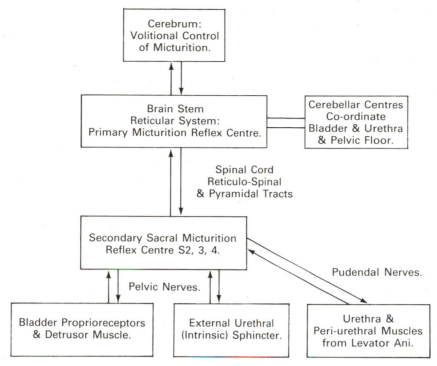

Fig. 24.1 Simplified the schematic representation of neurological pathways controlling bladder and urethral function.

1. System above sacral reflex centre: lesions are suprasacral, or upper motor neurone, and preserve the micturition reflex.
2. Sacral reflex centre: lesions damage or destroy the micturition
3. Peripheral Innervation: reflex (lower motor neurone).

Sympathetic outflow to bladder and urethra is localized in lower thoracic and upper lumber spinal segments.

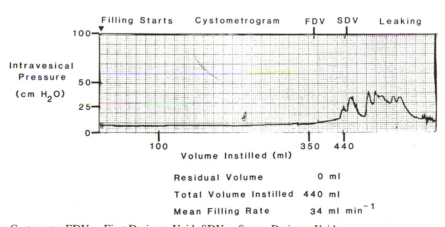

Fig. 24.2 Continuous Flow Cystometry FDV = First Desire to Void; SDV = Strong Desire to Void.
This is an overactive bladder, with marked increase in pressure at a low volume of 440 ml, leading to uncontrolled involuntary contraction and leakage. (Dept. of Medical Illustrations, Southern General Hospital.)

contraction, the term detrusor areflexia can be used. Autonomous bladder function results from lesions of the conus medullaris or sacral nerve outflow, the detrusor being termed decentralized since it no longer is influenced by higher centres. Lesions resulting from spinal injuries or tumour are often mixed in their effect and each patient requires careful assessment. When the bladder accepts very large volumes with little change in pressure, it demonstrates high compliance. Imprecise but commonly used terms such as autonic, atonic and hypotonic should be avoided.

TRIGONE

This is the triangular base plate with the ureteric orifices at two extremities and the internal urethral meatus at the third. The bulk of muscle in the trigone is a continuation of the detrusor muscle. The ureters pass obliquely through detrusor muscle, providing an anti-reflux valve as the bladder fills and also during micturition. The anti-reflux mechanism is reinforced by muscle specific to the trigone, a thin superficial layer with smaller muscle bundles than in detrusor. Gosling (1981) proposes that only this thin layer should be called trigonal muscle (Fig. 24.3). It passes through the internal urethral meatus into the proximal urethra where it is of little functional importance. It lacks acetyl cholinesterase, its parasympathetic innervation being minor.

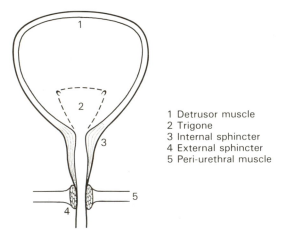

1 Detrusor muscle
2 Trigone
3 Internal sphincter
4 External sphincter
5 Peri-urethral muscle

Fig. 24.3 Scheme of bladder and urethra.
The internal sphincter is only recognizable in the male. However, the bladder neck in the normal female is capable of retaining urine. The peri-urethral muscle consists of fibres from levator ani. The male bladder neck and proximal urethra are supported by the prostate. The female structures are less well supported, relying mainly on pubo-urethral ligaments.

BLADDER NECK

There are striking differences between the male and female bladder neck mechanisms.

Bladder neck

The smooth muscle at the bladder neck forms a recognizable circle and extends to surround the upper urethra before merging with the muscle of the prostatic capsule. This bladder neck smooth muscle is different from detrusor muscle. Unlike the detrusor, it has a rich sympathetic innervation in common with the ejaculatory system. This internal sphincter contracts during ejaculation, preventing semen entering the bladder. Retrograde ejaculation can occur if innervation is defective. Prostat-

ectomy can also damage the internal sphincter and commonly produces retrograde ejaculation. Fortunately wedge excisions of the bladder neck are uncommon now, urologists having adopted more conservative approaches.

Bladder neck function is the subject of continuing controversy and its role in micturition and in the maintenance of urinary continence has not been resolved.

Female bladder neck

The smooth muscle in the female bladder neck is thinner and is not so well defined as in the male. Unlike the male, there is very little sympathetic innervation, supporting the view that the sympathetic is mainly involved in the male genital function. Identification of the bladder neck during clinical investigations can be difficult in the female, and measurements based on its location are suspect. The muscle fibres are longitudinal, probably shortening and widening the urethra during micturition. The posterior urethro-vesical angle has held an unduly prominent place in gynaecology. The loss of this angle demonstrated by stress cystography, has been an indication to restore the angle by surgery. It is considered important that the bladder and proximal urethra be held within the abdominal cavity, on the basis that increases of intra-abdominal pressure affecting the bladder content will also produce simultaneous increase in urethral closure pressure by contraction of levator ani, fibres of which form a peri-urethral closure mechanism. When the posterior urethro-vesical angle is normal, it has been assumed that this mechanism is preserved. However, the angle may be held rigidly by scar tissue, particularly following surgery. Scarring may reduce the passive closure of bladder neck leading to leakage. Emphasis has moved away from the posterior vesico-urethral angle to the preservation of mobility in bladder neck and urethra.

The pubo-urethral ligaments consist of two strong posterior and one rather weaker anterior collection of elastic and collagen tissue. These ligaments suspend the urethra from the pubic bone, fusing with the urethra at the junction of its middle and distal thirds. The ligaments hold the upper third of the urethra within the abdominal cavity so that changes of intra-abdominal pressure are exerted on this part of the urethra simultaneously with rises in intravesical pressure, thus preventing leakage of urine.

URETHRA

The urethra serves two functions. It maintains continence but during micturation it opens to form a channel for the passage of urine. In the male, the flow takes the form of a jet with good directional quality. Distortion of the urethra by stricture, oedema or other conditions produces

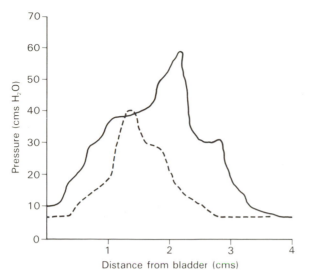

Fig. 24.4 Urethral Closure Pressure Profile: ——— 340 ml in bladder --- 130 ml in bladder. This urethra improves in functioning length and pressure exerted along that length when the bladder fills. An incompetent urethra tends to deteriorate as the bladder fills. If the urethra is fibrosed, for example, following multiple surgery, the profile tends to remain poor as the bladder fills.

birth. Deterioration is particularly common after the menopause and can be corrected by the application of hormone cream or oral hormone replacement therapy.

The female urethra is attached to the anterior wall of the vagina and as a result is susceptible to repeated minor trauma. Urethral irritation produces urgency, frequency and pain during or after micturition. These symptoms are commonly interpreted as indicating cystitis or the urethral syndrome. Careful history and examination of the urethra can usually identify the problem.

Urethral muscle

Smooth

This consists of a continuation of the detrusor, thinning out around the external meatus.

Striated

This muscle is distributed in a circular fashion on the outer surface of the urethral smooth muscle. Its maximum concentration is at the middle third of the urethra and it extends over the anterior wall of the proximal and distal urethra. The posterior component is only present in the middle third and even there it is thin. This muscle is slow twitch in type and is the intrinsic sphincter. It is innervated from S2, 3 and 4, fibres being distributed along branches of the pelvic (splanchnic) nerve, and not the pudendal nerve as described in earlier accounts. The nerve supply to this sphincter therefore runs in bundles of fibrous tissue above the pelvic floor, and is at risk during pelvic surgery. The pudendal nerve of course runs below the pelvic floor, and in the past surgeons were taught that its preservation would protect sphincteric function. This comforting thought can no longer be sustained.

Peri-urethral striated muscle

This contains fast and slow twitch fibres and contributes to the closure mechanism. Unlike the intrinsic sphincter it is supplied by the pudendal nerve.

spattering. The quality of the jet is dependent upon the expelling force but it is also influenced by the rather transverse shape of the main length of the urethra, and in the male the vertical slit formed by the external urethral meatus.

The urethral closure mechanism is complex and only partially dependent on sphincteric muscle. Indiscriminate use of the word sphincter has caused confusion. The concept of a complex closure mechanism is more useful, and encourages greater accuracy in diagnosis. Continence is also dependent on inhibition of the micturition reflex (Fig 24.4). The components of the closure mechanism are:

1. Urethral:
   a. Elastic and Vascular tissue
   b. Mucus
   c. Muscle: smooth and striated
2. Peri-urethral: This is made up by contributions from the striated muscle in the pelvic floor
3. Pubo-urethral ligaments, and in the male the prostate. These support the urethra.

Female urethral closure mechanism

The female bladder neck does not have the accumulation of muscle that forms the internal sphincter in the male although it remains closed in normal women until micturition is initiated.

Urethral elasticity, vascularity and mucus production contribute to a soft inner layer resistant to the leakage of urine. Mucus also protects against infection. All these components deteriorate with age and after multiple child

Male urethral closure mechanism

This is altogether a more robust system, supported by the prostate and protected by its greater length. Elasticity, vascularity and mucus production all play a part and are less susceptible to ageing and trauma than in the female.

Smooth muscle

The arrangement in bladder neck has already been described. It is responsible for closing the bladder neck during ejaculation. The muscle extends downwards to merge with that of the prostatic capsule.

Striated muscle

This is concentrated around the urethra distal to the verumontanum to form the distal intrinsic sphincter. This is commonly referred to as the external sphincter. As in the female, this is a slow twitch muscle innervated by branches from the pelvic nerves.

Peri-urethral striated muscle

This is stronger than but otherwise similar to the female arrangement.

Measurement of urethral closure pressure profile (UCPP)

UCPP demonstrates the intraluminal pressure exerted along the length of the urethra with the bladder at rest. Again the zero reference point for pressure measurement is the level of the superior edge of the symphysis pubis. The measurement is invalidated if detrusor contraction occurs, since this may be associated with reflex relaxation of the urethral closure mechanisms as micturition develops. The urethral closure pressure profile is also affected by the volume of fluid in the bladder. The normal urethra tends to improve its profile as the bladder fills, whereas the deficient urethra may show deterioration. A fibrosed rigid urethra has a more constant profile.

Measurement of UCPP with concomitant cystometry is particularly helpful in the assessment of incontinent women prior to surgery. However, it must be combined with cystometry (Fig. 24.4).

NORMAL MICTURITION

The normal infant initially voids reflexly subsequently developing voluntary control first during waking hours and then subconscious control at night. This acquired ability is subject to individual variation and may be affected by psychological factors. Deterioration in control is common in the elderly, especially if cerebral degeneration occurs. Regular voiding can prevent or diminish incontinence in both age groups.

Boyarsky estimated that micturition involves 15 reflexes. It is certainly a complex mechanism and even now our knowledge of innervation and mechanisms of voiding is incomplete. Observation of one's own voiding patterns gives clear evidence that micturition is influenced by the volume in the bladder, environment (including ambient temperature) and psychological status. The basic mechanisms are listed in Figure 24.5. Bed wetters tend to be deep sleepers and it is possible that they simply do not respond to the normal bladder sensation. It is also possible that there is an immaturity of the control over reflex voiding. A few wet because of psychological problems, but of course once wetting is established, psychological disturbance rapidly follows both in the patient and relatives. Conscious control can be strengthened by suitable training methods including the enuretic alarm.

Evaluation of micturition

The bladder and urethra constitute a functioning unit during micturition, and disorders may be complex. Diagnostic investigation has greatly improved in recent years.

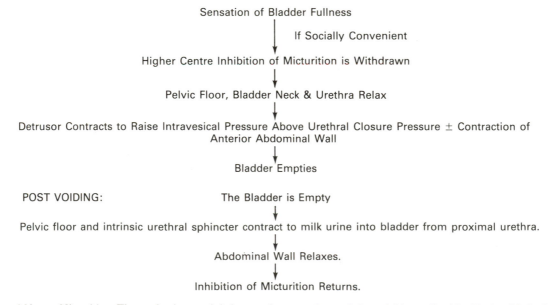

Fig. 24.5 Normal Mature Micturition. The mechanisms and their control are complex, and the activities outlined in this simplified scheme may occur simultaneously. At times and especially in women, the anterior abdominal wall may play a more significant role than the detrusor, by raising intra-abdominal pressure to produce voiding. Babies do not have higher centre control and some children are slow to develop mature inhibition of micturition, a common cause of bed wetting.

Measurement of voiding

The least invasive method is to observe the stream as the patient voids. Unfortunately this is scarcely possible with females, and many men find difficulty in voiding on demand and in public. Flowmeters are now available commercially. Manufacturers have become aware of the developing market and there is a increasing variety of equipment. Potential buyers should seek the advice of established urodynamic referral centres.

It is important to record the pattern of voiding as well as measuring maximum flowrate, flowtime and volume voided (Fig. 24.6). A single measurement is of very doubtful value. The subject should avoid distending the bladder beyond the normal for that individual, since over-distension can produce deterioration in flowrate and flowtime. Overdistension can cause prolonged effects on voiding and should be avoided in the postoperative or bedridden patient, otherwise retention may result. Since sensation tends to be reduced following overdistension the patient may not become aware of the problem. Obviously the risk is greater when there is a pre-existing defect of innervation. Over-distension of the bladder is used in the treatment of bladder overactivity, but the results are not very predictable and improvement may be transient.

Pressure flow measurement

It is important to determine whether poor micturition is due to an overactive closure mechanism, underactive detrusor or both. Physical obstructions can be detected by long-established urological endoscopic examination, but functional disturbances may not. Pressure flow measurements combine cystometry with flowmetry. It is essential to determine detrusor pressure (intravesical pressure minus intra-abdominal pressure) to distinguish between voiding due to detrusor activity, and voiding produced by increases

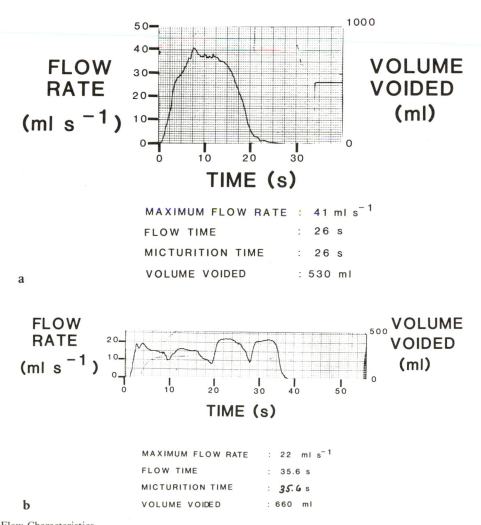

a.
MAXIMUM FLOW RATE : 41 ml s^{-1}
FLOW TIME : 26 s
MICTURITION TIME : 26 s
VOLUME VOIDED : 530 ml

b.
MAXIMUM FLOW RATE : 22 ml s^{-1}
FLOW TIME : 35.6 s
MICTURITION TIME : 35.6 s
VOLUME VOIDED : 660 ml

Fig. 24.6 a. Normal Flow Characteristics
b. Normal Maximum Flow Rate but obviously Prolonged Flow Time. Voiding has been aided by straining to increase intra-abdominal pressure, producing an irregular pattern of voiding. (Dept. of Medical Illustrations, Southern General Hospital.)

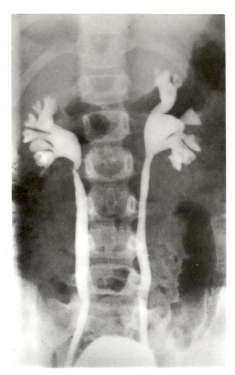

Fig. 24.7 Bilateral ureteric reflux (courtesy of Dr. E.M. Sweet, Royal Hospital for Sick Children). Reflux can be caused by simple infection and adequate treatment can restore normal function. A similar appearance results from defective ureterovesical muscle activity in neurological conditions. Micturating cystography and/or descending ureterography may be required to distinguish between the dilatation of reflux and of ureteric obstruction.

in the intra-abdominal pressure. Adequate voiding in the absence of detrusor contraction can be produced by abdominal straining, especially in women. However, this is not always effective since straining can also increase intra-urethral closure pressure via the peri-urethral muscles of the pelvic floor.

Micturition cystourethrography provides visual information about the bladder and urethral function including the presence or absence of reflux into ureters. It is fashionable to combine this examination with pressure flow studies, but the procedure can be overwhelming, adversely affecting the patient's performance (Fig. 24.7).

NEUROLOGICAL ABNORMALITIES AFFECTING BLADDER AND URETHRAL FUNCTION

With such a complex system of reflex and higher centre control, it is not surprising that many conditions can affect micturition, continence and male sexual function. Until the recent explosion of interest in urodynamics and subsequent classification of nomenclature, terminology of bladder and urethral dysfunction has been based on the site and degree of neurological damage. The level of damage is not always easy to identify. The classical

descriptions of the bladder in paraplegia were influenced by the inadequacies and complications of treatment. In recent years greater concern and respect for the preservation of bladder function following spinal injury has brought the realization that some of the earlier defects were based on bad management and subsequent urinary tract infection producing abnormalities of the bladder and urethra. It has become clear that lesions are seldom well circumscribed, and each patient must have individual assessment. At the other extreme, many abnormalities of bladder and urethral function exist without detectable neurological disease. The overactive bladder may be the first indication of multiple sclerosis, and it may take several years for the definitive diagnosis to be made.

Urodynamics has focused on detrusor-sphincter dysfunction regardless of site and degree of neurological damage. Of course neither approach in isolation is sound, but exact description is to be encouraged. We should no longer accept the nonsense of terms like non-neurogenic neurogenic bladder, a description given to an over- or underactive bladder: without evidence of neurological disease elsewhere. When there are exaggerated tendon reflexes, and the bladder is shown to be overactive with 'uninhibited' contractions, it may well be hyper-reflexic, especially in the female. The male is more complex in that obstruction to the flow can cause detrusor overactivity and this may co-exist with neurological disease. It is essential to keep an open mind, investigate adequately using urodynamic procedures and all other means available for the assessment of the patient as an individual. In this way, it should be possible to preserve residual function with the prospect of some recovery particularly following regeneration of nerves. That regeneration can occur is demonstrated by the temporary effect of denervation procedures employed in the management of overactive bladders.

The use of urodynamics then has lead to a functional approach to management. However, diagnosis and localization of the underlying pathology should also be attempted both for the benefit of the patient and to further understanding of this complex mechanism.

ELECTROMYOGRAPHY (EMG)

Where gross disorders occur, EMG is relatively easy to interpret and is much used in the investigation of spinal cord injuries and other neurological conditions. Measurement is made by means of surface or needle electrodes connected to a sound transmitter or to a recording chart. Surface electrodes are non-specific and the information obtained from them is of doubtful value. Needle electrodes are more accurate, but the muscle groups are so close and their interplay so complex that exact positioning and subsequent interpretation of signal is difficult. Movement at the electrodes is difficult to avoid and leads to artefact. In some equipment, the recording apparatus is incapable of adequate response thus introducing further artefact to an investigation that is already highly subjective in its evaluation. An anal plug EMG electrode commonly is used to estimate urethral closure activity, particularly in children in whom the insertion of needle electrodes into the urethral sphincter is especially difficult and painful when there is normal or residual sensation. Until recently it was thought that anal and urethral sphincter E.M.G. activity was comparable. However, it has now been shown that dissociation of these muscle groups can occur in suprasacral or sacral-spinal cord injury, and therefore the technique can provide misleading information.

NEUROLOGICAL PATHOLOGY

It is accepted that disorders of bladder and urethral function can exist in absence of apparent obstruction, outlet damage or recognizable neurological disease. However, recognizable neurological disease is common and examples are shown in Table 24.3. This is not the place for detailed description but an outline will be given.

Age

At the extremes, there is the immaturity of higher control of continence common in the enuretic, and the deterioration seen in the senile or cerebral degenerate.

Supranuclear (i.e. above the sacral micturition centre)

There are many possible factors affecting this area. Psychological disturbance commonly affects micturition and continence, producing a mixed and sometimes varying picture. Trauma, tumours and vascular lesions can affect bladder and urethral function. The consequences in this group have been referred to as being upper motor neurone lesions, but it is now recognized that the clinical conditions may reflect both upper and lower motor neurone abnormalities. In general the bladder is overactive, with preservation of the micturition reflex but voluntary micturition may be impaired. Surgery should not be contemplated until the individual is fully assessed.

The overactive bladder will respond to anticholinergic and other pharmacological agents such as tricyclic antidepressants, musculotrophic drugs such as Flavoxate and prostaglandin synthetase inhibitors like Indomethacin. Individual response and tolerance are very variable, and treatment should be altered accordingly. Denervation techniques include bladder overdistension, transection and vesical or selective sacral denervation. When poor compliance has resulted from fibrosis or interstitial cystitis, bladder capacity can be increased by caecocystoplasty or similar operation. This may also be combined with denervation techniques. Critical reviews of these techniques supersede anecdotal reports and will be found in the bibliography.

The closure mechanism may be spastic with poor or absent co-ordination between detrusor contraction and urethral relaxation. This is commonly called detrusor-

Table 24.3 A simplified account of neuropathology affecting bladder and urethral function.

Region affected	Effect	Examples
Cerebrum	Overactivity of bladder	Psychological including anxiety
Brain stem	Intact micturition reflex	Multiple sclerosis
Cerebellum	Impaired or absent voluntary micturition.	Parkinsonism
Spinal cord, above	Possible spasticity pelvic floor producing	Vascular insufficiency
Spinal reflex centre	detrusor-urethral dyssynergia and poor voiding.	and cerebral degeneration.
	= 'Upper motor neurone' effect, producing frequent, urgent micturition with urge incontinence.	Trauma to brain and/or spinal cord
Spinal micturition	Underactive or inactive detrusor	Protruded lumbar disc and lesions of cauda equina
Reflex centre S2, 3, 4	Absent micturition reflex	and conus medullaris
	Possibly weakness of paralysis of pelvic floor.	Trauma
	= 'Lower motor neurone' effect: poor voiding with overflow dribbling incontinence.	
Peripheral neuropathy	Impaired sensation and defective proprioception	Diabetes
Distal to spinal reflex centre	Poor voiding leading to painless retention and overflow incontinence.	Pernicious anaemia
	'Lower motor neurone' effect: Lack of sensation means symptoms are slow to appear.	Pelvic surgery Tabes dorsalis

Mixed lesions are common. Co-ordination of bladder and urethral activity may be lost, leading to poor and incomplete or inappropriate voiding. The neurology of micturition and control is not yet fully understood. Intermediate controlling transmitter-like substances are thought to exist. Sympathetic inhibition of detrusor activity probably is achieved by modulation of ganglionic transmission in the pelvic plexuses. (Gosling in Urologic Clinics of North America). Further elucidation is important for the development of effective pharmacological treatment. Study of transmitters and receptors is continuing, for example, the role of β-adrenergic receptors in bladder vault and α adrenergic receptors in the base of bladder, bladder neck and proximal urethra.

urethral dyssynergia. When this occurs, high intravesical pressure is produced with poor voiding and there is increased risk of damage to the upper urinary tract from back pressure. The ureterovesical mechanism may also be defective, increasing the risk of kidney damage from reflux.

Pharmacological treatment should be attempted and a more effective range is likely in view of current interest. Sphincterotomy may be necessary to improve emptying in order to protect ureters and kidneys. Rendering the individual totally incontinent is no longer considered a desirable aim but is sometimes inevitable. It is of interest that sphincterotomy does not necessarily result in incontinence. Spinal fractures at T10 damage the spinal cord in the region of the conus. To use current nomenclature, the results may be a mixture of upper and lower motor neurone lesions. When the fracture is at or above T5–6, filling the bladder to its capacity may produce severe hypertension, vascular responses demonstrating autonomic hyper-reflexia. In these patients care must be exercised during urodynamic studies involving filling of the bladder.

Stimulation of the urethra or bladder neck by catheter movement can induce spasm in leg muscles and urodynamic findings may then be difficult to interpret.

Sacral spinal lesions

These include damage to cauda equina and conus medullaris by tumour or trauma, for example pressure from a lumbar disc. In these conditions, the micturition reflex is defective or absent, leading to chronic retention. Usually this will be a low pressure bladder, since the pelvic floor and urethral closure mechanisms are also defective in most cases. The end result is retention with overflow incontinence.

Peripheral lesions

The nerve supply to bladder and urethral closure mechanisms can be damaged during pelvic surgery, leading to retention with or without incontinence. Provided this complication is detected and chronic overdistension prevented, bladder function can often be restored by regular and double voiding. Nerve regeneration can occur producing further improvement. The concomitant impairment of sexual function in the male can also be transient but strong psychological support is required for its recovery.

The peripheral neuropathy found in diabetes, pernicious anaemia and the uncommon condition of tabes dorsalis can also produce impairment of bladder awareness leading to painless chronic retention. Initially the micturition reflex is present, but subsequently is damaged by the effects of prolonged bladder distension unless the individual is trained to void regularly and completely. As in postpelvic

surgery damage, the bladder problem presents late usually with retention and overflow.

Sacral reflex testing

Causes of bladder and urethral dysfunction should be localised when possible and assessment is made more accurate by testing sacral reflexes.

1. *Anal reflex*: The normal anus contracts when a finger is inserted into the rectum. This reflex may be absent in active homosexual males.
2. *Anal cutaneous reflex*: The anus contracts when the peri-anal skin is stimulated, for example by pin prick.
3. *Bulbocavernosus reflex*: The anal sphincters contract when the glans penis or clitoris is squeezed, or when a urethral catheter is pulled down into the bladder neck. It is thought that perineal and anal stimulation causes inhibition of detrusor, a possible explanation for retention following operations like haemorrhoidectomy.

Trick stimulation of micturition

In some individuals with lesions above S2, 3, 4, voiding can be produced by stroking or tapping the lower anterior abdominal wall or stimulating the anus by touch or by inserting a finger into the rectum. Voiding can also be aided by coughing or other techniques to raise intra-abdominal pressure. Application of suprapubic pressure sometimes helps. Individual response to these various methods is variable and each individual should be encouraged to experiment until the most efficient trick stimulant technique is found.

Bladder pain

Samuel Pepys in his Diary gives a good account of the intractable, overwhelming nature of bladder pain experienced when he had a stone in his bladder. Obviously removal of the cause and simple analgesics will first be used. When pain persists and cannot otherwise be treated, the denervation procedures previously described can at least diminish the intractable pain although the effects may be transient. Cordotomy can be more effective but requires specialist skill and may interfere with bladder and other function. Pain following radiation for bladder tumour can be diminished by urinary diversion.

Bladder response to indwelling catheters

The commonest indwelling catheter is retained in the bladder by balloon (Foley type catheter). Even the normal bladder and urethra commonly are irritated by both the catheter and its balloon, responding by overactivity. When the bladder is kept empty by continuous drainage, the tip of the catheter erodes the mucosa and increases detrusor activity. The further the catheter projects into the bladder and the greater the volume in the balloon, the greater the stimulus to the detrusor. As a result urine tends to bypass the catheter and the individual who still has sensation will describe spasmodic pain. These problems can be reduced by allowing the bladder to fill and float away from the tip of the catheter, using intermittent drainage. This also preserves bladder capacity, preventing fibrotic contraction from chronic infection and possibly disuse atrophy of detrusor. The stimulus to the bladder and urethra can be reduced by using the smallest possible catheter, with the minimum amount in the balloon. A size 16FG is usually sufficient, and a 10 ml balloon will keep the catheter in place unless the bladder neck is widely open or the individual allows undue traction on the catheter.

Modern suprapubic cannula avoid these problems and are invaluable when bladder function is expected to return. The cannula can be closed by a tap, enabling the patient free opportunity to attempt voiding without the worry of the physical and psychological trauma produced by repeated urethral catheterization when voiding is unsuccessful. This is the ideal method of drainage in patients with spinal or head injury, if only during the initial assessment.

Therapeutic electrical stimulation

Micturition

Direct stimulation of the detrusor produces contraction but poor voiding. Attempts have been made to produce a stimulator for the spinal cord micturition centre. This is more logical since micturition requires relaxation of the urethral closure mechanisms as well as detrusor contraction. However, fibrosis around implanted electrodes is common, and long term results have been disappointing.

Continence

Electrical stimulation probably has a dual role, firstly by stimulation of the urethral closure mechanisms and secondly, by reflex inhibition of detrusor muscle. Considering the widespread acceptance of electrical stimulation in standard physiotherapeutic practice, it is surprising that patient-operated miniature stimulators for use at home are not more popular, especially since they cost less than 1 week of outpatient physiotherapy treatment in hospital. More complex stimulators requiring surgical implantation have been effective in carefully selected patients.

PHARMACOLOGY

As our knowledge of the mechanisms of bladder and urethral function increases, appropriate and specific pharmacological treatment should become more readily available. Even now, the overactive bladder can usually be controlled by anticholinergics. Unfortunately, it is more difficult to stimulate voiding.

At present, few drugs have been developed specifically for their effect on bladder and urethral function. Clinicians and experimental pharmacologists have borrowed from other specialities, scanning the list of side effects to determine which preparations are likely to be effective. With increased awareness of the potential market, this must be a growth area in the near future.

The multidisciplinary approach to bladder and urethral function has advanced our understanding of micturition and continence. It is to be hoped that there will be a similarly rapid improvement in our methods of treatment.

FURTHER READING

Bates et al 1970 Synchronous cine-pressure-flow cystourethroscopy with special reference to stress and urge incontinence. British Journal of Urology 42:714

Caldwell K P S 1975 Urinary Incontinence. Pitman Medical Publishing, Kent

Cantor E B 1979 Female urinary stress incontinence. Charles C Thomas Springfield, Illinois.

Glen E S, Rowan D 1973 Continuous flow cystometry and urethral pressure profile measurement with monitored intravesical pressure. A diagnostic and prognostic investigation. Urological Research 1: 97–100

Glen E S 1979 Diagnostic techniques for defining types of urinary incontinence and therapeutic use of electrical muscle stimulators. Acta Urologica Belgica 47: 162–167

Glen E S 1984 Urodynamics. In: Taylor S, Chisholm G, O'Higgins N, Shields R (eds) Textbook of Surgery, Heinemann, London p 332–341

Glen E S 1980 Urodynamic investigation of urinary incontinence. Forum, Proceedings European Association of Urology, 4th Congress, Athens, Abstracts p 69

Gosling J A, Dixon J S, Critchley H O D, Thompson S 1981 A comparative study of the human external sphincter and peri-urethral levator ani muscles. British Journal of Urology 53: 35–41

Griffiths D J 1980 Medical Physics Handbook 4. Adam Hilger Ltd, Bristol

Percy J P, Neill M E, Swash M, Parks A G 1981 Electro physiological study of motor nerve supply of pelvic floor. Lancet i: 16–17

Rowan D 1986 The study and control of bladder-urethral function, Uro-lit available from Diss Elektronik A/Ss, DK-2740 Skovlunde, Denmark

Stanton S L, Tanagho E A 1980 Surgery of Female Incontinence. Springer-Verlag, New York

Turner-Warwick, Whiteside C G 1979 The urology clinics of North America Vol. 6, W.B. Saunders, London

Walter S, Olesen K P, Nordling J, Andersen J T, Meyhoff H H, Hald T 1980 Neurogenic Bladder. Acta Obstetrica and Gynecologica Scandinavia 57: 337–347

International continence society

The Standardisation of Terminology of Lower Urinary Tract Function: Collation of First 3 reports of the International Continencê Society Committee for Standardisation of Terminology. Bates P, Bradley W E, Glen E, Griffiths D, Melchior H, Rowan D et al 1979 The Journal of Urology 121: 551–554

N.B. These reports separately were published in most urology journals, including the British Journal of Urology.

Fourth Report on the Standardisation of Terminology of Lower Urinary Tract Function: Terminology relating to neuromuscular dysfunction of the lower urinary tract. Bates P, Bradley W E, Glen E, Melchior, Rowan D, Sterling A HM, Sundin T, Thomas D, Torrens M, Turner-Warwick R, Zinner N, Hald T, British Journal of Urology 1981 Vol 53: 333–335, Acta Urologica Japonica 1981 Vol 27: 1568–1571, Scandinavian Journal of Urology and Nephrology 1981 Vol 15: 169–171, Urology 1981 Vol 17: 618–620

Proceedings

1st Annual Conference — not published, and in recent years the proceedings have consisted of preprints issued to participants.

2nd Annual Conference — Paris 1974 Glen E S (ed) Urologia Internationalis 29: 163–248

3rd Annual Conference — Copenhagen 1975 Glen E S (ed) Urologia Internationalis 30 (i): 1–108

4th Annual Conference — Mainz 1976 Glen E S (ed) Urologia Internationalis 31 (1–2): 1–136

5th Annual Conference — Glasgow 1977 Glen E S (ed) Urologia Internationalis 32: 77–268

6th Annual Conference — Antwerp 1978 Coolsaet B (ed) Urologia Internationalis 33: 3–204

Testis

The testes are paired organs with the double but inter-related functions of spermatogenesis and sex hormone production. An understanding of spermatogenesis is important when trying to help the infertile couple, in the development of new methods of contraception and in assessing hazardous working environments. The hormonal function of the testes is relevant when considering disorders of puberty, the management of the undescended testes and the hormonal treatment of prostatic cancer. Incorrect management of the common condition of undescended testes can render the patient liable to subsequent infertility and an increased chance of testicular malignancy. The proper development of the vas deferens, seminal vesicles and prostate is under the influence of sex hormones and the function of these organs is also necessary for fertility. Vasectomy is now one of the most frequently performed minor operations and the systemic or testicular sequelae are of importance. Knowledge of the neurophysiology of the male reproductive tract allows an understanding of referred testicular pain and aids the treatment of sexual disability in patients with disorders of ejaculation or paraplegia.

TESTICULAR DESCENT

Testicular descent usually takes place at the end of the seventh month of fetal life and it has been shown that if the testes do not lie in the scrotum by 1 year of age, spontaneous descent is unlikely (Scorer & Farrington, 1971). The process of descent and the differentiation towards the male state is under the influence of androgens secreted by the fetal testes in response to placental gonadotrophins. Ovarian activity is not necessary for female fetal development as evidenced by the fact that radiation castration of male fetal mice results in regression to the female state (Raynaud, 1958) and in cases of adrenocortical hyperplasia inappropriate androgens cause scrotal development in female babies (female pseudohermaphrodism (Maxted et al, 1965). Tissues arising from the mesonephric duct (body

and tail of the epididymis, vas deferens and seminal vesicles) grow in response to fetal testosterone whereas tissues of mullerian duct origin that would normally develop into female internal genitalia are suppressed by another hormone, mullerian inhibitory factor (MIF) which is thought to be secreted by the fetal Sertoli cells. There is some evidence that testicular undescent and the risk of subsequent testicular malignancy can result from an excess in the mother of oestrogens and perhaps progesterone in the seventh fetal week when the testes are developing (Henderson et al, 1979).

SPERMATOGENESIS

The seminiferous tubules at birth are small in diameter with no cell differentiation. At 5 years they elongate and become more tortuous; the tubule diameter increases but there is still no differentiation of cells. From the age of 9–15 years there is an increase in tortuousity and cell differentiation occurs into the various spermatogenic layers (Charney et al, 1952). Thus, testicular enlargement which is one of the first signs of puberty is mainly accounted for by differentiation and growth of the seminiferous tubules. This testicular enlargement is partly in response to increased secretion of follicle-stimulating hormone (FSH) and luteinizing hormone (LH). The first sperm appear in the urine at the age of 12 years and this potential fertility before the appearance of mature secondary sex characteristics has led to this time of development being called the fertile eunoch stage. In old age the tubules no longer appear uniform, the diameter decreases and there is great variation in the germinal epithelium with patchy spermatogenesis.

Two types of cell are found lining seminiferous tubules, the spermatogonium and the Sertoli cell.

The Spermatogonium (Fig. 25.1)

The spermatogonium divides by mitotic division to give

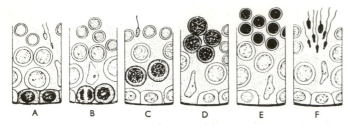

Fig. 25.1 Successive stages in the maturation of spermatogonia to spermatozoa (Garven H S D 1967 Student's Histology Livingstone, Edinburgh)

rise to spermatocytes, the first in the line of cells leading to spermatozoa. The spermatocytes then undergo two stage meiotic division to form spermatids. During the first division of meiosis there is no reduction in chromosomes, the resulting cells are known as secondary spermatocytes. These undergo reduction division to form haploid spermatids. Two of the four spermatids carry the X chromosome and two carry the Y (male-determining chromosome). The four spermatids resulting from meiosis are then formed into spermatozoa by a process known as spermateliosis. During this process the nucleus condenses to form the head of the sperm and this is capped by the achrosome which is a condensation of the golgi granules (Mann, 1964).

The duration of human spermatogenesis is important to the clinician planning treatment. Groups of spermatogonia develop synchronously and pass through the various stages in a cyclical manner. The time required for this has been studied by autoradiography; human testes were injected with tritiated thymidine and testicular biopsies examined. This revealed labelled spermatocytes at 16 days, immature spermatids at 32 days and formed spermatozoa at 64 days (Heller & Clermont, 1963).

Sertoli Cell

The Sertoli cell acts as an intermediary between cells of spermatogenesis and the blood and this function has been termed the blood testis barrier (Setchell & Waites, 1975). Evidence for this barrier is the presence of tight junctions between adjacent Sertoli cells when examination is made with the electron microscope and also the difference in composition between the seminiferous tubular fluid and the plasma. Potassium is higher than in plasma, sodium and chloride lower, the sugar inositol is 100 times higher, testosterone 30 times higher and gamma globulin is absent. The intact barrier is also immunological in that spermatozoa are not recognised by the immune system as self and injected spermatozoa will induce 'an immune response (Mancini et al, 1965). A breakdown in this barrier seems to result in some cases of auto-immune infertility (Rumke, 1980). The Sertoli cell is also important in synthesizing and metabolizing steroid hormones and may be the target for the gonadotrophic stimulus of spermatogenesis (Lofts,

1978). In addition, in infancy the Sertoli cell is thought to secrete mullerian inhibitory factor.

HORMONAL SECRETION

The testis has an endocrine function in addition to spermatogenesis. Testosterone is produced in the Leydig cells (Fig. 25.2) which lie in groups in the stroma between the seminiferous tubules. The Leydig cell nucleus tends to be vesicular with one or two prominent nucleoli and with most of the remaining chromatin condensed under the nuclear membrane. In infancy cells are small with scanty non-vacuolated cytoplasm. In adult life the cells are much larger and the cytoplasm contains vacuoles filled with lipoid material. In old age the cells are scanty and again small and non-vacuolated; many histiocytes are present and appear yellow because of their content of lipoid debris.

One of early events in the change towards puberty is an increase in the circulating level of LH and FSH but the trigger for this is not known. The Leydig cells hypertrophy in response to LH secretion and produce testosterone; secretion is not constant, but is characterized by a series of pulses mainly at night. This pulsed secretion continues throughout reproductive life, gradually diminishing in old age.

The main effects of androgen secretion are the development of the secondary sex characteristics and the accessory sex glands but both testicular androgens and FSH are necessary for normal spermatogenesis. The testes also secrete a small amount of oestrogen and this may play a part in negative feedback. Although the secondary sex characteristics develop in response to hormones there is in addition a genetic component, e.g. baldness is more marked in some families than others. Enlargement of the seminal vesicles and prostate cannot occur in the absence of androgen secretion but can be induced prematurely by large doses of androgens. It might be supposed that the relationship between puberty and testosterone production is a simple one; however, in the bull the androgen content of the testes shows only a gradual increase through the first (2–3 years of life without any sudden increase at the time

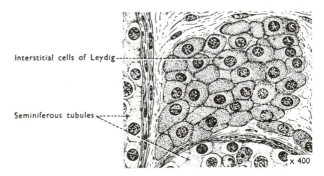

Fig. 25.2 The interstitial cells of the testis (Garven, loc. cit).

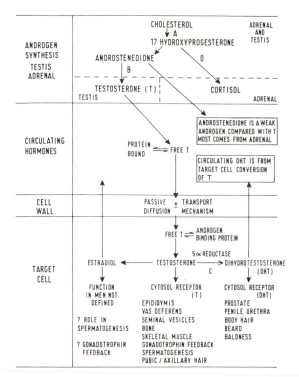

Fig. 25.3 Androgens in the male (the scheme is simplified and several intermediate compounds are omitted).

of sexual maturity which is reached at about 9 months. In humans the secondary sex glands and testes start to develop before there is any marked increase in testosterone. These facts suggest that the relatively abrupt onset of puberty may be due to increased sensitivity of the target organs in addition to any increase in androgens. In Figure 25.3 the relationship between testicular testosterone and the effects on the target cell is shown. Points to note from Figure 25.3 are:

1. Testosterone is secreted by the testis. Testosterone synthesis from cholesterol shares a common pathway with adrenal cortisol. The adrenal secretes a weak androgen (androstenedione).

2. Blood testosterone measurement includes protein bound and free testosterone but free testosterone only is available for uptake by the target cells. Plasma testosterone levels are in the region of 20 pmol/l and plasma DHT levels 2.5 pmol/l.

3. The mode of entry of steroid hormones into the target cell is not yet understood; specific transport mechanisms have been described for some cells e.g. rat uterus, the pituitary and the prostate gland.

4. Intracellular androgen binding protein probably provides an intracellular reservoir of hormone

5. Different target cells have specific cytosol receptors for testosterone and dihydrotestosterone.

6. The hormone receptor complex is translocated to the nucleus where it attaches to specific sites within the chromosome. As a result previously dormant genes become available for transcription of RNA and new messenger RNA and ultimately new proteins appear.

7. Evidence suggests that testosterone receptor complex regulates gonadotrophin secretion, wolfian duct tissue differentiation during sexual development and spermatogenesis whereas dihydrotestosterone receptor complex is responsible for external virilisation as the embryo develops and for adult sexual maturation and adult sexual life. How do we know this? One way is by studying patients with inborn errors of metabolism: lack of 20, 22 desmolase and other enzymes (A) results in adrenal insufficiency and female genitalia despite male chromosome complement and rudamentary testes (male pseudo hermaphrodism). Lack of 17β hydroxysteroid dehydrogenase (B) and lack of 5α reductase (C) also result in male pseudo hermaphrodism. On the other hand, lack of 11 and 21 hydroxylase (D) in a chromosomal female results in adrenal insufficiency and male external genitalia because of an excess of adrenal androgens (female pseudo hermaphrodism).

It can be seen that many steps are necessary for the normal androgen effect and that specific inborn errors of metabolism can occur both in the pathways of synthesis and in the metabolism of androgen in the target cell. Androgens are partly broken down in the liver and conjugated with glucuronic acid which renders them water soluble allowing excretion by the kidney.

Hypothalamic pituitary control of the testes

The hormones promoting testicular function, luteinizing hormone (LH) and follicle stimulating hormone (FSH) are the same in men and women. In Figure 25.4 the main influences acting on the secretion of these gonadotrophins are shown. FSH, LH releasing factor (FSH, LHRF) is synthesized in the hypothalamus and carried by the pituitary portal system to the anterior pituitary. This releasing hormone is also secreted in a pulsatile fashion and the pulse frequency deteetermines the relative amounts of FSH and LH released. Luteinizing hormone induces the Leydig cell to secrete testosterone which in turn has a negative feedback effect on hypothalamic secretion. Some testosterone is converted to oestrogen and this also has a negative feedback effect. FSH promotes spermatogenesis probably by stimulating the Sertoli cells to produce local androgens. The feedback from spermatogenesis has not been fully elucidated. It is known that, following castration, the output of gonadotrophin in the urine rises and remains high, suggesting that the pituitary has escaped from restraint imposed by the testes. In addition, in rats, a cell free extract of the testes from which steroid hormones have been removed will also suppress FSH output. In the extract there are a number of polypeptides and it has been shown that these are responsible for this effect. The name inhibin has been given to the hormone responsible for this feedback and recently assays have been

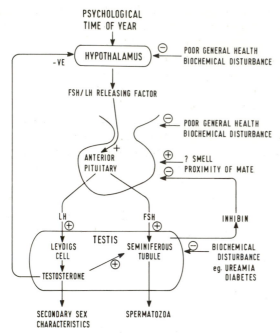

Fig. 25.4 Hormonal control of the testis

developed. It is possible, however, that more than one polypeptide may be involved but nevertheless the new assays should give us a better understanding of spermatogenesis and the effects of any treatment.

There are many other influences on the pituitary hypothalamic control of the testes. Some animals have a breeding season; man in contrast seems to have become adapted towards continuous breeding as judged by the small storage areas in the epididymis and the constancy of the hormonal state throughout the year. There is some evidence, however, that human sexual activity is greater in April and less in November (Titmar, 1978) and there may be some seasonal variation in sperm production (Tjoa et al, 1982). Whether smell influences the pituitary is a matter of conjecture; experiments have been conducted where nuns were given pillows which had been previously used by men and this produced a marked disturbance in their normal menstrual cycle; it is also possible to administer synthetic releasing factor as a snuff. Thus the physiological mechanisms exist for scents to influence the pituitary gonadal axis and certainly in animals this is an important mechanism. Disturbed cell metabolism as a result of biochemical disturbance such as uraemia or diabetes will affect the system at many levels; thus patients with kidney failure on dialysis often had impaired gonadotrophin secretion and impaired target organ sensitivity and such patients are often infertile.

THE EPIDIDYMIS

This gland consists of convoluted tubules surrounded by muscle and lined by secretory epithelium. The epididymis is the main reservoir for sperm in most mammals but in man the sperm stores are smaller and more towards the head (Glover, 1981). Spermatozoa leave the testes through the efferent tubules to enter the head of the epididymis and undergo a period of maturation lasting 10–14 days. The sperm tail increases in rigidity and the result is a change from corkscrew motility to progressive motility (Bedford et al, 1973). The ability of sperm to fertilize also undergoes maturation. The composition of the rete testes fluid undergoes change in the epididymis; the concentration of carnitene increases markedly. This substance is synthesized in the liver and concentrated in the epididymis. At low concentrations it promotes sperm motility but higher concentrations inhibit motility. Another compound, glyceryl phosphoryl choline (GPC), is also secreted by the epididymis and both carnitene and GPC are sometimes used as markers of epididymal function.

The blood testis barrier is not present in the epididymis and theoretically this is a site where sperm may be 'seen' by the immune system. It should be remembered that sperm are not normally recognized by the immune system as 'self' because the first sperm appear at an age when the immune system has already fully developed. One possible mechanism to prevent autosensitization in the epididymis is the presence of suppressor/cytotoxic lymphocytes in the mucosa of the epididymal ducts (Ritchie et al, 1984).

VAS DEFERENS

This duct is lined by columnar, non-ciliated epithelium and has a thick muscle coat. Sperm passage through the duct is a result of constant peristalsis which increases 100-fold during ejaculation. The mucosa of the vas is particularly rich in supressor/cytotoxic T-cells and these may help prevent sensitization at this site.

SEMINAL VESICLES

These consist of muscular convoluted tubules lined by epithelium which secretes up to 80% of the volume of the ejaculate. This fluid contains fructose, fibrinogen-like protein and prostaglandins.

Fructose is important as a source of energy for spermatozoa. Although fructose in semen is derived from the vesicles, the actual amount is inversely proportional to sperm density; the normal range being 1200–4500 μ/sml (Schirren, 1963). Values below the lower limit may indicate androgen deficiency or disease of the seminal vesicles and the presence of fructose in the ejaculate can be used clinically as a marker of seminal vesicle function. Fructose production is a true secondary sex characteristic as it disappears after castration or hypophysectomy but is capable of being restored by the administration of androgens. The fibrinogen like protein is coagulated by prostatic enzyme. The clot of seminal fluid sticks to the cervical mucus allowing time for sperm to colonise cervical mucus. The role of prostaglandins is not understood.

Some spermatozoa may enter the vesicles and this explains why after vasectomy there is a delay before all sperm are cleared from the ejaculate.

THE PROSTATE

The prostate contributes up to 20% of the volume of the ejaculate and consists of glandular follicles opening into epithelial ducts surrounded by smooth muscle. Prostatic fibrinolysins are important for the subsequent liquefaction of the semen clot which normally occurs 20 minutes after ejaculation. Prostatic fluid is acid and is rich in acid phosphatase, calcium, ascorbic acid, citric acid and lactic acid. Both semen and seminal fluid have a high zinc content, higher levels being found only in the eyes and cornea. Zinc may have a role in inhibiting microbiological organisms and in stabilizing sperm membranes. Hundreds of compounds have been isolated from seminal fluid (Mann & Lutwak Mann, 1981) but the function of most is not understood. Disorders of these compounds almost certainly account for some cases of unexplained infertility. The area is of considerable immunological interest because invading bacteria must be repelled yet highly antigenic sperm have to be tolerated. How this immunological balance is achieved is not understood but it is known that seminal fluid has a potent suppressive effect on many of the cells of the immune system including macrophages (James & Hargreave, 1984).

The prostate gland, like the seminal vesicle, is hormone-dependent. In older men there is often a gradual enlargement secondary to hyperplasia of both glandular and muscular tissue. The changes are similar to benign mammary hyperplasia and both conditions are thought to result from changes in the hormonal milieu. It has recently become possible to study intracellular hormones and it has been shown that carcinomatous prostatic tissue contains a greater proportion of intracellular testosterone compared with benign prostatic tissue (Habib et al, 1976). Studies of the intracellular compartment are important because prostate cancer is often hormone-dependent and oestrogen treatment or castration will in most cases suppress tumour growth for a time. It is thought that this effect is by depriving the still sensitive tissue of testosterone stimulation rather than any direct effect on the cancer tissue and it is hoped that better understanding of the intracellular hormonal milieu will allow better selection of patients who will respond and not escape from hormonal treatment. Stilboestrol was commonly used because this oestrogen is active when taken by mouth and measurements have shown that a dose of 1 mg, three times per day is enough to suppress testosterone production. However, it is being replaced by new synthetic oestrogens because it is very difficult to prevent the workforce in stilboestrol-making factories from suffering unacceptable oestrogenic side effects and because even at the low dose of 1 mg, three times a day some patients may suffer cardiovascular side effects. Alternative hormonal management is orchiectomy or equally effective subcapsular orchiectomy. This latter operation has the advantage that the sense of mutilation is less.

Secretion of acid phosphatase by prostatic cancer tissue is a useful tumour marker and when elevated usually indicates that the tumour has spread beyond the prostatic capsule.

SPERMATOZOA

The ultrastructure of the spermatozoon is shown in Figure 25.5. This has largely been determined by electron microscopy. The nucleus in the head carries the parental genetic material. As a result of meiotic division sperm contain 23 chromosomes which is half the normal cell complement of 46. Repeated attempts have been made to separate X- and Y-bearing sperm because this would be of great economic benefit to cattle breeding programmes but no practical method has yet been found. The nucleus is capped by the achrosome which contains enzymes necessary for ovum penetration. After ejaculation spermatozoa undergo a change called capacitation. During this ill-understood process the achrosome becomes less distinct and the sperm then becomes capable of fertilizing. Capacitation can be

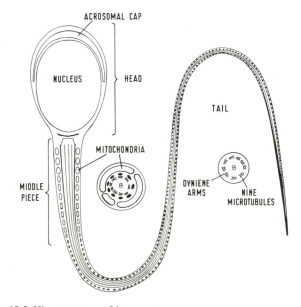

Fig. 25.5 Ultrastructure of human sperm.

induced artificially by exposing sperm to ionophores; these are substances which induce ion transfer across the cell membrane. This technique may be important in the future to optimise conditions for in vitro fertilization.

The mid-piece is an area rich in mitochondria and is thought to be concerned with the metabolism of fructose to provide energy for motility although Rothschild (1962) points out that the estimated work done on propulsion accounts for only a very small fraction of the fructose and oxygen that is consumed. The tail consists of nine pairs of microtubules arranged in a circle around two central microtubules. Swimming action is produced by contraction of the microtubules to produce two-dimensional bending waves of constant amplitude passing from the middle piece to the tip of the tail. Transient connections are made between adjacent microtubules by dyniene arms enabling control of sliding movements between tubules. This structure is similar to all cilia in the body. There is an interesting although rare condition called Kartagener's syndrome where the cilia are defective. The condition can be diagnosed by examining sperm tails under the electron microscope and the finding that the microtubules are missing their dyniene arms. Patients with Kartagener's syndrome have chronic chest disease, sinusitis and immotile sperm. They usually also have dextrocardia.

DEEP FREEZING OF SEMEN

In many cases there is no effective treatment for men with damaged spermatogenesis and there has been increasing demand for help in this situation using artificial insemination with donor sperm. In veterinary practice liquid nitrogen storage of bull sperm has been widely used and these techniques have been applied to banking of human sperm. Freshly ejaculated semen are mixed with egg yolk and glycerol and placed in liquid nitrogen vapour for 10 minutes before finally being immersed in liquid nitrogen. The egg yolk and glycerol protect the sperm from intracellular crystal formation during freezing. Many successful human pregnancies have resulted following artificial insemination using donor sperm (Hargreave, 1985) with the same success rates with fresh or frozen semen. Human sperm are relatively fragile, compared with those of domestic animals and only selected human donors have samples that can be stored satisfactorily but the reasons for this are not yet clear.

ASSESSMENT OF MALE FERTILITY

Assessing the couple's fertility

When a man has no sperm in the ejaculate (azoospermia) it is easy to label that man as infertile but in most cases when some sperm are present it is much more difficult to define the couple's problem. It is reasonable to regard an infertile marriage as one where the couple have had intercourse for 2 years without contraception and without any pregnancy resulting and to investigate the problem at this stage. Because two people are involved both must be assessed and it must always be remembered that both may have problems. The most frequently encountered problem is in fact a disorder of ovulation and this must be remembered before the infertility is ascribed to a poor sperm count.

Collecting semen samples

Examination of semen samples is necessary to diagnose defects in spermatozoal structure or activity. Because of day-to-day variation more than one sample should be examined. Samples can be produced either by masturbation or coitus interruptus following a period of abstinence corresponding to the couple's normal coital frequency. If analysis is abnormal the results should be compared with specimens collected after abstinence of 3 days and this may indicate that the primary fault has been nothing more than incorrect frequency of intercourse. Another cause for a temporary depression in sperm quality is febrile illness during the preceding 2–3 months. If this is suspected, a further sample should be tested after an interval of a month.

Semen analysis

Volume

Routine semen analysis includes estimation of volume normally between 2 and 5 ml. Volumes consistently below 1.0 ml indicate possible androgen deficiency, damage to accessory glands (post-inflammatory) or reflux of semen into the bladder.

Motility

Sperm motility is the most important measurement. Often poor motility is associated with poor sperm concentration and morphology and generalized damage to spermatogenesis. Absent motility in the presence of good numbers of sperm may be found in cases of infection, immobilizing antisperm antibodies, prostaglandin deficiency, and in Kartagener's syndrome. It is generally accepted that 50% of sperm should show active progressive movement for up to 4 hours after ejaculation.

Concentration

Sperm density is the second most useful measurement. The lower limit of normal sperm concentration is usually quoted as 20×10^6 ml. This figure is derived from

Table 25.1 The chances of conception related to sperm density and motility. The figures in the box represent the percentage chance of the couple reporting a pregnancy during the following 12 months. This analysis has been restricted to couples where the wife had known normal investigation results. This table can be used to give a couple a prognosis. (From Hargreave & Elton 1983, by permission of the editor of the British Journal of Urology)

		Months already trying to conceive			
		12	24	48	96
	Azoo	0	0	0	0
	0	0	0	0	0
	0.5	16	12	9	6
Millions of motile sperm per ml	*1.0*	25	19	14	9
	2.0	34	26	19	13
	5.0	36	28	21	14
	10.0+	37	28	21	14

comparison between fertile and infertile populations (MacLeod, 1951). However, if sperm concentration figures are examined from a population of infertile men in relation to the subsequent chance of pregnancy it is found that the prognosis deteriorates substantially only when the sperm concentration and motility fall below 1×10^6 motile sperm per ml (Table 25.1). This figure is very much lower than is conventionally accepted but is independently corroborated by results of treatment of azoospermic men with hypogonadotrophic hypogonadism when pregnancies occur with as few as 2×10^6 sperm in the ejaculate (Sherins, 1982). The clinical implications of these findings are that problems of ovulation should not be neglected on account of an apparently poor sperm count; it is unwise to counsel a man as infertile unless there are no sperm in the ejaculate but rather it is better to talk in terms of reduced chances.

Morphology

Sperm morphology may also be assessed but this measurement is time consuming and does not correlate well with clinical prognosis. This lack of correlation is probably because both man and the gorilla differ from all other animals in having a wide variation in normal sperm forms and it is difficult to know which variations are abnormal.

Immature forms

The presence of more than 3% immature sperms is considered to be a sign that spermatogenesis is under stress and this is usually accompanied by a marked rise in the percentage of tapering forms. These tapering forms of sperm head also appear in the ejaculate 14–21 days after the onset of acute viral illness or other testicular insult.

Zona-free test

It is now possible to fertilize human or animal eggs in

vitro. This technique seems likely to change our understanding of human fertility and revolutionize treatment of both male and female infertility. Hamster eggs from which the zona pellucida, the species specific barrier, has been removed are readily penetrated by heterologous sperm (Aitken, 1983) but why this is so is not understood. The property which as far as is known is particular to hamster eggs has allowed the development of a new test of sperm function which may give better prognostic clinical information than conventional sperm measurements as well as opening a new field of research into defects of fertilizing ability.

In vitro fertilization

Fertilization of the wife's or donor eggs in the test tube with subsequent reimplantation of the fertilized egg into the uterus is used to treat female infertility when the fallopian tubes are blocked and also male infertility when the chances of fertilization are thought to be very poor. This technique may be particularly valuable when the defect is poor sperm motility because placing selected sperm near the egg reduces the need for motility over long distances in the female genital tract.

Antisperm antibodies

Approximately 7% of infertile men have circulating and seminal plasma antibodies against sperm. The aetiology of these antibodies is not understood but there are two theories: either there is a breech in the blood testis barrier, probably in the epididymis, or infection in the prostate and seminal vesicles triggers autosensitization. One way antibodies interfere with fertility is by binding the antibody-coated sperm to cervical mucus so that the sperm, although motile, become trapped. Better understanding of the mechanisms of antisperm antibody induction and action may one day lead to new treatment for male infertility and possibly a new method of contraception.

AZOOSPERMIA

If there are no sperm in the ejaculate this is either because of severe damage to spermatogenesis or because of functional or mechanical obstruction. These two categories can be distinguished by examination of testicular size and by measurement of follicle stimulating hormone (FSH). Testis damage bad enough to cause azoospermia will result in small testes and will cause disturbance of feedback to the pituitary resulting in a high level of circulating FSH and testis biopsy is not necessary to define the problem (Hargreave & Jequier, 1978). If the FSH is normal then azoospermia is secondary to functional or mechanical obstruction. In cases with mechanical obstruction secondary to gonococcal epididymitis the operation of epididymovasostomy is very successful. In most cases in the UK there is no evidence of postgonnoccocal obstruction and the nature of the obstruction is not well defined. Some cases may be because of a congenital failure of fusion of ducts derived from the mesonephric duct (body and tail of the epididymis) and those which derive from the urogenital fold (the head of the epididymis). Some patients with obstructive azoospermia give a history of sinusitis or chest disease and investigation will reveal defects in mucociliary clearance. These cases are likely to be the result from an as yet undefined inborn error of metabolism. In 10% of cases of obstructive azoospermia there is congenital absence of both vasa; this is commonly missed on clinical examination. Unilateral absence of the vas is much rarer but when found is nearly always associated with an absent or ectopic kidney on that side.

DAMAGE TO SPERMATOGENESIS

The common situation in the infertility clinic is the man with poor sperm concentration and motility and an elevation of FSH. If testicular biopsy is done this usually shows generalized damage to spermatogenesis with hyalinization of seminiferous tubules. What causes this testicular damage? The germinal epithelium is known to be one of the most sensitive tissues in the body and indeed this property is exploited by the pharmaceutical industry in the mouse sperm test which is used as a toxicity screening test for mutagenic or carcinogenic compounds. Some proven causes of testicular damage are listed in Table 25.2 but in

Table 25.2 Damage to spermatogenesis

Trauma
   Tortion of the testis
Undescended testis
   May be related to maternal hormones
Orchitis
   Bacterial, fungal, viral (mumps)
Toxic chemicals
   Organic chemicals
   — Solvents
   — Pesticides
   Heavy metals
   — Lead
   — Cadmium
   — Mercury
Toxic environments
   Radiation at work
Treatment-related
   Cytotoxic agents
   Radiation therapy
   Dialysis
Over indulgence
   Alcohol
   ? smoking
Chromosomal abnormality

this age of environmental hazards there are likely to be many more; the epidemiology of infertility is still largely unresearched. In most cases it is impossible to define the problem but occasionally a dramatic situation arises where the whole work-force of a particular factory is affected. For example 76 men out of 133 making the pesticide kepone developed an illness characterized by nervousness, tremor, pains and oligozoospermia (Cannon et al, 1978).

There are some well known causes of damaged spermatogenesis. Mumps orchitis may result in infertility but remains an uncommon cause. Two other well-known causes are considered in more detail, chromosomal disorders and undescended testes.

Chromosomal disorders

Sperm fall into two categories—those carrying an X chromosome and those carrying a Y chromosome. Ova on the other hand all carry an X chromosome. As a result, subsequent zygotes may be XX (female) or XY (male). Anomalous combinations are possible and the resulting zygote may be viable. All but one of the X chromosomes in each somatic cell undergoes inactivation at an early stage in development and forms the sex chromatin body. Cytological studies have shown that in the cells of various tissues in different female animals, including the human, one chromosome appears darkly stained and is seen at the periphery of the nucleus underlying the nuclear membrane (Fig. 25.6). This sex chromatin body is interpreted as being the inactivated X chromosome. It is known that when an individual has two or more X chromosomes all but one of them become inactivated so that the number of chromatin bodies is alaways one less than the number of X chromosome. No chromatin bodies will therefore be found in the normal male XY or in Turner's syndrome in the female XO but one chromosome body will be detectable in cells of the normal female XX and in Klinefelter's syndrome in the male XXY. Nuclear sexing by means of

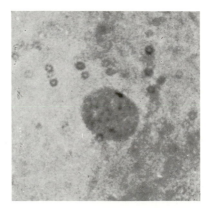

Fig. 25.6 From a buccal smear, stained only for nuclear material. At the periphery of the nucleus note the small densely stained chromatin body. (Courtesy of Dr P D Stewart, Vale of Leven Hospital.)

blood smears and scrapings of buccal mucosa (Barr & Bertram, 1949) is still widely used. Klinefelter's syndrome, XXY, is one of the commonest found in men presenting with infertility and is always associated with damaged spermatogenesis, usually azoospermia and often reduced testosterone output.

Testicular maldescent

The importance of testicular maldescent lies in the later complications of infertility and malignancy. There are three types of maldescent; retractile testes (migratory), ectopic testes and testes with arrested descent (undescended testes).

Retractile testes (migratory)

This is the commonest form of maldescent if indeed it can be called such for retraction of the testes to the external inguinal ring at the age of 5–6 years is physiologically normal. The testes lie in the scrotum at birth but when the cremasteric muscle reflex contractions develop they are pulled to the external inguinal ring. This reflex is most marked in 5- to 6-years which is unfortunately when school medical examinations are usually carried out. It would be better to screen new-born babies and to consider surgical correction in those babies where descent to the scrotum has not occurred by 1 year of age. Retractile testes will descend spontaneously at the age of 10.

Ectopic Testes

Ectopic testes are those which have been diverted from the normal pathway of descent by a mechanical barrier. The barrier is the result of inappropriate fibrous tissue growth into the developing gubernaculum and the commonest site is at the scrotal neck (Backhouse, 1964) Most ectopic testes lie in the superficial inguinal pouch just outside the external inguinal ring but more rarely they are found in the femoral or pubic region. Histological section of an ectopic testis will often show normal spermatogenesis and providing surgery is carried out before puberty fertility should be normal (Mack et al, 1962).

Arrested descent (undescended testes)

The testes may arrest at any point on the normal pathway of descent between the posterior abdominal wall and the scrotum. The surgical problem with this type of maldescent is that the testicular vessels and vas deferens will be shorter than the length required to reach the scrotum. This type of maldescent may be caused by a failure of the proper hormonal milieu during the later months of pregnancy or by an insensitivity of the target tissues to these hormones. Some defects of testes with arrested descent

have been described by Lackgren and Ploen (1984). Scott (1961) noted that in patients with unilateral undescent the opposite testis although palpably normal and fully descended was often histologically abnormal; hence the unexpectedly high incidence of sterility and subfertility in patients with unilateral testicular descent. Intra-abdominal and impalpable testes account for between 5 and 20% of cases but it must be remembered that although the sensitive process of spermatogenesis will be damaged, the Leydig cells and male hormone production will be normal wherever the testes, and thus patients with bilateral undescended testes will have normal male secondary sex characteristics and sex drive.

Complications of testicular maldescent

Undescended testes are more liable to trauma because they do not lie within the protection of the abdominal cavity nor are they free in the scrotum to move before a blow. The risk of malignancy in a patient with maldescent is 35 times the normal risk. The annual incidence of testicular tumour is 2.1–2.3 per 100 000 males so that the actual risk in the presence of a maldescended testis is still very low. It seems likely that the only testes subject to this increased risk are those with arrested descent (undescended testes) but because it is not always easy to distinguish from case records ectopic testes from those with undescent this is not absolutely certain. Possibly the same inherent tissue abnormality accounts for the arrested descent, the subsequent infertility and any tendency towards malignancy. Scott (1962) reported bilateral undescended testes resulting in complete sterility as well as finding impairment in unilateral cases. If the potential for fertility is to be conserved then orchiopexy should be performed before the developing seminiferous tubules can be damaged. The seminiferous tubules start to grow at 6 years with spermatogenesis being established by about the age of 11; thus ideally orchiopexy should be performed before the age of six particularly in those cases of arrested testicular descent. It is also possible that early orchiopexy may give some protection against subsequent malignancy but because of the difficulties in mounting prospective studies of sufficient duration and because of the difficulties with retrospective analysis of case records, this has not yet been proven.

EFFECTS OF CASTRATION

Orchidectomy removes the source of both spermatozoa and testicular hormones; sterility is invariable but the somatic changes vary with age. Much of our knowledge of the male accessory organs stems from experiments by John Hunter who was the first to note postcastrate recession of the prostate and seminal vesicles.

Before puberty

If castration is performed before puberty secondary sex characteristics fail to develop. The penis, seminal vesicles and prostate remain small and immature; the voice remains high-pitched, hair does not grow on the face, trunk or axillae and pubic hair is of feminine distribution. Abnormal deposits of fat may appear in the breasts, buttocks and hips but generalized obesity is not invariable. Fusion of the epiphyses is delayed but growth in length may also be retarded, so whilst some will become long-limbed giants, others will develop normal stature. The skin is pale and exposure to sunshine seldom produces a tan. Sexual desire is absent. Intellectual power is rarely impaired but a sense of mutilation may produce profound psychological disturbance.

After puberty

Castration after puberty is followed by atrophy of the seminal vesicles and prostate as these glands rely on testosterone for their maintenance but the extragenital secondary sex characteristics are not affected. Sexual desire and reaction frequently disappear but in many cases successful coitus has continued. The psychological trauma of adult castration may be profound. Because of the involution of the hormone-dependent, secondary sex glands there is a diminution in the volume of seminal fluid and all its constituents. These changes can be reversed by the administration of testosterone. The most common indication for bilateral orchiectomy is in the treatment of prostatic cancer usually in elderly men when these effects may be less marked.

EFFECTS OF VASECTOMY

Bilateral vasectomy for contraceptive purposes is now one of the most frequently performed minor operations in the UK. This has in part resulted from worry about the use of long-term oral contraceptives and because of the lack of other aesthetically acceptable methods. In the majority of cases azoospermia will be achieved 3 months after operation. Dodds (1972) found 10.5% of 1600 cases had some sperm at 3 months and one patient in his series continued to produce sperm until 17 months after operation. One explanation for this is infrequent ejaculation; Marwood and Beral (1979) reported that coital frequency of less than once per week in men aged 40 or over was associated with longer periods before azoospermia was achieved. Occasionally the vasa regain patency months or even years after vasectomy and it is therefore unwise to guarantee vasectomy as a method of absolute contraception although the chances of late failure are very low.

In most experimental animals there is temporary depression of spermatogenesis immediately after vasectomy followed later by a gradual return to normal. Biochemical changes are more profound there being a marked reduction in free amino acids and an increase in fructose and citric acid (Mann, 1964). These results might suggest increased androgen activity but no endocrine consequences following vasectomy has been reported despite careful search (Hargreave, 1983). Up to 50% of men develop antisperm antibodies following vasectomy. These antibodies do not cross-react with other somatic antigens so there is no direct risk to other cells but secondary effects could occur. Post-vasectomy patchy orchitis has been reported in cats, mice, rats, guinea pigs, rabbits and man, but in most cases it is not known whether this orchitis is the result of immune response against testicular tissue or whether it is simply the result of reabsorption of sperm. In rabbits, the lesion has been shown to be secondary to immune complex orchitis (Bigazzi et al, 1976). Vasectomy has also been reported to increase the incidence of diet-induced atherosclerosis in the cynomolgus monkey (Alexander & Clarkson, 1978). In this experiment monkeys were fed on a diet containing twice as much cholesterol as that consumed by the average North American male and plasma cholesterol levels in the monkeys of 500 mg/dl were at least twice as high as those found in North American men. This atherosclerosis is thought to result from interaction between the high cholesterol levels and deposition of immune complex on the vessel walls. Does this happen in man? Circulating immune complexes have been found in man following vasectomy (Helleman et al, 1979), but so far epidemiological studies have not recorded any differences in auto-immune, cardiovascular or endocrine disease in man following vasectomy (Goldacre et al, 1978). Antibodies may prejudice attempts at vasectomy reversal because if they are present in the seminal plasma they interfere with fertility.

PHYSIOLOGY OF ERECTION

Erection and orgasm are the result of co-ordination between parasympathetic and sympathetic nervous systems. There is also a rich supply of peptigenic nerves to the erectile tissue. Erection of the penis is brought about by the nervi erigentes S2, 3 and 4 relaxing the muscle coats of the penile arteries and allowing greater blood flow into the erectile tissue. In addition to the augmentation of blood flow, there is some constriction of outflow (Brindley, 1983). The erectile tissue consists of the right and left corpora cavernosa which freely communicate with each other and the corpus spongiosum around the urethra and communicating with the erectile tissue of the glans. In addition to the haemodynamic component of erection the erectile tissue is largely comprised of smooth muscle (Meehan & Goldstein, 1983) and contraction of this smooth muscle against the column of blood further increases the efficiency of the erection.

At orgasm, semen is ejaculated by rhythmical contractions of the epididymis, vasa, seminal vesicles, prostate, bulbo and ischiocavernosus muscles; at the same time the bladder neck closes to prevent reflux into the bladder. This muscular action is the result of sympathetic activity mediated by the hypogastric nerve and can be simulated by electrical stimulation per rectum to the presacral area. Electro-ejaculation has been widely used to collect semen from cattle and in some cases from paraplegic men; if sensation is normal however, the procedure is too painful without general anaesthesia.

Presacral neurectomy or bilateral sympathectomy below L2 will prevent ejaculation but has no effect on erection. Ganglion blocking drugs such as hexamethonium by inhibiting both sympathetic and parasympathetic pathways, will reduce both ejaculation and erection and this effect is seen after many of the older antihypertensive drugs. Lesions affecting all the sacral nerves below S1, by severing the parasympathetic outflow, will abolish erections but ejaculation is still possible.

The female menopause has no such dramatic corollary in the male. Spermatogenesis as discussed above may continue in a patchy fashion into old age and likewise potency. 50% of men aged 65 coming for the operation of prostatectomy will be potent (Hargreave & Stephenson, 1977) and it is worthwhile bearing this in mind when counselling these men prior to operation. The cause of impotence in older men is not understood; in general the nerve pathways are intact although in rare cases there may be autonomic neuropathy secondary to diseases such as diabetes. In some cases arterial thickening is sufficient to prevent blood flow for erection. Primary psychological impotence is not so common as is often thought. Organic as opposed to psychogenic impotence can usually be distinguished by the presence of normal sleep erections or by the presence of an erection following intra-corporeal injection of papavarine. It should be remembered however that many men with organic impotence have psychological sequelae, the most common being anxiety about their failing performance. Erections can be measured by penile plethysmography; penile blood flow can be estimated by Doppler analysis and anatomy of the corpora can be demonstrated by injection of contrast and radiology.

TESTICULAR PAIN

The testicle and its coverings are sensitive to pain. The scrotum, tunica vaginalis and testes derive their sensory nerves from different sources. The scrotum is supplied by cutaneous branches of the pudendal nerves, from spinal segments S2 to S4. The tunica vaginalis is supplied by the genital branch of the genitofemoral nerve from segments LI and L2. The opportunity to scratch the tunica vaginalis with the point of a needle arises during the aspiration of hydrocele fluid, as noted by Brown (1949). When the

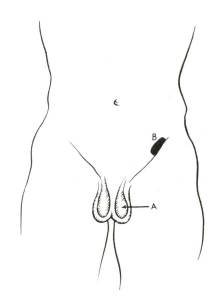

Fig. 25.7 Pain, induced by injecting hypertonic saline into the testicle at A, is experienced above the inguinal ligament at B. (After Brown, 1949.)

scrotal skin has been anaesthetized with procaine the blindfold patient is unaware of the needle puncture but experiences pain when the visceral or parietal portions of the tunica vaginalis are scratched. The pain is located in the scrotum but is not severe. It can be abolished by filling the tunica vaginalis with procaine solution (Fig. 25.7).

Sensory nerves from the testicle accompany the sympathetic nerves and enter the spinal cord between segments D10 and L2. Pure testicular pain can be elicited after anaesthetizing the scrotal skin and tunica vaginalis with procaine by injecting hypertonic saline into the testes (Brown, 1949). The pain experienced is severe, sickening and located within the scrotum but above the inguinal ring. The position corresponds with the site of origin of the testicle. Brown points out that it is a mistake to consider that the testicle takes origin in the loin, the final position of the kidney, since the upward migration of the kidney takes place after the testicle has become differentiated. The clinical application of this site of referred pain is amply demonstrated in tortion of the testes (Robb, 1956) and in tortion of the hydatid of Morgani (McNair, 1961).

Segmental pain arising naturally in the renal tract or artificially after the injection of hypertonic saline into the supraspinatous ligaments which range between D12 and L2, can radiate in the male to the scrotum and in the female to the labium. The nervous pathway involved is the genitofemoral nerve which is distributed in the male to the tunica vaginalis and in the female to the ligamentum teres.

Acknowledgement

In the previous editions of this book the chapter on the testis was written by the late Stuart Scott. I would like to acknowledge my debt to Mr Scott, who was my teacher.

REFERENCES

Aitken J 1983 The zona-free hamster egg penetration test. In: Hargreave T B (ed) Male Infertility Springer Verlag, Berlin p 75–86

Alexander N J, Clarkson T B 1978 Vasectomy increases the severity of diet-induced atherosclerosis in macaca fascicularis. Science 201: 538–541

Backhouse K M 1964 The gubernaculum testis Hunteri: testicular descent and maldescent. Annals of the Royal College of Surgeons 35: 15–33

Barr M L, Bertram E G 1949 A morphological distinction between neurone of the male and female, and the behaviour of the nucleolar satellite during accelerated nucleoprotein synthesis. Nature 163: 676–677

Bedford J M, Calvin H, Cooper G W 1973 The maturation of spermatozoa in the human epididymis. Journal of Reproduction and Fertility (Suppl.) 18: 199–213

Bigazzi P E, Kosuda L L, Hus K C, Andres G A 1976 Immune complex orchitis in vasectomised rabbbits. Journal of Experimental Medicine 143: 382–404

Brindley G S 1983 Sexual physiology in normal and paraplegic men. In: Hargreave T B (ed) Human Male Infertility. Springer-Verlag, Berlin. p 261–279

Brown F R 1949 Testicular Pain. Its significance and localisation. Lancet, i: 994–999

Cannon S B, Veazey J M, Jackson R S, Burse V W, Hayes C, Straub W E et al 1978 Epidemic kepone poisoning chemical workers. American Journal of Epidemiology 107: 529–537

Charney W C, Conston, A S, Meranze D R 1952 Development of the testes. A histological study from birth to maturity with some notes on abnormal variations. Fertility and Sterility, 3: 461–477

Dodds D J 1972 Reanastomosis of the vas deferens. Journal of the American Medical Associations 220:1498

Glover T D 1981 The Epididymis. In: Chisholm G D, Williams D I (ed) Scientific foundations of Urology, 2nd edn. Heineman Medical Books, London. p 544–555

Goldacre M J, Clarke J A, Heasman M A, Vessey M P 1978 Follow up of vasectomy using medical record linkage. American Journal of Epidemiology 108: 176–180

Habib F k, Lee I R, Stitch S R, Smith P H 1976 Androgen levels in the plasma and prostatic tissues of patients with benign hypertrophy and carcinoma of the prostate. Journal of Endocrinology 71 99–107

Hargreave T B 1983 Vasectomy. In: Hargreave T B (ed) Springer-Verlag, Berlin. p 297–308

Hargreave T B 1985 Artificial insemination by donor. (Leading article) British Medical Journal, 291: 613–614

Hargreave T B, Elton R A 1983 Is conventional sperm analysis of any use? British Journal of Urology 55: 774–779

Hargreave T B, Jequier A M 1978 Can follicle stimulating hormone estimation replace testicular biopsy in the diagnosis of obstructive azoospermia? British Journal of Urology 50: 415–418

Hargreave T B, Stephenson T P 1977 Potency and prostatectomy. British Journal of Urology 49: 683–688

Helleman H W J, Samuel T, Rumke Ph 1979 Sperm autoantibodies as a consequence of vasectomy. ii: Long term follow-up studies. Clinical and Experimental Immunology 38: 31–36

Heller, C G, Clermont Y 1963 Spermatogenesis in man: an estimate of its duration. Science, 140: 184–186

Henderson B E, Benton B, Jing J, Yu M C, Pike, M C 1979 Risk factors for cancer of the testes in young men. International Journal of Cancer, 23: 598–602

James K, Hargreave T B 1984 Immunosuppression by seminal plasma and its possible clinical significance. Immunology Today, 5: 357–363

Lackgren G, Ploen L 1975 The morphology of the human undescended testis with special reference to the sertoli cell and puberty. International Journal of Andrology 7: 23–38

Lofts B 1978 Testicular function: a comparative viewpoint. Journal of the Royal College of Surgeons (Edin.), 23: 67–80

MacLeod J 1951 Semen quality in 1000 men of known fertility and in 800 cases of infertile marriage. Fertility and Sterility 2: 115–139

McNair T J 1961 Torsion of the hydatid of Morgani with special reference to the site of pain. Journal of the Royal College of Surgeons (Edin.), 7: 48–54.

Mack W S, Scott L S, Ferguson Smith M A, Lennox B 1962. Ectopic testes and true undescended testes: a histological comparison. Journal of Pathology and Bacteriology 82: 439–443

Mancini R E, Andrada J A, Saraceni A, Bachmann A E, Lavieri J C, Nemridousky 1965. Immunological and testicular response in man sensitised with human testicular homogenate. Journal of Clinical Endocrinology 25: 859–875

Mann T 1964 The biochemistry of semen and the male reproductive tract. John Wiley and Sons, New York

Mann T, Lutwak Mann C 1981 Male reproductive function and semen. Themes and trends in physiology, biochemistry and investigative andrology. Springer-Verlag, Berlin

Marwood R P, Beral V 1979 Disappearance of spermatozoa from the ejaculate after vasectomy. British Medical Journal 1:87

Maxted W, Baker R, McCrystal H, Fitzgerald E 1965 Complete masculinization of the external genitalia in congenital adrenocortical hyperplasia. Presentation of two cases. Journal of Urology 94: 266–270

Meehan J P, Goldstein A M B 1983 High pressure within the corpus cavernosum in man during erection—its probable mechanism Urology 21: 385–387

Raynaud A 1958 L'appareil gubernaculaire du fetus de souris et ces modifications experimentales. Bulletin de la société zoologique de France 83: 340–347

Ritchie A W S, Hargreave T B, James K, Chisholm G D 1984 Intra-epithelial lymphocytes in the normal epididymis. A mechanism for tolerance to sperm auto-antigens? British Journal of Urology 56: 79–83

Robb W A T 1956 Torsion of the spermatic cord. Journal of the Royal College of Surgeons (Edin.) 2: 71–76

Rothschild L, 1962 Spermatozoa. British Medical Journal 2: 743–749

Rumke, Ph. (1980). Can oligozoospermia be induced by autoimmunity? In: Frajese G (ed) Proceedings of the International Symposium on Oligozoospermia: Recent Progress in Andrology. Raven Press, New York: p 185–197

Schirren C 1963 Relation between fructose content of semen and fertility in man. Journal of Reproduction and Fertility 5: 347–358

Scorer C G, Farrington G H 1971 Congenital deformities of the testis and epididymis. Butterworths, London

Scott L S, 1961 Unilateral cryptorchidism subsequent affects on fertility. Journal of Reproduction and Fertility 2: 54–60

Scott L S 1962 Fertility in cryptorchidism. Proceedings of the Royal Society of Medicine, 55: 1047–1050

Setchell B P, Waites G M H 1975 The blood testis barrier. In Hamilton D W, Greep R O (eds) Male reproductive system, section 7, Endocrinology. Handbook of physiology, Vol v. American physiological society, Washington DC, p 143–172

Sherins R J 1982 Treatment of hypogonadotrophic hypogonadism. In: Garcia C R, Mastroanni L, Dubin L, Amelar R D (eds), Current therapy of Infertility 1982–83. P14 Pub C V Mosby, New York

Tittmar H G 1978 Seasonal fluctuation in condom retrieval. IRCS Medical Science Anatomy and Human Biology 6:135

Tjoa W S, Smolensky M H, Hsi B D, Steinberger E, Smith K D 1982 Circannual rhythm in human sperm count revealed by serially independent sampling. Fertility and Sterility 38: 454–459

Ovary

The ovary has two main functions, the production of germ cells (gametogenesis) and the secretion of sex hormones. It cannot be considered, however, as an independent organ; it is a link in a complex chain which extends from the hypothalamus and pituitary to the external genitalia.

FETAL DEVELOPMENT

The ovary, like the testis, develops as a thickening of the coelomic epithelium over the urogenital ridge. The gonad, until 6 weeks of fetal life, is undifferentiated but is made up of a cortical and medullary part. In females the cortex becomes the main substance of the ovary whereas in males the medullary portion develops to become the testis. It is not yet fully understood how the bisexuality of the gonad at this very early stage of development is changed; it is due to some complex, sex-determining mechanism, dependent upon genetic and not hormonal factors because, in the human, hormones have no effect on fetal gonadal differentiation although they may have some effect on the developing genitalia.

The germ cells, which are present in the undifferentiated gonad, probably arise near the yolk sac and travel via the mesentery to the gonads (Witschi, 1948). In the past it was thought that the germ cells arose from the coelomic epithelium which accounts for the term germinal epithelium, applied to the layer of cells surrounding the ovary. This is now know to be a complete misnomer. As early as 6–8 weeks of fetal life the testis can be recognized by its complex pattern of sex cords containing medullary germ cells (Pryse-Davies, 1974). If these cords are not apparent the gonad is a rudimentary ovary.

During embryological development there is a considerable increase in the number of germ cells (now called oogonia) in the ovary (700 to 7 000 000). These oogonia eventually become the oocytes within primordial follicles. Primordial follicles can be recognized in the ovary after 20 weeks of foetal life. The germ cells are surrounded by coelomic epithelium which in adult life will be the gran-ulosa cells of developing follicles, while mesenchyme from the urogenital ridge gives rise to the theca interna and ovarian stroma (Pryse-Davies, 1974). During the latter part of pregnancy there is a decrease in the number of germ cells present within the ovary. This decrease is due to atretic degeneration leaving about 2000 primordial follicles present in the ovary at birth (Baker, 1963).

It is surprising that the maternal hormones have much less effect on the fetal ovary than on other parts of the genital tract of the fetus. The development of an ovarian cyst or the presence of cystic ovaries are rare events in the newborn.

At birth the main part of the cortex of the ovary is made up of primordial follicles, stroma cells and blood vessels. The medulla lies deep to the developing follicles and consists of loose, vascular stroma containing mesonephric ducts and tubular remnants.

During the neonatal period and childhood there is further regression or atresia of many of the primordial follicles. Only a small number, probably a few hundred, are destined to reach maturity during the reproductive life of the female. These follicles develop by proliferation of pregranulosal epithelial cells to form a multilayered granulosa. Condensation of stromal cells surrounding these primary follicles form what are called the thecal layers. Once the granulosa cavitates to form an antrum the development of what is known as the Graafian follicle is complete (named after Regner de Graaf who first described them in 1672).

Ovarian function is centred on the Graafian follicle. From it the ovum is extruded and the various cellular components of the follicle are responsible for the production of the principal ovarian hormones.

THE OVARIAN CYCLE

Hormone production by the ovary is responsible for the menstrual cycle of the female. Although the menstrual cycle is the outward manifestation of female reproductive function, similar cyclical changes take place both in the pituitary gland and in the ovary during the reproductive years.

Gonadotropins secreted by the anterior lobe of the pituitary have a direct effect on the ovary. These gonadotropins are known as follicular-stimulating hormone (FSH) and luteinizing hormone (LH). Follicular-stimulating hormone is responsible for commencing maturation of the ovarian follicles. To begin with, several follicles start to ripen under its influence. The factors determining which follicle should ripen completely, and why that follicle is the one from which the ovum is shed are not completely understood. Prior to ovulation taking place there is a burst of luteinizing hormone secretion which probably triggers off ovulation and is responsible for the development of the corpus luteum. Coincident with this LH surge there is a smaller peak of FSH production, the significance of which is not clear (Midgley & Jaffee, 1968). There is also a burst of oestradiol production prior to the rise in LH (Diczfalusy & Landgren, 1977). If fertilization of the ovum does not occur, the ovarian cycle continues.

The action of FSH and LH is not the only determining factor in ovarian function since the release of these gonadotrophic hormones from the anterior pituitary is controlled by the hypothalamus by means of a direct vascular connection, the hypophysioportal system. Polypeptide chemical transmitters, thought to be produced by the arcuate nucleus of the hypothalamus, are considered to be the mechanism by which gonadotropic hormone release is brought about. How many of these releasing hormones exist is not known. Luteinizing hormone-releasing hormone (LHRH) is now well recognized and has been synthesized. Doubt exists as to whether there is a separate follicular stimulation releasing hormone which provokes FSH production as well as LH RH stimulation and LH output from the anterior pituitary. It is possible that the one transmitter fulfils both functions and would

be better termed GRH (gonadotrophin releasing hormone). From experimental and clinical observation LH RH is normally secreted in episodic bursts at hourly intervals which is sufficient to stimulate LH secretion. The basis of cyclical activity throughout the female reproductive system is probably due to what is called the hypothalamic clock (Beck et al, 1973).

Hypothalamic activity can be modified by external influences such as emotional or psychological events and also by a feedback mechanism determined by the level of circulating oestrogen or progesterone. Similarly, there may be a short-loop feedback mechanism directly concerned with the production of FSH and LH (Fig. 26.1).

As the Graafian follicle matures under the influence of FSH and later LH, the developing ovum is surrounded by the zona pellucida and an accumulation of granulosa cells known as the cumulus oophorus. This protrudes into the cavity of the follicle now filled with fluid (Fig. 26.2). The innermost lining of the follicle still consists of granulosa cells which make up the membrana granulosa.

Just before ovulation takes place the ovum with its surrounding cumulus oophorus floats free. Outside the membrana granulosa the cells of the ovarian stroma give rise to a well vascularised layer known as the theca interna.

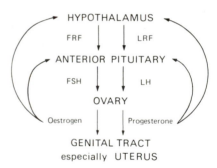

Fig. 26.1 Hormonal control of ovarian function.

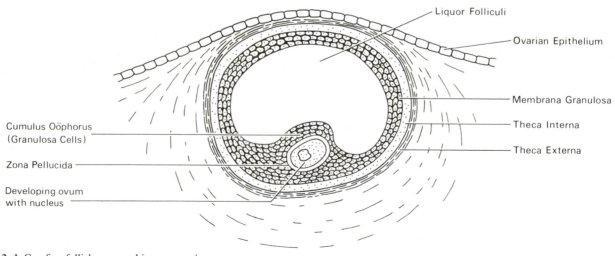

Fig. 26.2 A Graafian follicle approaching maturation.

The theca externa surrounds the theca interna and is formed by tissue compression as the follicle increases in size; it is composed chiefly of connective tissue.

To allow ovulation to take place the projecting surface of the follicle, covered by ovarian (germinal) epithelium breaks down and the ovum is released with the liquor folliculi. The mechanism controlling the actual follicular rupture is not apparent but proteolytic enzymes may be involved (Rondell, 1970). The free ovum passes into the Fallopian tube. If it is to be fertilized it must be penetrated by a spermatozoon within 12 hours of extrusion, otherwise it undergoes degenerative changes and is incapable of normal development. This is the basis of the so-called 'safe period' which, as a means of contraception, is only 'safe' provided the day of ovulation can be forecast accurately.

When ovulation has occurred the wall of the follicle collapses inwards and fills the space left by the escaped ovum. A small blood clot is usually present as well. Hypertrophy of the cells of the membrana granulosa eventually replaces the clot and forms a mass of lipid-filled granulosa lutein cells. There is also proliferation of the theca interna giving rise to theca lutein cells. Thus the corpus luteum is formed; it can be recognized on inspection of the ovary by its yellow appearance due to the large amount of lipid in the cells.

If pregnancy occurs the corpus luteum continues to enlarge and may reach 3 or 4 cm in diameter. At this stage it can be palpated on bi-manual pelvic examination and is liable to be misdiagnosed as an ectopic pregnancy or as an ovarian cyst. Operative interference should be avoided and further enlargement does not occur after the third month of pregnancy.

In the absence of conception the corpus luteum degenerates and forms a corpus albicans, a small mass of scarred tissue which can be seen on the ovary. When present these signify that ovulation has taken place at some time or other. Simple atresia of follicles which never reach maturity cannot be seen so easily. In the investigation of the infertile female patient it is important to be able to recognize on macroscopic examination of the ovary or on microscopic examination of an ovarian biopsy a corpus luteum, corpora albicantes or atretic follicles.

Hormones produced by the ovary

Ovarian metabolism of steroid hormones is exceedingly complex. After synthesis by the ovary the steroid hormones are secreted into the peripheral circulation mostly bound to plasma proteins (Williams-Ashman & Reddi, 1971) and thus reach the target tissues. The mechanism by which steroid hormones act on target cells is not clearly understood (Grant, 1969).

Although a large number of steroid hormones are produced by the ovary, for practical purposes the three main ones are oestrogen, progesterone and androstene-dione. Though the last is important if its output is increased thus reflecting a degree of abnormality, the first two are essential to normal reproduction in the female.

Oestrogen

Oestrogen is produced by the granulosa cells, the cells of the theca interna of the ripening ovarian follicle and from the corpus luteum. Small amounts of oestrogen may be produced by the adrenal which could account for the oestrogen found in the urine of prepubertal girls and of women who have had their ovaries removed surgically.

Oestradiol 17β is the major oestrogen secreted by the ovary and is the most potent (Fig. 26.3).

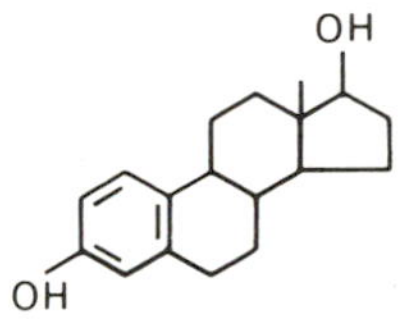

Fig. 26.3 Oestradiol 17-β.

Oestrone and oestriol, metabolized from oestradiol 17β, are also found in substantial amounts in the plasma. In the liver oestrogens are oxidized or converted to glucoronide and sulphate conjugates. These may be secreted in the bile and reabsorbed back into the blood stream. In the presence of liver disease such as cirrhosis oestrogen metabolism can be impaired. High circulating oestrogen levels may result, which can give rise to postmenopausal bleeding or the development of skin lesions. About a 10th of the total ovarian secretion of oestrogen is recovered in the urine (Keele & Neil, 1971).

At least 10 metabolites of oestrogen appear but the three main ones — oestradiol, oestrone and oestriol — can be assayed separately. Oestrogens are excreted throughout the menstrual cycle rising after the end of menstruation to a peak about the time of ovulation and diminishing gradually thereafter, except for a small peak late in the luteal phase just a few days before the onset of menstruation (Brown et al, 1958). The first peak of oestrogen production corresponds to the active phase of follicular ripening while the second peak is associated with the corpus luteum and does not occur in the absence of ovulation. The cyclical variation of oestrogen production is not found in premenarcheal (Pennington & Dewhurst, 1969) or postmenopausal females, but a wide variation of oestrogen excretion levels may be found at these times.

Effect of oestrogen on different tissues and organs. The closer to the age of puberty a girl becomes the more oestrogen is excreted and cyclical variations occur. It is at this time in the life of the female that the effects of oestrogens on various organs are best observed. At the climacteric when oestrogen levels fall, various changes due to lack of oestrogen also become apparent. The naturally-occurring oestrogens have an effect on many tissues and organs and even on the ovary itself. Oestrogen by some means facilitates the growth of the Graafian follicle. In contrast it is responsible for a decrease in secretion of FSH and LH by a feedback mechanism through both the hypothalamus and pituitary. Actual enlargement of the pituitary can be caused by high circulating oestrogen levels; if there is any evidence to suggest enlargement of the pituitary, whatever the cause, a patient should be warned of the dangers of pregnancy, because of the marked increase in circulating oestrogen; for the same reason the administration of exogenous oestrogen for either contraception or menopausal symptoms should be avoided.

Oestrogen is responsible for the growth and duct development of the breasts at puberty, as well as pigmentation of the nipple areola (Goodman & Gilman, 1970).

It is difficult to determine the part played by oestrogens in female configuration apart from breast development. The narrow shoulders and broad hips, converging thighs and diverging arms and the fat distribution peculiar to the female over the buttocks and breasts may be due to lack of androgen rather than the effect of oestrogens, since similar characteristics are found in castrate males.

The various parts of the genital tract are very responsive to oestrogen. The effects are most apparent on the endometrium of the uterus since oestrogen is responsible for the proliferative phase of the endometrium and, together with progesterone, maintains the secretory phase. Without the effect of progesterone the endometrium continues to proliferate and the condition of cystic glandular hyperplasia develops. This is most commonly found at the beginning and the end of female reproductive life.

Oestrogen causes a hyperaemia and hypertrophy of the uterine smooth muscle most obvious during pregnancy; however, the role of oestrogens in the initiation of labour remains as obscure as ever.

The effect of oestrogen on the cervix of the uterus is reflected in the cervical mucus which becomes thinner, less viscid and more alkaline. The survival and transport of spermatozoa are accordingly enhanced.

The vaginal epithelium becomes cornified under the influence of oestrogen and cornified cells can be seen in vaginal smears. Lack of cornification, as seen in the postmenopausal patient, renders the vaginal mucosa more liable to infection and the condition can be termed true oestrogen-deficiency vaginitis rather than senile vaginitis as it is commonly called. The use of oestrogen locally as a cream not only causes the vaginal epithelium to show improved cornification but also restores the normal pH of the vagina.

Lack of circulating oestrogen also causes senile changes in the vulva. There is loss of fat in the labia majora and the labia minora tend to disappear or coalesce. This can cause pruritis which will respond to local oestrogen therapy. Oestrogens may increase Fallopian tube motility.

General skin manifestations associated with abnormally high oestrogen levels are seen in patients with liver disease when the red 'liver palms' and spider angiomas are almost certainly due to an increase in circulating oestrogen consequent to poor liver function. A similar appearance may be seen during pregnancy.

The effect of oestrogen on different tissues may vary according to the oestrogen receptors in the particular tissue. Insufficient is as yet known about these receptors and their variations to be certain what part they do actually play.

Oestrogen induces retention of sodium and consequently water. Weight gain during the second half of the menstrual cycle is due to increase in body fluid and women at this time may experience generalized discomfort, swelling of the ankles, irritability and a feeling of fullness in the abdomen and breasts. Mental depression is occasionally present as well. This is known as the premenstrual tension syndrome. Unfortunately, not all cases are alleviated either by the use of progestogens to counteract the effect of oestrogen or the use of diuretics to get rid of retained fluid. The use of spirolactone, pyridomine, bromocriptine and Primrose oil in attempting to relieve such symptoms indicates how poorly understood the condition really is; that it is entirely due to oestrogens would seem unlikely.

Oestrogen is thought to lower plasma cholesterol levels. The effect is almost certainly due to the action of the hormone on the lipoproteins associated with cholesterol. This may account for the lower incidence of myocardial infarction and other complications of atherosclerotic disease found in women before middle age. After the menopause, when the ovary no longer produces oestrogen, the prevalence of atherosclerotic disease increases and becomes similar to that in the male.

When ovarian production of oestrogen wanes, the female is much more liable to osteoporosis, which can cause scoliosis and backache (Nordin et al, 1968) and fractures become more common (Smith et al, 1969). Oestrogen exerts an anticatabolic effect on skeletal tissue and thus prevents the excess bone reabsorption that usually starts during the female climacteric. It has been shown that the osteoporotic effect may start even a decade before the actual cessation of menstruation, but proving that this is due to oestrogen deficiency would be difficult (Aitken et al, 1973).

Progesterone

Unlike other ovarian steroids which may be produced even if in limited quantities by the adrenal, in the non-pregnant female, progesterone is almost exclusively of ovarian origin. Circulating progesterone levels reflect

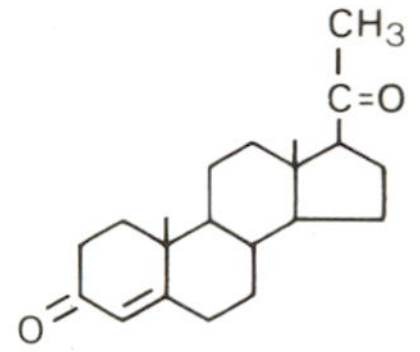

Fig. 26.4 Progesterone.

therefore true ovarian function better than any other steroid. Progesterone (Fig. 26.4) is secreted by theca lutein and granulosa lutein cells of the corpus luteum of the ovary. It is converted in the liver to pregnanediol which is conjugated with glucuronic acid and excreted in the urine. The output in the urine is probably 10–40% of the total production and therefore it is of value to determine the amount of urinary pregnanediol if attempting to assess the function of the corpus luteum. During the follicular phase of the menstrual cycle the output of progesterone is scarcely above that found in the male but after ovulation the output increases significantly and only diminishes towards the end of the cycle if pregnancy has not occurred. If fertilization takes place the level of progesterone secretion rises with the development of the corpus luteum of pregnancy and continues to rise throughout pregnancy due to production by the placenta.

Effect of progesterone on different tissues and organs. Unless very large amounts of progesterone are in circulation it has no action on organs not previously primed by oestrogen. The action of progesterone is basically antagonistic to oestrogen and therefore a fine balance of both hormones is required to produce maximum effects. Progesterone and oestrogen are responsible for the endometrial changes found in the second half of the menstrual cycle. This secretory phase of the endometrium is indicative of ovulation having taken place. Accordingly, in the investigation of the infertile female, endometrial biopsy carried out in the premenstrual phase should establish whether ovulation is taking place or not. If there is no evidence of secretory activity it merely means that ovulation has not taken place during that one cycle and may not necessarily be a constant feature. The corollary is also true.

Progesterone decreases the excitability of myometrial cells as well as their sensitivity to oxytocin and their spontaneous electrical activity. The clinical use of progesterone, however, in attempts to arrest uterine activity has been disappointing.

The action of progesterone on cervical mucus is to cause it to become thicker and more viscid with an increase in its cellular content. If cervical mucus is spread on to a glass slide to dry and then examined microscopically, these cellular elements are recognized if there is adequate circulating progesterone. If progestational activity is not present or greatly diminished the cervical mucus dries out in the so-called ferning pattern due to its crystal content. This test is of help in establishing whether ovulation is taking place or whether menstrual cycles are anovulatory with no progestational phase.

Progesterone is thought to evoke epithelial proliferation in the vagina and an increase in mucus secretion.

In the breast, development of lobules and alveoli are brought about by progesterone. This activity is greatly increased during pregnancy when the level of circulating progesterone is much higher than normal, due to the contribution from the placenta.

It is not certain whether the rise in basal body temperature consequent to ovulation is due to the action of progesterone. Secretion from the developing corpus luteum would hardly have such an immediate effect. The rise in body temperature is of value to couples wishing to increase the chance of conception since it will indicate when intercourse should take place. In contrast, if a patient can establish when ovulation takes place by studying her daily temperature, it can be used to indicate when intercourse should not take place if pregnancy is to be avoided; this however, is an unreliable method of contraception.

Progesterone has an indirect effect on the ovary; it is antagonistic to follicular development and can inhibit LH secretion. These actions are either through the hypothalamus or directly on the anterior pituitary.

It is interesting that alveolar P_{CO_2} falls during pregnancy as the circulating progesterone increases. This phenomenon is seen to a lesser extent in the luteal phase of the menstrual cycle. If progesterone alone is involved in producing this effect it must have the properties of a respiratory stimulant.

Androstenedione

Androstenedione is secreted in small amounts by the ovary. It is produced by the cells of the ovarian stroma. Tissue remnants from the undifferentiated ovary may be responsible for this although it has been suggested that cyclical changes occur in the stroma of the ovary. Androstenedione is converted in the liver to testosterone. Increase in ovarian androgen production means either the presence of a virilising tumour or the patient is suffering from the Stein-Leventhal syndrome. (see below)

Relaxin

It is thought that the ovary secretes, especially during pregnancy, a non-steroid polypeptide hormone known as relaxin. Its chemical structure is complex although in some ways it resembles human insulin. The cells of the ovary responsible for its secretion are probably in the corpus luteum of pregnancy.

Its main function is to help parturition by its 'relaxing' effect on the symphysis pubis and sacro-iliac joints. It may also have a softening effect on the cervix and may decrease uterine motility. In the non-pregnant, it is thought to enhance the effects of oestrogen and progesterone on the genital tract.

INVESTIGATION OF OVARIAN FUNCTION

Because of the complex relationships between the hypothalamus, the pituitary and the ovary, assessment of ovarian function alone can be very difficult. Symptoms which seem to indicate malfunction of the ovary may be due to lack of stimulation by higher centres, or failure of response of target organs.

Ovarian activity may require to be investigated in clinical conditions such as primary or secondary amenorrhoea or oligomenorrhoea, infertility and some cases of menorrhagia. Precocious puberty, virilisation or suspicion of a hormone secreting tumour may also call for further investigations.

There are three methods of assessing ovarian function:

1. Appropriate hormone assay
2. Histological examination of the endometrium
3. Laparoscopy and ovarian biopsy
4. Examination of the ovaries using ultrasound

Other investigations such as the taking of basal body temperature daily, examination of cervical mucus and cytological examination of desquamated vaginal epithelium may indicate ovulation but cannot be regarded as wholly reliable.

Hormone assay

Estimations of the urinary excretion of oestrogen and pregnanediol throughout a menstrual cycle can, of course, indicate whether ovulation is occurring (Pepperell et al, 1975). Unusually low oestrogen excretion may indicate ovarian failure. Pregnanediol excretion at the level of that in the male is found with anovulatory cycles, whereas the oestrogen output may rise significantly. Serum oestrogen and progesterone levels are reasonably simple assays and have largely replaced the need for urine collections, except in special circumstances when diurnal variations may be important. If estimations of FSH and LH are carried out following menstruation, the exact time of ovulation may be pinpointed, especially if an LH surge is seen. Studies of serial measurements of LH correlated with direct inspection of the ovaries and histological examination of luteal tissue indicate that in the majority of women ovulation takes place 24–48 hours after the LH peak (Yussman & Traynor, 1970; Croxatto et al, 1974).

All these hormonal assays taken together are helpful in determining whether the primary fault causing anovulation is in the hypothalamus, the pituitary or the ovary.

Virilism is seldom due to malfunction of the ovary unless associated with a masculinising tumour such as an arrhenoblastoma. In these cases raised 17-ketosteroid excretion may be found.

Failure of end-organ response is present if urinary excretion of oestrogen and pregnanediol shows a cyclical change without menstruation. End-organ failure, however, is a relatively uncommon condition if the uterus is present and of normal size.

Evidence of ovulation is most frequently looked for in patients suffering from primary infertility.

Histology

Secretory changes in the endometrium indicate that ovulation has taken place, at least in the particular cycle under review. Evidence of anovulation should be confirmed as a regular occurrence before considering treatment. Patients who suffer from puberty menorrhagia or menopausal menorrhagia may have failure of ovulation as the basis for their condition. In these cases the endometrium is seen microscopically to show cystic glandular hyperplasia. This is indicative of excessive oestrogen production without the antagonism of progesterone. Similar histopathological changes may be observed in patients (especially those after the menopause) who have oestrogen producing tumours of the ovary or who have ingested large doses of exogenous oestrogen without progestogens.

Laparoscopy

The use of the laparoscope to visualize the ovaries directly without the need to do a formal laparotomy has helped greatly in the diagnosis of abnormal conditions of the ovary. The naked eye appearance of a corpus luteum on one or other ovary is evidence that ovulation has taken place. If the ovary is seen to contain multiple follicular cysts without a corpus luteum the lesion is not necessarily primarily ovarian. Lack of a corpus luteum indicates failure of ovulation which is reflected in a high level of circulating oestrogen and negligible progesterone.

If the ovary is not polycystic and lacks a corpus luteum a biopsy should be carried out through the laparoscope. An adequate amount of tissue must be obtained for histopathology to assess whether the ovary is still capable of responding to outside influences, i.e. FSH and LH, or has become atrophic as in a premature menopause. Primordial follicles should be apparent in the biopsy material if the ovary is still capable of response.

Examination of the ovaries using ultrasound

Ultrasound was used initially to detect different cysts of

the ovaries (Donald et al, 1958) but more recently, using real-time or static equipment through a full bladder, normal or polycystic ovaries maybe recognized. The developing Graafian follicle can be serially studied until the time of ovulation. The technique correlates well with endocrinological assessments (Hackelaer et al, 1979) and has the advantage over hormone assays of getting immediate results. It is also non-invasive, apparently harmless and can be repeated frequently with little extra cost. The development of in vitro fertilization and the necessity to retrieve an ovum just prior to ovulation makes the technique of great value in this field.

LESIONS AFFECTING OVARIAN FUNCTION

Ovarian function may appear to be upset though the actual lesions affect the hypothalamus, the pituitary or the uterus. In many such cases the ovaries themselves are perfectly normal and their activity is impaired purely due to lack of proper stimulation. General conditions which give rise to upsets of menstrual function are often erroneously believed to be due to malfunction of the ovary. These include cases of anorexia nervosa, poorly controlled diabetics and patients with marked hyperthyroidism. In these instances it is hypothalamic or pituitary function that is affected and not the ovary per se. Similarly failure of the uterus to respond to cyclical oestrogen and/or progesterone is purely the fault of the target organ and not the ovary, although such a condition is unusual if the uterus is in fact present.

Ovarian function is upset in the clinical condition known as the Stein-Leventhal or polycystic ovary syndrome, although it is uncertain whether the lesion is in the ovary or in the ovarian hypothalamic feedback mechanism. Hypersecretion of androgen by the ovarian stroma may be found and circulating androstenedione levels are raised. Erratic bursts of LH secretion occur but never the normal mid-cycle surge which evokes ovulation; consequently the ovary becomes polycystic. Ovulation is induced infrequently; the patient complains of irregular periods, hirsutism, increasing acne or infertility. On bimanual pelvic examination the ovaries may be appreciably enlarged. Clomiphene (see below in relation to ovarian stimulation) is now the treatment of choice for this condition since it corrects the fault in the hypothalamic-pituitary-ovarian axis. Prior to the availability of clomiphene, wedge resection of the ovary was the most widely used treatment.

Ovarian tumours seldom present with symptoms of abnormal ovarian function except before puberty or in the postmenopausal patient. Hormone-secreting tumours however, can upset normal ovarian hormone production. The granulosa cell tumour and the thecoma, arising from the cells of the theca interna, produce oestrogen. These tumours can present with symptoms of precocious puberty or postmenopausal bleeding. Unusually, in the reproductive period of life they may be present when the patient complains of menorrhagia or polymenorrhoea. Urinary oestrogen excretion is markedly increased (Brown & Beischer, 1972). Other manifestations of high oestrogen levels may be apparent if vaginal and cervical cytology is carried out. If there is an increase of pregnanediol in the urine as well as increased oestrogen, the tumour may be arising from the cells of the corpus luteum. This type of tumour is known as luteoma.

The androgen-producing tumour which arises from the ovarian stroma is called an arrhenoblastoma. Urinary excretion of 17-ketosteroids is raised due to the increased production of androstenedione. If should be remembered that females with symptoms of virilism are more liable to have upsets of other endocrine organs rather than the ovary, but it is worthwhile excluding the presence of a palpable ovarian tumour before proceeding to further investigations in such cases.

Brenner tumours of the ovary, although usually benign and non-functioning, can produce increased amounts of either oestrogen or androgen; this is due to their possible origin from Walthard inclusions which may contain cells potentially capable of secreting either hormone.

CONTROL OF OVARIAN FUNCTION

Control of ovarian function is most important when either suppression or stimulation of ovulation is required. The most widespread control of ovarian function is employed by women using the contraceptive pill. The first clinical trials started in 1956 (Pincus et al, 1958) and by the mid 1960s its use was widespread. It is estimated that at least 50 000 000 women now use oral contraceptives (Piotrow & Lee, 1974). There are three main types of pill which suppress ovulation; the combined pill, which contains both oestrogen and progestogen, is taken from the fifth to the 25th day of each cycle; the sequential pill which is taken for the same time but the first 15 pills contain oestrogen alone while the last 10 contain both oestrogen and progestogen and the triphasic pill which varies the relative amount of oestrogen and progesterone during the 21 days for which the contraceptive is taken.

The choice of pill is dependent on the possible adverse effects of oestrogen or progestogen therapy on the individual patient but they are all efficient methods of suppressing ovulation. It is not clear how these preparations actually do this but they probably act on the hypothalamic-pituitary axis preventing gonadotropin release (Pincus, 1965). Recent work indicates that they may also directly affect the hypothalamus to inhibit luteinizing hormone releasing factor and can also cause direct suppression of the pituitary gland (Spellacy et al, 1980; Mishell et al, 1977). Release of LH does not occur in mid-cycle and a decrease in FSH secretion is usually found. It is important to appreciate that the hormonal content of the pill does not act directly on the ovary but their effects are on other parts of the female reproductive system.

The so-called mini-pill which contains progestogen alone does not owe its contraceptive action to suppressing ovulation.

The menstrual cycle, while the patient is on oestrogen and progestogen therapy, is an artificial cycle since the uterus is merely reacting to exogenous hormones. Giving preparations such as the contraceptive pill to produce periods either in primary or secondary amenorrhoea or in oligomenorrhoea is of no value except to prove that the uterus responds to hormonal stimulation. Such patients should be investigated to determine which part of the complex mechanism associated with menstruation is at fault.

There is no evidence to suggest that subsequent ovarian function is in any way affected by suppression of ovulation. Amenorrhoea following the use of the pill is the result of gonadotropin suppression. Menstruation may restart spontaneously or can be encouraged by giving a preparation such as clomiphene (Shearman, 1975). Clomiphene is an anti-oestrogen substance which may either block oestradiol uptake by the pituitary or reduce its uptake by the anterior hypothalamus (Mahesh & Greenblatt, 1964; Kobayashi et al, 1967). The success in treating post-pill amenorrhoea with clomiphene proves that the ovary is not responsible in the first place for the suppression of menstruation.

One cause of infertility in the female is failure of ovulation. In these cases with careful selection ovulation can be induced in about 70% of patients (MacNaughton, 1973). Several methods are currently employed.

Clomiphene which acts on the hypothalamic-pituitary axis, as indicated above, regulates the output of pituitary gonadotropins. Although it is claimed that ovulation has been achieved using clomid in as many as 91.4% of cases (Rust et al, 1974), the percentage of pregnancies subsequent to this has only been about 38%. Therapy with clomiphene can cause the development of large multiple ovarian cysts as well as signs and symptoms of excessive ovarian stimulation (Greenblatt, 1965) if the drug is given in high dosage for too long. Such complications are minimal if the dosage is kept to between 100–200 mg for 5 days only per cycle (Murray & Osmond-Clarke, 1971). The incidence of multiple pregnancy after clomiphene citrate therapy is about six times higher than the normal incidence (Hack et al, 1970).

Injections of gonadotropin are given sequentially. The preparations most widely used are human menopausal gonadotropin (HMG) extracted from the urine of post-menopausal women, and human chorionic gonadotropin (HCG) obtained from the urine of pregnant women. Both these preparations contain FSH and LH but HCG is predominantly luteinising and when given after a course of HMG should induce ovulation. Various regimens for such treatment have been employed (Shearman, 1972; Bettendorf et al, 1977; Hull et al, 1982). More recently pulsed GNRN has been used by means of a special pump and in some cases has proved effective (Mason et al, 1984). Whatever drug or regimen is used, the treatment must always be carefully monitored. Stimulating ovulation requires very careful supervision and should only be undertaken at centres where there are facilities for accurate hormonal assay of oestrogen and progesterone. Also such treatment should only be employed where it is certain that failure of ovulation is the only demonstrable abnormality to account for failure of conception and that the ovary will respond if stimulated.

When using direct stimulation of the ovaries with gonadotropins great care should be taken not to overstimulate them. If carefully controlled by withholding HCG, if urinary oestrogen is produced in excess of 120 mg/24 h (WHO, 1973), mild degrees of hyperstimulation is found in less than 5% of cases and severe degrees in less than 1% (Elles & Williamson, 1975). By such means the incidence of multiple pregnancy caused by multiple ovulation should also be reduced, though it still happens in about a third of pregnancies. Hopefully the disasters of five or six pregnancies at one time which occurred when such therapy was first introduced are now anecdotes of iatrogenic errors.

Since suppression of ovulation gives rise to anovulatory cycles which are pain free, primary dysmenorrhoea can be treated by giving the contraceptive pill. This has practically replaced surgical treatment of the condition. The only cases to be avoided are those in which menstrual irregularity is associated with dysmenorrhoea.

Hyperprolactinaemia may be a factor in female infertility. It is thought that corpus luteum function is impaired by high prolactin levels and eventually anovulatory cycles occur. The clinical syndrome of amenorrhoea and galactorrhoea known as the Chiari-Frommel syndrome has been considered to be due usually to raised levels of circulating prolactin.

For many years it has been considered that abortion, especially in the early weeks of pregnancy, may be due to failure of the corpus luteum to produce adequate progesterone for the maintenance of the pregnancy. This has been the rationale for giving progesterone in cases of recurrent abortion. It is very doubtful whether exogenous progesterone is of any value (Brown & Beischer, 1972) and its widespread use should be condemned. Probably only a small number of cases of habitual abortion are due to an inadequate corpus luteum. Chorionic gonadotropin containing LH may help such patients. The alternative is to give a clomiphene-like substance to improve endogenous LH production.

PUBERTY AND THE FEMALE CLIMACTERIC

The ovary is not the organ responsible for initiating puberty whereas ageing of the ovary is responsible for the female climacteric.

The output of oestrogen in the urine of prepubertal girls varies considerably but the closer the girl gets to the age of puberty the more oestrogen is excreted. A marked increase in gonadotropic activity seems to be mainly responsible for the onset of puberty which usually occurs between 10 and 15 years in the female. The cyclical release of FSH and LH brings about maturation of the ovary with subsequent increase in oestrogen output. Girls may pass through a stage of regular fluctuation in ovarian oestrogen excretion which in time is sufficient to produce an LH surge with consequent ovulation (Winter & Faiman, 1973). This would account for the gradual development of the female secondary sex characteristics, the eventual start of an anovulatory menstrual cycle at about 13 years and finally ovulation.

Apart from tumours of the ovary, precocious puberty is almost always associated with intracranial lesions indicating that the ovaries are merely acting in response to the gonadotropic hormone. Such lesions may be tumours or cysts which produce hypothalamic stimulation or may be due to postencephalitic or postmeningitic effects.

Delay in the onset of puberty may be due to gonadal dysgenesis (Turner's syndrome). The 'streak' gonads fail to respond to gonadotropin stimulation and consequently a low oestrogen output will be found in the urine although FSH and LH levels will be raised. Raised levels of gonadotropins are found in individuals lacking functional ovaries (as in Turner's syndrome) years before puberty which indicates that normal prepubertal ovaries must be capable of depressing gonadotrophic hormone secretion.

In patients with primary amenorrhoea it should never be assumed that the ovary is primarily at fault since the cause may have its basis anywhere from the hypothalamus to the uterus. A careful history and complete physical examination may give a correct provisional diagnosis. Final confirmation can usually be made using hormone assays, chromosome karyotypes, laparoscopy and, if necessary, ovarian biopsy.

The term menopause by definition refers to cessation of menstruation whereas the female climacteric is the period of time during which female reproduction ceases. This lasts between 1 and 5 years. The process is a gradual one as at puberty. Menstrual cycles become anovulatory; menstruation is irregular and finally ceases. The ovaries no longer respond to gonadotropic stimulation and there is lowering of oestrogen and progesterone production. In premenopausal patients oestradiol derived from the maturing follicle is the main circulating oestrogen, whereas after the menopause it is oestrone which is produced by extraglandular conversion in fat and liver tissue of adrenally secreted androstenedione (McDonald et al, 1978). Raised levels of FSH and LH are found for many years after the menopause (Chakravarti et al, 1976).

The symptoms related to the climacteric are mainly brought about by the fall of circulating oestrogen. The menopause usually occurs between 45 and 55 years. If it occurs before the age of 40 it can be considered as premature, whereas menstruation lasting beyond 55 years should be considered abnormal and requires investigation.

Oestrogen deficiency gives rise to signs such as atrophic changes in the vulva and vagina and diminution in size and tone of breast tissue (unless excess fat is laid down). It also upsets calcium metabolism with consequent osteoporosis. Reduction in circulating oestrogen diminishes its inhibiting influence on the pituitary and in consequence there is likely to be a greater output not only of FSH, which is always a valuable indicator of ovarian failure, but also of other pituitary hormones. Excess production of growth hormone gives rise to obesity and acromegalic changes. Increase in thyrotropic hormone may be responsible for the vasomotor upsets (hot flushes) and some of the emotional upsets, and overproduction of adrenocorticotropic hormone induces a degree of virilism.

Although oestrogen deficiency may be the basic cause of many of the symptoms complained of during the female climacteric, it is impossible to separate the organic from the psychosomatic. Symptoms such as forgetfulness, lack of libido, headaches, insomnia, ringing in the ears, precordial pain and changes in appetite are all difficult to ascribe to hormone deficiency.

Recently much attention has been focused on the giving of oestrogens as replacement therapy once menstruation has ceased (Greenblatt, 1965). The main arguments in favour of such therapy are that it may delay the development of osteoporosis, will keep the prevalence of coronary artery disease to that of the female in the reproductive period of life, and will prevent the senile changes taking place in the vulva and vagina. Dyspareunia due to vaginitis or actual tissue contraction will be avoided. Against these benefits the increased incidence of thromboembolism associated with oestrogen therapy must be considered and also the effects of prolonged oestrogen therapy are possibly not yet fully appreciated. Some reports (Smith et al, 1975; Ziel & Finkle, 1975) suggest that the risk of endometrial cancer was substantially enhanced by oestrogen replacement therapy. Though this is difficult to prove it is advisable to give progestogen as well as oestrogen to ensure regular shedding of the endometrium (Greenblatt, 1976).

Ideally replacement therapy should start when ovarian function begins to ebb, which is almost certainly several years before complete cessation of menstruation. Variation in the actual time of the menopause would make it difficult to know when to start replacement therapy in each individual.

Oestrogen must not be considered as a drug giving the properties of eternal youth; the process of ageing is inevitable. Replacement therapy may help some of the symptoms.

Although for logistic and financial reasons it would seem impractical to prescribe oestrogen replacement therapy for all patients, it may be of value in patients who have had surgical removal of the ovaries, especially if carried out before the age of 45 years or if menopausal symptoms are distressing. Care should be taken to give the smallest amount of oestrogen which will suppress the menopausal symptoms and should be used for a limited period of time. A conjugated oestrogen preparation combined with progesterone is preferred.

SURGICAL REMOVAL OF THE OVARIES

Ovarian function suddenly ceases if the ovaries are removed surgically or are ablated by irradiation. The latter is usually associated with the treatment of genital cancer although uncommonly it may be employed as a means of inducing the menopause.

Frequently the surgeon is faced with the problem of whether to remove or to conserve the ovaries at the time of hysterectomy for benign lesions. After the age of 45 years, when ovarian function is almost at an end, there seems little point in conservation; before 45 years, if the ovaries macroscopically appear normal, most surgeons believe that they should not be removed. The main argument against leaving the ovaries is based on the fact that a patient with her ovaries removed will not subsequently develop ovarian carcinoma, a significant cause of death in the female. The use of hormone replacement therapy after surgical removal of the ovaries would seem to satisfy all points of view, though whether exogenous oestrogens have all the benefits of endogenous hormones is not known.

The operation of oophorectomy is practised too frequently for the removal of ovarian cysts especially in younger women before 35 years. If an ovarian cystectomy is carried out, even if only a small amount of ovarian tissue is conserved, that ovary can function adequately. The hormonal and gametogenic properties are maintained for the time being irrespective of what may happen in the future either to it or to the contralateral ovary. If a young woman has an oophorectomy and within a few years her remaining ovary requires removal, she is left with no hope of fertility and undergoes a premature menopause. Similar arguments apply in favour or conserving the ovary in cases of ectopic pregnancy or bleeding from a corpus luteum.

REFERENCES

Aitken J M, Hart D M, Anderson J B, Lindsay R, Smith D A, Speirs C F 1973 Osteoporosis after oophorectomy for non-malignant disease in premenopausal women. British Medical Journal 2: 325–328

Baker T G 1963 A quantitative and cytological study of germ cells in human ovaries. Proceedings of the Royal Society of London, Series B. Biological Sciences 158: 417–433

Beck F, Moffat D B, Lloyd J B 1973 Control of reproductive rhythm. In: Beck F (ed) Human Embryology and Genetics 1st edn. Blackwell, Oxford, pp 105–110

Bettendorf G, Lehmann F, Leidenberger F 1977 Hormonal treatment of female infertility in regulation of human fertility. In: Diczfalusy, E (ed) World Health Organisation Symposium, Moscow 1976, Scriptor, Copenhagen, pp. 155–179

Brown J B, Beischer N A 1972 Current status of oestrogen assay in gynaecology and obstetrics: Part 1. Estrogen assays in gynaecology and early pregnancy. Obstetrical and Gynecological Survey 27: 205–235

Brown J B, Klopper A, Loraine J A 1958 The urinary excretion of oestrogens, pregnanediol and gonadotrophins during the menstrual cycle. Journal of Endocrinology 17: 401–410

Chakravarti S, Collins W P, Forecast J D, Newton J R, Oram D H, Studd J W W 1976 Hormonal profiles after the menopause. British Medical Journal 2: 784–787

Croxatto H B, Carril M, Cheviakoff S, Patriti N, Pedroza E, Croxatto H D et al 1974 The interval between LH peak and ovulation in women. In: Proceedings of the VIIIth World Congress of Fertility and Sterility, Buenos Aires. Excerpta Medica International Congress Series

Diczfalusy E, Landgren B M 1977 Hormonal changes in the menstrual cycle. In: Diczfalusy E (ed) Regulation of Human Fertility — World Health Organisation Symposium, Moscow 1976 Scriptor, Copenhagen, pp 21–71

Donald I, MacVicar J, Brown T G 1958 Investigation of abdominal masses by pulsed ultrasound. Lancet i: 1188–95

Ellis J D, Williamson J G 1975 Factors influencing the pregnancy and complication rates with human menopause gonadotrophin therapy. British Journal of Obstetrics and Gynaecology 82: 52–57

Goodman L S, Gilman A 1970 The Pharmacological Basis of Therapeutics, McMillan, London, p 1539

Grant J K 1969 Action of Steroid Hormones at Cellular and Molecular Levels. Essays in Biochemistry 5: 1–58

Greenblatt R B 1965 Estrogen therapy for postmenopausal females. New England Journal of Medicine 272: 305–308

Greenblatt R B 1976 Estrogens and endometrial cancer. In: Beard R J (ed) The Menopause MTD Press, Lancaster, pp 247–263

Hack M, Brish M, Serr D M, Insler V, Lunenfeld B 1970 Outcome of pregnancy after induced ovulation. Journal of the American Medical Association 211: 791–797

Hackeloer B J, Fleming R, Robinson H P, Adam A H, Coutts J R T 1979 Correlation of ultrasonic and endocrinological assessment of human follicular development. American Journal of Obstetrics and Gynecology 135: 122–128

Hull M G R, Savage P E, Bromham D R 1982 Anovulatory and ovulatory infertility — Results with simplified management. British Medical Journal 284: 1681–1685

Keele C A, Neil E 1971 Samson Wright's applied physiology. Oxford University Press, London, p 541

Kobayashi T, Kato J, Villee C 1967 In: Wood C (ed) Proceedings of Vth World Congress of Gynaecology and Obstetrics, Butterworth, Sydney, p 351

Macnaughton M C 1973 Treatment of female infertility. Clinics on Endocrinology and Metabolism 2: 545–560

Mason P, Adam J, Morris D V, Tucker M, Price J, Voulgaris Z et al 1984 Induction of ovulation with pulsatile luteinising hormone releasing hormone. British Medical Journal 288: 181–185

Mahesh V B, Greenblatt R B 1964 Steroid secretions of the normal and polycystic ovary. Recent Progress in Hormone Research 20: 341–394

McDonald P C, Edman C D, Hemsell D L, Porter J C, Sliteri P K 1978 Effect of obesity on conversion of plasma androstenedione to estrone in post-menopausal women with and without endometrial cancer. American Journal of Obstetrics and Gynaecology 130: 448–455

Midgley A R Jr, Jaffee R B 1968 Regulation of human gonadotropins. Journal of Clinical Endocrinology and Metabolism 28: 1712–1718

Mishell D R Jr, Kletsky O A, Brenner P F, Roy S, Nicoloff J 1977 The effect of contraceptive steroids on hypothalamic-pituitary function. American Journal of Obstetrics and Gynaecology 128: 60–70

Murray M, Osmond-Clarke F 1971 Pregnancy results following treatment with clomiphene citrate. Journal of Obstetrics and Gynaecology of the British Commonwealth 78: 1108–1114

Nordin B E C, Young M M, Bentley B, Ormondroyd P, Sykes J, 1968 Lumbar spine densitometry methodology and results in relation to the menopause. Clinical Radiology 19: 459–464

Pennington G W, Dewhurst C J 1969 Hormone excretion in premenarcheal girls. Archives of Disease in Childhood 44: 629–636

Pepperell R J, Brown J B, Evans J H, Rennie G C, Burger H G 1975 The investigation of ovarian function by measurement of urinary oestrogen and pregnanediol excretion. British Journal of Obstetrics and Gynaecology 82: 321–332

Pincus G, Rock J, Garcia C R, Rice-Wray E, Paniagua M, Rodriguez I 1958 Fertility control with oral medication. American Journal of Obstetrics and Gynaecology 75: 1333–1346

Pincus G 1965 The Control of Fertility. Academic Press, New York

Piotrow P T, Lee C M 1974 Oral Contraceptives Population Report Series A No 1, p 28

Pryse-Davies J 1974 The development, structure and function of the female pelvic organs in childhood. Clinics in Obstetrics and Gynaecology 1: 483–508

Rondell P 1970 Biophysical Aspects of Ovulation, Biological Reproduction Supplement 2: 64–89

Rust L A, Israel R, Mishell D R 1974 An individualised graduated therapeutic regimen for clomiphene citrate. American Journal of Obstetrics and Gynecology 120: 785–790

Shearman R P 1972 In: Dewhurst C J (ed) Integrated obstetrics and gynaecology for postgraduates. Blackwell, London, p 498

Shearman R P 1975 Secondary amenorrhoea after oral contraceptives — treatment and follow up. Contraception 11: 123–133

Smith D A, Anderson J B, Shimmins J, Spiers C F, Barnett E 1969 Changes in metacarpal mineral content and density in normal male and female subjects with age. Clinical Radiology 20: 23–31

Smith D C, Prentice R, Thomson D J, Herrman W L 1975 Association of exogenous estrogen and endometrial carcinoma. New England Journal of Medicine 293: 1164–1167

Spellacy W N, Kalra P S, Buhi W C, Birk S A 1980 Pituitary and ovarian responsiveness to a graded gonadotropin releasing factor stimulation test in women using a low-estrogen or a regular type of oral contraceptive. American Journal of Obstetrics and Gynecology 137: 109–115

Williams-Ashman H G, Reddi A H 1971 Actions of vertebrate sex hormones. Annual Review of Physiology 33: 31–82

Winter J S D, Faiman C 1973 The development of cyclic, pituitary-gonadal function in adolescent females. Journal of Clinical Endocrinology and Metabolism 37: 714–718

Witschi E 1948 Migration of the germ cells of human embryos from the yolk sac to the primitive gonadal folds. Contribution to Embryology 32: 67–80 Washington: Carnegie Institute

World Health Organisation 1973 Agents stimulating gonadal function in the human. World Organisation Technical Report Series No 514

Yussman M A, Traynor M L 1970 Serum levels of follicle stimulating hormone and luteinising hormone and of plasma progesterone related to ovulation by corpus luteum biopsy. Journal of Clinical Endocrinology and Metabolism 30: 396–399

Ziel H K, Finkle W O 1975 Increased risk of endometrial carcinoma among users of conjugated estrogens. New England Journal of Medicine 293: 1167–1170

Immunology and surgery

An appreciation of immunological concepts is necessary, or at least desirable, in those involved in the practice of modern surgery. In general surgical practice the immune system is crucial in combating infection, whereas in the expanding field of organ transplantation, immunological rejection of the graft is the major incompletely solved problem. The immune system is of relevance to aspects of cancer research and of importance in the aetiology of other diseases met in surgical practice, in particular some endocrine and intestinal diseases. However, the impact of immunology on surgery goes far beyond this. Advances such as the development of monoclonal antibodies have led to the increasing use of immunological methods for both diagnosis and monitoring in a wide spectrum of diseases. Currently much research is being directed into the use of immunological methods to aid treatment of disease and in the long term it may be possible to manipulate specific aspects of the immune system for therapeutic purposes.

BASIC IMMUNOLOGY

Before the more applied aspects of immunology can be considered it is first necessary to review current concepts of the immune response. The field of immunology is progressing rapidly and to the non-specialist may present a daunting prospect to keep pace with, especially since the nomenclature often appears complex and confusing. Fortunately, familiarity with the details of much of the nomenclature is unnecessary in order to appreciate the important immunological principles and their clinical relevance.

The immune system can conveniently be divided into the innate (or non-specific) immune system and the adoptive (or acquired) immune system. Innate immunity is the body's major defence against most infecting organisms and its principal components are phagocytic cells, natural killer cells and a variety of soluble factors released by these and other types of cell. This part of the immune system has little specificity and no ability to 'learn', i.e. it does not become more effective on repeated exposure to the same infection. In marked contrast, the adoptive immune system, in which the principle components are lymphocytes and their soluble products, produces a highly specific response to an infection and has the ability to 'learn', so that on subsequent exposure to the same infection, there is a more rapid and effective (secondary) response. Innate and adoptive immune mechanisms do not always operate entirely independently and, as will be seen, there are various interactions between the two components.

THE INNATE (NON-SPECIFIC) IMMUNE SYSTEM

The body's first line of protection against the entry of pathogenic organisms is the skin and the mucosal surfaces. Together these provide an effective mechanical barrier which is supplemented by the protective effects of secretions such as lysosyme in tears and acid in the stomach, both of which destroy bacteria. In addition, the mucinous secretions of the respiratory and gastrointestinal tract trap and expel organisms and also contain anti-microbial substances. If organisms succeed in penetrating these local defences then they are faced with the more generalized components of innate immunity outlined below, which act rapidly to destroy them.

Phagocytes

Circulating neutrophils and monocytes rapidly accumulate at sites of infection. These phagocytic cells are attracted into infected tissue by the presence of chemotactic factors (such as complement components or bacterial products) and are able to ingest and destroy microorganisms. The ability of phagocytes to attach to and ingest bacteria is greatly facilitated by the presence of opsonins which may be either complement activation products or specific antibody. In its role as an opsonin, antibody is an example of an important interaction between the innate and acquired immune system. Organisms which gain access to the circulation are cleared by the fixed phagocytic cells of the reticuloendothelial system such as hepatic Kupffer cells, alveolar macrophages and macrophages in the spleen and lymph nodes.

Complement

Complement (C) consists of a group of serum proteins the complexities of which are only now being appreciated. The nine main components (C1–C9) of the complement system act in sequence in much the same way as the process of blood coagulation. Complement activation occurs when antigen-antibody complexes activate the C1 component and trigger the cascade (the classical pathway of complement activation) or when the cell surfaces of microorganisms cause the conversion of the C3 component to C3b, thereby triggering the system (the alternative pathway).

Complement activation products have a wide range of biological effects. Their role as both opsonins and chemoattractants in phagocytosis has already been described. In addition they may lyse target cells, increase vascular permeability, cause smooth muscle contraction and bring about mast cell degranulation.

Acute phase proteins

The levels of a number of serum proteins increase rapidly during infection or following injury. These 'acute phase' proteins include a variety of transport proteins, proteinase inhibitors and coagulation and complement proteins. Their effects are varied but some undoubtedly play a role in non-specific defence, e.g. C-reactive protein reacts with the C protein of pneumococci and thereby activates the complement system as well as acting directly as an opsonin.

Interferon and natural killer (NK) cells

Both interferon and natural killer (NK) cells are of special importance in the defence against viral infection. The interferons are a family of glycoproteins which are released from cells when they become virally infected. Their effect is to make nearby cells resistant to viral infection. Natural killer cells are circulating leukocytes of unknown cell lineage which are able to recognise and destroy virally infected cells without prior sensitization. The cytotoxic activity of NK cells is greatly augmented by the presence of interferon. As will be seen later, interferon has other important roles in adoptive immunity and both interferon and NK cells may play a role in destroying cells which have undergone malignant transformation.

THE ADOPTIVE OR ACQUIRED IMMUNE SYSTEM

Adoptive immunity, unlike innate immunity, is found only in higher animals. It is a very sophisticated system which, through a complex series of cellular interactions, is able to produce a highly specific and effective response to a foreign substance (antigen). The specificity of this response allows the immune system to deal with innumerable different foreign antigens, without the danger of mistaking the body's own cells and proteins as foreign and inadvertently mounting a response against them. As already noted, the adoptive immune system has 'memory' so that a repeated exposure to a particular antigen produces a more effective secondary response. This latter feature forms the rationale for the use of vaccination as a method of protecting the body from subsequent infection.

The immune response initiated when an antigen is introduced into the body may be of two kinds.

1. Antibodies may be produced against the antigen. This is termed humoral immunity and occurs, for example, when an individual is injected with tetanus toxoid. Specific antibodies are formed which give protection against infection by the tetanus bacillus. Humoral immunity can be adoptively transferred by serum alone.

2. A group of sensitized cells may be produced which are capable of attacking and destroying the antigen. This response is known as the cell-mediated immune response and is mediated by lymphocytes, either directly or indirectly by the recruitment of other non-specific effectors such as macrophages. Cell mediated immunity can be adoptively transferred by sensitised lymphocytes but not by serum alone. Responses of this kind are important for protection against certain intracellular pathogens such as tubercle bacilli, for killing virally infected cells and for immunity to protozoal infection. As will be seen, cell mediated responses play an essential role in graft rejection and may also be involved in tumour immunity.

THE ROLE OF THE LYMPHOCYTE

The lymphocyte plays a central role in all adoptive immune responses. This was clearly shown by the work of Gowans in which rats which had been depleted of lymphocytes, by drainage of lymph from the thoracic duct, were unable to mount a significant immunological response against an antigen challenge. When the animals were given lymphocyte injections, their ability to mount both humoral and cell mediated responses was fully restored. A further major advance in the understanding of the immune system came with the discovery that there are two major populations of lymphocytes, namely B lymphocytes and T lymphocytes. Both types of lymphocyte originate in the bone marrow from a common lymphoid precursor cell. T cells are processed in the thymus (hence T cells) and are subsequently able to proliferate in response to an antigen into effector cells with a variety of functions, including those concerned with cell mediated responses. B cells differentiate in the bone marrow (in birds B cells differentiate in a cloacal organ called the bursa of Fabricius, hence B cells) and are not directly influenced by the thymus. Following antigenic stimulus, B cells differentiate further into antibody producing plasma cells and are therefore concerned with humoral immunity.

After leaving the primary lymphoid organs (bone marrow and thymus) the majority of lymphocytes are to be found in the secondary lymphoid tissue, i.e. lymph nodes, spleen and gastrointestinal associated lymphoid tissue. It is in these secondary lymphoid tissues that the most important immune responses occur. The lymphocytes are not permanently resident in such tissue, but continuously circulate from the blood, to all the body tissues, into the lymphatics, through the lymph glands and then back into the blood via the thoracic duct. This lymphocyte traffic ensures wide distribution of both 'virgin' and 'memory' lymphocytes, therefore maximising their chances of encountering 'new' or 'previously met' antigens, and allowing them ready access to other lymphocytes which have the potential to participate in an immune response.

Although B and T lymphocytes appear identical on light microscopy they can be readily distinguished by certain surface characteristics. Traditionally the presence of surface immunoglobulin on B cells (but not T cells) or the presence of receptors for sheep red blood cells on T cells (but not B cells) was used to differentiate between B and T lymphocytes. However, it is now possible to identify not only B and T lymphocytes, but also different T cell subpopulations by using monoclonal antibodies to label specific marker glycoproteins which the different lymphocyte subsets carry on their cell membrane. These surface markers or antigens are associated with functional differences, for example T cells with a helper/inducer function (Th/i) carry the CD4 antigen whereas T cells with a cytotoxic/suppressor function (Tc/s) carry the CD8 antigen. Other surface antigens may be identified which play a role in cellular regulation or define the degree of maturation of the lymphocyte. An increasing number of lymphocyte surface antigens (and the monoclonal antibodies which label them) are being discovered, although there is, as yet, no known antigenic determinant which distinguishes T suppressor cells from T cytotoxic cells.

ANTIBODY PRODUCTION

When an antigen such as a pathogenic bacterium is introduced into the body, it is recognised as foreign by B

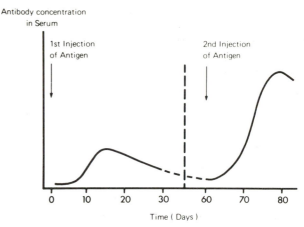

Fig. 27.1 Primary and secondary immune responses

lymphocytes. As a result, a population of these B cells divides into large blast cells which then differentiate into plasma cells. These plasma cells synthesize the highly specific antibody.

An individual is capable of making specific antibodies against an almost unlimited number of antigens. The basic mechanism underlying such great diversity is clonal selection as proposed by Jerne and Burnet. This may be summarized as follows. Each B lymphocyte has the genetic information available to make only one particular antibody. The molecules of that antibody are built into the surface of the lymphocyte as receptors (surface immunoglobulin) for the appropriate antigen. The antigen acts essentially as a trigger, stimulating the production of a clone of sensitised cells. Different B lymphocytes have different specificities and, because of genetic diversity, all antibody specificities are covered by the lymphocyte population.

The first contact with antigen initiates the primary response which is characterized by a delay of a few days before antibodies are detected in the blood. If, after an interval, the individual is subjected to a second challenge by the same antigen the rise in antibody levels is faster, and higher blood values are obtained. This secondary response (Fig. 27.1) is related to the retention in the body of long-lived 'memory' lymphocytes capable of a rapid response to antigenic stimulation.

CELLULAR CO-OPERATION IN ANTIBODY PRODUCTION

In all adoptive immune responses there are complex interactions between the different types of cell involved. The principles of cellular co-operation, outlined below in relation to antibody production and shown diagramatically in Fig. 27.2, also apply to cell mediated immunity.

The presence of free antigen may not by itself be suffi-

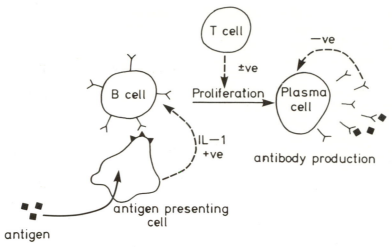

Fig. 27.2 Cellular co-operation in antibody production

cient to cause an immune response. Before an antigen can be recognised as foreign by a lymphocyte, the antigen must be taken up, processed and presented on the surface of a specialised antigen presenting cell. These antigen presenting cells are derived from bone marrow and are found predominantly in lymphoid tissue (dendritic cells and macrophages) in the skin (Langerhans cells) and in the liver (Kupffer cells). When the modified antigen is displayed on the surface of an antigen presenting cell, in close association with other 'self' cell surface molecules, it is recognised as foreign by immunoglobulin receptor molecules on the surface of B cells, or by T cell receptor molecules on the surface of T cells. In addition to presenting antigen to lymphocytes in a highly immunogenic form, the antigen presenting cell also releases the monokine interleukin-1 (IL-1). This soluble factor has a non-specific stimulatory effect on the already activated lymphocytes which differentiate into plasma cells and begin secreting antibody. Although T lymphocytes are unable to produce antibody themselves they still participate in many antibody responses by producing lymphokines. For example, antigen activated T helper cells may release B cell growth factor, which augments B cell activation and differentiation.

Once activated, the antibody response to an antigen would, if unchecked, proceed like a chain reaction in the immune system and result in almost unlimited antibody production which would be both unnecessary and harmful. All immune responses are, therefore, closely regulated. The presence of newly produced antibody directly inhibits the production of excess antibody by B cells and, in addition, suppressor T lymphocytes are activated which exert a controlling influence on the immune response.

ANTIBODY STRUCTURE AND FUNCTION

Antibody molecules are able to combine specifically with

an antigen. This enables them to neutralize the antigen molecules of a toxin (antitoxins), to combine with antigens on, for example, bacteria and either destroy them by activating complement or coat their surface and thereby facilitate their ingestion by phagocytes (opsonisation). Antibodies are also involved in 'antibody-dependent cell mediated cytotoxicity' (ADCC), a term used to describe the in vitro ability of 'Killer' (K) cells to lyse target cells coated with specific antibody. Both lymphocytes (a subpopulation known as null cells) and macrophages may be capable of mediating K activity. The in vivo role of this phenomenon is unclear but may be important for destroying protozoa.

Antibody activity is associated with the gamma-globulin fraction of serum and consequently antibodies are known as immunoglobulins. The major class of immunoglobulin in serum is IgG and this represents the predominant antibody formed in the secondary response. Four other classes of immunoglobulin can be recognized, namely immunoglobulin A, M, E and D.

Immunoglobulin G (IgG)

The basic structure of IgG is shown in Figure 27.3. Each molecule comprises two heavy and two light polypeptide chains linked by disulphide bonds. By enzymatic and chemical means the molecule can be split into various subunits which have allowed analysis of its structure and function.

The enzyme papain splits the molecule into two Fab fragments (the antigen binding sites) and an Fc (crystallizable) fraction which is the portion of the molecule which binds to receptors on macrophages or lymphocytes. In contrast, pepsin splits the molecule in a different position giving a $F(ab)_2$ fragment, which like the original molecule is divalent and hence will combine with two antigen molecules. The Fab fragments contain the highly variable portions of the molecule which determine the specificity. Antibody molecules should not be thought of

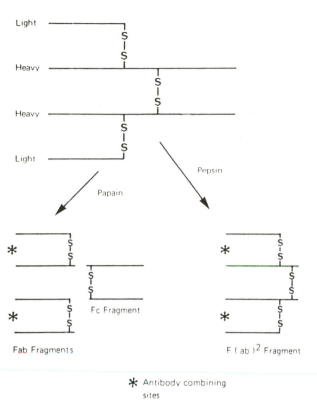

Fig. 27.3 Molecular structure of antibody

as static compounds. They are able to modulate their shape and can be seen on electron microscopy as a Y-shaped structure.

Immunoglobulin A (IgA)

This is present in saliva, tears and gastrointestinal and bronchial secretions. Its function appears to be in the primary defence of the external and internal surfaces of the body. It forms dimers spontaneously by association with a polypeptide known as the J-chain.

Immunoglobulin M (IgM)

This high molecular weight immunoglobulin is a pentamer of the basic four chain immunoglobulin unit linked by J-chains. IgM appears early in the primary response and its structure gives it a high antigen combining valency making it very efficient at fixing complement and causing agglutination.

Immunoglobulin E (IgE)

These antibodies are present in blood in extremely low concentrations and are primarily associated with mast cells in the skin. When exposed to specific antigen, degranulation of mast cells occurs. They probably play a role in protection of body surfaces but they are also associated with the allergic responses seen in atopic dermatitis and

hay fever. The levels also rise following infection with parasites.

Immunoglobulin D (IgD)

The role of this immunoglobulin is not clear.

CELL MEDIATED IMMUNE RESPONSES (CMI)

These are immune responses in which antibody does not play a major role. Instead, antigen activated T cells mediate the response either directly by the generation of cytotoxic T cells or indirectly by the release of lymphokines which recruit non-specific effector cells (Fig. 27.4). This latter response is exemplified in vivo by the delayed type hypersensitivity reaction in which the intradermal injection of an antigen (e.g. tuberculin or purified protein derivative) leads to local induration and oedema 24 hours later.

As previously noted, T lymphocytes are activated by antigen which has been processed and displayed on the surface of an antigen presenting cell. The T cell recognises the foreign antigen, in association with other 'self' surface glycoprotein molecules of the antigen presenting cell, via a specific antigen receptor molecule. This leads to the development of antigen specific cytotoxic T cells or specifically activated clones of T cells which release lymphokines. All cell mediated responses are regulated by the development of suppressor T cells and the soluble suppressor factors which they release.

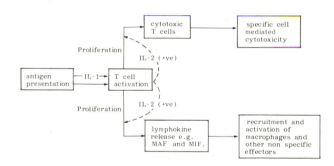

Fig. 27.4 Cell mediated immune response

Cytotoxic T cells

Cytotoxic T lymphocytes are able to kill 'target' cells by attaching themselves to their targets via specific antigen receptors and then causing cell lysis by enzymes released from cytotoxic cell granules. These lymphocytes are able, after prior sensitisation, to kill virally infected cells, hence limiting the spread of virus in the body. They are also important because of their ability to recognise foreign transplant antigens and thereby cause graft rejection.

Lymphokine release by T cells

Lymphokines are biologically active molecules capable of mediating many of the cellular interactions of an immune response. Since they are not antigen specific, the specificity of their response is at the level of the activated T cell which produces them. Because the various lymphokines have usually been described according to their biological activity (which often overlaps), their nomenclature has unfortunately become unnecessarily complicated.

Some of the more important lymphokines are described below. So far the precise molecular structure of only a small number of these is known.

(a) *Interleukin 2 (IL-2)*. This was originally named 'T cell growth factor' because it is a potent stimulator of T cell proliferation. It promotes the expansion of clones of activated T cells and is an integral part of most immune responses.

(b) *Interferon gamma*. This was previously called immune interferon. Like the other types of interferon it has anti-viral activity but it also exerts powerful immuno-regulatory effects on the function of T and B lymphocytes, NK cells and macrophages.

(c) *Lymphokines involved in antibody responses*. B cell growth factor and B cell differentiation factor help in the development of plasma cells and hence antibody production.

(d) *Lymphokines acting on macrophages*. Macrophages are attracted to sites of lymphocyte activation by the release from T cells of chemotactic factors. Migration inhibition factor (MIF) prevents them from leaving and macrophage activating factor (MAF) increases their ability to kill target cells. In this way macrophages make an important contribution to immune responses. They are able to secrete a large number of inflammatory substances including enzymes, oxygen radicals, interferon and prostaglandin.

(e) *Lymphotoxin*. Some activated T cells are capable of secreting a soluble lymphokine called lymphotoxin. The role of this non-specific toxin is unknown but it may play a part in killing virally infected cells or in tumour cell destruction.

Given the wide-ranging effect of the above lymphokines, it is readily apparent that as well as being able to mediate cell mediated immune responses by recruiting nonspecific effectors, particularly macrophages, they are involved in all aspects of the adoptive immune response.

PRESENT CONCEPTS OF THE IMMUNE RESPONSE

Our understanding of the interaction between the different cells involved in adoptive immune responses is far from complete. The essential role played by non-lymphoid antigen presenting cells in initiating most immune responses has been emphasized and the role that non-specific cells such as macrophages and NK cells play as effector cells under lymphokine direction has been described. In addition, the ability of the different lymphocyte populations to interact directly or indirectly by the release of different kinds of lymphokine has been alluded to. In the light of current knowledge, it is apparent that the division of adoptive immunity into well-defined cell-mediated and humoral components, although convenient, is an oversimplification and most antigens produce an integrated response with contributions and interactions from both of these divisions.

CLINICAL ASSESSMENT OF THE IMMUNE SYSTEM

Based on the information described above a number of tests are available which can be used to assess the immune system of an individual. These tests may be used in clinical research to determine whether a particular disease process or treatment causes impaired immune function. Since most of these investigations only assess a particular aspect of the immune system, it is common practice to include a selection of such tests to obtain an overall assessment or immune profile. Many of these tests are difficult and expensive to perform and therefore, with the exception of some of the more simple screening tests, they are only used in routine clinical practice when there is a strong clinical suspicion of a defect in a particular aspect of the immune system. A limitation of most of the measurements of immune function is that they are made from only one anatomical compartment of the lymphoid system, namely, peripheral blood.

A range of the currently available tests is listed and briefly discussed below.

Humoral response (B-cell response)

1. Estimation of B lymphocytes (both absolute numbers and percentage).
2. Estimation of serum immunoglobulin (IgG, IgM and IgA) levels.
3. Lymphocyte transformation. Stimulation of lymphocytes by antigens or mitogens (complex molecules often derived from plants) causes them to develop into lymphoblasts. This process of lymphocyte transformation can be assessed during in vitro culture by the uptake of radio-labelled thymidine, a nucleotide precursor incorporated in DNA synthesis. Certain polyclonal mitogens (e.g. pokeweed mitogen) preferentially activate B cells whereas others (e.g. concanavalin A and phytohaemagglutinin) selectively stimulate T cells. This test can be performed in the presence of either a standard normal serum or in the presence of the patient's own (autologous) serum in order

to show whether any observed impairment in lymphocyte transformation is due to an intrinsic cellular defect or due to serum inhibitory factors.

4. Specific antibody response e.g. by determining tetanus antibody levels in the blood after injecting tetanus toxoid into a non-immunised individual (primary response) or a previously immunised individual (secondary response).

Cell mediated immune response (T-cell response)

1. Estimation of T lymphocytes and subpopulations (absolute numbers and percentage) using monoclonal antibodies.

2. Lymphocyte transformation.

3. Delayed hypersensitivity skin testing. The simple technique of skin testing remains an effective method for the overall assessment of cellular immunity. A battery of recall antigens (commonly PPD, *Candida albicans*, mumps and streptokinase) are injected intradermally and the resulting erythema and induration assessed at 24–48 hours. Inability to react to this test is termed anergy. If anergy to recall antigens is present then a sensitising compound, such as DNCB can be applied to the skin, followed after several days by a further challenging dose in an additional attempt to elicit a delayed type hypersensitivity response.

4. Measurement of lymphokine production. There are a number of in vitro assays aimed to examine the release by lymphocytes of lymphokines, e.g. macrophage migration inhibitory factor (MIF).

Phagocyte function

1. Estimation of neutrophils and monocytes (absolute numbers and percentage).
2. Nitroblue tetrazolium (NBT) test.
3. Ingestion and killing of *S. aureus* or *C. albicans*.
4. In vivo leukocyte migration (Rebuck skin window).

Complement

1. Measurement of total haemolytic complement activity (CH_{50}) by lysing of sensitised sheep red cells.
2. Measurement of specific complement components.

IMMUNOLOGICAL TOLERANCE

Under certain circumstances when an experimental animal is exposed to an antigen it may, instead of mounting an immune response, develop a state of specific immunological unresponsiveness towards the antigen. This phenomenon is known as immunological tolerance. An important observation in our understanding of tolerance, made in the 1940s, was that non-identical cattle twins which had shared the same blood supply via a common placenta permanently retained in their bloodstream red cells from each other which had been naturally exchanged across the placenta. These twins were thus chimaeras (i.e. had cells of genetically different tissue types) and were shown to be able to accept blood cells (and tissue grafts) from each other. However, in twins which did not have a common placenta (and hence no natural blood exchange), blood cells or tissue grafts exchanged between each other were rapidly destroyed by immunological mechanisms. In subsequent experiments Billingham, Brent and Medawar showed that specific tolerance to skin grafts could be induced in mice by injecting adult lymphoid cells into embryonic or neonatal animals. This suggested that if an animal was exposed to an antigen before a certain stage in its development, then it could 'accept' that antigen as 'self' and acquire tolerance to it. Further work has shown that although the immune system of embryo and neonatal animals is particularly susceptible to the induction of tolerance, it is also possible to induce tolerance to a variety of different antigens in adult animals. The dose of antigen given is of critical importance and whereas a particular dose of antigen may initiate a strong immune response, a much smaller or much higher dose may induce tolerance ('low dose' and 'high dose' tolerance).

The lymphocyte is undoubtedly the key cell in the induction of tolerance but as yet the precise cellular mechanism of tolerance is unclear. In the clinical setting, the induction of tolerance to specific antigens is not yet possible though the implications of being able to do so are very great.

ALTERED IMMUNOLOGICAL RESPONSIVENESS

Under normal conditions antigenic stimulation produces an immune response which is beneficial to the host and results in destruction or inactivation of the antigen. Excessive or inappropriate stimulation (immunostimulation) of the lymphoid system with continued activity of the response or inability to mount a proper immunological reaction (immunodeficiency) may both be detrimental to the host.

Excessive stimulation of the immune response

This may occur due to chronic exposure to the antigen. For example, a contact dermatitis is a typical delayed hypersensitivity reaction but because the individual reacts specifically to the allergen, chronic dermatitis results. Allergic responses, as in rhinitis, hay fever and some forms of asthma, are again excessive responses to antigenic stimulation, occurring in particularly sensitive individuals. In all of these conditions removal of the antigen results in a diminution of the response and is associated with clinical improvement.

A group of conditions, the autoimmune diseases, occurs because of stimulation of the individual's immune response against its own body components. A wide variety of diseases are associated with the presence of autoantibodies, including Hashimoto's thyroiditis, thyrotoxicosis, pernicious anaemia, primary biliary cirrhosis, chronic active hepatitis, Sjögren's syndrome, rheumatoid arthritis and systemic lupus erythematosis. These diseases tend to be associated in the one individual and may run in families.

Immunodeficiency states

Immunodeficiency may occur because of a fundamental defect in the immune system, usually present from birth (primary immunodeficiency) or because of the depressive effect produced by surgical operations, malignant disease, chemotherapy and radiotherapy or a variety of other factors (secondary or acquired immunodeficiency states). These will now be discussed separately.

PRIMARY IMMUNODEFICIENCY DISEASE

These rare diseases are usually genetically determined and frequently manifest in early childhood by recurrent and severe infections sometimes resulting in death. They may be classified according to the particular aspect of the immune system which is affected and this determines the pattern of infection seen in affected individuals.

Defects in innate immunity

In chronic granulomatous disease, the neutrophils and monocytes have a congenital enzyme deficiency and are unable to kill ingested bacteria, particularly staphylococci. Affected children are, therefore, prone to recurrent suppurative infections. Chediak-Higashi syndrome is another rare condition in which phagocytes are unable to kill ingested bacteria, this time because of defective lysosomes.

Defects in innate immunity may also occur because of deficiency in the complement components. Depending on which component is deficient the susceptibility to infection may be minimal or severe.

B cell deficiency

In Bruton's agammaglobulinaemia (infantile sex-linked agammaglobulinaemia) there is a congenital immunoglobulin deficiency. Affected infants are, therefore, susceptible to severe bacterial infections but since they have normal cell mediated immunity their resistance to many viral infections is normal. Treatment of these children is by giving repeated injections of human gammaglobulin. Transient hypogammaglobulinaemia is a similar but less serious condition which spontaneously disappears in early childhood. Sometimes immunoglobulin deficiency may not become apparent until adult life, so called late onset or common, variable immunodeficiency.

T cell deficiency

This may result from complete or partial failure of the thymus gland to develop (DiGeorge syndrome). Children affected by this rare condition are unable to mount an effective cell mediated response and therefore suffer from severe viral and fungal infections. Their resistance to pyogenic bacteria is relatively normal although they have an impaired antibody response to many antigens because of the requirement for T helper cells. Treatment of this fatal disease by neonatal thymus grafting has been tried but unfortunately the resulting T lymphocytes recognise the thymus graft as 'foreign' and proceed to destroy it.

Combined B cell and T cell deficiency

In severe combined immunodeficiency (which includes Swiss-type), the absence of humoral and cell mediated immunity renders affected individuals susceptible to infection by all types of pathogen and early death results. Since this is a stem cell deficiency, bone marrow transplantation from a sibling may effectively restore the immune system but unless the transparent is well matched, graft-versus-host disease occurs.

SECONDARY OR ACQUIRED IMMUNODEFICIENCY DISEASE

This is much more common than primary immunodeficiency but the nature of the immune defects and the pattern of infection are not as clear cut. There are usually multiple contributing factors and the degree of immunodeficiency is very variable. The main importance of secondary immunodeficiency is an awareness by the clinician that it may exist and that affected patients are more susceptible to infection. Unfortunately there is as yet no effective form of immunotherapy available.

Post-operative depression of the immune response

The immunosuppressive effect of anaesthesia and surgery in healthy individuals was clearly demonstrated in the classic study by Slade and co-workers. Healthy renal transplant donors giving a kidney to a relative were found to show a transient depression of immunity after surgery. Blood levels of total B and T cells, lymphocyte transformation and delayed hypersensitivity skin testing were all depressed for several days. The clinical significance of this immune depression is not clear though there are two important theoretical implications: (i) the susceptibility to infection may be increased and (ii) in cancer patients, cells disseminated at the time of operation may not be subject to normal immunological control.

Shock, trauma and burns

In these situations depression of the immune response is even more pronounced. Impairment in aspects of innate, humoral and cell mediated immunity have all been recognised and it seems likely that these contribute to the development of infection which is often the major cause of death in such patients.

Surgical operations involving immunological organs

A great deal of our knowledge of the immune response is related to the measurement of reactions which occur in blood. However, the lymphoid system involves the thymus, spleen, lymph node and gut in addition to the blood and lymphatic vessels. Surgical removal of any one of these organs may, therefore, be expected to have an effect on the immune response.

Thymectomy

The earlier work in mice showed that thymectomy at the time of birth resulted in a profound depression of cell mediated immunity. The clinical counterpart of this is congenital thymic aplasia (Di George's syndrome) in which a similar syndrome occurs. In adults, however, the immunological effects of thymectomy are as yet unclear. In many cases the thymus is removed because of myasthenia gravis and, as these patients may already be immunologically abnormal, the results are difficult to interpret.

Splenectomy

The spleen is an important immunological organ and it might be expected that its removal would be associated with a depressed immune response. In children there does appear to be an increased susceptibility to infection following splenectomy. In adults, however, apart from the well known consequences on the platelet count, no accepted immunological complication occurs, though there may also be an increase in the incidence of infections.

Lymphadenectomy

In the experimental literature related to cancer immunology, some reports suggest that removal of the local or draining lymph nodes of the tumour results in dissemination of malignant cells and decreased survival rates, hence the clinically important argument relating to whether local draining lymph nodes should, or should not,

be excised. Evidence for and against this in the human tumour situation is conflicting and a final decision on this awaits the results of properly controlled clinical trials.

Resection of bowel

In birds, the bursa of Fabricius, a gut-associated lymphoid organ, is important for B cell differentiation. However, there is no such gut associated organ in man and although the human gastrointestinal tract contains a large amount of lymphoid tissue, surgical resection of a segment of bowel is not usually associated with an altered immune response.

Effect of radiation on the immune system

Lymphoid tissue is very sensitive to the effects of radiation. Observations in victims of accidental total body irradiation and animal studies have shown that after lethal or near lethal doses of irradiation, there is a rapid disappearance of circulating lymphocytes. However, the consequences of this lymphopaenia are overshadowed by the profound neutropenia, thrombocytopenia and gastrointestinal effects which are the main cause of morbidity and mortality. Total body irradiation undoubtedly results in profound immunosuppression and attempts were even made to make use of this in the early days of organ transplantation in order to prevent graft rejection but it was quickly abandoned because of the serious side effects.

The radiosensitivity of lymphocytes led to the successful use of radiotherapy to treat Hodgkin's disease. In contrast to whole-body irradiation, it was found that patients could tolerate relatively high doses of total lymphoid irradiation using an inverted Y field. Patients treated in this way were shown, when tested, to have severe impairment of both humoral and cellular immunity although the presence of Hodgkin's disease and concurrent treatment, e.g. chemotherapy, may have contributed to this observation. Surprisingly, in view of these findings, the increased susceptibility of these patients to serious infection or to the development of other types of malignancy was not dramatic.

Whether the effects of regional or local radiotherapy have any clinically significant effect on the immune system is unclear. There is no clinical support for this and although such treatment may, for example, be associated with decreased response to skin testing, this may be a reflection of the underlying malignancy or other unrelated factors.

Chemotherapy and immunodepression

A number of drugs have profound immunosuppressive effects. In particular, the chemotherapeutic agents used to treat malignancy are cytotoxic for both neutrophils and lymphocytes. Steroids, in addition to their powerful anti-inflammatory effects also depress many different aspects of immune function, hence their use in organ transplantation to prevent rejection. Along with the other commonly used immunosuppressants in transplantation (azathioprine and cyclosporin A) their non-specific effect on immune function enhances the risk of opportunistic infection in the graft recipient.

Nutritional status and the immune response

There is abundant evidence from Third World studies that nutritional deprivation is associated with impaired immunological function and risk of infection. Disturbances of both humoral and cell mediated immunity occur in malnutrition. A degree of nutritional impairment is a common occurrence among many surgical patients, especially those who are seriously ill and an awareness of this has led to the increased use of nutritional support, e.g. by intravenous feeding, in those surgical patients most affected. Whether such attempts to correct the nutritional deficiency in these patients can lead to improved immunological responsiveness is, however, controversial.

Immune depression and malignancy

Many types of malignant disease may be associated with depression of immune responses. The degree of immune depression assessed, for example, by delayed hypersensitivity skin testing has been shown in some studies to relate to the stage of the malignant disease. Whether or not the observed immune depression is directly due to the tumour or to other related factors such as malnutrition in these patients is not clear.

The acquired immune deficiency syndrome (AIDS)

The presence of infection, especially by viruses, may lead to secondary immune depression. An extreme and dramatic example of this is AIDS which is due to the human immunodeficiency virus (HIV) and is transmitted from affected individuals by body fluids. This disease became prevalent in the last decade and was seen mainly in male homosexuals, intravenous drug abusers and haemophiliacs receiving factor VIII derived from pooled plasma. AIDS produces a deficiency in cell mediated responses. Humoral responses are less affected and neutrophil function is normal. The peripheral blood from affected individuals shows a lymphopenia, predominantly due to a decrease in T cells. The number of cytotoxic T cells is relatively normal but there is a severe reduction in T helper cells, giving a grossly decreased CD4/CD8 ratio. AIDS patients are prone to severe opportunistic infections and to a high incidence of Kaposi's sarcoma, an otherwise uncommon tumour. The disease is invariably fatal.

MONOCLONAL ANTIBODIES

Conventional immunisation results in the production of an antiserum comprising a heterogeneous group of antibodies (i.e. polyclonal antibodies) each directed at different antigenic determinants, of different subclasses and of different affinity. Köhler and Milstein achieved a major scientific breakthrough when they devised a technique which allowed the production of monoclonal antibodies, i.e. antibodies of identical molecular structure and hence the same highly specific properties. The essential step in this technique is the fusion of a normal antibody producing lymphocyte with a myeloma cell, which confers immortality to the resulting 'hybridoma'. Using cloning techniques, a single clone of the 'hybridoma' producing the desired monoclonal antibody is obtained and by propagating this clone either in tissue culture or as ascitic fluid, an endless supply of monoclonal antibody can be made available (Fig. 27.5).

The current and potential clinical applications of monoclonal antibody technology are enormous and only an indication of these can be given here. They may be used to label lymphocyte subpopulations, thus allowing analysis, isolation or depletion of the various cell subpopulations. In clinical organ transplantation the in vivo-administration of such antibodies to cause immunoregulation is being explored whereas in bone marrow transplantation they can be used in vitro to eliminate T cells from the marrow transplant and prevent graft versus host disease. Monoclonal antibodies are proving increasingly useful in many types of immunoassay, in blood grouping and tissue typing, in the immunohistological diagnosis of cancer and in the diagnosis and typing of pathogenic

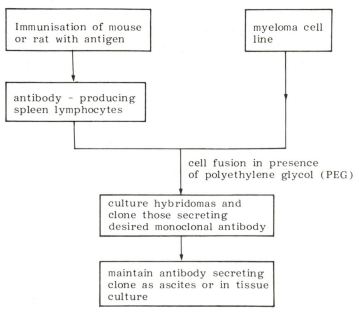

Fig. 27.5 Production of monoclonal antibody

organisms. Exciting, but as yet unobtained goals, are the use of monoclonal antibodies in imaging techniques to localize primary and metastatic tumours and to target cytotoxic agents coupled with antibody to tumours — the so-called 'magic bullet'.

The majority of monoclonal antibodies being used are the product of mouse or rat hybridomas but much effort is now being made to produce human monoclonal antibodies. Although this is proving technically difficult, if successful this technology would allow antibodies to be produced against human antigens which are only poorly antigenic in rodents. Human monoclonal antibodies would also be of greater clinical use since they could be administered in vivo without the risk of sensitisation that injecting rodent antibodies carries.

TRANSPLANTATION IMMUNOLOGY

The transplantation of organs from unrelated donors into recipients to replace damaged or diseased organs is now widely established. Cadaveric renal transplantation has become a routine treatment for end stage renal failure and transplantation of the heart, liver and pancreas, are being carried out with increasing frequency. Unless suitable and reliable artificial support systems become available or great advances in the prevention or early treatment of the original disease occur, neither of which seem likely in the foreseeable future, then the practice of organ transplantation will continue to increase. The major barrier to effective organ transplantation is rejection of the transplant by the recipient's immune system. Before discussing the immunological aspects in detail it is important to outline the terminology involved.

Autograft. A graft taken from one part of an individual and transplanted to another site in the same individual, e.g. a skin graft in a burned patient.

Isograft. A graft between genetically identical individuals e.g. renal transplantation between identical twins or inbred animals of the same strain.

Allograft. A graft between genetically non-identical individuals of the same species (syn. Homograft), e.g. a cadaveric renal transplant from an unrelated donor.

Xenograft. A graft between individuals of different species, e.g. a monkey kidney into a human.

Orthotopic transplant. A transplant grafted into its normal site.

Heterotopic transplant. A transplant placed into an abnormal site, e.g. kidney transplantation into the iliac fossa and not the loin.

Immunological basis of allograft rejection

Tissue and organs transplanted between genetically disparate individuals are, in the absence of immunosup-

pressive therapy, rejected within a few days of grafting. This rejection process shows the characteristic features of an immunological response, i.e. specificity and memory. Consequently, a second graft from the same donor undergoes accelerated (second set) rejection, whereas a second graft from an unrelated (third party) donor is rejected at a normal (first set) tempo.

Early work by Gibson and Medawar (1943) with skin grafts showed that rejecting grafts become heavily infiltrated by lymphocytes and monocytes, suggesting that cell mediated responses rather than antibodies were involved in graft rejection. Support for this hypothesis was provided from animal studies in which it was shown that sensitivity to grafted tissue (i.e. second set rejection) could be transferred by lymphocytes but not serum obtained from a graft recipient. That the T lymphocyte plays an essential role in graft rejection is clearly shown by the inability of congenitally athymic or neonatally thymectomised animals to reject an allograft. Restoring such animals with normal T cells readily restores their ability to reject a graft.

In clinical renal transplantation the picture of graft rejection is less clear because of the possibility of previous sensitisation and the necessity for immunosuppressive treatment. Three main categories of graft rejection are recognised.

Hyperacute rejection

This occurs almost immediately after transplantation. It is due to the presence in the recipient of preformed cytotoxic antibodies because of previous sensitisation to graft antigens by blood transfusion or an earlier graft. The complement fixing antibodies rapidly damage the graft vasculature with platelet aggregation, thrombosis and infarction. Fortunately careful pre-transplant screening has almost eliminated this type of rejection.

Acute rejection

This is due to classical cellular immune mechanisms and occurs to some extent during the first few weeks of most transplants. The graft becomes heavily infiltrated with T cells, B cells, macrophages and NK cells. Both cytotoxic T cell lysis and delayed type hypersensitivity responses appear to be capable of causing graft damage but in the majority of cases any such rejection episode can be reversed by the immunosuppressive therapy.

Chronic rejection

If a graft is not acutely rejected within the first few weeks the chances of long term survival are much improved. Nevertheless, a small proportion of grafts steadily succumb to chronic rejection many months after transplantation. Humoral responses appear to be involved in late chronic rejection. The glomerular capillaries become coated with antibody and gradual fibrosis and loss of renal function occur.

Tissue typing

Close matching of donor and recipient with respect to transplantation antigens is an essential requirement for bone marrow transplantation to avoid rapid graft rejection or graft-versus-host disease. By contrast, matching for corneal graft is unnecessary since the cornea appears to be an immunologically privileged site. In renal transplantation (and possibly for other transplanted organs) attempts to match the tissue types of donor and recipient produce a definite, though relatively small, increase in graft survival.

The first requirement in organ matching is to match ABO blood group antigens, since these antigens are expressed not only on red blood cells but on most cells of the body, and if mismatched will elicit a strong immune response in the recipient due to the presence of naturally occurring antibodies to the ABO antigens. Tissue typing is employed to identify an individual's leukocyte antigens or HLA type. These transplantation antigens are expressed on most cells of the body and they are coded for by a cluster of genes — the Major Histocompatibility Complex (MHC) — situated on chromosome 6. The MHC codes for the alleles of the HLA-A, HLA-B and HLA-C loci (class I MHC antigens), and for the alleles of the HLA-DR, -DP and -DQ loci (class II MHC antigens). The HLA-A and -B loci and in particular the DR loci are considered to code for the most important transplant antigens. To date, there are 20 well defined A locus alleles, 33 B locus alleles and 10 DR alleles. An individual possesses two alleles for each locus (one inherited from each parent), but may be homozygous at one or more loci. Logistically, for the majority of renal transplants, perfect matching of donor and recipient at all loci is not possible. In practice, it is common to attempt to match both or at least one of the DR loci (since there are fewer DR types than HLA-A and -B types) and thereafter, where possible the HLA-A and -B loci. Retrospective studies after renal transplantation show that with an increasing number of HLA DR, A and B mismatches there is a progressive decrease in the graft survival rate.

An individual's tissue type is determined in the laboratory from a preparation of peripheral blood lymphocytes. These are tested serologically, using typing antisera prepared from blood obtained from patients who have received previous blood transfusions or from multiparous women who have developed specific antibodies against paternal HLA antigens. More recently, monoclonal antibodies are becoming available to identify particular antigens. In addition to tissue typing, as part of the organ matching procedure it is essential to perform a 'cross match' prior to transplantation, using recipient serum and donor lymphoid cells, in order to exclude the presence in the recipient of pre-formed cytotoxic antibodies. Such antibodies may occur in multiparous women or in previously transfused or transplanted patients and if present could result in hyperacute rejection of the graft. It should be emphasised that despite a complete match of the HLA-A, -B, and -DR locus antigens, rejection episodes may still occur in response to 'minor histocompatability antigen' differences, but these tend to be more amenable to immunosuppressive therapy.

Apart from their role in transplantation immunology, it is apparent that a number of specific HLA types are associated with a predisposition to certain diseases, especially those with an immunological basis and in particular autoimmune disease. The best known example is the association between ankylosing spondylitis and possession of the HLA-B27 phenotype in which around 95% of sufferers possess this antigen, while autoimmune insulin-dependent diabetes is associated with the DR-3 and DR-4 phenotypes.

Methods of preventing rejection

Although tissue typing reduces the chances of graft rejection, it is essential to give immunosuppressive drugs after organ grafting and these have to be continued indefinitely to prevent rejection. Until recently the most widely used immunosuppressive regimen was a combination of azathioprine and prednisolone which act by non-specifically ablating the immune response. Recently, cyclosporin A, a newer drug, has been used increasingly. This important drug is a metabolite of a fungus and its action is more specifically directed at lymphoid cells than conventional immunosuppressive drugs. Cyclosporin A exerts its powerful immunosuppressive effect mainly through its action on T cell activation, preventing the development of cytotoxic T cells. Unfortunately, its side effects include nephrotoxicity and hepatotoxicity.

If signs of rejection occur, despite the presence of the above immunosuppressive drugs, then additional immunosuppressive measures may be introduced. These include the use of anti-lymphocyte serum (ALS). This serum is raised by injecting an animal (commonly a rabbit or horse) with human lymphocytes. When the globulin fraction of the resulting antiserum is injected into the transplant recipient, it selectively destroys lymphocytes. A drawback of this treatment is that it may cause hypersensitivity reactions to the injected animal proteins. Recently the administration of monoclonal antibodies directed at T lymphocytes has also been tried with some success. After injection, the monoclonal antibody binds to T cells which are rapidly depleted (probably by opsonisation) from the body. Both of the above agents may be successful in reversing a graft rejection episode.

Two other supplementary immunosuppressive treatments which have been tried are thoracic duct drainage and total lymphoid irradiation. Although both methods effectively deplete the body of circulating lymphocytes, they are serious undertakings and neither has been widely adopted in clinical practice.

Immunological enhancement

Following the early successes in the use of preimmunisation to prevent infectious disease, attempts were also made to treat cancer in the same way. Unexpectedly, preimmunisation of an animal with killed tumour cells allowed *prolonged* survival of a subsequent tumour challenge. This phenomenon, known as enhancement, although harmful in the context of tumour immunology, is also applicable to transplantation immunology where it may prolong allograft survival.

In experimental transplantation, enhancement may be brought about by either pretreating the recipient animal with serum containing antibodies directed against the graft (passive enhancement) or by immunising the recipient with cells of the same strain as the donor (active enhancement).

Despite a great deal of experimental work, the precise mechanism of immunological enhancement is not understood. Proposed mechanisms include:

1. Coating of graft antigens by antibody which blocks the rejection response.
2. Binding of antibody to and elimination of 'passenger leukocytes' in the graft.
3. Elimination by phagocytosis of specifically activated helper T cells which have bound graft antigen-antibody complexes.
4. Induction of suppressor T cells which specifically suppress the cell mediated response against the allograft.

Although the effectiveness of enhancement has been shown in a variety of experimental conditions its application to clinical transplantation has produced disappointing results. An exception is the beneficial effect that blood transfusion, prior to cadaveric renal transplantation confers on graft survival. Because patients who have not received blood transfusion prior to renal transplantation are more likely to reject a renal graft, it is now standard practice to give elective blood transfusions to patients on the transplant waiting list. Unfortunately, this sometimes results in the development of cytotoxic antibodies which may give a positive crossmatch test against lymphocytes from a prospective kidney donor, precluding the use of the kidney in that particular recipient.

Bone marrow transplantation

This offers a chance of cure in an increasing number of patients with otherwise fatal malignant or non-malignant conditions. It is most often used in the management of haematological malignancy and occasionally in patients with certain solid tumours, but also has a role in non-malignant diseases such as severe combined immune deficiency, severe aplastic anaemia and thalassaemia major. In essence, the patient is given a very high dose of chemotherapy or total body irradiation to destroy completely the malignancy and also the patient's own lymphoid tissue and bone marrow which would otherwise rapidly reject the graft. Bone marrow from a well-matched donor, invariably a sibling since this offers the best chance of a good match, is then transplanted at the appropriate time and the transplant recolonizes the recipient's bone marrow. Although the technique is relatively simple, marrow grafting is a hazardous procedure. Complications related to graft rejection, infection and bleeding may be difficult to control and even when the donor is an HLA identical sibling and in the presence of immunosuppressant drugs, graft-versus-host disease is still common. The risk of graft-versus-host disease can be reduced if T cells can be eliminated from the donor marrow prior to transplantation. A promising way of achieving this involves incubating the harvested marrow with anti-T-cell monoclonal antibodies, either with complement or bound to a toxin, in an attempt to destroy any T cells.

CANCER IMMUNOLOGY

For many years it has been postulated that the immune response plays a role in preventing the development, growth and spread of cancer. Convincing clinical proof of this is still awaited but a number of observations suggest that immune reactions to tumours are important in humans.

1. Spontaneous regression of tumours. This is rare but there are numerous well documented cases.
2. Patients who are immunosuppressed either by drugs, radiotherapy or because of primary immunodeficiency disease, have an increased risk of malignancy. The tumours seen are not the types frequently found in non-immunosuppressed patients. Often they are lymphoid tumours which may be because immunosuppression reduces the normal control of lymphoid proliferation and thus predisposes to lymphoid malignancy.
3. Malignant tumours are often infiltrated by lymphocytes and macrophages and in some studies this finding has been correlated with improved prognosis.
4. In several large post mortem series, the incidence of latent cancers, especially thyroid and prostate, is much higher than would be expected from the clinical incidence of these tumours. This suggests that tumours may develop and be destroyed before they become clinically evident.

These clinical observations, taken together, are in keeping with a role for the immune system in cancer control.

Tumour antigens

The proposal that immune responses are able to destroy malignant cells implies that tumour cells have specific antigens on their surface which allow them to be distinguished from normal cells. There is abundant evidence that experimental tumours in animals may express such tumour specific antigens which are able to induce an immunological response. However, many of these animal tumours are virally or chemically induced and, at present, no truly tumour specific antigen has been identified on spontaneously occurring human malignancies.

It is important to appreciate that many so-called 'tumour specific' antigens are not exclusively specific to tumour cells. Some tumour antigens, although not normally found on the type of cell from which the tumour was derived, may be found on other normal cell types. Furthermore, some tumour antigens may be differentiation antigens, i.e. antigens only occurring transiently during the normal differentiation of a cell, and hence only expressed on a minority of normal cells, e.g. 'stem-cell' antigen in lymphoblastic leukaemia.

Some malignant tumours express antigens which are only normally found in significant amounts on foetal tissue. The two best known of the increasing range of these oncofoetal antigens are alpha fetoprotein (AFP) and carcinoembryonic antigen (CEA). These two tumour markers are of limited use in the diagnosis of some forms of cancer, but more importantly, serum levels of AFP and CEA may be used to monitor the progress of the tumour and the response to treatment. Attempts have also been made to localise metastatic disease by the in vivo use of radiolabelled monoclonal antibody to CEA.

Immunity to tumours

It is unclear which of the many components of the immune system are responsible for tumour immunity. The popular view is that this may depend on the nature of the tumour. Since NK cells are able to lyse certain tumour cells in vitro it has been suggested that they may function as an immunosurveillance system or first line of defence against the development of a tumour. Interferon gamma, in addition to stimulating NK cell lysis, also inhibits cell growth, suggesting that it may have direct antitumour activity. Antibody activated macrophages and cell mediated cytotoxicity may also be capable of contributing to tumour immunity.

Immunotherapy of cancer

This refers to the use of immunological methods to try and adversely affect the growth of an established tumour. Many methods have been tried but most have been disappointing. Non-specific immunological adjuvants such as BCG (Bacillus-Calmette-Guerin) or *Corynebacterium parvum* have been given empirically to try and stimulate an antitumour response but clinical trials have shown little benefit. More recently, Interferon gamma (derived from recombinant DNA technology) has been tried. Again its effects to date have been disappointing with some evidence for partial response but also significant side effects. However, trials of Interferon gamma as well as other lymphokines (notably Interleukin 2) in cancer chemotherapy are continuing. Another possibility is the use of tumour specific immunotherapy. Methods tried include vaccinating a cancer patient with killed tumour cells or, alternatively, stimulating an aliquot of peripheral blood monocytes and lymphocytes by in vitro culture with tumour, prior to re-injecting them into the patient. None of the above methods are likely to be used routinely in the near future.

FURTHER READING

General immunology

Hanson L A, Wigzell H 1985 Immunology. Butterworths, London
Playfair J H L 1984 Immunology at a glance. Blackwell, Oxford
Roitt I M 1984 Essential immunology. Blackwell, Oxford
Weir D M 1983 Immunology. Churchill Livingstone, Edinburgh

Clinical applications

Calne R Y 1984 Transplantation immunology: clinical and experimental. Oxford University Press, Oxford

McMichael A J, Fabre J W 1982 Monoclonal antibodies in clinical medicine. Academic Press, London
Lennox E S 1984 Clinical applications of monoclonal antibodies. British Medical Bulletin. Churchill Livingstone, Edinburgh.
Christou N V 1985 Host defence mechanisms: systemic responses. In: Meakins, J L (ed) Clinics in Critical Care Medicine. Churchill Livingstone, Edinburgh
Mitchison N A 1982 Protective immunity (to tumours) in vivo. In: Lachmann P, Peters D K (eds) Clinical Aspects of Immunology. Blackwell, Oxford.

Shock

The syndrome of hypotension, tachycardia, pallor, sweating, peripheral cyanosis, hyperventilation, clouding of consciousness and oliguria is universally accepted as the clinical expression of the shock state. The full-blown presentation is usually preceded by more subtle physiological and metabolic disturbances which are not so easily measured by the bedside but of greater significance from the point of view of effective treatment. Thus whilst changes in arterial blood pressure and heart rate, for example, are readily recognized and routinely recorded, earlier alterations in blood volume, blood flow and oxygen consumption are likely to have occurred, correction of which may lead to rapid restoration of normal cardiovascular and respiratory status. In the absence of appropriate early treatment shock leads to a progressively widening gulf between oxygen supply and demand, the final effect of which is to produce irreversible changes in cell metabolism.

This chapter summarizes current views on the main physiological and biochemical disturbances of shock. A short account of the precipitating factors and their general consequences leads on to more detailed consideration of the haemodynamic, neurohumoral and cellular disturbances. Organ dysfunction and failure are described and a short note on the principles of treatment is also included.

PRECIPITATING FACTORS

Almost any insult to the body can lead to shock and when the syndrome is fully developed few physiological processes remain unaffected. For these reasons any *general* description of the syndrome inevitably tends to emphasize the final common pathway of tissue hypoxia rather than the earlier, readily reversible, stages. It is also clear that the duration of onset of the shock state is quite variable and its initial pattern and character are influenced not only by the primary aetiology but also by the pre-existing condition of the patient and the nature of coincident treat-

ment. Interpretation of these various factors is not always easy and uncertainty about the precise sequence of pathophysiological events has led to differences of opinion that may be more apparent than real.

It is convenient to consider shock under three primary aetiological groupings — cardiogenic, hypovolaemic and distributive — always accepting that overlap between the groupings is common clinical experience and that their metabolic consequences may be indistinguishable and may influence the pattern of haemodynamic response.

Cardiogenic shock

Failure of the heart as a pump may be due to:

1. Primary myocardial dysfunction from
   a. Myocardial infarction
   b. Serious cardiac arrhythmias
   c. Myocardial depression from a variety of causes, e.g. drugs
2. Miscellaneous causes which include
   a. Tension pneumothorax
   b. Vena caval obstruction
   c. Cardiac tamponade

Hypovolaemic shock

Reduction in the circulating fluid volume (blood volume) in the form of loss of whole blood, plasma or extracellular fluid or a combination of the three.

Distributive shock

Changes in resistance vessels may be brought about by specific disorders which include:
1. Decrease in resistance
   a. Spinal anaesthesia
   b. Neurogenic reflexes, as in acute pain
   c. Possibly the end stages of hypovolaemic shock
2. Septic shock
   a. Change in peripheral arterial resistance

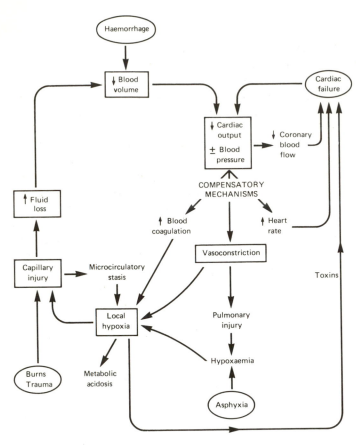

Fig. 28.1 Mechanisms leading to reduced cardiac output and inadequate tisue perfusion (from Hackel et al, 1974)

b. Change in venous capacitance

c. Peripheral arteriovenous shunting

Whatever the cause, shock is associated with a reduction in blood flow through the vessels of the microcirculation to a level which is incompatible with normal tissue oxygen consumption. The fall in oxygen consumption is variable in degree and in time of onset, apparently occurring earlier in some forms of shock, e.g. septic shock, than in others. Once the shock process becomes established it tends to be self-perpetuating (Fig. 28.1) and leads to progressive disturbance of cellular function.

HAEMODYNAMIC DISTURBANCES

Changes in blood pressure, heart rate, peripheral perfusion and urine output are usually the first features to draw the surgeon's attention to the possibility of shock. The central nervous system initiates the body's homeostatic responses to acute injury (including fluid loss) by mechanisms which are complex and ill-understood. Multiple afferent stimuli (arterial and venous pressure and volume, osmolality, pH, hypoxia, pain and anxiety, tissue damage and sepsis) are, with few exceptions, integrated in the medullary vaso-motor centre, either directly or via higher centres such as the mid-brain, hypothalamus and cerebral cortex. Thence efferent stimuli are relayed to the sympathetic nervous system and adrenal medulla. On this basis it might be supposed that the haemodynamic response to shock should be constant and predictable but such is not the case (Table 28.1).

The degree of hypotension is quite variable, depending inter alia on the severity and duration of shock and the magnitude of cardiovascular compensatory responses. Indeed, in the early stages of traumatic shock excessive vasoconstriction may occur such that the ensuing hyper-tension may mislead the inexperienced observer and cause delay in appropriate treatment. This is particularly common in previously fit young males. The changes in heart rate are equally unreliable and the reported frequency of tachycardia may be more a reflection of the body's response to fluid repletion used in treatment than of the normal physiological response to hypovolaemia. In a recent study (Sander-Jensen et al, 1986) of 20 consecutive patients with hypotension due to haemorrhage (mean blood loss corresponding to 36% of estimated blood volume), only two patients showed an increase in heart rate prior to resuscitation. The remainder had a mean heart rate of 9 beats/min lower than the steady state value. The bradycardia, whose mechanism probably involves a reflex relayed through vagal afferent C fibres from the left ventricle, is thought to serve as a protective mechanism allowing for improved diastolic filling when venous return is critically reduced.

In hypovolaemic and cardiogenic shock peripheral perfusion is generally reduced, giving rise to the charac-

Table 28.1 Clinical features of the three main types of shock

	Cardiogenic shock	Hypovolaemic shock	Distributive shock
Systemic arterial pressure	Decreased	Decreased	Decreased
Heart rate	Increased/(Decreased)	(Decreased)/Increased	Increased
Central venous pressure	Increased	Not increased	Variable
Urine output	Decreased	Decreased	(Increased)/Decreased
Core/peripheral temperature gradient	Increased	Increased	Decreased/Increased
Cardiac output	Decreased	Decreased	Increased/(Variable)
Pulmonary capillary wedge pressure	Increased	Decreased	Variable

teristic mottled pallor and cyanosis of the extremities; the skin becomes intensely cold to the touch. In the early stages of septic shock, on the other hand, or during the phase of resuscitation, the skin of the periphery may be flushed and warm. This 'hyperdynamic' response reflects the presence of vasodilator substances secondary to the septic process (but does not necessarily indicate that the response is adequate to meet increased tissue requirements for oxygen).

One of the most constant clinical observations in shock is oliguria although again, the magnitude of reduction in urine output varies with the rapidity of onset of the shock process. Urine formation ceases when the systemic arterial pressure falls to 50 mmHg but in septic shock, for example, other mechanisms (e.g. endotoxaemia) may cause reduction in glomerular filtration at higher perfusion pressures.

In recent years technological advances have allowed the measurement of some additional haemodynamic variables (Swan & Ganz, 1983) and thus helped to elucidate further the mechanisms of shock and the individual patient's response to treatment. Notable amongst these newer measurements are central venous pressure, pulmonary artery pressure and cardiac output.

Cardiac output

Changes in cardiac output (and therefore oxygen availability) are central to the disturbances of shock and the ability to measure this parameter has been particularly valuable in determining optimum haemodynamic goals for restoration and maintenance of normal oxygen consumption. The ready availability by the bedside of continuous information relating the factors contributing to cardiac output and its distribution (Fig. 28.2) has become increasingly rewarding as advances in treatment have emerged. In the case of pharmacological agents, for example, separate manipulation of preload (pulmonary capillary wedge pressure) and afterload (systemic vascular resistance) using selective vasoactive drugs (see below) has considerably improved the effectiveness of acute resuscitation of the shocked patient.

Acute cardiac failure may arise as a primary disturbance of one of the integral functions of the heart or secondary to some disturbance elsewhere in the body. The shock state itself may induce cardiac failure and thereby contribute to the vicious cycle of haemodynamic disturbance which has already been described (Fig. 28.1). The heart was first implicated in the shock syndrome when

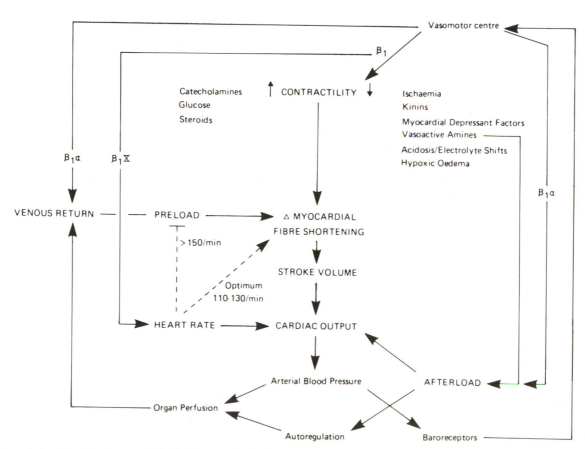

Fig. 28.2 Interrelationships of intrinsic variables in the systemic circulation and ways in which extrinsic factors may exert their influence (After George & Tinker, 1983)

Wiggers (1950) demonstrated that dogs subjected to sustained haemorrhagic hypotension eventually required increasing transfusion of the shed blood to maintain blood pressure. Initially left atrial pressure rose followed by elevation of right atrial pressure and death finally supervened with a progressive fall in cardiac output in spite of replacement of all the shed blood. In the 35 years since Wigger's original work many laboratory and clinical investigations have shown that cardiac failure is an important component of the shock state although its onset and severity in an individual animal or patient is difficult to predict.

One problem is to assess myocardial function independent of other cardiovascular variables. Changes in arterial blood pressure in response to changes in central venous pressure (induced by fluid administration) may be used as a rough guide to cardiac performance but a more reliable relationship is that between left ventricular stroke work and left ventricular end-diastolic pressure, being less dependent on changes in heart rate and peripheral vascular resistance. The changes in stroke work and end-diastolic pressure in response to the central venous administration of a standard fluid load may be used to construct left ventricular function curves and comparison made of the latter before and after shock. In such a study on anaesthetized, spontaneously breathing dogs (MacDonald et al, 1975), one group of animals (Group I) was bled to a mean arterial blood pressure of 40 mmHg over a period of 15–20 minutes when the shed blood was immediately re-infused over a period of 40–45 minutes. In a second group of

animals (Group II) the tube leading to the bleeding reservoir was clamped when the mean arterial pressure reached 40 mmHg, preventing any further transfer of blood from the animal to the reservoir; during the subsequent 2 hours mean arterial blood pressure rose spontaneously to over 100 mmHg when the shed blood was re-infused again over a period of 40–45 minutes. In a third group of animals (Group III) the mean arterial blood pressure was maintained at a level of 40 mmHg for a 2-hour period by bleeding off or re-infusing blood as required, after which the blood was re-infused in similar fashion. Figure 28.3 shows representative left ventricular function curves from each group before and after shock. In Groups I and II these curves were similar before and after shock. In Group III, the post-shock curve is markedly depressed. Using such haemorrhagic shock models the effect of certain pharmacological agents commonly used in the treatment of established shock may be assessed. The apparent improvement in left ventricular function after the administration of ouabaine and isoprenaline may thus be demonstrated (Figs 28.4 and 28.5). Interpretation of these curves is complicated by the fact that changes in compliance of the left ventricle may occur secondary to administration of these drugs.

The clinical relevance of these laboratory studies is that rapid transfusion of blood or other fluids following haemorrhage or trauma in patients may be associated with the onset of cardiac failure and the more prolonged the period of shock the more pronounced is this effect. In the management of shocked patients a rough assessment of

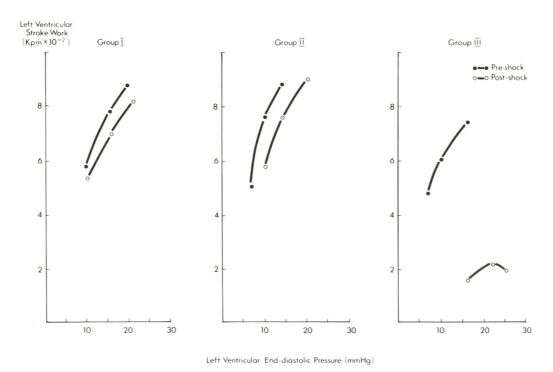

Fig. 28.3 Representative ventricular function curves from each group obtained during fluid loads before and after shock

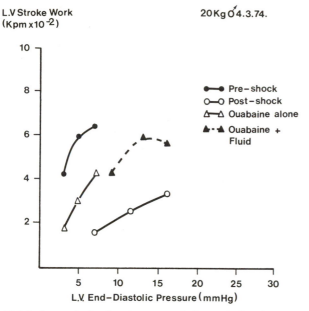

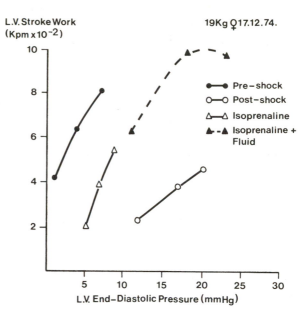

Fig. 28.4 Left ventricular function curves before and after shock. Post-shock ventricular function was improved by the administration of ouabaine and the effect enhanced by additional intravenous fluid

Fig. 28.5 Left ventricular function curves before and after shock. Post-shock ventricular function was improved by isoprenaline and additional intravenous fluid

cardiac function may be obtained by noting the relationship between changes in central venous pressure and arterial blood pressure produced by rapid transfusion of small amounts of colloid fluid; the presence of cardiac failure as distinct from hypovolaemia may thus be determined. In one study of a large group of shocked patients suffering from trauma, sepsis and haemorrhage, but without evidence of a primary cardiac defect, 20% responded to a test fluid load of 500 ml of dextrain in such a way as to indicate cardiac insufficiency, and another 20% had a combination of cardiac insufficiency and peripheral circulatory failure (Shoemaker et al, 1971).

The cause of cardiac failure in shock has evaded precise definition. Since the myocardium has a high oxygen consumption, a discrepancy might be expected to occur between myocardial oxygen availability and consumption during severe hypotension. However, the work of the heart, and therefore myocardial oxygen consumption, falls in most forms of shock. Moreover, the normal heart is able to protect itself to a remarkable degree by autoregulatory vasodilatation during hypotension. These factors account for the difficulty in producing biochemical evidence of myocardial ischaemia. On the other hand, the electrocardiogram during severe hypotension frequently shows changes consistent with ischaemia and, in long-term recovery experiments, patchy necrosis of myocardial cells has been demonstrated (Hackel et al., 1974). Another possible explanation of the heart failure present in patients with shock has recently come to light, in the form of a circulating myocardial depressant factor (MDF) (Lefer, 1973). This substance is thought to originate in the

ischaemic pancreas and may reach the systemic circulation via the lymphatic system. In a group of shocked patients who later died of cardiac failure, increased levels of this substance were found in plasma ultrafiltrates (Fisher et al, 1973). It is also possible that endotoxin may directly damage myocardial cells but clearcut evidence of this effect is lacking and, in any case, is likely to occur only after prolonged endotoxaemia (Hinshaw et al., 1972). In septic shock, oedema of cardiac muscle consistent with compartmental fluid shifts, has been observed in experimental studies (Postel & Schleorb, 1977). This change occurred early and did not recover for some time in spite of prompt and adequate resuscitation.

In patients with long-standing atheromatous coronary artery disease, cardiac failure may be more readily explained after a period of shock. The patient with diseased coronary arteries may be unable to dilate his vessels in response to hypotension (see Fig. 28.6) and myocardial ischaemia of greater severity may occur in these patients than in patients with normal coronary arteries for an equivalent degree of hypotension.

The possibility of unsuspected myocardial infarction contributing to the clinical presentation should always be borne in mind in shocked patients, particularly if arrhythmias occur during or after hypotension. The acute onset of myocardial infarction may explain an unexpected failure to respond to resuscitation. Other causes of primary cardiogenic shock include the drugs and agents used by the anaesthetist, e.g. barbiturate and halothane, and, in the late post-operative period, the risk of pulmonary embolism arises.

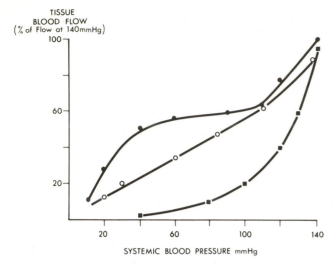

Fig. 28.6 The relationship between systemic arterial perfusion and tissue bloodflow in organs demonstrating either a passive pressure-flow pattern (■–■; e.g., skin) or a vascular autoregulation (●–●; e.g., heart and brain). Autoregulation is probably absent in the heart and brain when the major arteries are atheromatous; under these conditions the pressure-flow relationship is probably linear (○–○)

Drugs which stimulate cardiac action are often advocated in shock and there is little doubt that cardiac output can be increased in this way. Indeed digitalisation is not infrequently specifically indicated to correct uncontrolled artrial fibrillation. Ouabain may be preferred to digoxin if a rapid action is imperative; in either case the intravenous route should be used because of uncertain absorption by other routes. Isoprenaline has the advantage that, in addition to its inotropic action, it dilates the peripheral blood vessels, but its tendency to produce tachycardia and even tachyarrhythmias is a disadvantage. A number of new inotropic drugs are being eveluated, e.g. dobutamine, glucagon and dopamine; some of these are already proving valuable (see below).

Microcirculatory disturbances

Under normal physiological conditions the proportion of the cardiac output available to individual organs is dependent upon the perfusion pressure and the degree of smooth muscle tone in the supplying vessels. This is usually considerable and is due to the activity of sympathetic vasoconstrictor fibres to the arterioles (precapillary resistance vessels) and to the venules (postcapillary resistance vessels) and veins (capacitance vessels). The relationship between perfusion pressure and tissue blood flow varies greatly in individual organs and is illustrated in Figure 28.6. Some tissues (e.g. skin and, to a certain extent, skeletal muscle) have a passive pressure-flow relationship (convexity towards the pressure axis). Quite a different relationship is seen in the renal, cerebral and coronary vascular beds; steady-state pressure-flow curves

are almost horizontal until a pressure of about 50 mmHg is reached when flow decreases precipitously (and the convexity is then towards the flow axis). This ability of an organ to maintain flow despite changes in perfusion pressure is termed autoregulation. It occurs in the absence of vasomotor nerves and is an intrinsic property of the vascular smooth muscle of the organ concerned. Basically autoregulation is a protective mechanism by which the body attempts to compensate for a reduced perfusion pressure to 'vital' organs. Reduction in tissue blood flow in response to a reduced systemic arterial blood pressure (to levels commonly observed in shocked patients) will clearly be much more marked in tissues and organs that do not exhibit vascular autoregulation. In addition, autoregulation is altered when the major supplying arteries become diseased. In experimental animals rendered hypertensive (Fitch et al, 1976), the normal autoregulatory pattern is retained but is shifted to the right with the result that haemorrhage produces a sharp reduction in blood flow at a higher than normal mean arterial blood pressure. Autoregulation is almost certainly reduced when the arterial cross sectional area is reduced by atheroma; this is probably the reason why the manifestations of reduced coronary and cerebral blood flow in circulatory shock are more common in older patients.

A second compensatory mechanism available to the body during acute cardiac failure or hypovolaemia is increased sympathoadrenal discharge. This not only increases myocardial contractility but also leads to constriction of the arterioles (thereby tending to restore blood pressure towards normal) and of the capacitance vessels (hence maintaining venous return to the heart) The magnitude of vasoconstriction in some of the 'non-vital' areas of the body is not reflected in any of the routine clinical haemodynamic measurements and thus is often not appreciated. In a recent experimental study, for example, a 10% reduction in blood volume produced negligible changes in arterial pressure and heart rate, but an almost 30% reduction in colon blood flow and oxygen availability (Gilmour et al, 1980). The profound decrease in splanchnic blood flow has important implications for liver function, since approximately 70% of hepatic blood flow normally traverses the portal vein.

The responses of the vessels of the microcirculation in skeletal muscle to increased sympathetic discharge are summarized in Table 28.2. Under normal conditions, and early in shock, the effect of sympathetic stimulation results in constriction of the resistance vessels on both sides of the capillary bed. However since precapillary resistance (arteriolar constriction) is increased to a greater extent than postcapillary (venular) resistance mean capillary pressure is decreased and there is a tendency for fluid to move into the circulation from the tissue spaces by osmosis. Late in shock there is a marked change in vascular reactivity; despite the continued release of noradrenaline the response of

Table 28.2 Effects of stimulating peripheral vasoconstrictor fibres to skeletal muscle

	Pre-capillary resistance vessels (arterioles)	Sphincter activity	Post-capillary vessels (venules, capacitance)	Mean capillary pressure	Fluid movement
Normal response and response early in shock	Marked constriction (++++)	Increased (+++)	Marked constriction (+++)	Decreased	Inward
	There is a decrease in blood flow and transcapillary fluid movement is into the circulation; survival is favoured				
Response late in shock	(+ or −)	(−)	(++)	Increased	Outward
	This change is due to declining vascular reactivity, especially of pre-capillary segment, and to accumulation of metabolites. Fluid leaves circulation and this, with pooling in capacitance vessels, decreases venous return.				

arteriolar smooth muscle declines much more rapidly than does that of venular smooth muscle. This 'fade' is accentuated by the accumulation of metabolites such as lactic acid which have more profound vasodilator effects on arterioles than on venules. The result of this change in vascular reactivity is that mean capillary pressure is increased which favours transudation of fluid from the plasma into the tissue spaces. Fluid loss is also accentuated by circulating vasoactive substances (such as histamine and the plasma kinins) which increase capillary permeability. From their animal experiments, Mellander and Lewis (1963) estimated that in a 70 kg man in shock (with 30 kg skeletal muscle mass) this change in vascular reactivity could result in a decrease of circulating blood volume of more than 600 ml/hour. This would be achieved by filtering only 2 ml of fluid into the interstitial spaces of every 100 g of muscle — a volume hardly detectable as oedema.

One of the consequences of continuing postcapillary vasoconstriction and loss of intravascular fluid is haemoconcentration; this leads to an increase in blood viscosity and therefore a higher resistance to blood flow, from the Poiseuille relationship

$$\text{flow} = \frac{\pi(P_1 - P_2)r^4}{8l\eta}$$

where $P_1 - P_2$ is the pressure drop across vessels of length l and radius r; η is the viscosity of the perfusing fluid.

Additional factors which influence blood viscosity are the fibrinogen level and the haematocrit, both of which are raised in the early stages of shock. These changes in the characteristics of the blood lead to widespread aggregation ('sludging') of red cells and of platelets. Platelet aggregation can be induced by the presence of thrombin, noradrenaline, endotoxin and particulate matter (for example, fibres of collagen released from injured vessels). These appear to release adenosine diphosphate (ADP) from the platelets themselves and this substance is known as the most active platelet aggregating agent. Although platelet aggregation may be beneficial to the organism (haemostasis, phagocytosis of foreign material and interaction with bacteria and viruses) under conditions of decreased tissue perfusion platelet aggregation may obstruct flow (by mechanical plugging of key vessels) and this may lead to infarction of the tissue supplied by the obstructed vessel. Platelet agglutination is accelerated by bacterial endotoxins and hence the deposition of intravascular fibrin is particularly marked in septic shock. The presence of intravascular fibrin stimulates the process of fibrinolysis whereby fibrin is broken down by plasmin, a protease of broad specificity, to produce several degradation products. If the process of intravascular coagulation is protracted, the blood clotting factors may become depleted producing thrombocytopoenia and occasionally afibrinogenaemia. A bleeding diathesis may emerge which can be fatal. Intravascular coagulation may be present throughout the tissues but in man, the lung, liver and kidney are particularly vulnerable.

A further consequence of increased blood viscosity and resistance to blood flow in the vessels of the microcirculation is a reduction in flow velocity. When velocity in the smaller vessels is reduced to 0.1–0.2 mm/sec (about 20% normal) erythrocytes tend to form long continuous chains of 20–30 cells (rouleaux formation). If the endothelium is damaged wall-adhering thrombi (consisting of fibrin, platelets, erythrocytes and granulocytes) may also form which may obstruct the vessel or be released into the circulation to form emboli. A characteristic feature following injury to the blood vessel wall is the occurrence of wall-adhering granulocytes which have been demonstrated in the human skin under conditions of low perfusion.

No description of the microcirculatory response to shock would be complete without mention of the interstitial fluid compartment. The fluid volume within this phase is substantial (almost four times the plasma volume) and the bulk is found in the skin, viscera and skeletal muscle. A decrease in the 'functional' extracellular fluid volume follows sustained haemorrhage (Shires et al, 1973). In the early stage of hypovolaemic shock, much of this volume loss is accounted for by transfer to the vascular compartment, with involvement of both the gel and free-fluid phases of the interstitium (Fig. 28.7) (Haljamäe, 1984). Later, as microvascular pressure relationships alter, transport of fluid from the vascular compartment into the interstitium occurs; a proportion of this fluid enters the hypoxic cells, to a degree which is dependent on the severity and

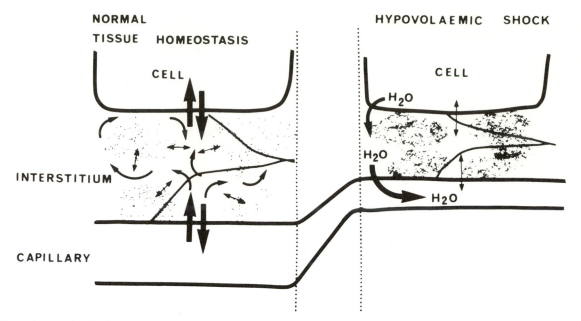

Fig. 28.7 Effects of hypovolaemic shock on the interstitial fluid phase. The capillary surface area available for blood-tissue exchange processes is decreased. Fluid is mobilized from the interstitial phase (resetting of pre- to post-capillary resistance ratio) and from cells (glucose-osmotic factors). The result is an increased interstitial colloid density and reduction of the free-fluid phase (after Haljamäe, 1984)

duration of the shock. The gastrointestinal tract may be more vulnerable to these effects than the muscle mass and, ultimately, disintegration of the organism may be largely influenced by absorption of toxic factors from the gut (Haglund & Lundgren, 1978).

NEUROHUMORAL MECHANISMS

Shock is associated with the release into the circulation of a variety of substances, many of which have vasoactive properties.

Vasopressin (AVP) and adrenocorticotrophic hormone (ACTH) are commonly regarded as the principal 'stress hormones'. Increased production of these hormones follows a variety of different stimuli, principally increased osmolality (detected by osmoreceptors in the hypothalamus), decreased arterial pressure and volume (detected by vascular mechanoreceptors and relayed via the tractus solitarius) and psychological stress (relayed via the limbic system). ACTH is released into the blood stream in response to corticotrophin releasing factor (CRF), the composition of which is still uncertain, but would appear to comprise several components including a 41-residue peptide (CRF-41), vasopressin and adrenaline (Buckingham, 1985). ACTH stimulates the production of cortisol, which plays a major role in protecting the organism from the effects of hypovolaemia. Another anterior pituitary peptide, β-endorphin (derived from the same precursor as ACTH), is also released during stress and is thought to mediate longer-term neuronal and endocrine changes. It was thought to have been implicated in producing cardiovascular depression in shock (Holaday et al, 1983), but a recent study (Watson et al, 1984) has suggested that another endogenous opiate, met-enkephalin, may be more important in this connection (see below).

The basic endocrine activation in shock involves release of the catecholamines and angiotensin, with related later increases in the plasma concentrations of such hormones as cortisol, growth hormone, glucagon, antidiuretic hormone and aldosterone; the main metabolic action of several of these hormones is mediated by the 'cell messenger' or intermediate cyclic adenosine monophosphate. The combined effect is to mobilize energy reserves and conserve salt and water. In the short term these mechanisms may be regarded as protective, but ultimately they lead to the breakdown of cellular integrity.

There is a massive outpouring of catecholamines in all forms of shock; plasma adrenaline concentrations exceed noradrenaline concentrations in hypovolaemic shock (Benedict & Grahame-Smith, 1978) while the reverse is true in septic shock (Griffiths, 1972). In a recent study in patients with traumatic shock, plasma catecholamine concentrations were found to correlate positively with Injury Severity Score; plasma noradrenaline concentrations were significantly higher on admission in non-survivors than in the casualties who survived serious injury (Davies et al, 1984). Angiotensin II, the most potent vasoconstrictor known, is also released into the blood following

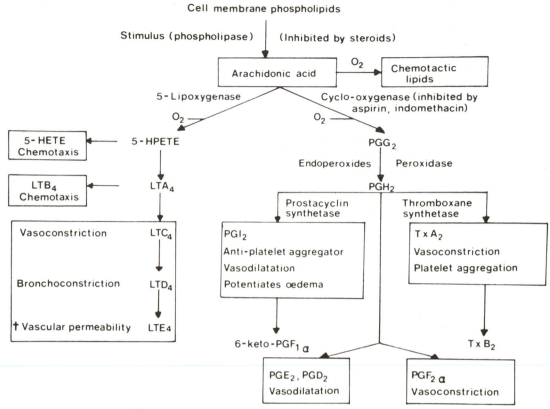

Fig. 28.8 Arachidonic acid metabolites in inflammation

shock and has been incriminated as a cause of heart failure after prolonged severe haemorrhage (Morton et al, 1977); another extracardiac cause of heart failure is the presence in the blood of myocardial depressant factor (MDF), a circulating peptide released from hypoxic pancreatic acinar cells (Lefer, 1978). Catecholamines and angiotensin II stimulate secretion of one another and blockade of both would appear to be necessary if complete abolition of vasoconstriction is desired. A possible further inter-reaction is with enkephalins, which are stored with catecholamines in adrenal chromaffin cells and which may suppress cholinergic-dependent catecholamine release from the adrenal glands (Kumakura et al, 1980). Opiate antagonists, for example naloxone, might act either by blocking this suppression locally or by antagonizing central enkephalinergic inhibition.

Other substances released into the blood during shock include histamine, plasma kinins, complement components and arachidonic acid metabolites. Histamine has long been thought to have a role in the aetiology of shock and its presence in large quantities has been demonstrated in the blood of shocked septic patients (Griffiths, 1972). This vasodilator substance is derived partly from the mast cell granule, but there is also evidence that endotoxin stimulates the rate of production of histamine by activating histidine decarboxylase. The weight of present evidence would suggest that histamine does not play an important part in initiating hypovolaemic shock but is of undoubted significance in septic shock.

Plasma kinins are vasodilator polypeptides which increase capillary permeability. They are released by both hypoxia and endotoxaemia from inactive precursors (kininogens) present in the α_2-globulin fraction of the plasma protein. The initial step appears to be activation of the Hageman factor (factor XII) which leads to conversion of kininogen to kinin by proteolytic enzymes (kallikreins) released from leucocytes and injured tissues. In addition to their systemic vasoactive properties, other important effects characteristic of major sepsis may be attributed to high plasma kinin levels including an increase in cardiac output, elevated pulmonary vascular resistance, and hypercatabolism. Resolution of haemodynamic disturbances coincident with a fall in kinin levels has been observed following relief of sepsis in patients suffering from septic shock (O'Donnell et al, 1976). Activation of the Hageman factor also promotes complement activation, with the subsequent release of a number of pharmacologically active substances which appear to be responsible for leucocyte aggregation and endothelial cell damage. (Further reference to local mediators of microvascular injury is made in the later section dealing with the lung). These various effects are unusual following uncomplicated hypovolaemia, but readily occur in the presence of shock compounded by trauma or sepsis (Whaley et al, 1979).

Prostaglandins and leukotrienes are synthesized by cellular microsomes from arachidonic acid via the cyclo-oxygenase and lipo-oxygenase pathways respectively (Fig. 28.8). Macrophages, neutrophils, platelets and mast cells are all involved in the generation of these substances, which have a wide range of pharmacological effects on the cardiovascular system. Prostaglandins of the E and F groups exert directly opposing physiological actions in the microcirculation; the ratio of the concentrations of these metabolites in response to injury thus appears to be of considerably greater importance than their absolute values. The same is true for the thromboxane: prostacyclin ratio in organs such as the heart and lung (see below). These observations may help to explain the indifferent results obtained from early pharmacological attempts (using, for example indomethacin and aspirin) to block the adverse effects of the prostaglandins in shock. The recent emergence of more selective blocking agents may well improve this situation. Leukotrienes are potent chemotactic factors and, in addition, cause bronchoconstriction, vasoconstriction and microvascular exudation of protein (Piper, 1983). There are no clinically applicable selective inhibitors of the lipo-oxygenase pathway; glucocorticoids induce inhibition of the common arachidonate precursor, phospholipase A_2, thus blocking the production of both metabolic pathways.

The presence of tissue injury or sepsis complicating hypovolaemia is likely to promote the production of inter-leukin 1 from macrophages. This recently identified lymphokine appears to depend on arachidonate metabolism for its capacity to induce fever and regulate immune function. Its importance in injury metabolism is only beginning to be explored (Fleck et al 1985).

It is impossible to predict the effects at the microcirculatory level of the combined release of the above humoral agents; however, it is clear that a massive release of such potent vasoactive agents must have important consequences in shock states and the ultimate response in individual patients presumably depends on the relative amount and potency of each agent in blood and tissues. The initial hypotension that gives rise to the high output/low resistance shock seen in patients with sepsis may well be owing to the release by bacterial products of plasma kinins, histamine and PGE. These agents may also contribute (by direct effects on capillary permeability) to the transudation of fluid from capillaries. The increased peripheral resistance observed in haemorrhagic, cardiogenic and the later stages of septic shock is almost certainly caused by the release of catecholamines and angiotensin II.

CELLULAR DYSFUNCTION

At the cellular level, three important features of cell injury may be considered: altered cell volume regulation; altered energy metabolism; and the suicide-bag concept of lyso-

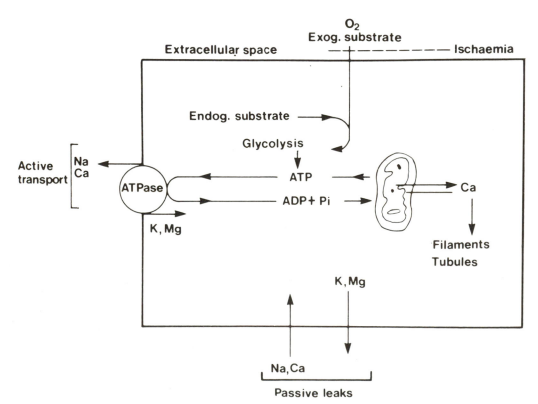

Fig. 28.9 Diagram showing some important factors in cell volume and ion regulation in mammalian cells. (After Trump et al, 1980)

somes (Trump et al, 1980). One of the earliest consequences of reduced oxygen availability is a decrease in cellular adenosine triphosphate (ATP) content (Fig. 28.9). This essential energy source for the ionic pump of the plasma membrane is normally broken down to adenosine diphosphate (ADP) and phosphate in the presence of ATPase. The absence of the high energy phosphate bonds leads to depression of pump function and cell swelling, the cells tending to approach Gibbs-Donnan equilibrium with an increase in intracellular sodium, calcium and water content and a loss of potassium and magnesium. In spite of these observations, evidence of membrane dysfunction in the face or *normal* tissue ATP concentrations suggests that energy depletion is only one of a number of factors involved (Shires & Shires, 1984). When oxygen tension decreases to a critical value within the mitochondrion (thought to be of the order of 0.1 kPa ($<$ 1 mmHg) (Nunn, 1977)), the electron transfer mechanism, which accounts for 90% of the body's oxygen consumption, becomes defective. Oxidative phosphorylation is uncoupled and ATP production gradually ceases. Associated structural changes, visible on light and electron microscopic examination, include mitochondrial swelling and disruption of the lining membrane, initially involving only the outer layer. Eventually the inner membrane also deteriorates as a result of continued low ATP concentrations. ATP deficiency also contributes to two other metabolic consequences of importance in hypovolaemic shock — abnormalities of calcium flux within the cell (Sperelakis & Schneider, 1976) and lactic acidosis. Persistence of high intracellular calcium concentrations leads to myocardial cell fatigue failure and asystolic cardiac arrest. Lactic acidosis, stimulated by increased phosphofructokinase activity, augments calcium slow channel inhibition at pH less than 6.8, as well as having adverse effects on other enzyme systems. The hypothesis that lysosomes contribute to the downward spiral of refractory shock by dissemination of destructive enzymes is undoubtedly attractive and, indeed, there is good evidence that lysosomal disruption does occur, but this would appear to follow, rather than cause, cell death (Trump et al, 1976). Likewise, significant structural changes in other cellular organelles tend to occur late in the ischaemic process.

The aforementioned pattern of pathophysiological disturbance occurs in all cells, but the susceptibility of different cells to hypoxia and ischaemia is very variable. Astrocytes, for example, cease to function after seconds, whilst skeletal muscle will function anaerobically for 30 min and hepatic cells for several hours; increased supplies of glucose are required to provide adequate substrate for anaerobic glycolysis, which may be a problem in low flow states. Clearly, in the presence of complete ischaemia the progress of cellular disintegration will be more rapid, but (depending on a variety of factors) the kidney and liver, for example, have survival times, at 37°C, of 1–2 h. The plasma membrane and early mitochondrial changes are readily reversible if the cause of shock is promptly eliminated, and several pharmacological agents are known to attenuate or even reverse some of the adverse metabolic effects, for example ATP-MgCl$_2$ (Peitzman et al, 1981; Chaudry et al, 1983), glucose-insulin-potassium (Bronsveld et al, 1984), calcium channel blockers (Hackel et al, 1981) and steroids (Goldfarb & Glenn, 1983). None of these agents is of proven clinical value.

ORGAN DYSFUNCTION IN SHOCK

Laboratory studies have shown that there is a large species variation in the physiological and metabolic response to shock. In the dog, for instance, the administration of endotoxin produces a raised portal venous pressure and a low central venous pressure while, in the cat, pulmonary vasoconstriction and a raised central venous pressure with early cardiac failure are more likely to occur. In baboons and probably man, the lung, the liver and the kidney appear particularly susceptible to shock. These observations have led over the years to the belief that the failure of a specific organ may account for the eventual refractory nature of shock. There is little evidence to substantiate this 'target organ' concept since it is clear that almost every cell in the body is adversely affected by the shock process. There is merit, however, in appreciating that the shocked patient is susceptible, for example, to respiratory or renal failure and that precautions should be taken to reduce the risks of further damage to these organs. This is particularly relevant when there is pre-existing cardiopulmonary or renal disease.

THE LUNG

The shocked patient normally has an increased respiratory rate with a variable change in tidal volume. In the early stages a fall in arterial carbon dioxide tension usually occurs with minimal changes in arterial oxygen tension. The increased respiratory rate results from an increase in peripheral chemoreceptor activity and from the stimulant effect of systemic metabolic acidosis.

Investigation of the hyperventilatory response in shock has revealed a discrepancy between the increase in minute ventilation and the decrease in arterial carbon dioxide tension. The arterial carbon dioxide tension which frequently falls to 25–30 mmHg should fall considerably further if there was a corresponding increase in alveolar ventilation. The discrepancy is due to an increase in dead space ventilation, i.e. ventilation of alveoli with diminished or absent blood supply. The diminution in blood flow leads to widespread inequalities in the ventilation/perfusion ratios. In those alveoli where the ventilation greatly exceeds perfusion, alveolar carbon dioxide tension falls to low levels and dilutes the carbon dioxide concentration of more normally perfused alveoli. Thus it is characteristic in shock for the difference between the arterial carbon dioxide tension and the mixed expiratory or end-tidal carbon dioxide tension to increase and this measurement is a useful reflection of changes in pulmonary blood flow. In the early stage of haemorrhagic shock there is remarkably little change in lung mechanics.

In the normal lung up to 3% of the blood reaches the left side of the heart effectively without coming in contact with alveolar gas — so-called pulmonary venous admixture. This includes blood passing through poorly ventilated alveoli, through completely unventilated alveoli and by-passing the alveoli altogether (i.e. the bronchial and thebesian circulations). A combination of these effects produces the normal alveolar-arterial oxygen tension difference. The proportion of this difference which may be attributed to true shunt, i.e. blood passing through completely unventilated alveoli or normal anatomical vascular shunts is revealed when the patient breathes 100% oxygen; this manoeuvre readily corrects the hypoxaemia of ventilation/perfusion inequalities and is another useful measurement of gas exchange in shock. Such measurements have revealed that in the early stages of shock true shunt may fall, although later a substantial rise may occur as a result of pulmonary oedema or alveolar collapse. Pulmonary oedema may be produced by left heart failure or by the direct effects of poor perfusion on the integrity of the pulmonary capillaries; alveolar collapse may also result from poor perfusion leading to diminished production of surfactant, from medullary hypoxia or indirectly from the effects of various drugs which decrease compensatory hyperventilation.

As a result of diminished systemic blood flow during shock, oxygen is extracted in large amounts from the blood returning to the heart with a consequent fall in mixed venous oxygen tension. Normally, the level of mixed venous oxygen tension does not significantly influence arterial oxygen tension but when a large shunt is present, as in the later stages of shock, the mixed venous oxygen tension becomes increasingly important as a cause of arterial oxygen desaturation.

The pulmonary circulation is less accessible for the purpose of measurement than the systemic circulation and only in the past few years have the pulmonary vascular responses to shock been studied in any depth. Clinical studies have shown that pulmonary vascular resistance increases during hypotension, often more than systemic vascular resistance, and the rate of its return towards normal relates to the clinical outcome (Shoemaker et al, 1973). The mechanisms regulating pulmonary vascular resistance in the acutely shocked patient are being extensively investigated but amongst those already identified are central autonomic neuroregulatory processes, local factors such as acidosis, alveolar hypoxia and hypercarbia, circulating substances such as catecholamines, serotonin and thromboxane and rheological factors such as cellular aggregates, microthrombi and fat emboli.

The disturbances of gas exchange in the lung tend to disappear, or at least improve, on restoration of normal blood flow. In a few instances, however, gas exchange may again or further deteriorate, giving rise to the condition commonly termed 'shock lung'. This is probably only one of a number of clinical descriptions grouped under the collective term 'acute respiratory distress syndrome' (ARDS). The primary abnormality of ARDS is widespread increased permeability of the alveolocapillary membrane to larger molecules such as albumen and other proteins; this causes increased fluid flux and, when the compensatory mechanisms are exceeded, flooding of the interstitial and alveolar spaces occurs (Demling, 1980). The normal alveolar stabilizing properties of surfactant are impaired by the alveolar flooding. Within a few hours of injury, coagulation of intra-alveolar protein occurs and necrosis of the alveolar epithelial cells (type I pneumocytes) becomes evident. This is followed by hyperplasia of the surfactant producing type II pneumocytes and the accumulation of interstitial inflammatory cells, including fibroblasts. Fibrosis, which tends to focus on the alveolar ducts, begins within seven days of the onset of ARDS. Within the pulmonary microcirculation, thrombotic and/or microembolic occlusion may occur in association with vasoconstriction, interstitial compression and leucocyte aggregation.

The precise mechanisms which lead to ARDS are uncertain. Complement activation (see above) would appear to be involved and, in the presence of reduced blood flow, is responsible for leucocyte aggregation and the capillary permeability defect. Putative local mediators of the microvascular injury include arachidonic acid metabolites, plasma or phagocyte-derived proteases, fibrinogen degradation products (particularly the fibrin D monomer) and toxic oxygen radicals released by activated leucocytes. Serotonin and histamine may play a secondary role in the pulmonary vascular response to shock.

THE KIDNEY

The kidney is vulnerable to ischaemia although there is not necessarily a close relationship between the severity of shock and the prevalence of acute renal failure. A number of factors modify this relationship including, on the one hand, the speed and adequacy of treatment and, on the other, the presence of sepsis, crush injury, or pre-existing renal disease.

Under normal circumstances the kidney receives as much as 25 per cent of the cardiac output. During shock there is a substantial reduction in renal blood flow and urine output ceases altogether at an arterial blood pressure of about 50 mmHg. Glomerular filtration rate also falls in proportion to the fall in blood pressure, but the filtration fraction rises, presumably as a result of more marked vasoconstriction of the efferent glomerular arterioles. The fall in renal blood flow is particularly marked in the cortex although there may be some sparing of the inner cortical zone; the slower the onset of shock, the greater the opportunity for 'autoregulation' and diversion of flow to juxtamedullary glomeruli. The mechanism by which these changes in renal blood flow are effected is uncertain, but catecholamines and angiotensin II are known to constrict renal cortical vessels and local formation of angiotensin may account for the persistence of renal ischaemia after resuscitation. PGE_2, originating in the renal medulla, may oppose the vasoconstrictor action of the catecholamines and angiotensin and its absence may contribute to the initiation of acute renal failure. Ischaemia may not be the only basis for acute renal failure but it does seem to play a key role (Fig. 28.10).

Coincident with the fall in blood flow during shock is a fall in oxygen consumption as a result of which sodium reabsorption from the tubules is reduced with a corresponding increase in urine sodium. In most cases these changes are reversed following prompt treatment of shock but patchy ischaemia may persist and acute renal failure may result (Brown, 1977). The advent of modern haemodialysis techniques has shown that this is a reversible process and restoration of normal renal function among survivors is the rule (Chapman, 1979). In the absence of complications a patient survival rate of around 70% may be expected.

In addition to these direct sequelae of shock on the kidney, other indirect effects succeed renal ischaemia, of which perhaps the most important is the release of aldosterone by the adrenal cortex. The juxtaglomerular apparatus in the renal cortex responds to blood volume depletion and sodium deficiency by producing renin which acts in the blood to form angiotensin II. This potent vasopressor stimulates the adrenal cortex to release aldosterone, the function of which is to conserve body sodium and thus blood volume.

Like aldosterone, both cortisol and corticosterone are produced in excess during shock and even when hypotension is severe and prolonged, adrenal cortical failure has been demonstrated only rarely. Thus administration of hydrocortisone is not indicated on physiological grounds; nevertheless large doses of steroids have been shown by some to exert a beneficial influence in experimental shock although only if given within a few minutes of the onset of shock. In the dose recommended (50 mg/kg of hydrocortisone), steroids exert a vasodilatory action, increase the production of adenosine triphosphate (ATP), increase the conversion of lactic acid to glycogen and stabilize lysosomal membranes. The adrenal medulla has already been shown to play an important role in the cardiovascular response to shock and it seems that low blood volume is more important than low blood pressure in initiating catecholamine release.

THE LIVER

In spite of its central role in metabolism, the liver has not been as extensively studied in relation to shock as have other organs. Nevertheless, hepatic dysfunction following hypovolaemic and septic shock is well recognized and persistence of jaundice is a gloomy sign (Banks et al, 1982).

Hepatic blood flow and oxygen consumption fall during hypotension. In low output septic shock the high pressure hepatic arterial circulation appears to be more affected than the low pressure portal circulation (Imamura and Clowes, 1975). If hypotension persists for more than 24 hours hepatic necrosis is common (Sherlock, 1975); the

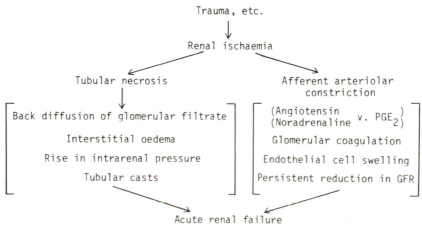

Fig. 28.10 Mechanisms involved in acute renal failure.

injury affects the perivenular hepatocytes (MacSween & Scothorne, 1979) which undergo coagulative necrosis usually with only a mild inflammatory response. Hypotension of less than 10 hours duration rarely causes hepatic necrosis although the parenchymal cells may become oedematous, swollen and vacuolated (George et al, 1978). With adequate resuscitation these changes begin to regress after 1–3 days.

In high output septic shock total hepatic blood flow is increased but not in proportion to cardiac output and the greatly increased oxygen demand of the liver may not be met. The problem may be further complicated by the presence of various toxic substances in the blood which contribute to liver damage. Escherichia coli endotoxin, for example, may selectively inhibit the bile-salt/independent bile secretory mechanism (Utile et al, 1977). Histological examination of the liver in patients dying of septic shock shows a number of non-specific changes comprising varying degrees of cholestasis, venous congestion, focal liver cell necrosis and reactive inflammatory changes with Kupffer cell hyperplasia and portal tract inflammation. In a small number of instances, cholestasis may be accompanied by a striking and peculiar pattern of cholangiolitis but without major duct obstruction (Banks et al, 1982).

The 'standard' liver function tests reveal mild jaundice and prolonged prothrombin time in response to hypovolaemic shock. The changes are usually transient and rarely accompanied by enzyme disturbances. The incidence of these features is greatly increased in septic shock — 63 per cent in one survey of 57 patients (Banks et al, 1982) and all of 22 patients in a report of the recently recognized toxic-shock syndrome (Gourley et al, 1981).

The prognostic inadequacy of the standard liver function tests has led to evaluation of alternative techniques including indocyanine green clearance (as an indication of hepatic blood flow) and antipyrine elimination (as a reflection of hepatocellular oxidative function). Both techniques are proving to be of considerable therapeutic and predictive value in shocked patients.

Hypotension and sepsis may produce a disturbance of the normal detoxifying role of the liver. In particular, Kupffer cell injury impairs handling of endotoxin which may then gain access in large quantity to the systemic circulation with profound effects on the host. Furthermore, injury to the Kupffer cells may render the hepatocytes susceptible to damage by endotoxins or other toxic substances. A recent report (Scovill et al, 1978) indicated that a humoral factor playing an important part in hepatic reticuloendothelial function can now be detected in blood. This factor (fibronectin or opsonic α_2 surface-binding glycoprotein), if present in a low quantity, may point to impaired Kupffer cell function. Restoration of normal values of the glycoprotein appears to be of value in the treatment of septic shock.

SEPTIC SHOCK

Although sharing many of the clinical features of other forms of shock, septic shock presents problems that are sufficiently distinctive to merit separate mention. Treatment is often protracted and mortality remains high even in centres with specialized facilities. There are probably two main explanations for these facts — delay in diagnosis until after the onset of the refractory stage of the syndrome and uncertainty as to the precise mechanisms whereby bacteria (or bacterial products) produce shock.

The commonly held view that septic shock is easily recognized and readily distinguished from other forms of shock is, in many cases, erroneous. Certainly the young otherwise healthy individual in whom bacteraemia occurs secondary to urological intervention, will manifest fever and hypotension, the cause of which is obvious. The majority of patients who develop septic shock, however, are either older or have some associated systemic disease, may be frankly hypovolaemic and, not infrequently, have latent cardiac disease. The pathophysiological basis of shock in these patients is a complex mixture of factors, only one of which is the presence of infection.

Shock occurs in association with both Gram-positive and Gram-negative infections — less frequently in the former (about one in ten patients) than in the latter (about one in three patients). In the past, it was believed possible to discriminate between Gram-positive and Gram-negative septic shock on clinical grounds, but recent evidence makes it clear that this is untrue. In a study of 59 patients, Wiles and his colleagues (1980) were unable to detect a difference in any physiological variable between organism group, or indeed between specific organisms. After initial resuscitation, all patients exhibited a hyperdynamic cardiovascular response with abnormal vascular tone; some degree of myocardial depression was evident in most patients. Mortality was over 70% in both Gram-positive and Gram-negative septicaemia. The conclusion reached in this study was that while the exact pathogenesis of the septic response remained unclear, it did not seem to be peculiar to a specific microorganism. This supports the contention that the fate of patients suffering from septic shock is determined by the speed and adequacy of initial resuscitation and, thereafter, by the nature of the underlying disease process.

In the early stages of septic shock (the hyperdynamic phase), cardiac output is often high and the skin warm and dry. Urine output may be elevated and some patients may exhibit an inappropriate polyuria at the expense of effective circulating plasma volume. These effects are related to the presence in the circulation of various pyrogens and to the release by bacterial products of plasma kinins, histamine and prostaglandins of the E series. These agents may later contribute (by direct effects on capillary permeability) to the transudation of fluid from capillaries. The primary respiratory response is hyperventilation, mediated by both central and peripheral mechanisms, and arterial blood gas analysis may reveal only some reduction in P_{CO_2}. Metabolic acidosis in septic shock is more variable than in other forms of shock and, therefore, less reliable as a prognostic indicator.

In the later stages of septic shock (the hypodynamic phase), cardiac output falls and there is marked hypotension, peripheral vasoconstriction and oliguria. These effects are almost certainly caused by the release of catecholamines and angiotension II. More recently discovered substances such as thromboxane B_2, derived from damaged platelets, may augment this reaction particularly in the pulmonary circulation and contribute to a deterioration in pulmonary gas exchange with a progressive fall in arterial P_{O_2}.

Metabolic disturbances appear earlier in septic than in other forms of shock. Characteristically, the arteriovenous oxygen difference falls and in some patients' oxygen consumption may be very low (Wilson & Gibson, 1978). There is agreement that the most likely explanation for this observation is impaired cell metabolism. This metabolic defect interferes with capillary and cell membrane function and prevents the cells from utilizing oxygen and energy substrates properly to form ATP. Lipolysis occurs with high circulating levels of free fatty acids and serum triglycerides (Wardle, 1979). In muscle there is a block to the intracellular oxidation of glucose, which, together with an inability to utilize ketone bodies, leads to increased catabolism of branched-chain amino acids. The disturbance in carbohydrate metabolism may be due to inhibition of certain of the reactions within the citric acid cycle which may account for the lower than expected levels of lactate in septic shock. Hypophosphataemia and hypocalcaemia are also common.

Many of the haemodynamic and metabolic effects which have been described may be attributable to circulating endotoxin, the complex lipopolysaccharide coating of Gram-negative bacteria, and in particular the lipid-A moiety. Endotoxin causes aggregation of platelets by direct damage to the cell wall, and of white cells by an indirect action via activated complement. Platelet aggregation leads to the formation of thrombi in the microcirculation at a rate which may swamp fibrinolytic and reticuloendothelial phagocytic mechanisms. White cell aggregation may also cause plugging of the microvasculature with damage of the capillary endothelium resulting from direct contact with toxic oxygen radicals, such as superoxide anion and hydrogen peroxide, released from the leucocytes (Jacob et al, 1980).

These microcirculatory disturbances may be observed widely throughout the body and may result in focal necrosis in the lung, kidneys and liver, as well as other organs.

In the lung, damage to the capillary endothelium leads to the development of protein-rich pulmonary oedema which, if not arrested early, may progress to the fully developed adult respiratory distress syndrome. In the kidney, endotoxaemia may cause an already reduced glomerular filtration rate to fall further and precipitate acute renal failure. If the source of sepsis can be successfully eradicated recovery is possible.

Jaundice may occur in the presence of extrahepatic Gram-negative infection. The jaundice is of a cholestatic type, typically reflected in elevation of conjugated serum bilirubin and alkaline phosphatase, with modest increases in serum transaminases. The histological appearances in the liver are those of intercellular and intra-canalicular bile stasis with little or no evidence of parenchymal damage. The observed cholestasis in sepsis may be caused by the inhibitory effect of endotoxin on the active sodium transport mechanism of hepatocytes.

Failure of liver function abnormalities to return to normal within a few days of a septic insult often indicates a persisting source of major infection (Royle & Kettlewell 1980). Attention has once again begun to centre on the role of the hepatic Kupffer cells in the removal of bacteria and their breakdown products, including endotoxin, from the circulation. The activity of these cells is inhibited during an episode of septic shock (Scovill et al, 1978) and the success of treatment may well be determined by the degree of functional recovery which ensues after the phase of resuscitation.

TREATMENT

The importance of prompt and adequate resuscitation in the early stages of shock is clear, often before the diagnosis can be confirmed. In practice, acute resuscitation of a patient suffering from *any* form of shock is influenced more by the nature of the associated physiological disturbances than by specific aetiological factors. Success of subsequent treatment, on the other hand, is largely dependent on detection and elimination of the underlying cause. In many patients, considerable overlap will exist between the two processes.

Initial resuscitation

The objective of treatment is to restore adequate oxygen availability for the metabolic requirements of the tissues. The immediate aims are to augment intravascular volume, optimize cardiac output and its distribution, and ensure adequate pulmonary gas exchange. These aims are achieved by minimizing further fluid loss and replacing estimated loss with either colloid or crystalloid solutions and transfusion with concentrated red cells to a haematocrit of 30–35%; by the judicious use of pharmacological agents; and by the administration of oxygen together with mechanical ventilation when indicated.

The wise counsel, found in all first aid manuals, of reducing the risk of further fluid loss in the hypovolaemic patient appears to carry less weight once the patient has crossed the hospital threshold (Waddell, 1975). It should be realized that avoidance of unnecessary movement, immobilization of broken limbs, gentle handling of damaged tissues and maintenance of pressure dressings are as important in the accident and emergency department, the operating theatre or the intensive therapy unit as during pre-hospital transportation. The practice of tilting the hypovolaemic patient head-down in an attempt to augment venous return is less frequently utilized than formerly. There is certainly no evidence that this manoeuvre achieves any consistent haemodynamic improvement (Sibbald et al, 1979) and adverse pulmonary and cerebral effects have been reported. Raising the legs is an adequate and safe first aid procedure.

Fluid administration/oxygenation

Strange to relate, perhaps, the type of fluid loss in shocked patients does not influence the choice of initial fluid replacement as much as the perceived nature of the underlying physiological disturbance. Successful resuscitation, however, is dependent more on the rapidity and adequacy of fluid repletion than on the composition of the regimen. Dispute as to the selection of fluid for resuscitation (the 'colloid v. crystalloid' controversy) centres mainly on issues relating to philosophy, side-effects and economics.

Crystalloid solutions have been recommended on the basis that in hypovolaemic or haemorrhagic shock fluid is lost from the interstitial compartment as well as from the intravascular compartment (Carrico et al, 1976). Losses from both compartments may be repleted by the rapid administration of up to 2 l of balanced salt solution after which the need for blood may be assessed with reference to packed cell volume and evidence of further haemorrhage. Colloid solutions have been advocated primarily because they restore plasma volume without overloading the interstitial compartment (Shoemaker, 1976). Reconstituted plasma, dextran and some of the more recently developed colloid solutions all fulfil this requirement although each has its own individual properties, the details of which are beyond the scope of this chapter.

The criticism has been levelled at both crystalloid and colloid solutions that they have a tendency to promote the formation of pulmonary oedema, particularly in septic shock and severe haemorrhagic shock. If colloid escapes into the pulmonary interstitial compartment it may encourage progressive oedema formation (Holcroft & Trunkey, 1975) and is less readily cleared from the lungs than crystalloid. The final answer to these various problems has yet to emerge but it is agreed that a 20% deficit of blood volume may be replaced adequately by buffered electrolyte solution. Loss in excess of 20% of the blood volume may also be corrected using electrolyte solutions but plasma or some form of plasma substitute is usually added to restore normal colloid osmotic pressure. Many clinicians believe that the best results in shock resuscitation are achieved using a combination of colloid and crystalloid solutions and there is some evidence that oxygen consumption is higher with the combination than with either regimen alone (Smith and Norman, 1982). Blood is administered as soon as indicated and available. There is good evidence that optimal oxygen transport to the tissues is achieved when the haematocrit is maintained around 30% (Gruber et al, 1976).

It goes without saying that any acid-base abnormality should be corrected although the restoration of a normal blood pH may have little immediate effect on cardiovascular and respiratory function. Electrolyte disturbances should also receive prompt attention after acute fluid deficit has been corrected when the true extent of these disturbances will be more easily assessed. Hyperkalaemia is common in shock but hypokalaemia may rapidly occur if large volumes of intravenous fluids are administered. Such disturbances in serum potassium concentrations complicate resuscitation, especially in the presence of cardiac failure when the administration of such drugs as digitalis may be considered necessary.

The beneficial effect of fluid repletion will be attenuated if hypoxaemia is present. Rapid restoration to normal of the oxyen capacity of the blood is imperative. In the first instance this may be achieved by an increase in the inspired oxygen concentration. When shock has been severe or protracted, there may be a progressive deterioration in pulmonary gas exchange with a substantial increase in the work of breathing. Under these circumstances one of the more important recent advances in treatment has been the early use of intermittent positive pressure ventilation. The need for ventilation may continue for a day or two after the phase of acute resuscitation and, on occasion, positive end-expiratory pressure (10–15 cm of water) is of additional value (Falke et al, 1972).

Pharmacological agents

If elimination of surgical factors together with restoration of blood volume and red cell mass fails to restore cardiac output, then pharmacological assistance may be required. Unquestionably, the drugs most commonly used in these circumstances are the inotropic agents (to increase myocardial contractility) with or without the use of vasodilators (to decrease afterload) (Foëx, 1983). Dopamine has proved attractive for its effects on both cardiac output and urine output. If administered by i.v. infusion at a rate ($2-20$ μg kg^{-1} min^{-1}) such that systolic arterial pressure does not increase above 80–100 mmHg, dopamine will normally induce a gratifying diuresis. If the rate is increased, the α-adrenergic agonist action of the drug emerges and arrhythmias occur. The risk of intrapulmonary shunting should be noted, and that toxic side-effects increase with the passage of time, although withdrawal of this agent has been successfully achieved after many days of administration. Dobutamine, acting directly on β_1-adrenergic receptors, may have a more pronounced inotropic action on the heart than dopamine, with less marked effects on heart rate and excitability. A manoeuvre which is gaining popularity is to use dopamine by low-dose infusion during the early stages of resuscitation to maintain renal perfusion and — if cardiac output requires to be augmented — either to increase the dose of dopamine or to add dobutamine (with the aim of achieving the best combination of pharmacological actions). Commonly used vasodilators are chlorpromazine, nitroprusside and nitroglycerin; selection should be based on the predominant cardiovascular disturbance.

Two further drugs are worthy of mention. Corticosteroids have been given to shocked patients after severe trauma (Rokkanen et al, 1974; Svennevig et al, 1984) and sepsis (Sprung et al, 1984). A variety of beneficial effects was noted, but mortality was unaffected. In the recovery phase, particularly after shock of traumatic origin, persistent sympathetic overactivity is sometimes observed. Such patients are at risk of increased intracranial pressure and recurrent haemorrhage. The use of a drug such as labetalol, which combines α- and β-adrenergic blocking actions, has proved to be of value in this situation (Morel et al, 1984).

Further treatment

In general, patients should be adequately resuscitated from shock before surgery, but in some instances this may not be possible. Haemorrhage may be severe from the outset or may become severe during fluid repletion; either way it is best to commence surgery as soon after initiation of resuscitation as possible. In the presence of sepsis, normal cardiovascular function may be difficult to restore until the source is eliminated.

REFERENCES

Banks J G, Foulis A K, Ledingham I Mc A, MacSween R N 1982 Liver function in septic shock. Journal of Clinical Pathology 35:1249

Benedict C R, Grahame-Smith D G 1978 Plasma noradrenaline and adrenaline concentrations and dopamine-B-hydroxylase activity in patients with shock due to septicaemia, trauma and haemorrhage. Quarterly Journal of Medicine 47:1

Bronsveld W, van Lambalgen A A, van den Bos G C, Thijs L G, Koopmans P A R 1984 Effects of glucose-insulin-potassium (GIK) on myocardial blood flow and metabolism in canine endotoxin shock. Circulatory Shock 13:325

Brown C B 1977 Shock and the kidney: pathophysiology and pharmacological support. Intensive Care Medicine 3:1

Buckingham J C 1985 Hypothalamo-pituitary responses to trauma. British Medical Bulletin 41:203

Carrico C J, Canizaro P C, Shires T 1976 Fluid resuscitation following injury: rationale for the use of balanced salt solutions. Critical Care Medicine 4:46

Chapman A 1979. In: Chapman A (ed) Acute Renal Failure. Churchill Livingstone, Edinburgh

Chaudry I H, Ohkawa M, Clemens M G, Baue A E 1983 Alterations in electron transport and cellular metabolism with shock and trauma. In: AM Lefer W. Schumer (eds) Molecular and Cellular Aspects of Shock and Trauma. Liss, New York p 67

Davies C L, Newman R J, Molyneux S G, Grahame-Smith D G 1984 The relationship between plasma catecholamines and severity of injury in man. Journal of Trauma 24:99

Demling R H 1980 The pathogenesis of respiratory failure after trauma and sepsis. Surgical Clinics of North America 60:1373

Falke K J, Pontoppidan H, Kumar A, Leith D E, Geffin B, Laver M B 1972 Ventilation with end-expiratory pressure in acute lung disease. Journal of Cinical Investigation 51:2315

Fisher W D, Heimbach D M, McCardle C S, Maddern M, Hutchison M M, Ledingham IMcA 1973 A circulating depressant effect following canine haemorrhagic shock. British Journal of Surgery 60:392

Fitch W, Jones J V, MacKenzie E T, Harper A M 1976 Autoregulation of cerebral blood flow in chronically hypertensive baboons. Circulation Research 39:555

Fleck A, Colley C M, Myers M A 1985 Liver export proteins and trauma. British Medical Bulletin 41:265

Foëx P 1983 Inotropic and vasodilator agents. In: Ledingham I McA Recent Advances in Critical Care Medicine. Vol 2 Churchill Livingstone, Edinburgh p 45

George B C, Ryan N T, Ullrick C, Egdahl R H 1978 Persisting structural abnormalities in liver, kidney, and muscle tissues following haemorrhagic shock. Archives of Surgery 113:289

George R J D, Tinker J 1983 Pathophysiology of shock. In: Tunker J, Rapun M (eds.) Care of the critically-ill patient. Springer Verlag, Berlin p 174

Gilmour D G Aitkenhead A R, Hothersall A P and Ledingham IMcA 1980 The effect of hypovolaemia on colon blood flow in the dog. British Journal of Surgery 67:82

Goldfarb R D, Glenn T M 1983 Regulation of lysosomal membrane stabilization via cyclic nucleotides and prostaglandins: the effects of steroids and indomethacin. In: Molecular and Cellular Aspects of Shock and Trauma (A.M. Lefer, W. Schumer eds) Liss, New York p 147

Gourley G R, Chesney P J, Davis J P, Odell G B 1981 Acute cholestasis in patients with toxic shock syndrome. Gastroenterology 81:928

Griffiths J 1972 The sequential assay of plasma catecholamines and whole blood histamine in early septic shock. In: eds I. McA. Ledingham and T.A. McAllister, Conference on 'Shock'. Kimpton, London p. 76

Gruber U F, Sturm V, Messmer K 1976 Fluid replacement in shock. In: Shock, Clinical and Experimental Aspects, ed. Ledingham I. McA. Excerpta Medica, Amsterdam p 231

Hackel D B, Mikat E M, Reimer K, Whalen G 1981 Effect of verapamil on heart and circulation in hemorrhagic shock in dogs. American Journal of Physiology 241:H12

Hackel D B, Ratliff N B, Mikat E M 1974 The heart in shock. Circulation Research 35:805

Haglund U, Lundgren O 1978 Intestinal ischemia and shock factors. Federal Proceedings 37:2729

Haljamäe H 1984 Interstitial fluid response; in Clinical Surgery International. Vol. 9. Shock and Related Problems (ed. G T Shires), p 44 New York: Churchill Livingstone

Hinshaw L B, Greenfield L J, Owen S E, Black M R, Guenter C A 1972 Precipitation of cardiac failure in endotoxin shock. Surgery, Gynecology and Obstetrics 135:39

Holaday J M, D'Amato R J, Ruvio B A, Feverstein G, Faden A L 1983 Adrenalectomy blocks pressor responses to naloxone in endotoxin shock. Evidence for sympatho-medullary involvement. Circulatory Shock 11:201

Holcroft J W, Trunkey D D 1975 Pulmonary extravasation of albumin during and after hemorrhagic shock in baboons. Journal of Surgical Research 18:91

Inamura M, Clowes G H 1975 Hepatic blood and oxygen consumption in starvation sepsis and septic shock. Surgery, Gynecology and Obstetrics 141:27

Jacob H S, Craddock P R, Hammerschmidt D E, Muldow C F 1980 Complement-induced granulocyte aggregation: an unexpected mechanism of disease. New England Journal of Medicine 302:789

Kumakura K, Karoum F, Guidotti A 1980 Modulation of nicotinic receptors by opiate receptor antagonists in cultured adrenal chromaffin cells. Nature (London) 283:489

Lefer A M 1973 Blood-borne humoral factors in the pathophysiology of circulatory shock. Circulation Research 32:129

Lefer A M 1978 Properties of cardioinhibitory factors in shock. Federal Proceedings 37:2734

Mellander S, Lewis D H 1963 Effects of haemorrhagic shock on the reactivity of resistance and capacitance vessels and on capillary filtration transfer in cat skeletal muscle. Circulation Research 13:105

Morel D R, Forster A, Suter P M 1984 Evaluation of i.v. labetalol for treatment of post-traumatic hyperdynamic state. Intensive Care Medicine 10:133

Morton J J, Semple P F, Ledingham IMcA, Stuart B, Tehrani M A, Reyes A, McGarrity G 1977 Effect of angiotensin-converting enzyme inhibitor (SW20881) on the plasma concentration of angiotensin I, angiotensin II and arginine vasopressin in the dog during hemorrhagic shock. Circulation Research 41:301

MacDonald J A E, Milligan G F, Mellon A, Ledingham IMcA 1975 Ventricular function in experimental hemorrhagic shock. Surgery, Gynecology and Obstetrics 140 572

MacSween R N M, Scothorne R J 1979 Developmental anatomy and normal stricture. In: MacSween R N M, Anthony P P, Scheuer P J (eds) Pathology of the liver. Churchill Livingstone. Edinburgh p 1–31

Nunn J F 1977 Applied Respiratory Physiology 2 Edn, p 378. London: Butterworths

O'Donnell T F, George H A, Clowes G, Talamo R C, Colman R W 1976 Kinin activation in the blood of patients with sepsis. Surgery, Gynecology and Obstetrics 143:539

Peitzman A B, Shires G T III, Illner H, Shires G T 1981 Effect of intravenous ATP-MgCI$_2$ on cellular function in liver and muscle in hemorrhagic shock. Current Surgery (Philadelphia) 38:300

Piper P J 1983 Pharmacology of leukotrienes. British Medical Bulletin 39:255

Postel J, Schleorb P R 1977 Cardiac depression in bacteraemia. Annals of Surgery 186:74

Rokkanen P, Alho A, Avikainen V, Karaharju E, Kataja J, Lahdensuu M, Lepisto P, Teruo T 1974 The efficacy of corticosteroid in severe trauma. Surgery, Gynecology and Obstetrics 138:69

Royle G T, Kettlewell M G W 1980 Liver function tests in surgical infection and malnutrition. Annals of Surgery 192:192

Sander-Jensen K, Secher N H, Bie P, Warberg J, Schwartz T W 1986 Vagal slowing of the heart during haemorrhage: observations from 20 consecutive hypotensive patients. British Medical Journal 292:364

Scovill W A, Saba T M, Blumenstock F A, Bernard H, Powers S R 1978 Opsonic 2 surface binding glycoprotein therapy during sepsis. Annals of Surgery. 188:521

Sherlock S 1975 in Disease of the Liver and Biliary System, 5th edn. (edited by Sherlock S.). Blackwell Scientific, London p 490

Shires G T, Carrico C J, Canizaro P C 1973 Shock; in Major Problems in Clinical Surgery, Vol 13 Philadelphia: Saunders

Shires G T, Shires G T III 1984 In: Clinical Surgery International, Vol 9: Shock and Related Problems (ed. G T Shires), pp 19, 127. London: Churchill Livingstone

Shoemaker W C 1976 Comparison of the relative effectiveness of whole blood transfusions and various types of fluid therapy in resuscitation. Critical Care Medicine 4:71

Shoemaker W C, Brown R S, Mohr P A, Manson D O, Carey J S 1971 The cardiovascular system. In: Cortico Steroids in the Treatment of Shock, eds Schumer W, Nyhus L M p 16 Chicago: University of Illinois Press

Shoemaker W C, Monson D O 1973 Effect of whole blood and plasma expanders on volume-flow relationships in critically ill patients. Surgery, Gynecology and Obstetrics 137:453

Sibbald W JP, Paterson N A M, Holliday R L, Baskerville J 1979 The Trendelenburg position: hemodynamic effects in hypotensive and normotensive patients. Critical Care Medicine 7:218

Smith J A R, Norman J N 1982 The fluid of choice for resuscitation of severe shock. British Journal of Surgery 69:702

Sperelakis N, Schneider J A 1976 A metabolic control mechanism for calcium ion flux that may protect the ventricular myocardial cell. American Journal of Cardiology 37:1079

Sprung C L, Caralio P V, Marcial E H, Pierce M, Gelbard M A, Long W M, Duncan R C, Tendler M D, Karpf M 1984 The effects of high-dose corticosteroids in patients with septic shock. A prospective controlled study. New England Journal of Medicine. 311:1137

Svennevig J L, Bugge-Asperheim B, Vaage J, Geiran O, Birkeland S 1984 Corticosteroids in the treatment of blunt injury of the chest. Injury 16:80

Swan H J C, Ganz W 1983 Techniques for investigating cardiovascular function; in Care of the Critically Ill Patient (eds J. Tinker and M. Rapin), p 933. Berlin: Springer-Verlag

Trump B F, McDowell E M, Arstila A U 1980 Cellular reaction to injury. In: Hill, R B, LaVia M F (eds) Principles of Pathobiology, 3rd edn. Oxford University Press, New York p 37

Trump B F, Mergner W J, Kahng M W, Saladino A J 1976 Studies on the subcellular pathophysiology of ischemia. Circulation 53 (suppl. 1), 17

Utili R, Abernathy C O, Zimerman H J 1977 Studies on the effects of E. Coli endotoxin on canalicular bile formation in the isolated perfused rat liver. Journal of Laboratory and Clinical Medicine. 89:471

Waddell G 1975 Movement of critically ill patients within hospital. British Medical Journal 2:417

Wardle N 1979 Shock: bacteraemic and endotoxin shock. British Journal of Hospital Medicine 1:223

Watson J D, Varley J G, Hinds C J, Bouloux P M, Tomlin S, Rees L H 1984 Adrenal vein and systemic levels of catecholamines and metenkephalin-like immunoreactivity in canine endotoxin shock; effects of naloxone administration. Circulatory Shock 13:47

Whaley K, Yee Khong T, McCartney A C, Ledingham IMcA 1979 Alternate pathway complement activation and its control in gram-negative endotoxin shock. Journal of Clinical and Laboratory Immunology 2:117

Wiggers C J 1950 The Physiology of Shock. Commonwealth Fund, New York

Wiles J B, Cerra F B, Siegel J H, Border J R 1980 The systemic septic response: does the organism matter? Critical Care Medicine 8:55

Wilson R F, Gibson B S 1978 The use of arterial-central venous oxygen differences to calculate cardiac output and oxygen consumption in critically ill surgical patients. Surgery 84:362

Index